PRIMARY CARE GERIATRICS

A Case-Based Approach

Department of Family
& Community Medicine
College of Osteopathic Medicine
Michigan State University
West Fee Hall
East Lansing, MI 48824-1315

PRIMARY CARE GERIATRICS
A Case-Based Approach

RICHARD J. HAM, M.D.
Distinguished Chair in Geriatric Medicine
Professor of Medicine, Professor of Family Medicine
State University of New York Health Science Center at Syracuse
Syracuse, New York

PHILIP D. SLOANE, M.D., M.P.H.
Professor
Department of Family Medicine
University of North Carolina School of Medicine
Chapel Hill, North Carolina

THIRD EDITION

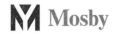 Mosby

St. Louis Baltimore Boston Carlsbad Chicago Naples New York Philadelphia Portland
London Madrid Mexico City Singapore Sydney Tokyo Toronto Wiesbaden

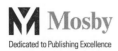

A Times Mirror
Company

Vice President and Publisher: Anne Patterson
Editor: James Shanahan
Developmental Editor: Laura Berendson
Project Manager: Patricia Tannian
Production Editor: Heidi Fite-Crowley
Book Design Manager: Gail Morey Hudson
Manufacturing Manager: Dave Graybill

THIRD EDITION

Printed in the United States of America
Composition by Clarinda Company
Printing/binding by Von Hoffmann Press, Inc.

Mosby–Year Book, Inc.
11830 Westline Industrial Drive
St. Louis, Missouri 63146

Library of Congress Cataloging in Publication Data

Primary care geriatrics :   a case-based approach / [edited by] Richard
    J. Ham, Philip D. Sloane. — 3rd ed.
           p.   cm.
      Includes bibliographical references and index.
      ISBN 0-8151-4188-2
      1. Geriatrics—Case studies.   I. Ham, Richard J.   II. Sloane,
    Philip D.
      [DNLM: 1. Geriatrics—case studies. 2. Primary Health Care—case
    studies.   WT 100 P952 1996]
    RC952.7.P75   1996
    618.97—dc20
    DNLM/DLC
    for Library of Congress   96-12932
                                                            CIP

96 97 98 99 00 / 9 8 7 6 5 4 3 2 1

To
Doris Gilpin and **Leonore Sloane**
devoted readers of the second edition
who have given us encouragement in completing the third

PDS

In memory of
Dr. John Ham
(1914–1995)

RJH

Contributors

PATRICIA P. BARRY, M.D., M.P.H.

Chief, Geriatrics Section, Department of Medicine
Director, Gerontology Center
Boston University School of Medicine
Boston, Massachusetts

DOUGLAS B. BERKEY, D.M.D., M.P.H., M.S.

Associate Professor and Chair
Department of Applied Dentistry
University of Colorado School of Dentistry
Denver, Colorado

SHARON A. BRANGMAN, M.D., F.A.C.P., A.G.S.F.

Assistant Professor of Medicine
Program in Geriatrics, Department of Medicine
SUNY Health Science Center at Syracuse
Syracuse, New York

KENNETH BRUMMEL-SMITH, M.D.

Medical Director
Long-Term Care Division
Providence Health Systems, Oregon
Portland, Oregon

JAMES W. CAMPBELL, M.D.

Assistant Professor, Fellowship Director
Medical Director, Alcoholism Services of Cleveland
Case Western Reserve University School of Medicine
Metro Health Medical Center
Cleveland, Ohio

PATRICK P. COLL, M.D.

Director, Geriatric Medicine
St. Francis Hospital and Medical Center
Assistant Professor
Departments of Family Medicine and Medicine
University of Connecticut Health Center
Hartford, Connecticut

MARIA FEDOR, M.D.

Board Certified Geriatrician
Private Practice
Fort Lauderdale, Florida
Norristown, Pennsylvania

MARY KANE GOLDSTEIN, M.D.

Chief, Section of General Internal Medicine
VA Palo Alto Health Care System
Palo Alto, California
Clinical Assistant Professor
Stanford University School of Medicine
Stanford, California

NEIL K. HALL, M.D.

Director of Geriatrics, Clinical Campus at Binghamton
SUNY Health Science Center at Syracuse
Binghamton, New York
Medical Director, Ideal Senior Living Center
Endicott, New York

RICHARD J. HAM, M.D.

SUNY Distinguished Chair in Geriatric Medicine
Professor of Medicine, Professor of Family Medicine
Director, Program in Geriatrics, Department of Medicine
SUNY Health Science Center at Syracuse
Syracuse, New York

FRANKLIN HARGETT, M.D.

Clinical Assistant Professor
Department of Family Medicine
University of North Carolina
Chapel Hill, North Carolina

JOHN M. HEATH, M.D.

Assistant Professor, Geriatric Division and Fellowship
  Director
Department of Family Medicine
Robert Wood Johnson Medical School
University of Medicine and Dentistry of New Jersey
New Brunswick, New Jersey

KENNETH W. HEPBURN, Ph.D.

Assistant Professor
Department of Family Practice and Community Health
University of Minnesota
Minneapolis, Minnesota

JOHN A. HOEPNER, M.D.

Chairman, Department of Ophthalmology
SUNY Health Science Center at Syracuse
Syracuse, New York

J. CHRISTOPHER HOUGH, M.D.

Associate Clinical Professor, Family Medicine
Wayne State University School of Medicine
Medical Director, Family and Adult Medicine
MidMichigan Stratford Village
Midland, Michigan

DONNA LIND INFELD, Ph.D.

George Washington University
Department of Health Services Management and Policy
Washington, D.C.

TIMOTHY J. IVES, Pharm.D., M.P.H.

Associate Professor, School of Pharmacy
Clinical Associate Professor
Department of Family Medicine, School of Medicine
University of North Carolina
Chapel Hill, North Carolina

DENNIS W. JAHNIGEN, M.D.

Director, Center on Aging
Goodstein Professor of Geriatric Medicine
Head, Division of Geriatric Medicine
University of Colorado Health Science Center
Denver, Colorado

JOSEPH M. KEENAN, M.D.

Professor
Department of Family Practice and Community Health
University of Minnesota
Minneapolis, Minnesota

J. EUGENE LAMMERS, M.D., M.P.H.

Medical Director, Geriatrics/Medicare HMO
Methodist Medical Group
Clinical Assistant Professor, Department of Medicine
Indiana University School of Medicine
Indianapolis, Indiana

DEBORAH M. LASTINGER, B.S.N.

Director of Cancer Home Care Program
Department of Health Care Sciences
George Washington University School of Medicine and
  Health Sciences
Washington, D.C.

DEBORAH A. LEKAN-RUTLEDGE, M.S.N., R.N.C., C.C.C.N.

Clinical Nurse Specialist, Wellcare Dynamics
Adjunct Assistant Professor, School of Nursing
University of North Carolina
Chapel Hill, North Carolina

ROBERT J. LUCHI, M.D.

Professor and Chief, Section of Geriatrics
Department of Medicine
Director, Huffington Center on Aging
Baylor College of Medicine
Houston, Texas

MARLENE J. MASH, M.D.

Clinical Associate Professor of Dermatology
Temple University
Philadelphia, Pennsylvania
Private Practice
Yardley, Pennsylvania

DARLYNE MENSCER, M.D.

Geriatric Education Coordinator
Carolinas Medical Center, Department of Family Practice
Charlotte, North Carolina

JAMES Q. MILLER, M.D.

Alumni Professor of Neurology
University of Virginia, Health Sciences Center
Charlottesville, Virginia

ARSHAG D. MOORADIAN, M.D.

Professor of Medicine
Director, Division of Endocrinology
Department of Internal Medicine
St. Louis University Medical School
St. Louis, Missouri

LEONARD W. MORGAN, M.D.

Professor and Chairman
Department of Family Medicine
Texas Tech University Health Science Center at Odessa
Odessa, Texas

LAURA MOSQUEDA, M.D.

Training Director, Rehabilitation Research and Training
  Center
Rancho Los Amigos Medical Center
Director of Geriatrics
St. Luke's Medical Center
Pasadena, California

JOHN B. MURPHY, M.D.

Residency Director and Director, Division of Geriatrics
Department of Family Medicine
Brown University/Memorial Hospital of Rhode Island
Pawtucket, Rhode Island

BONNY NEYHART, M.D.

Associate Clinical Professor, Department of Family Practice
School of Medicine
University of California, Davis
Sacramento, California

JAMES G. O'BRIEN, M.D.

Director of Geriatrics
St. Lawrence Hospital and Health Care Services
Interim Associate Dean for Community Programs
Michigan State University
East Lansing, Michigan

L. GREGORY PAWLSON, M.D., M.P.H.

Professor and Chairman
Department of Health Care Sciences
George Washington University School of Medicine
  and Health Sciences
Washington, D.C.

GARFIELD C. PICKELL, M.D.

Associate Professor
University of California at Davis School of Medicine
Hughson, California

ALICE K. POMIDOR, M.D., M.P.H.

Assistant Professor of Family Medicine
Case Western Reserve University
Medical Director
MetroHealth Center for Skilled Nursing Care
Cleveland, Ohio

JOEL POTASH, M.D.

Medical Director, Hospice of Central New York
Clinical Associate Professor
Department of Family Medicine and Program in Medical
  Humanities
SUNY Health Science Center at Syracuse
Syracuse, New York

RICHARD L. REED, M.D., M.P.H.

Geriatric Program Coordinator
Associate Professor
Department of Family Practice and Community Health
University of Minnesota Medical School
Minneapolis, Minnesota

PETER J. RIZZOLO, M.D.

Professor, Department of Family Medicine
University of North Carolina
Chapel Hill, North Carolina

RICHARD G. ROBERTS, M.D., J.D.

Professor of Family Medicine
University of Wisconsin, School of Medicine
Madison, Wisconsin

BRUCE E. ROBINSON, M.D., M.P.H.

Professor and Director, Geriatrics
Department of Medicine, College of Medicine
University of South Florida
Tampa, Florida

HAROLD RUBENSTEIN, D.P.M., F.A.C.F.A.S.

Clinical Assistant Professor
Department of Orthopedic Surgery
Department of Medicine
SUNY Health Science Center at Syracuse
Syracuse, New York

PHILIP D. SLOANE, M.D., M.P.H.

Professor
Department of Family Medicine
University of North Carolina School of Medicine
Chapel Hill, North Carolina

JEFFREY L. SUSMAN, M.D.

Associate Professor and Vice Chair of Family Medicine
Director of Primary Care, College of Medicine
University of Nebraska Medical Center
Omaha, Nebraska

GEORGE E. TAFFET, M.D.

Assistant Professor, Section of Geriatrics
Department of Medicine
Baylor College of Medicine
Houston, Texas

JEAN M. THIELE, R.N., G.N.P.

Geriatric Nurse Practitioner
Michigan Regional Medical Center
Family Practice Residency Program
Midland, Michigan

JAKOB ULFARSSON, M.D.

Private Practice
Internal Medicine and Rheumatology
Hollywood, Florida

INGRID H. VALDEZ, D.M.D.

Director, Geriatric Dentistry
VA Medical Center, Denver
Clinical Assistant Professor, Department of Applied Dentistry
University of Colorado School of Dentistry
Denver, Colorado

HELEN M. WATERS, M.S., C.C.C-A.

Acting Director
Coordinator, Audiology
Communication Disorder Unit
SUNY Health Science Center at Syracuse
Syracuse, New York

JANE V. WHITE, Ph.D., R.D.

Professor, Department of Family Medicine
University of Tennessee at Knoxville
Knoxville, Tennessee

HENRY M. WIEMAN, M.D.

Medical Director ESP,
A PACE Replication at Fallon,
Geriatrician, Fallon Health Care Systems
Worcester, Massachusetts

DOUGLAS C. WOOLLEY, M.D.

Associate Professor
Department of Family and Community Medicine
University of Kansas School of Medicine at Wichita
Wichita, Kansas

Preface

The changing emphases in U.S. health care (generalism and primary care the priority; cost containment the bottom line) are already powerful influences on the evolution of medical education and clinical practice. Geriatrics has always been a central and vital component of primary care medicine; it is now more clearly defined than ever as a primary care discipline. Generalist physicians already find their services in considerable demand, and physicians in training are being encouraged to enter primary care. During this period of upheaval and transition, it is more important than ever that all the providers of geriatric medical care and all the teachers of it maintain continuous awareness of the principles of geriatrics, both in individual patient situations and in broader matters of developing the health care system, health policy, practice patterns, and medical education. As the health care system changes, it is vital that we, as clinicians and educators, involve ourselves in ensuring that the system becomes more appropriate for the elderly patients we serve: individuals who may be overwhelmed by "freedom of choice" or who may be too ill and frail to make "informed choices" or to judge the quality of providers and treatments. Many of our assumptions about patients, even now as the health care system is changing, are based on the needs and abilities of literate, well-informed, motivated, decisive individuals typified by successful, middle-class, well-educated, working people. We must recognize the amazing heterogeneity of elders, and be cautious never to patronize or demean. Many are highly articulate, want to be involved in making their own decisions, and will assert their right to do so; many others are more fragile and in need of care and will not be well served by a system that treats only those who declare themselves to be patients and can present themselves in a functional and well-organized fashion at a physician's office at the appointed time. As well as recognizing that elders differ in these broad characteristics, we realize now that in just the next few decades a vastly increasing proportion of elders will be minorities: individuals with ethnic, cultural, and other characteristics (including prevalence of disease states) that differ from the "majority" norms.

As the demographic changes predicted throughout the 1960s and 1970s come to pass and the "baby-boom" generation experiences firsthand the aging of parents and other older relatives, their wellness or illness, and their death, and as dynamic and politically active Americans experience aging firsthand in themselves, the pressure to provide health care that is appropriate is becoming more intense. There is growing societal consensus on sensitive and emotional issues, such as the intensity of treatment that is appropriate at a given stage of illness. Family members are more aware than ever of their responsibilities, not only in attempting to achieve what their older relative would have wished but also in considering society as a whole and priorities for the distribution of society's resources; few are now unaware that resources are not limitless and that inappropriate, costly care is, in reality, billed to all of us.

Against this background, the fact that there is so much more that can and should be done to prevent, treat, and facilitate recovery from many of the most common problems that afflict the old and the fact that we sometimes do more than we should in maintaining cardiopulmonary support and nutrition, for example, make it vital that everyone understand the breadth and potential of our field. As health professionals, all of us have an educational role, not only in teaching those who are learning to be health professionals but in sharing our knowledge and ideas with our colleagues in many other disciplines: political representatives, administrators, lawyers, and judges.

Our clinical knowledge is advancing at an exciting rate—the demonstration of how much can be achieved through exercise and rehabilitation; advances in both high-tech and low-tech feeding and nutritional techniques that have an immediate impact on clinical practice; the dynamism of Alzheimer's research, with the beginnings of some specific treatment; better definition of the roles of medication, environment, and specific behavioral therapies in patients with dementia; the reduced side effect profiles and the increased specificity of the newer antidepressants and much greater societal awareness of the frequency of depression and the effectiveness of its treatment; and the continually advancing technology for noninvasive investigation. However, the exponential increase in numbers of patients with Alzheimer's disease alone far outweighs this excitement: we must make immediate improvements in our handling of such patients. Mental health services have essentially been withdrawn from this patient group, and the challenge to the general medical and long-term care system presented by patients who need a high level of expert behavioral mental health handling by nursing and physician staff is not being met. Basic principles as espoused by Marjorie Warren decades ago ("Why is this patient in bed?") still need to be emphasized. "High-tech" still immobilizes patients; deconditioning from immobilization is a real phenomenon (perhaps one of the geriatric "giants"), and physicians still miss the forest while concentrating on one tree, getting one organ system "tuned up" while the person slips into dependency. Every health care professional needs to be a geriatrician at times! All of us need to be able both to look at the "big picture" (functional independence, mobility, continence, clarity of cognition, appropriateness of mood, nutrition, and quality of life) and to look painstakingly at the details, the little things that can override all of our other efforts: the mouth, feet, vision, hearing, sleep, the bowel and bladder, skin care, etc.

The revisions to our book have attempted to address all of these things, and although much of the book remains organizationally the same and the principle remains the same (that it is most stimulating and meaningful to learn from real cases that can be encountered in real life), most of the text has been rewritten, and many of the chapters have been completely redone, with new authorship and a fresh approach.

All of us learn how to care for patients from our involvement with and observation of real cases. The exciting part of our medical education—the apprenticeship of intern and resident days—is "case-based learning." When the committee designing the curriculum for the first edition of this book, back in the early 1980s, enthusiastically endorsed the principle that the curriculum we designed and the materials we produced would be built around exemplary cases, we were only formalizing and setting down the way in which most clinicians who have evolved into educators generally feel most comfortable: the case at hand sparks discussion of the principles, data, and facts. These principles and data, when applied, demonstrate their relevance by helping the patient or family.

Even more than in the previous editions, we have emphasized the primary care interaction between you, the physician, and the patient and family members, concentrating in the text (as well as in the cases) on the information that you will actually need to use with the patient and family. We have deliberately included less of the historical or histopathological background than was included in previous editions. We have concentrated on knowledge the family and patients will need to acquire from you and on skills that you must possess in order to do as good a job as possible in the time available. This book is designed to complement rather than rival the heavier textbooks in geriatric medicine, internal medi-

cine, and family medicine, but it is vital to realize that *any* textbook only complements the current literature. In reediting this book we have often needed to advise our readers to be sure to keep one step ahead of their best-informed families (if they can!) or, alternatively, to be appropriately humble (but critical, too) when family members bring in "news" from the media. Much is happening that is both relevant to our field and of general interest because everyone is experiencing aging and its effects on health.

Following feedback from some of our readers, we have reinstituted the literary (and sometimes not so literary) quotations in the unit openers, and we have also added clinical "pearls." These are intended to be the succinct "truths" that can get hidden in the text and hidden in the complexities of the patients that we see. The best of these pearls are brief, memorable, and straightforward enough that they are useful in our own role as clinicians who are educators of families and others; some of the pearls merely highlight or emphasize things that are covered in the text. We believe that they will work to lighten the text and add to the uniqueness and memorability of our book.

Chapter 1 is a succinct introduction to primary care and its relationship to geriatrics that everyone using this book should read first. Sections and chapters dealing with the health care system have been updated, of course, but in addition, we have added specific chapters on the special characteristics of the several different sites of geriatric care. There is a new chapter on terminal care, and the chapters on nutrition, health maintenance, and ethics reflect changed thinking and new guidelines that have evolved recently. In the clinical sections, we have expanded the chapter on depression to be more problem oriented and to reflect that depression is often part of the broader syndrome of "failure to thrive." Both that chapter and the one on dementia have been modified to reflect DSM-IV terminology as well as the many advances in management and clinical and scientific knowledge. Consideration of all the other major syndromes has been updated, with a fresh approach to falls and falling and a more interdisciplinary approach to incontinence. We welcome other health care disciplines among our many new authors to bring their specific wisdom to the sections on the mouth and the feet, for example. Unit III of the book is modified in that the attempt to be "site specific" for the various clinical problems has been removed: the clinical problems can occur in any setting, and the cases and text reflect the need for all of us to be able to manage these many challenging diagnoses in every setting, from the streets of the city through to the intensive care unit.

We hope this book conveys an active, intervening, anticipatory approach, with the health professional energetically working with the patient and family, even if one or the other is not pressing for care. In geriatrics (as in pediatrics), our patients frequently do not realize their needs and are therefore not the willing participants that we sometimes assume. This is why we have to be prepared to go to the patient's home if necessary and to use every interaction as comprehensively as possible. We hope our book counters the view some still have of geriatrics being a passive, merely psychosocial, branch of medicine; there is a huge amount of *real* medicine (as well as *real* psychosocial care) to do in this field. Practitioners of the art of geriatrics should never believe that "nothing can be done"; never lose the sense of the centrality and autonomy of the patient; realize that medical decision making is not only between the patient and the physician but in a broader context of family circumstance and environment; look for the nonpresented "hidden" problems that can represent major disabilities (cognitive impairment, incontinence, depression); focus on maintaining function, relieving pain, and maintaining mobility in order to fulfil the objective that underlies all we do—reducing or postponing dependency; and look for the many "smaller" details that, unaddressed, can negate more dramatic efforts while at the same time looking at the "big picture."

To whom, then, is this book addressed? Clearly, primary care physicians in practice and training are central to our readership, but we know that both prior editions were widely used by nurse practitioners and physician assistants in training as well as those from other disciplines, including non–health care ones; we are all part of a common team, and we welcome their readership. The language of the cases has been edited to maintain the sense that "you are the physician"; the idea is to have the reader feel the challenge of being in the central medical role. Bearing in mind how many nonphysicians use our text, we did consider using less specific language, but it reduces some of the power of language to involve the reader if we use all generic, health professional terms. We share with many other health care disciplines the perception that physician education is particularly important in our field. We hope that many health professionals who would not regard themselves as "in primary care" will read this book, despite the title. In our opinion every health professional interacting with elders has to take on some of the characteristics of the primary care physician. All must understand the art of involving other disciplines when appropriate and of managing the many transitions from site to site and professional team to professional team that geriatric medical practice necessitates in our currently fragmented system.

This book, then, is an attempt to teach the principles and the majority of the important information that must be understood and incorporated by all of us into clinical practice if we are to ensure the optimal management of our elderly population, particularly during this time of dramatic and far-reaching change in medical knowledge and health care organization. We hope you enjoy it, and we welcome your comments.

Richard J. Ham, M.D.
Philip D. Sloane, M.D., M.P.H.

Acknowledgments

We acknowledge with gratitude the patience and helpfulness of our editorial advisors at Mosby Year–Book, Inc. (Stephanie Manning, Laura Berendson, and Heidi Fite-Crowley) and multiple colleagues and friends who have contributed to this book and have made suggestions both formally and informally about it, especially Sharon Brangman, John Heath, Adam Klausner, William Pendlebury, and William Reichel. The book has evolved from previous editions. Isadore Rossman's original leadership and encouragement with the first edition remains with us in spirit, along with the many other editorial advisors who first got us going on the "case-based approach" that has clearly been so applicable to this particular part of medical education. The enthusiastic secretarial help and the efficiency of Deborah Menifee, Anne Bucci, and Pamela Newton were essential. Thanks, too, to the Sloane and Ham families for giving up many family nights and weekends to get this done.

Introduction: How To Use This Book

This book is described as having a "case-based approach." Although many other texts of geriatric medicine have appeared since our first edition, this book is still unique in its approach. We hope that you will find it an enjoyable way not only of acquiring skills and knowledge concerning geriatric health care, but also of experiencing the *enjoyment* that the editors and authors of this book all share as they assist their elderly patients and families to make the best of the many challenges that life and society have handed them.

Our book is designed on the assumption that learning medicine from real cases is much more vivid, practical, memorable, and meaningful than reading fact-filled texts. In most of the chapters, the initial presentation, progress, and management of illustrative cases are integrated into the text. As you, the reader, work through the cases, the text reviews the illnesses and syndromes exemplified by them. The text itself is completely updated and generally takes a problem-oriented approach. We have tried to exemplify, or to "role model," in general, the optimal approaches to the many situations and syndromes that fill our text. Not all the cases are managed correctly; where things should have been done better, the case discussion says so: after all, it is the cases where we could have done better from which we learn most.

We have attempted to maintain a problem-oriented approach, although the necessity of having individual chapters on individual diseases has forced us to vary our approach somewhat; still, a problem-oriented approach is implied. After all, this is an important principle of geriatric medicine: focus on the problems as they affect the patient's life, define them, figure out all the diagnoses and influences that cause them, prioritize them, and address them. Thus, we hope that at the end of each chapter our readers will have a refreshing and up-to-date fund of knowledge, some of the skills needed to apply the information to future cases, and a sense of the current consensus on treatment, its intensity, and breadth. This is all based on the principle that Professor Brocklehurst and others have espoused: that involvement breeds enthusiasm and that enthusiasm is what we must feel as health professionals for our elderly patients and what we must communicate to those around us.

In organizing and writing this text, we have used the approach we would use for a midday case conference in a primary care training program. A resident or student might present the opening part of a particular case. A faculty member or visitor would be available to cover the topic concerned. After the initial presentation, the faculty person would stop and comment on the mode of presentation and the considerations going through his or her mind at that point. Then the case would continue with extra details. After further specific comments on the case, more broad and general comments, amounting to a formal presentation regarding the main syndrome or problem illustrated by the patient, would be given. At the end, to give a sense of completion, the resolution of the case would be presented, with some closing comments about the application of the generic material to that particular situation. It is to this ideal, "case-based" approach that we have devoted ourselves. By using real cases, we hope that practicality and application of the material are immediately seen and dryness is avoided.

The chapters are all similarly organized. There are formal objectives so that the reader will know what we wish to achieve in each chapter. There are pretest and posttest questions (as well as study questions after the cases in the text) to stimulate creativity and active learning. The pretests and posttests are not formally validated and are not intended to be used as quantitative assessments of knowledge. In general, the posttest is more rigorous than the pretest. If the reader has trouble with the pretest, he or she certainly needs to read the chapter. If the reader has trouble with the posttest, he or she needs to read it again. But the main objective of the questions is to encourage involvement.

Generally, the next item in the chapter is the first part of one case (or several). All are identified by a fictitious name, and all were real patients (sometimes modified to illustrate certain points). The opening case descriptions are followed by study questions, which are questions the health care professional should be asking at that point in the presentation of the patient.

Following these initial parts of the case(s), the text begins. It is typographically differentiated from the cases, so that it can be easily referred to separately for later review and reference. In general, the text describing each syndrome, illness, or situation is organized in the same sequence in which information is obtained in primary care settings. Thus the text alternates with the cases and is related to them as they evolve, but it is organized to stand alone as well.

In general, we have tried not to have more than two cases in progress at once—it would get confusing. Occasionally, the cases are mere vignettes, but often the cases progress over months and sometimes many years (as in the chapters on dementia and on normal aging). The cases in this book, as in primary care practice, are seen in many sites—the emergency room, the hospital, the nursing home, the office, the home, and elsewhere in the community.

Each chapter has a brief summary of the main principles or content and their significance from the perspective of primary care practice, and each chapter ends with posttest questions and references (which include authorative reviews to enable further reading).

The book is divided into three units. The first outlines the principles of geriatric primary care and the characteristics of older persons from which these principles arise. The second provides detailed, case-based approaches to the major geriatric syndromes, which have been called the "giants" of geriatric medicine. The third section is more of a potpourri of common conditions and situations that we felt required separate consideration. This is not a fully comprehensive textbook. We gave much thought to what should be excluded, since this book is not intended to be encyclopedic. We believe that application of the principles outlined in Unit I and demonstrated in Unit II to *any* condition presenting in an older patient would result in better care.

Although the first edition of this book was originally based on materials for medical students, it would be a rare medical student who would graduate knowing everything in this text. Both prior editions were widely used in primary care residency training programs, in the training of nurse practitioners and physician assistants, and by many other health professionals in training. It has also been useful, gratifyingly for us, to our own peers: faculty in academic geriatric programs and practicing physicians, who daily face the challenge of providing optimal geriatric care despite the limitations of our system and of our societal response to those in need. We know of others, including clergy and other non–health care professionals, who have enjoyed and learned from the book; this is good, since many other individuals (not all health professionals) are essential to an effective team. Even so, the language of the book is directed toward physicians in practice and physicians in training; we have retained that emphasis in order that the text may be as involving as possible to the principal readership of this book. In fact, as you will see, the cases continually imply that *you* are the physician, and that it is *your* decisions that are influencing the case.

We hope that you enjoy this book and that you will find it refreshing, "different," and a practical way to learn or update your knowledge of geriatric health care.

Preparing already for the fourth edition, we always appreciate suggestions, comments, and ways in which this text can be improved.

Richard J. Ham, M.D.
Philip D. Sloane, M.D., M.P.H.

Contents

PRIMARY CARE GERIATRICS
A Case-Based Approach

UNIT I
PRINCIPLES AND PRACTICE

"Get along and doctor your sick," said Granny Weatherall. "Leave a well woman alone. I'll call for you when I want you. . . . Where were you forty years ago when I pulled through milk-leg and double pneumonia? You weren't even born. . . . I pay my own bills, and I don't throw my money away on nonsense!"
—Katherine Anne Porter, *The Jilting of Granny Weatherall*

I must create a system or be enslaved by another man's.
—William Blake, "Jerusalem"

If I'd known I was going to live this long, I'd have taken better care of myself.
—Eubie Blake, on reaching his 100th birthday

Grow old along with me!
The best is yet to be,
The last of life, for which the first was made.
—Robert Browning, "Rabbi Ben Ezra"

It ought to be lovely to be old
to be full of peace that comes of experience
and wrinkled ripe fulfillment.
—D.H. Lawrence, "Beautiful Old Age"

I do not want two diseases, one nature-made and one man-made.
—Napoleon Bonaparte

Why is this patient in bed?
—Marjorie Warren, pioneer geriatrician, 1940s, Britain

We're only being selfish; she would never have wanted to keep going like this.
—Daughter of advanced dementia patient, Syracuse, 1994

Now more than ever seems it rich to die,
To cease upon the midnight with no pain. . . .
—John Keats, "Ode to a Nightingale"

CHAPTER 1

Primary Care

PHILIP D. SLOANE and RICHARD J. HAM

In the late nineteenth century Kaiser Wilhelm chose the age of "three score and five" to identify Prussians who qualified for "old age" benefits. Now, more than a century later, it is the norm rather than the exception among Western populations to reach that age. Yet our culture clings to the concept that the sixty-fifth year marks the end of productivity and the beginning of decrepitude.

In truth, the modern equivalent of Kaiser Wilhelm's three score and five is probably around 80 years of age. When we think about older populations, we should divide them into two groups:

- The relatively healthy elderly, most of whom are between the ages of 65 and 80 and whose health care needs are not very different from those persons of late middle age
- The frail elderly, most of whom are 75 years and older and require special monitoring and services

Primary care geriatrics concerns itself with both of the above population groups, in other words, everyone aged 65 and older. *Specialty* or *consultative geriatrics* tends to focus on the frail elderly.

PRIMARY CARE DELIVERY TO OLDER PERSONS

The term *primary care* emerged in the late 1960s, when it became clear that the U.S. health care system was overspecialized.[1] A definition of primary care should include the following elements[1-5]:

- Provision of a point of entry into the health care system
- Management of the majority of health problems of individual patients
- A sense of ongoing responsibility for the patient's overall health care, including emergency services, preventive care, coordination of visits to other providers, and continuity of care over time
- An approach that considers biological, psychological, and social factors
- A sense of responsibility for the health of the community within which patients live, including surveillance of health problems and provision of health services to the community

Most primary care is delivered in physicians' offices. According to the National Ambulatory Medical Care Survey (NAMCS), there were 155,870,000 office visits by persons aged 65 and older to all physicians in 1991.[6] Of these, approximately 21% were to general and family practitioners and approximately 25% were to internists. Among the specialties, these two provide the vast majority of geriatric primary care. Therefore about half of all office visits by older persons are to primary care physicians. Of the specialists, those registering the most visits by older persons were ophthalmologists (approximately 14% of all office visits by older persons to any physician) and dermatologists (5% of all office visits by older persons).[6]

Table 1-1 lists the most common presenting complaints and primary diagnoses for all office visits (primary care and specialist) by older persons, according to the NAMCS. It indicates that the most common problems of older persons involve chronic diseases and health maintenance. Thus a large part of primary care geriatrics is the management of chronic illness and the prevention of increased disability. This is different from primary care of younger populations, in which acute conditions predominate.

In addition to the physician's office, sites for primary care for older persons include long-term care settings. Nearly 10% of older persons live in nursing homes or domiciliary care facilities (which include board and care facilities and supervised assisted living), and most of these persons are the frail elderly, who have sizeable health needs. Institutions providing long-term care are important sites of primary geriatric care.

Nonphysician health professionals are also important providers of primary care for older persons.[7] Nurse practitioners, physician assistants, and gerontological nurse specialists provide significant primary care services under physician supervision. Social workers play a key role in managing psychosocial problems and in helping patients negotiate the health care system. In the home, the other core site of geriatric primary care (after the office and long-term care institutions), care is provided almost entirely by nurses.

PRACTICING PRIMARY CARE GERIATRICS

Primary care physicians for older persons face a challenging and perhaps daunting task. Physicians must accept responsibility for overseeing all aspects of the complex health needs of older persons. They must set priorities among a multitude of health and psychosocial problems. Physicians must do all this with limited time, limited compensation, and the danger that any action may lead to adverse consequences.

In this context, a physician's first priority is usually to respond to the patient's concerns, in other words, to the patient's presenting problems. Often a stated concern is merely the symptom of a more obscure problem (such as alcoholism or fear of cancer), and it is up to the physician to try to uncover the actual reason for the patient's visit. Any illness in old age can be associated with cognitive impairment, and dementing illnesses are much more common with increasing age. Because of these possibilities, presentation of the problems by other concerned surrogate individuals, such as family members and neighbors, is frequent and welcome, although it may complicate the patient's care: such individuals inevitably color their input with their own attitudes and fears.

A second priority is to monitor known health problems. Diabetes, hypertension, chronic heart disease, osteoarthritis, and other chronic illnesses require frequent

Table 1-1   Most Common Reasons for Office Visits and Final Diagnoses Among Older Patients (All Physicians, 1991)

	Age (yr)	
	65-74	75 and Older
10 Principal Reasons for Visit		
	1. Postoperative visit	1. General medical examination
	2. General medical examination	2. Vision dysfunction
	3. Vision dysfunction	3. Postoperative visit
	4. Glaucoma	4. Glaucoma
	5. Cough	5. Blood pressure check
	6. Diabetes mellitus	6. Cough
	7. Back symptoms	7. Cataract
	8. Hypertension	8. Vertigo or dizziness
	9. Blood pressure check	9. Hypertension
	10. Skin lesion	10. Back symptoms
10 Most Common Diagnoses		
	1. Essential hypertension	1. Essential hypertension
	2. Diabetes mellitus	2. Glaucoma
	3. Glaucoma	3. Cataract
	4. Cataract	4. Diabetes mellitus
	5. Chronic ischemic heart disease	5. Chronic ischemic heart disease
	6. Osteoarthritis	6. Osteoarthritis
	7. Dermatoses	7. Cardiac dysrhythmias
	8. Cardiac dysrhythmias	8. Organ or tissue replaced by other means
	9. Lipid disorders	9. Dermatoses
	10. Bronchitis	10. Heart failure

From US Department of Health and Human Services, Public Health Service: National Ambulatory Medical Care Survey: 1991 Summary, *Vital and Health Statistics*, Series 13, No 116, May 1994.

reexamination. Diseases affecting cognition or mood, such as dementia and depression, require especially proactive monitoring. Medications must be reviewed, and adverse effects sought. Primary care involves regular assessments of chronic problems, often within the context of a visit for an acute illness or a "regular checkup."

Beyond managing acute and chronic problems, physicians often must advise patients and their families on issues related to health maintenance and disease prevention. The patient whose health is failing may need encouragement to consider a new living option, or a patient with arthritis may need help confronting the need to lose weight. All patients need to be offered regular health monitoring (such as mammography and vision screening) and recommended immunizations.

Finally, physicians must monitor each patient's psychological status, living situation, and sources of social support. These factors generally make the difference between subjective well-being and a sense of ill health. When a disabling illness develops, these factors play an important role in determining the individual's ability to regain some semblance of normality and independence. Physicians must get to know their patients' families and social environments and endeavor to treat their patients in the context of these aspects of their lives. It is espe-

cially important to engage family members, or the equivalent, and to ensure their sense of sharing in the care of the patient.

Geriatrics differs from traditional internal medicine because it emphasizes certain issues that are more prevalent among the elderly than among younger persons. These issues include *broad syndromes* such as confusion, falls, dizziness, dysmobility, and incontinence; a high prevalence of *disability,* with a concomitant need to maintain a *rehabilitative* focus; and an ever-present concern about *iatrogenesis* (see Box 1-1). Underlying all these issues is the presence of *multiple problems,* rather than only one or two, in elderly patients and the frequent presence of *multiple causes* for each problem. This interaction of multiple problems makes primary care geriatrics one of the most difficult (and intellectually challenging) fields in medicine.

RECENT TRENDS

During the 1990s several issues that relate directly to primary care geriatrics have emerged. There has been a call for "generalist" physicians and an attempt to position the field of geriatrics within this new movement. This has led to debate as to whether the field of geriatrics is a medical specialty or a primary care discipline. In addition, the

---

BOX 1-1
Key Features of Geriatric Medicine

Geriatric Syndromes

The following are common final pathways by which failures in a variety of organ systems can manifest themselves:

Confusion
Falls
Dizziness and imbalance
Immobility and dysmobility
Incontinence
Fatigue
Weight loss

Management of Disability

Management should focus on function rather than diagnosis, care rather than cure, and independence rather than freedom from disease.

Low Therapeutic Ratios with High Risk of Harming the Patient

The most common preventable condition in geriatrics is iatrogenic disease; its avoidance and detection are hallmarks of high-quality geriatric care.

---

rapid growth of managed care has necessitated the prompt modification of practice styles and the acquisition of new skills and approaches for primary care geriatricians.

Call for More "Generalist" Physicians

During the early 1990s, concern about rising health care costs spurred interest in reforming the health care system. As part of the move toward health care reform, attention once again became directed to overspecialization and the need for more primary care physicians. The word *generalist* became popularized to indicate physicians whose training and practice pattern contained the elements of good primary care. The Council on Graduate Medical Education (COGME), in a report to Congress and the Secretary of Health and Human Services, recommended that the nation set a goal that at least 50% of practicing physicians be generalists.[8] As had occurred two decades earlier, debate raged about which medical specialties were "true" generalists.

Is Geriatric Medicine a Primary Care Field?

The debate about generalists and primary care led to questions about the nature of geriatrics as a field. In 1992 the Board of the American Geriatrics Society (AGS) unanimously supported a resolution stating that geriatric medicine is first and foremost a primary care discipline. They noted that however a geriatrician is defined—whether as a physician who has received the Certificate of Added Qualifications (CAQ) in geriatric

medicine in internal medicine or family practice or as a physician member of the AGS—nearly all spend at least 95% of their clinical practice providing primary care services.[9] This statement represented a shift in the leadership of the AGS away from the model of geriatrics that had been popular in the 1980s, when geriatrics was seen as a consultative specialty. The need for specialized consultative services in geriatrics is still recognized; however, it is at present unclear how such consultative services will be provided in our changing health care milieu. One source might be (as it traditionally has been) the academic program; but as our health care system changes, it is not clear whether this will be a widespread pattern.

Managed Care

Early in the decade, discussion of federally mandated health care reform and the concern of third-party payers spurred the proliferation of managed care systems, whose cornerstone is the primary care physician. Health maintenance organizations (HMOs) for older persons began developing, supported by special Medicare and Medicaid authorization. All indications are that this trend will accelerate during the coming decade. Currently many Medicare HMOs do not employ geriatricians, and the role of geriatric medicine in guiding primary care practice in HMOs needs to be strengthened. Some ways that geriatricians can assist managed care organizations are by developing the following: (1) a standardized, general screen for functional impairment for all patients; (2) referral of complex geriatric cases to a multidisciplinary team for assessment and (in some cases) management; (3) protocols for common geriatric problems, especially chronic disease management; (4) appropriate health screening; and (5) use of standardized assessment instruments where available and well validated.[10]

The Future

Geriatricians do not have to worry about becoming obsolete. The continued "graying of America" and, indeed, the world will ensure the need for primary care physicians for the elderly. However, the current concern over national resource allocation will continue, and geriatric care will need to be practiced within significant resource constraints. Still, progress continues to be made and must persist in all areas, ranging from the understanding of basic biochemical and cellular mechanisms of disease to the provision of new and improved forms of health care. Participating in the acquisition of knowledge, translating medical advances to the clinical setting, and setting standards for the medical community are among the important roles for primary care geriatricians.

GOALS OF THIS BOOK

This book focuses on the needs of physicians who incorporate geriatrics into primary care practice. It emphasizes the primary care approach to geriatrics rather than the more specialized skills such as multidisciplinary geriatric assessment and inpatient consultation. It focuses on problems commonly encountered in the three major primary care settings: the physician's office, long-term care institutions, and the home. It also introduces common problems whose management includes hospitalization and rehabilitation, since the sites where these services are provided represent important components of the primary care physician's practice.

The book is case based because most physicians learn better in the context of patients. The book aims to introduce the range of primary care geriatric practice to students, residents, and practitioners in family medicine, internal medicine, nursing, and allied health fields.

REFERENCES

1. Golden AS, Carlson DG, Hagen JL: *The art of teaching primary care,* New York, 1982, Springer.
2. Alpert JJ, Charney E: *The education of physicians for primary care,* Washington, DC, 1973, US Department of Health, Education, and Welfare, Health Resources Administration.
3. Parker AW, Walsh JM, Coon M: A normative approach to the definition of primary health care, *Milbank Q* 54:415-438, 1976.
4. Silver HK, McAtee PR: A descriptive definition of the scope and content of primary health care, *Pediatrics* 56:957-959, 1975.
5. Mullan F: Community-oriented primary care: an agenda for the 80s, *N Engl J Med* 307:1076-1078, 1982.
6. US Department of Health and Human Services, Public Health Service: National Ambulatory Medical Care Survey: 1991 Summary, *Vital and Health Statistics,* Series 13, No 116, May 1994.
7. Levinson D: Getting the job done: helping hands in geriatric primary care, *Geriatrics* 45:58-65, 1990.
8. Rivo ML, Satcher D: Improving access to health care through physician workforce reform: directions for the 21st century: third report of the Council on Graduate Medical Education, *JAMA* 270:1074-1078, 1993.
9. Burton JR, Solomon DH: Geriatric medicine: a true primary care discipline (editorial), *J Am Geriatr Soc* 41:459-462, 1993.
10. Friedman B, Kane RL: HMO medical directors' perceptions of geriatric practice in Medicare HMOs, *J Am Geriatr Soc* 41:1144-1149, 1993.

CHAPTER 2

Demographics

RICHARD J. HAM

OBJECTIVES

On completion of this chapter, the reader will be able to:

1. Describe the current demographic trends and the way they will influence the relative age of the population over the next five to six decades.

2. Describe the current demographics of the aged population itself in relation to marital status, physical dependency, living arrangements, and financial resources and the directions which these differences are anticipated to change in the coming five to six decades.

3. Understand the influence that these demographics and the changes in them will have on the reader's own current and future clinical practice.

4. Straightforwardly describe the significance of these demographics in order to be able to authoritatively influence appropriate change in the health care delivery system.

5. Recognize the importance of not allowing the overall statistics to inappropriately effect the management of individual cases.

The "demographic imperative," as it has been called, is one of the most powerful reasons for all health professionals to fully understand the characteristics and needs of elderly patients and the current state of clinical knowledge and research about them in order to immediately incorporate suitable approaches into current (and future) clinical practice. There is considerable evidence, as well as anecdote and popular feeling (this last carrying much political weight) that the unique needs of elders are not well addressed by the current health care system. It is clearly not necessary for the individual clinician to be able to quote precise percentages (and in some instances such statistics can mislead) since each individual case is unique and will frequently prove to be "the exception to the rule." Nonetheless, individual clinicians must plan their own education and the organization of their practices in relation to the current and future needs of the population they serve. In addition, those serving elders must become active in ensuring that modifications in the patterns of delivery of future health care are influenced by knowledgeable clinicians to ensure that the direction of change appropriately reflects the aging of the population and its characteristics.

OVERALL AGING OF THE U.S. POPULATION

Since the turn of the century, the absolute number of Americans, and older Americans in particular, has increased considerably: an increase of 10 times the number of individuals over 65 and a tripling of the percentage of Americans who are over 65 (Fig. 2-1). Those over 65 currently represent 12.7% of our population (i.e., one in every eight Americans). This number, and the proportion of those over 65 in the total population, continues to increase. By the year 2000 13% of the U.S. population will be over 65, but only 30 years later, 20% of the population will be over 65. This particularly rapid increase in older Americans between 2010 and 2030 will occur because those persons in the "baby-boom" gen-

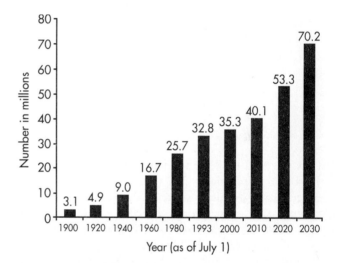

FIG. 2-1   Number of persons 65+, 1900-2030. Note: Increments in years on the horizontal scale are uneven. (Based on data from U.S. Bureau of the Census.)

eration will be reaching age 65. The growth of the older population is a little slower in the 1990s because of the reduced birth rate during the Depression of the 1930s. In total, by 2030 there will be *twice* as many individuals over 65 as there were in 1990.[1,2]

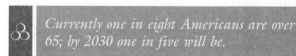

Currently one in eight Americans are over 65; by 2030 one in five will be.

GROWTH OF THE "OLD OLD"

The age of 65 is an arbitrary population cutoff. The need for special approaches because of increasing illness and frailty occurs much more often in the oldest of the old. Thus it is very significant that the older population is itself becoming older. Since the turn of the century, the "young old" (65 to 74) have increased by a factor of eight; the "middle old" (75 to 84) have increased by a factor of 14; and the "old old" (85+) have increased by a factor of 27.[1] It has been estimated that during this current 15-year period ending in the year 2000, the over 85 population is doubling in absolute numbers. This is of considerable significance since individuals over the age of 85 are much more likely to be ill, frail, or dependent.

This increase in the "old old" is in part because of increased life expectancy upon reaching the age of 65. Whereas a woman of 65 had a mean life expectancy of 19 years (and a man had one of 15 years) in 1987,[3] it is predicted that by 2050 women can anticipate 23 years as the mean survival, and men can expect 17 years. This means not only an exponential increase in the oldest of the old but also a continuing increase in the disparity between surviving women and surviving men, with an increase in female widowhood even beyond its striking existing preponderance.

> Current life expectancy at age 65 is about 19 years for a woman and 15 years for a man: already more years than many realize.

Thus the "old old" are the fastest growing segment of the older population, and it is their characteristics, rather than the less striking characteristics of the "young old," that should concern clinicians. Many authorities have emphasized that present preventive measures in early and mid life may well improve activity and independence and reduce morbidity in old age. But no amount of cardiovascular survival (which has been the major effect of preventive approaches on mortality so far) or cancer mortality and morbidity relief can counter the prevalence of dementia (50% of those over 85) or of degenerative arthritis (the most common chronic condition in the world).[4] These are just two of the conditions that produce progressive dependency on others in old age.

DEMOGRAPHICS OF THE ELDERLY POPULATION
Gender

For a combination of environmental, social, and genetic reasons, women out-survive men in most age groups. The increasing life expectancy of women at age 65 compared to men has been mentioned above. One result is a striking difference in the living arrangements and widowhood status of individuals over 65; these differences progressively increase with increasing age (Fig. 2-2). It is difficult to predict the future, but the current preponderance of men over 65 who are living with a spouse (75%) is striking when compared with the current proportion of women living with a spouse (41%), a proportion matched by the 43% of elderly women who either live alone or with nonrelatives (Fig. 2-3). Overall, older men are currently twice as likely to be married as older women, and half of older women are widows. In addition, the divorce rate for elders is apparently increasing, although it still only accounts for 5% of older persons.[5]

> Older men are twice as likely to be married as older women, and half of older women are widows.

Living Arrangements

The relatively high proportion of widowed women is but one factor leading to the striking difference between the genders in their living arrangements. Overall, 68% of older people not living in an institution do live in a family setting: 82% of older men and 57% of older women, the proportion living with a family decreasing with age. Of noninstitutionalized older people, 30% live alone: 41% of older women and 16% of older men (Fig. 2-3).[5]

The proportion of older individuals living in nursing homes increases with age: in 1990 1% of those aged 65 to 74, 6% of those aged 75 to 84, and 24% of the 85+ group lived in nursing homes. The disproportion of

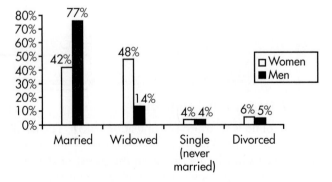

FIG. 2-2   Marital status of persons 65+, 1993. (Based on data from U.S. Bureau of the Census.)

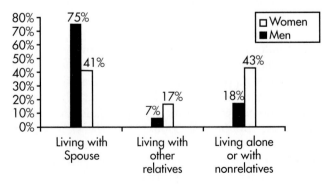

FIG. 2-3   Living arrangements of persons 65+, 1993. (Based on data from U.S. Bureau of the Census.)

women in such situations changes the social character and needs of the millions of Americans for whom such an institution is "home."[6,7]

Income and Poverty

The poverty rate for people over 65 is about the same as for the rest of the adult population (a little over 12%). However, with the additional 8% of elders living within 125% of the poverty level, the estimate is that one in five of the older population are poor or near poor.[2] Race makes a considerable difference: one in nine elderly whites, one in four elderly blacks, and one in five elderly Hispanics are currently poor. Gender also makes a difference: the poverty rate is almost double in women as compared to men. About the same proportion of older women live in poverty as do children in this country.

> *One in five elders are poor or near poor: one in nine whites and one in four blacks. The poverty rate is double in women.*

Despite these poverty figures, the net worth of many older individuals is such that individuals over 75 years of age on average have a median net worth well above the U.S. national average. Clearly there is considerable heterogeneity: some elders have considerable resources, especially in property, and yet a high proportion of elderly individuals currently have, and in the future will have, problems in maintaining basic living requirements such as shelter and food, with health care necessarily relegated.

Health and Functionality

As is emphasized throughout this text, health and functionality in all people decline with age, and reliable epidemiological research is gradually being carried out to establish the current level of functional disability and health care problems of our *current* aged population. Predicting trends in these issues and characteristics in the

future is difficult, although the optimism that much dependency and illness can be postponed has already turned out to be correct for certain conditions, especially those of cardiovascular origin. However, absent a "breakthrough," it is recognized now that the prevalence of not only dementia (to give just one disease-related example), but specifically dementia of Alzheimer's type, is higher in the very old population than had been previously suspected.[8] Many clinicians feel that there is much underreporting of chronic disability, and illness, so the figures quoted for the current prevalence of chronic diseases may well be underestimates.

In 1992 the most frequently occurring conditions per 100 individuals over 65 were as summarized in Table 2-1. The number of days of illness per year (days in which illness restricts activity) also increases with age. This is reflected in an increase in physician contacts (11 per year for those over 65, 5 per year for those under 65).[4] It is estimated that the current over 65 population uses approximately one third of the available physician resources, one fourth of the total medications prescribed, and constitutes more than two fifths of the acute hospital admissions. Clearly the impact on the costs of U.S. health care will be considerable.[9]

Studies of functional disability in ADLs (activities of daily living: personal self-care skills such as bathing, dressing, eating, transferring, walking, and toileting) and IADLs (instrumental activities of daily living: skills such as meal preparation, shopping, money management, telephoning, and house work) confirm increasing dependency with age. Fig. 2-4 summarizes the health-related difficulties by age group; the proportion of the popula-

Table 2-1 Most Common Chronic Conditions, 1992 in Older Americans

Diagnosis	Occurrence per 100 Elders over 65
Arthritis	48
Hypertension	46
Heart disease	32
Hearing impairment	32
Orthopedic impairment	19
Cataracts	17
Sinusitis	16
Diabetes	11
Tinnitus	9
Visual impairment	9

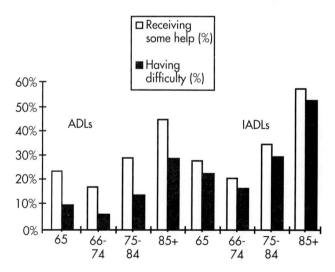

FIG. 2-4   Percent of persons having difficulty and receiving help with selected activities (by age), 1986. Note: Data refer to health-related difficulties only. *ADLs,* Activites of daily living; *IADLs,* instrumental activities of daily living. (Based on data from U.S. Department of Health and Human Services.)

tion receiving some help increases strikingly between the relatively independent "young old" and the relatively dependent "old old."[2] These figures alone justify the emphasis in geriatric medical care in general on the importance of the maintenance and enhancement of functional capability at all opportunities. This is one of the prime objectives of geriatric medicine; yet it must be recognized that there is an inevitability that increasing age and frailty will produce dependence on others, a nursing burden which all of society must share.

ETHNIC DIVERSITY

Whereas in 1990 approximately 13% of those over 65 were minorities, by 2030 one in four elders will be a minority. There are striking increases in the population of minority elders—greater increases than in the nonminorities. Between 1990 and 2030 the increase in older minorities will be more than 3 times the increase in white non-Hispanics: the percentage increase in minorities in the 65+ population compared with white non-Hispanics will be 7 times as much for Asians and Pacific Islanders; 2.5 times as much for American Indians, Eskimos, and Aleuts; more than 1.5 times as much for non-Hispanic blacks; and 6 times as much for Hispanics.[1] This greatly increased absolute number and proportionality of older individuals with different racial, ethnic, language, cultural, educational, and fiscal characteristics will profoundly influence future health care provision. The current needs of minority elders are not yet well defined.

However, it is established that minority elders are more likely to be in poverty, less likely to have completed high school, and, with the exception of Asians, have lower life expectancy.[10] Health status as well is reduced, with certain disease states having an increased prevalence in minorities (e.g., diabetes, hypertension, cancer, and cerebrovascular disease).[11] Ethnic, cultural, and language barriers to the care of these populations with their increased occurrence of illnesses pose special challenges in clinicians' attempts to initiate the proactive preventive approach that should be used to improve health in all patients as they age.

 By 2030 one in four elders will be a minority.

GEOGRAPHY OF OLD AGE

As is well recognized, certain states have a higher population of elders. Whereas most would recognize that the state with the highest proportion of elders is Florida, it is striking that many states (see Table 2-2) have an elderly population only a few percentage points behind this known "leader." In addition, in the last few years the elderly population has increased faster in other states than many would anticipate (Table 2-3). Of special significance is that the 13 states with the highest poverty rates for elders are in the South.[12]

Less well recognized is the fact that the absolute numbers of elders by state are highest in California (over 3 million), with Florida and New York tying for second place (over two million each) (Box 2-1).[12] Given the reorganization of health care services into ever more local networks and the significance of Medicaid as the source of support for the majority of elderly individuals so dependent that they require long-term institutional care, these state-by-state variations and their linkage to some of the states with the highest poverty rates is of importance.

Table 2-2   States with More Than 14% Aged over 65 in 1993

Florida	18.6%
Pennsylvania	15.8%
Iowa	15.5%
Rhode Island	15.5%
West Virginia	15.3%
Arkansas	15.0%
North Dakota	14.8%
South Dakota	14.7%
Nebraska	14.2%
Missouri	14.2%
Connecticut	14.1%
Massachusetts	14.0%

Table 2-3   Fastest Growing Elderly Population (More Than 8.5% Between 1990 and 1993)

Nevada	22%
Alaska	19%
Arizona	11%
Hawaii, Utah, New Mexico	10%
Wyoming, Colorado	9%

BOX 2-1
States with the Most Individuals over 65, 1993

Over 3 Million
California

Over 2 Million
Florida, New York

Over 1 Million
Pennsylvania, Texas, Ohio, Illinois, Michigan, New Jersey

SUMMARY

The logarithmic expansion of the elderly population, especially the oldest of the old, makes it vital that all possible efforts are made early in life to reduce dependency and increase health in old age. Although medical breakthroughs and changing technology may revolutionize the care of certain major conditions producing long-term dependency and illness in old age (such as Alzheimer's), such advances cannot be assumed. Therefore all individual clinicians and all those involved in the evolution of health care services must be aware, or be made aware, that a huge population of dependent elders in need of long-term care and not capable of producing the resources to care for themselves will represent the bulk of health care for the American population in the coming decades.[13] These aged individuals are our "future selves," so their needs are our needs. Having the medical, fiscal, and organizational resources in place is an urgent priority for all of society.

POSTTEST

1. Which one of the following statements is false?
   a. By the year 2000 one American in five will be over 65.
   b. Twenty-four percent of those over 85 live in nursing homes.
   c. One in five of those over 65 are poor or near poor.
   d. The fastest growing group among the elderly are those over 85.

2. Which one of the following statements is false?
   a. The poverty rate for the over 65 population is about the same as for the rest of the adult population.
   b. The life expectancy of all aging minority groups is less than that of non-Hispanic whites.
   c. The 13 states with the highest poverty rates for the old are in the South.
   d. Half of elderly women are widows.

REFERENCES

1. Spencer G: Projections of the population of the United States by age, sex, and race: 1988-2080, Current Population Reports, Series P-25, No 1018, Washington, DC, January 1989, US Bureau of the Census.
2. A profile of older Americans: 1994, Washington, DC, 1995, American Association of Retired Persons.
3. Vierck E: Aging America: trends and projections, Washington, DC, November 1989, US Senate Special Committee on Aging.
4. The current estimates from the National Health Interview Survey, United States, 1988, Vital and Health Statistics, Series 10, No 173, Hyattsville, Md, October 1989, National Center for Health Statistics.
5. Marital status and living arrangements, March 1989, Current population reports, Series P-20, No 433, Washington, DC, January 1989, US Bureau of the Census.
6. Hing E: Use of nursing homes by the elderly: preliminary data from the 1985 National Nursing Home Survey, Advanced data, No 135, Hyattsville, Md, May 1987, National Center for Health Statistics.
7. Ouslander JG: Medical care in the nursing home, JAMA 262(18):2582-2590, 1989.
8. Evans DA et al: Prevalence of Alzheimer's disease in a community population of older persons, JAMA 262(18):2551-2556, 1989.
9. Schneider EL, Guralnik JM: The aging of America: impact on health care costs, JAMA 263(17):2335-2340, 1990.
10. Estimates of the population of the United States, by age, sex, and race, Series P-25, No 485, Washington, DC, 1986, US Bureau of the Census.
11. US Department of Health and Human Services: Health status of minorities and lower income groups, ed 3, Rockville, Md, 1991, Government Printing Office.
12. State population and household estimates, with age, sex, and components of change: 1981-1987, Current population reports, Series P-25, No 1024, Washington, DC, May 1988, US Bureau of the Census.
13. Vierck E: Fact Book on Aging, Santa Barbara, CA, 1990, ABC-Clio.

PRETEST ANSWERS
1. d
2. b

POSTTEST ANSWERS
1. a
2. b

CHAPTER 3

Normal Aging

PHILIP D. SLOANE

OBJECTIVES

Upon completion of this chapter, the reader will be able to:

1. Describe the major biological theories of aging and their effects on observed phenomena of human aging.

2. Discuss and contrast three personality theories that discuss adjustments to aging: disengagement, activity, and continuity.

3. Discuss and give examples of the following principles of aging: the rule of thirds, functional reserve, and the distinction between average and healthy aging.

4. Identify and discuss common changes that occur with age in the following systems: muscular, skeletal, dental, skin, cardiovascular, respiratory, gastrointestinal, genitourinary, central nervous, special senses, and endocrine.

PRETEST

1. Which one of the following signs of aging occurs earliest in most adults?
   a. Difficulty reading fine print without glasses
   b. Inability to stay up all night and work the next day
   c. Radiological evidence of osteoarthritis of the spine
   d. Intense awareness that life is limited ("midlife crisis")
   e. Fixed wrinkling around the mouth
2. Which of the following statements is true about individuals at age 80 years?
   a. Vibratory sensation is equally reduced in distal and proximal joints.
   b. Over half of older persons report trouble sleeping at night.
   c. Renal perfusion is 75% to 80% of its value at age 30 years.
   d. Fewer than half of couples have been affected by death or disability of one or both spouses.
3. Which one of the following symptoms referable to the urogenital system is commonly reported by older persons?
   a. Increased vaginal mucus
   b. Reduced urinary frequency
   c. Vaginal bleeding
   d. Incontinence

Today's elderly grew up in a world so different from today's that it is often difficult for health care professionals to appreciate the setting in which their basic values developed. Many older persons grew up without electricity, running water, computers, Social Security, Medicare, Medicaid, nuclear weapons, television, radio, or refrigeration. Few adults went to college; the nation was predominantly rural; and strict racial segregation permeated Southern life. Opportunities for women were far more limited than today. Antibiotics were unknown, and hospitals were still largely places where people went to die. The generation gap separating elderly patients from students in the health professions can lead to misunderstandings because values and assumptions are different.

▼ MARTHA HILLIARD ROBINSON (Part I)
Childhood and Young Adulthood

Martha Hilliard Robinson was born on January 10, 1898, in a small rural community in eastern North Carolina called Tarboro. She had three older brothers, and her father owned a hog farm. Taking unusually well to "book learning," she was the first member of her family to complete high school. After graduation, Martha persuaded her father to allow her to attend Roth School of Nursing in Durham, North Carolina. Martha attended Roth for the year before the declaration of World War I, suffering at first from homesickness but gradually adjusting.

In the wave of patriotism after war was declared, Martha enlisted as an army nurse. She was sent to Base Hospital Number 165, north of Paris. There she met her first husband, Gerald Anthony Hilliard, a 27-year-old army physician from Raleigh who "had a gift for putting anyone at ease." Martha and Dr. Hilliard fell in love in France but decided to postpone marriage. Martha did not want to anger her father, who was furious that she had enlisted in the army without his permission. She and Dr. Hilliard also realized that during a time of war, perspectives are not always clear; so both felt it wise to wait until the war was over.

In 1918 Martha returned to Roth to complete her nursing education, and Dr. Hilliard resumed his appointment at Rex Hospital in Raleigh. They were married in 1920. Martha then worked for a private physician in Raleigh until she had a child, Gerald Junior. Thirteen months later, Jeremiah was born. Two years later, Martha had a third child, Rachel. Understandably, she did not consider returning to work. Her primary job was that of wife and homemaker, and wives of prominent physicians were expected to stay at home caring for the family.

Martha's life changed suddenly when Gerald Anthony Hilliard was killed on a rainy night in 1932. He had been returning home from the hospital when his car collided with a milk wagon, killing him instantly. Martha was 35 years old with three school-age children. Her father insisted that she move back to the family homestead in Tarboro, where she remained for 4 years. With her mother available to help care for the children, Martha resumed her nursing career by taking a part-time job in a local physician's office. Recalling this period of her life still causes Mrs. Robinson to weep.

In 1936 Martha applied for a staff nurse position at Roth Hospital because she "believed in what Roth was doing." Roth provided nearly three fourths of all free bedcare furnished to the destitute sick white citizens of Durham County (there was a separate black hospital at that time). Three months after Martha began working at Roth, her children joined her.

During 1936 Martha met her second husband, Benjamin Robinson III, an attorney. She had retained his services because of a problem with her first husband's death benefit. She was determined that the government not reduce her widow's pension, especially because she had three dependent children. She and Benjamin Robinson III were married in 1939 and remained together until his death in 1981, when Martha was 83.

STUDY QUESTION

- *How would knowledge of Mrs. Robinson's early life history assist a physician in providing sensitive, appropriate care for an acute illness at age 90 years?*

LIFE HISTORY, SOCIOECONOMIC CHANGES, AND COHORT EFFECTS

Only by listening carefully to their patients' personal life histories can physicians learn who their patients are, what they value, and how health care providers can best relate to them. It is often difficult in the face of acute illness for physicians to appreciate the patient's lifetime of experiences. Yet those experiences shape the values and perceptions of that individual, and knowing those values and perceptions can enable the physician to provide better care.

In response to the times in which its members have lived, each generation carries with it distinctive attitudes and health patterns. For example, even when they were younger, the elderly of today have tended to take fewer financial risks and to express depressive symptoms less often than succeeding generations. Such differences between generations are termed *cohort effects*.

CASE DISCUSSION

A physician seeing Mrs. Robinson for an episode of pneumonia or diverticulitis at age 92 years might not immediately appreciate the independence and self-reliance that she had demonstrated through her earlier life experiences. Her background in nursing, if known by her physician, would call for a more sophisticated level of communication about her illness than would be used with a poorly educated former laborer, for example.

▼ MARTHA HILLIARD ROBINSON (Part II)
Age 46

At age 46, Martha Robinson told her new family physician, Dr. Hensley, that she was worried about "getting decrepit." Dr. Hensley took each complaint seriously; Mrs. Robinson liked that. When his evaluation was complete, he explained each concern in language she understood, reassured her that her general health was excellent, and told her what she could do to stay healthy. He explained that the bright red spots on her abdomen, which had become prominent over the past 10 years, were cherry angiomata, benign clumps of blood vessels that commonly arise in the 30s and 40s. He explained that

the wrinkles around her eyes were normal by age 40; he called them "smile marks." He advised her, however, to avoid sun exposure, which accelerates wrinkling. He explained that her occasional right knee pain was osteoarthritis that had set in early because that knee had been injured playing baseball as a teenager. Finally, he explained that her problems reading fine print were normal, too, and caused by the lens of each eye losing its ability to change shape. He advised her to be fitted for reading glasses.

EARLY SIGNS OF AGING

Aging is a process that gradually leads to noticeable changes in many body systems. The most common early sign of aging is difficulty staying up all night and working the next day. Hair thinning in men begins early as well, often in the 20s. In the 30s come a variety of signs: graying hair, easier weight gain (as a result of decreased metabolism and reduced exercise), wrinkling of the forehead and the corners of the eyes, concern by many women about the "biological clock" of childbearing ability, and more frequent injury as a result of weekend athletic activities. Concern about financial security is common at this time as well, often because of family responsibilities.

Next, usually in the 40s, comes a period of gradual recognition of life's finite limitations. Reflection on personal mortality is often precipitated by a close friend who develops a serious illness or by aging parents. At the same time there is a developing awareness that many of the dreams and ambitions of youth will not be realized. These feelings lead to a reexamination of goals and attitudes toward living, a process popularly termed *midlife crisis*. In the best circumstances, this reflection continues for many years and leads to the adaptation of attitudes and habits that will promote good health in old age.

Skin Changes of Aging

The most visible signs of aging consist of changes in the skin and hair. Wrinkling, sagging of subcutaneous support, hair loss and graying, and a variety of benign and malignant skin conditions increase with frequency as individuals age. Many such changes occur more rapidly in whites and are accelerated by sun exposure. Although the pace varies, the sequence of changes is relatively uniform: sagging of the lateral aspects of the eyebrows, wrinkling of the forehead, horizontal skin lines at the lateral canthus of the eye, sagging of the tip of the nose, perioral wrinkling, and fat absorption of the buccal and temporal areas. Microscopic changes visible in aged skin include epidermal thinning, degeneration of the elastic fibers providing dermal support, thickening of collagen fibers in the dermis (often with pseudoscar formation), reduction in the numbers of sweat and sebaceous glands, and reduction in skin flow because of diminished vascularity.[1]

Presbyopia

Beginning in early adulthood, the ability of the lens to accommodate for near vision gradually diminishes. Eventually, the eye is no longer able to change the shape of the lens enough to focus on near objects, such as fine print. This gradual loss of lens elasticity, which is the most common age-related eye problem, is called presbyopia. By the 40s, most adults require reading glasses, and by age 55 years, nearly all persons have great difficulty focusing on close objects without glasses.

Osteoarthritis

Another ubiquitous aging change is osteoarthritis. By age 40 years, all adults have osteoarthritic changes visible in radiographs of the cervical spine. Similar progressive changes occur in most weight-bearing joints and in the hands as age increases. These physiological changes result from a wearing down of the articular bony surfaces that get frequent use. Reactive bone growth follows, with new bone extending laterally. This extra bone growth is visible radiographically as *spurs*.

Although all adults have osteoarthritic changes, most of these changes are not accompanied by significant symptoms. Severe osteoarthritis can be present without pain, although pain tends to mirror the severity of bony changes. Early symptomatic osteoarthritis tends to develop in joints that have undergone prior injury.

CASE DISCUSSION

Relatively early in Mrs. Robinson's adulthood, occasional osteoarthritic pain developed in her right knee, which had been injured when she was a teenager. That joint became an important source of physical impairment later in life.

SIGNS OF AGING IN THE 50S AND EARLY 60S

Certain events that commonly occur between the ages of 50 and 65 years foster a quickening sense of aging. These events include menopause, becoming a grandparent, experiencing the deaths of parents and friends, being the oldest at work, and having to face significant physical restrictions from one or more health problems. Many reminders of aging are social, such as qualifying for "senior citizen" discounts. Individuals in this age group typically feel on the threshold of old age. They often speak of a disparity between feeling young on the inside and appearing old to others. At the same time certain attitudes and activities develop that become more prominent in later years: a more philosophical approach to life, less irritation with minor issues, and reflection on life.[2]

▼ *MARTHA HILLIARD ROBINSON (Part III)*
  Ages 60 to 72

Mrs. Robinson was at the peak of her professional career at age 60. She had moved to Raleigh to become dean of the College of Nursing at Mercy Hospital. She recognized that her stamina had diminished, however, and she became fatigued particularly during out-of-town business trips. Routines had become important to maintain her energy. She exercised daily, and she was always in bed by 9:30 PM. She also noticed trouble reading in dim light and was frequently bothered by knee pain, especially when walking long distances or on stairs.

During the decade that followed, Mrs. Robinson's knee continued to be her biggest health problem. She stopped using the stairs, moved to a one-story house, changed her evening walks to avoid a downgrade, and frequently had pain at night. She took increasing doses of acetaminophen, occasionally with codeine, for pain. She began using a cane whenever she went outside the house. Her daily walks were replaced by swimming 3 times a week at the neighborhood pool.

At age 68, Mrs. Robinson saw Dr. Hensley because of vaginal bleeding after intercourse. He prescribed an estrogen cream, and the problem soon resolved. She was now retired and traveled frequently with her husband, Benjamin.

At age 72, she was placed on a diuretic for elevated blood pressure, which she attributed in part to her husband's heart attack the previous year.

STUDY QUESTIONS

- *To what extent are the above changes noted by Mrs. Robinson likely to be attributed to normal aging?*
- *To disease?*
- *To disuse or deconditioning?*
  List 10 environmental adjustments that may enhance the independence of an older person with severe osteoarthritis of the knee.

AGING CHANGES AND THE RULE OF THIRDS

In the past, considerable decline in major body systems was attributed to normal aging. In the last two decades, however, it has become increasingly apparent that much of what was previously ascribed to aging is the result of disease or disuse. In general, it is useful to consider a "rule of thirds" about decline in function that older patients report (Fig. 3-1). About one third of functional

"Aging changes" = Disease
                 + Disuse
                     + Normal aging

FIG. 3-1   Rule of thirds. Of changes in physiological function observed with advancing age, approximately one third is due to disease, one third to disuse, and one third to normal aging.

decline overall is due to disease, and another third is due to inactivity (disuse). This leaves approximately one third of the decline seen with age actually being caused by aging itself. For example, cardiac output declines by about 1% per year in "normal" subjects.[3] This alteration in physiology could be entirely due to the aging process. On the other hand, it is known that physical activity diminishes by at least 50% with increasing age and that occult cardiac disease is common in older persons and rare in young adults. Thus "normal" populations of older adults may manifest diminished cardiac function on the basis of deconditioning or occult disease, and those factors may be reflected as normative changes.

THEORIES OF BIOLOGICAL AGING

The basic mechanisms of aging are poorly understood. Although researchers can catalog physiological alterations that occur with age, they must turn to unproven theories to explain why aging occurs. Certainly, aging occurs at a biochemical and a cellular level. Two general theories, based on observations in laboratory animals and in humans, attempt to explain the phenomena that accompany aging.[4,5]

One line of reasoning suggests that aging results from gradual cellular damage through gene mutation, protein degradation, autoimmune processes, or the accumulation of toxic substances. Support for the gene mutation hypothesis is provided by the observation that liver cells from older mice have greater numbers of genetic mutations than similar cells from younger mice. Such mutations could arise from environmental exposure to radiation, free radicals, or other toxins. Free radicals are molecules produced as a by-product of normal metabolism; they are known to damage cellular elements, particularly membrane lipids and genetic materials.

Denaturation of proteins occurs through biochemical processes that lead to cross-link formation or nonenzymatic glycosylation. Such degenerative processes have been observed in a variety of proteins. Nonenzymatic glycosylation of proteins in the lens, for example, increases with age and appears to play a role in presbyopia and cataracts. If progressive over time, similar protein denaturation could widely impair cellular function. DNA repair could be affected; reduced DNA repair capabilities of older cells have been noted in the laboratory.

Immunological processes could also contribute to cellular aging. T-cell function declines with age. At the same time, abnormal monoclonal antibodies thought to represent autoimmune phenomena increase in frequency. These could lead to both cell damage and decreased resistance to infection or toxic damage.

There is also evidence that aging results from the accumulation of toxic substances, possibly by-products from cell metabolism. This is particularly applicable to cells that do not replicate, such as brain cells. Certain substances, such as lipofuscin pigment and amyloid, accumulate in these cells as people age.

The other general theory is that cell senescence is a genetically programmed phenomenon. Support for this hypothesis is provided by the observation that human fibroblast cells cultured in vitro gradually slow their rate of replication and, after about 50 mitoses, no longer replicate and therefore die. It now appears that all stem cells have similar finite proliferative capacities. Furthermore, long-lived organisms have more cell replications than short-lived organisms, and humans with the hereditary disease progeria, which is characterized by premature aging, contain cells with only two to four doublings. Genetically programmed decrements in mitotic capacity could contribute to age-associated declines in T-cell function, to degenerative vascular disease, and to producing a finite limit to the human life span.

ADAPTATION TO DISABILITY AND TO ROLE LOSSES

The decades of the 60s, 70s, and 80s involve physical, psychological, and social losses. By age 80, it is rare to be without one or more chronic disabling conditions (Table 3-1). In addition, significant psychological and social losses accompany advancing years (Box 3-1). Retirement, a spouse's illness, geographical separation from family members, relocation from a beloved home into a smaller apartment or retirement community, and many other common events during these years all represent losses. In the case of retirement, the older adult loses a sense of accomplishment, feelings of contribution to so-

Table 3-1 The Most Common Chronic Conditions in Adults 65 Years and Older

Problem	% Affected	Measures Available to Prevent Onset or Reduce Disability
Arthritis	46	Weight control, exercise
Hypertension	38	Salt restriction, weight control, antihypertensive medication
Hearing loss	28	Avoiding exposure to loud noises or wearing hearing protection
Heart conditions	28	Diet, control of hypertension, nonsmoking, low-fat diet
Chronic "sinus" problems	18	Nonsmoking
Visual loss	14	Wearing sunglasses in bright light
Bone problems	13	Adequate calcium intake, exercise, avoiding smoking and excessive alcohol use

ciety, and the opportunity to interact with peers in the workplace. Similarly, when a spouse becomes ill, the partner must make financial and life-style sacrifices to become a caregiver.

In spite of the potentially discouraging losses and limitations they face, men and women aged 65 to 70 years report greater happiness than adults in any earlier age group.[6] This reported happiness, which continues into the 70s, reflects in part certain advantages that older adults have over younger individuals: greater independence, fewer responsibilities, reduced concern about day-to-day inconveniences, and financial security (provided by Social Security and retirement programs). Such factors, especially when combined with good health, make older adults more capable of living for the day than they had been earlier in their lives. As articulated by one retired man, "I know that I'll never be happy if I can't enjoy what I have now."

SEXUALITY AND AGING

As a group, healthy older men and women often, but not universally, maintain an interest in and a capacity for sexual activity. The factors most strongly correlated with continued sexual intercourse beyond age 65 include prior sexual activity, physical health, and availability of a capable and interested partner.

Although the capacity for sexual activity exists beyond the age of 65, in general both physical responsiveness and ability to perform sexually diminish with age. Postmenopausal women often experience thinning of the vaginal mucosa and diminished vaginal secretions, largely as a result of estrogen deficiency. Erectile dysfunction, ranging from inability to maintain an erection to complete impotence, increases with age among men and is aggravated by many medications.

Many older couples give up sexual intercourse altogether, finding other ways to display physical affection. If a couple is not sexually active, however, the physician should ask both partners how they feel about the situation. Often, an inquiry into medical factors may identify remediable problems, such as drugs causing impotence in men or vaginal atrophy causing pain and bleeding in women.

▼ MARTHA HILLIARD ROBINSON (Part IV)
Age 78

Two months after her seventy-eighth birthday, Mrs. Robinson fell and broke her right wrist. She had been taking the garbage out to the compost pile in her backyard (a habit from her childhood days on the farm). It was dark, and she did not notice a piece of gravel on the uneven ground. "My ankle twisted, and I wasn't able to catch myself," she explained. Thinking back, she remembered that she had tripped several other times in the backyard since purchasing the house 14 years before, but this was the first time she had fallen.

Dr. Hensley felt that the accident might be a result of normal aging changes, but he followed up the incident with a thorough health evaluation. He noted that Mrs. Robinson had difficulty performing tandem gait but could maintain a standing position with her eyes closed (Romberg's test). Her heart, lungs, and kidneys were fine. Her right knee was considerably larger than the left, without an effusion, and a 10-degree flexion contracture was evident. Quadriceps, hip abductors, and hip extensors were all weak on the right side.

Laboratory test results included a hematocrit of 41%, a blood urea nitrogen of 14 mg/dl, a creatinine of 1.1 mg/dl, and a cholesterol of 234 mg/dl. Radiograph of her right wrist showed moderate osteoporosis and a displaced Colles' fracture. Her audiogram (see Fig. 3-2) showed bilateral high-frequency hearing loss, consistent with presbycusis.

Although he could not be certain that her severe knee osteoarthritis had caused Mrs. Robinson's fall, Dr. Hensley felt that it was the major treatable contributing factor. He arranged for her to see an orthopedic surgeon about a knee replacement. Several months later, she had the surgery. She worked hard to regain her strength and mobility during postoperative rehabilitation. By 6 months after surgery her knee mobility and strength were markedly improved and she was pain free.

STUDY QUESTION

■ *When an elderly patient is noted to have a functional problem such as weakness, recurrent falls, incontinence, or confusion, what general approach should the physician use to identify the relative contributions of disease, disuse, and normal aging to the problem?*

MULTIPLE PROBLEMS AND MULTIPLE ETIOLOGIC FACTORS

In the elderly, multiple problems are the rule. Illness generally results from several factors rather than from a single agent. Often several factors combine with a decrease in host resistance to lead to illness or injury. Thus problems that have been developing slowly often present acutely.

BOX 3-1
Common Social and Psychological Losses Among the Aged

Retirement
Death of a spouse
Death of a close family member
Children moving away
Friends dying, becoming disabled, or moving away
Moving into an apartment or retirement home
Inability to socialize resulting from sensory or physical impairments

CASE DISCUSSION

Mrs. Robinson's fall illustrates the principle that functional problems in the elderly tend to have multiple causes. Physiological studies demonstrate that dark adaptation declines with age, so Mrs. Robinson's vision was somewhat impaired as she walked to the compost pile. Furthermore, reaction times are slower, so she probably had more difficulty righting herself when she lost her balance. In addition, a disease process, osteoarthritis of the knee, had caused further impairment, leading to localized muscle atrophy and a mild contracture. One other physiological factor certainly contributed to her injury: reduced bone mass in the wrist from osteoporosis. In spite of all these physiological limitations, Mrs. Robinson did well until an environmental factor, a stone on uneven ground, created a challenge to her physiological reserves. Because of the multiple factors just cited and probably because of others as well, Mrs. Robinson was unable to prevent an injurious fall.

AGING CHANGES IN VITAL BODY SYSTEMS

Physiological decline with aging is a near-universal phenomenon among body systems but varies markedly from system to system. Table 3-2 summarizes findings for many body systems among healthy adults. Some of the most clinically vital systems—cardiovascular, pulmonary, urinary, gastrointestinal, musculoskeletal, and neurological—are briefly discussed below.[5,7,8]

Cardiovascular System

In the cardiovascular system, disease rather than normal aging appears to lead to most dysfunction. Blood pressure tends to rise with age, intrinsic cardiac contractile function declines, and cardiac reserve diminishes in nondiseased subjects. The cardiovascular system rarely fails, however, except as a result of disease or a severe physical challenge, such as perioperative overhydration. On the other hand, coronary artery disease is extremely common in older persons and remains the most common cause of death among adults 65 years and older.

Pulmonary System

A similar principle applies to pulmonary function. Some mild declines are noted with age, but physiological reserves are so great that aging alone rarely leads to significant impairment. Disease must always be sought as an explanation when disability results in pulmonary symptoms.

Urinary System

In contrast, physiological changes in the urinary system frequently lead to symptoms among healthy older adults. Among one group of elderly 65 years and older, 64% got up at night to urinate, 40% had little warning before needing to urinate, and 29% reported occasional loss of urine ("accidents").

With age, peak bladder capacity is reduced and the amount of residual urine modestly increases. In addition,

Table 3-2   A Summary of Selected Anatomical and Physiological Changes with Aging, Healthy Adults

System Affected	Change Noted	Age Span (yr)
Height	Average loss of 2 inches	40-80
Weight		
Men	Peaks in mid 50s, then declines	
Women	Peaks in mid 60s, then declines	
Total body water		
Men	Declines from 60% to 54%	20-80
Women	Declines from 54% to 46%	20-80
Muscle mass	30% decrease	30-70
Taste buds	70% decrease	30-70
Cardiac reserve	Decreases from 4.6 to 3.3 times resting cardiac output	25-70
Maximum heart rate	195 to 155 beats/min	25-70
Lung vital capacity	17% decrease	30-70
Renal perfusion	Reduced by 50%	30-80
Prostate gland (men)	Doubles in size	20-80
Cerebral blood flow	Reduced by 20%	30-70
Bone mineral content	Reduced by 25%-30% in women, 10%-15% in men	40-80
Brain weight	Reduced by 7%	20-80
Amount of light reaching the retina	Diminished by 70%	20-65
Plasma glucocorticoid levels	No change	30-70

Data from Kenney RA: *Physiology of aging: a synopsis,* Chicago, 1982, Year Book Medical Publishers; and Shock NW, Greulich RC, Andres RA et al: *Normal human aging: the Baltimore Study of Aging,* NIH Publication No 84-2450, Washington, DC, 1984, US Government Printing Office; and Williams ME: *The American Geriatric Society's complete guide to aging and health,* New York, 1995, Harmony Books.

renal blood flow is nearly halved and the renal tubules are less able to concentrate urine, requiring the kidneys to work into the night (when blood flow is best) to remove solutes from the blood. These factors combine to cause increased urinary frequency, including nocturia, in most older adults. Among men, prostatic hypertrophy is nearly universal, and with it come increased nocturia, urinary hesitancy, and decreased urinary stream. Finally, creatinine clearance steadily decreases with age, declining at a rate of approximately 1% per year beyond age 40, although there is wide variation among individuals. This reduced creatinine clearance increases the susceptibility of older persons to toxicity from renally excreted drugs.

Gastrointestinal System

Changes in the gastrointestinal system are uneven. Most universal are dental changes, particularly gum recession and tooth loss. One half of the population older than 65 years is edentulous, but poor oral hygiene and lack of dental care are more responsible than age. Peristalsis is diminished throughout the gastrointestinal tract, but symptoms of constipation rarely arise in the absence of poor diet, drug effects, decreased mobility, or disease. Similarly, gastric acid secretion is reduced (many elderly are achlorhydric), and moderate villous atrophy is present in the small intestine, but significant malabsorption does not occur in healthy elderly on adequate diets. The liver and the pancreas decrease in size with age, but the function of nondiseased organs remains adequate throughout life.

Musculoskeletal System

Musculoskeletal changes with advancing years are particularly significant, but disuse is probably as important a factor as aging itself. Muscle mass decreases by 30%, and decreases occur in muscular strength, endurance, and bulk. These decreases in function are accompanied by mi-

croscopic lipofuscin deposition, reduction in myofibrils, and marked reductions in glycolytic oxidative enzyme activity.[4] Deconditioning as a factor in muscular changes is supported by the observation that heart and diaphragmatic muscles are relatively spared of "aging" changes.

Changes in bone structure and composition are universal. Especially noteworthy is a decline in bone density. Both men and women achieve peak bone mass during their 30s or early 40s, after which there is a gradual decline. The rate of bone loss is more rapid among women than men, with the most rapid demineralization occurring during the 5 years immediately following menopause. When decreases in bone density become severe enough to result in fractures after minimal trauma, osteoporosis is said to be present. As noted previously, age-related degenerative changes in joints (osteoarthritis) are also extremely common.

Neurological System

Alterations in neurological function are also profound, particularly beyond age 75. Within the brain, neuronal loss, dendritic changes, pigment accumulation, decreases in neurotransmitters, and a modest lowering of brain weight have all been noted. The impact of these changes on function, however, is not understood well enough to affect the clinical management of patients.

Clinical findings of declines in performance measures, including common tests of neurological function, are more directly relevant. Table 3-3 summarizes some of these findings. Neurological function represents an area in which performance variability increases markedly with age, accompanied by a modest overall decline in function. For example, when a person is attempting to stand still with his or her eyes closed, the mean amplitude of body sway increases by approximately 30% between ages 20 and 30 years. This, combined with declines in pro-

Table 3-3   Decline in Performance on Standard Neurological Tests for Healthy Adults Between Ages 20 and 80

Test	Percent	
Handwriting speed	30	
Hand grip strength	22	
Coordination of finger grasp	27	
Vibratory sensation, toe	97	Decline on quantitative testing between ages 20 and 80 yr
Vibratory sensation, shoulder	58	
Foot reaction time	19	
Stability of body axis when attempting to stand still with eyes closed	32	
Palmomental reflex	21	
Pursuit eye movements	16	
Absent ankle jerk	9	Normal older adults with abnormalities
Finger-nose test	8	
Impaired pinprick perception	0	

Data from Kokmen E et al: *J Gerontol* 32:411-419, 1977; Potvin AR et al: *J Am Geriatr Soc* 28:1-9, 1980; and Maki BE, Holliday PJ, Fernie GR: *J Am Geriatr Soc* 38:1-9, 1990.

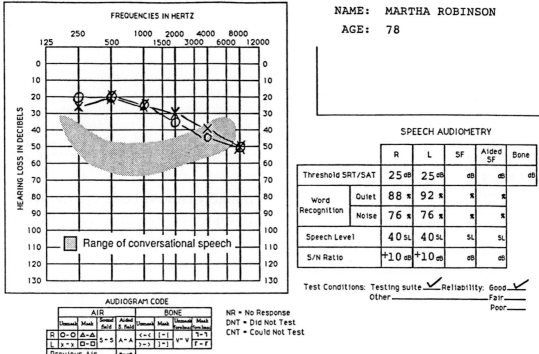

**UNC HOSPITALS
HEARING AND SPEECH CENTER**

NAME: MARTHA ROBINSON
AGE: 78

SPEECH AUDIOMETRY

		R	L	SF	Aided SF	Bone
Threshold SRT/SAT		25 dB	25 dB	dB	dB	dB
Word Recognition	Quiet	88 %	92 %	%	%	
	Noise	76 %	76 %	%	%	
Speech Level		40 SL	40 SL	SL	SL	
S/N Ratio		+10 dB	+10 dB	dB	dB	

Test Conditions: Testing suite ✓ Reliability: Good ✓
Other_____ Fair____
                       Poor____

AUDIOGRAM CODE

	AIR				BONE			
	Unmask	Mask	Sound field	Aided S. field	Unmask	Mask	Unmask forehead	Mask forehead
R	O–O	△–△	S–S	A–A	<–<	[–[	˅–˅	˥–˥
L	x–x	□–□			>–>	]–]		⌐–⌐
Previous Air			•–•					

NR = No Response
DNT = Did Not Test
CNT = Could Not Test

Case History: This 78-year-old woman reports difficulty understanding conversation in a group or when people "mumble and speak quietly." She has noticed this difficulty for several years and is not sure of any definite time of onset. She reports no associated dizziness, tinnitus, previous ear infections, or noise exposure.

Test Results: Audiological testing reveals a mild symmetrical sloping hearing loss bilaterally. Bone conduction thresholds (not demonstrated) are equal to air conduction thresholds, indicating that the hearing loss is sensorineural. Speech reception thresholds are 25 decibels bilaterally and are consistent with the pure tone thresholds in the 500-2000Hz range. Word recognition testing in quiet using monosyllabic word lists indicates a slight reduction in recognition of words presented at a comfortable listening level. In the presence of competing background noise, the patient experiences greater difficulty in understanding.

FIG. 3-2   Presbycusis. Audiogram of Mrs. Robinson at age 78. Hearing is progressively impaired at higher frequencies in both ears. Losses between 25 and 40 decibels constitute mild impairment; losses beyond 40 decibels are considered moderate impairment.

prioceptive function, results in a significant minority of older adults having difficulty performing Romberg's test, even in the absence of demonstrable disease.[7-9]

Special Senses

The special senses also show significant alterations with aging. Normal visual changes in aging include presbyopia, reduced contrast sensitivity, impaired adaptation to darkness or daylight, and delayed recovery from glare.[10] As noted earlier, crystalline changes in the lens impair near vision in the early 40s (presbyopia). Greater difficulty identifying objects in shadows or adjusting to a dark theater, for example, results from reduction in the number of retinal rod photosensitive discs. Between ages 20 and 80, several factors cut the amount of light reaching the retina by two thirds: reduced pupillary size, yellowing of the lens (making it more difficult to discriminate between blue and green), and opacification of the lens. Modest lens opacification scatters light, leading to glare sensitivity; severe lens opacification is called a *cataract*.

As a result of these changes, older adults require illumination that is bright but free from glare.

Another nearly universal finding in older persons is high-frequency hearing loss, termed *presbycusis* (Fig. 3-2). This pattern of hearing loss causes many older persons to have particular problems discriminating certain high-pitched sounds, such as *s, z, sh,* and *ch.* Speech discrimination is especially problematic when individuals with presbycusis are in noisy surroundings, such as a room with a slide projector fan blowing or a cocktail party.

CASE DISCUSSION

Mrs. Robinson's audiogram at age 78 (see Fig. 3-2) illustrates presbycusis. It shows that hearing is bilaterally impaired in the range beyond 3000 cycles per second. This means that Mrs. Robinson has particular difficulty discriminating high-pitched sounds and is likely to have problems understanding conversations in noisy environments.

MAINTENANCE OF HOMEOSTASIS

The kinds of impairments outlined, occurring over multiple organ systems, make it more difficult for the aging organism to maintain homeostasis efficiently. As a result, various homeostatic problems are seen with increasing frequency among older persons. Body fluid regulation is less precise, with elderly patients frequently demonstrating reduced thirst responses in the face of hypovolemia or hypernatremia. Thermoregulatory responses are also blunted, leading to increased susceptibility to hypothermia. Postural hypotension and vasovagal syncope are more common, arising from impairment of cardiovascular responses, decreased elasticity of blood vessels, and increased susceptibility to medications. Table 3-4 illustrates some common homeostatic impairments among older adults.

HOST DEFENSES AGAINST INFECTION

In the same manner that homeostasis is impaired, host defenses suffer from cumulative problems. The skin and mucous membranes—the body's primary barriers against infection—are thinner and receive diminished blood supply in the elderly. Mucociliary defenses and the cough reflex are less active, particularly in advanced age. Gastric achlorhydria removes an effective barrier against some pathogens. Prostatic hypertrophy, with increased residual urine volumes, reduces the natural process of flushing the bladder. Absence of fever in the face of bacterial infection is not unusual in older persons.

Polymorphonuclear lymphocyte numbers and function do not appear to diminish with age. Total lymphocyte counts also remain unchanged with advancing age, but certain subpopulations are altered, leading to reductions in cell-mediated immunity. In clinical examinations, reduced cellular immunity is evident as weakened reactions to common skin test antigens.

Table 3-4   Examples of Reduced Homeostatic Responses Common in Older Persons

Responses Commonly Reduced in Older Persons	Clinical Implications
Baroreceptor responsiveness	Increased susceptibility to postural hypotension
Thermoregulatory responses	Higher prevalence of hypothermia and hyperthermia
Cardiovascular reserve	Susceptibility to fluid overload
Thirst	Dehydration more common
Dark adaptation	Night driving more hazardous

COMMON LABORATORY TESTS AND AGING

As in other areas of medicine, distinguishing true physiological effects of aging from disease and disuse has also proven difficult in the area of laboratory testing. It appears, however, that most laboratory values change little if at all in normal healthy elderly. Notable exceptions are postprandial blood sugar, serum cholesterol in women, sedimentation rate, and serum triiodothyronine, or T_3 (because peripheral thyroxine, or T_4, is converted at lower rates in the elderly).[11] Table 3-5 summarizes aging changes in the median laboratory values of selected tests.

CASE DISCUSSION

Of the laboratory values obtained by Mrs. Robinson's physician, the hematocrit is clearly normal and should not change with age. The creatinine is in the high-normal range for that laboratory test. The test value probably represents significant reduction in creatinine clearance because creatinine clearance generally needs to be reduced by about half before the creatinine rises. Mrs. Robinson's serum cholesterol of 234 is probably normal, given the rise in median cholesterol with age seen in healthy women. The relative importance of cholesterol values in older adults, particularly women, remains controversial.

▼ MARTHA HILLIARD ROBINSON (Part V)
Age 84

During her annual physical examination at age 84 by Dr. Hensley, Mrs. Robinson expressed concern about not being able to sleep. "I'm in bed by 9:00 PM, read until 10:00 PM, and generally fall asleep," she said. "But by 2:30 AM I'm likely to be awake. Often, but not always, I go to the bathroom. Then, if I fall asleep, I wake up again at 4:30 or 5:00 AM. If only I could get a complete night's sleep!" With probing, Dr. Hensley was able to get Martha to talk about her husband's death of a stroke 8 months earlier. After determining that she was undergoing a normal adjustment to loss of a spouse, Dr. Hensley reassured her. He discussed the normal pattern of responses after losing a spouse. He also reviewed the physiol-

Table 3-5 Changes in the Median Value of Selected Common Laboratory Tests With Age

	Change During Ages 30 to 80	
Parameter	Men	Women
Hematocrit	5% fall	1% rise
White blood cell count	5% rise	5% fall
Westergren sedimentation rate	>100% rise	>170% rise
Sodium, serum	No change	No change
Potassium, serum	5% rise	1% rise
Creatinine, serum	2% rise	2% rise
Creatinine clearance	30% fall	30% fall
Blood glucose		
Fasting	5% rise	10% rise
1-hr postprandial	40% rise	40% rise
Albumin, serum	12% fall	9% fall
Calcium, serum	4% fall	No change
Cholesterol, total	5% rise	17% rise
Thyroxine, serum (T_4)	No change	2% fall
Triiodothyronine, serum (T_3)	20% fall	16% fall

From Dybkaer R: *Acta Med Scand* 209:1-9, 1981.

ogy of sleep and emphasized that her sleep pattern was normal.

At a later visit, Mrs. Robinson expressed concerns about her memory. "I can't remember the names of people I ought to know," she stated. "People I just met; people in church. I find myself writing notes to remember what to buy, even if I'm only going to the store for three or four items. I'm worried I might have Alzheimer's disease. What do you think, doctor?"

STUDY QUESTIONS

- How can a primary care physician effectively differentiate between benign forgetfulness and early dementia?
- Is sleep disturbance normal or abnormal in older persons?

CHANGES IN SLEEP PATTERNS

As many as 90% of older adults complain of some problems sleeping. In part, this is because physiological sleep patterns are altered in the elderly, causing them to spend a greater proportion of time in light sleep stages from which they are relatively easily awakened. In addition, older persons actually require less sleep than younger adults, although they generally spend more time in bed. Finally, nocturia, nocturnal dyspnea, arthritis pain, and a host of other physiological stimuli can awaken a sleeping elder. Often one or more trips to the bathroom are necessary during the night.

Thus the concept of an uninterrupted night's sleep is unrealistic for many older persons. When older adults complain of sleep problems, organic explanations such as paroxysmal nocturnal dyspnea or diabetes mellitus must

be ruled out, and depression should be considered. The majority of sleep problems, however, are best treated with reassurance that insomnia is not a progressive or fatal condition and with encouragement to accept nights that include a combination of wakefulness, resting, dozing, and sleep.

PSYCHOLOGICAL ISSUES IN THE 80S AND 90S

Few couples reach age 80 without the death or the significant disability of at least one spouse. Thus the years beyond age 80 invariably include dealing with disability, caregiving, bereavement, and loneliness. Sensory impairments, particularly hearing impairment, limit many individuals' ability to make new friends. Often physical impairments not only limit the ability to travel outside the home but impinge on activities of daily living. Beyond age 85, nearly 20% of older persons reside in nursing homes, and far more live in other caregiving settings.

Among individuals who remain independent, much of their energy is expended accomplishing daily activities, such as bathing, dressing, cooking, and eating. Friends and family are sources of strength. Visits to the physician's office are required more frequently, and the doctor and office staff provide important psychological support.

Death tends to be regarded without fear. Having faced these issues with loved ones and close friends, and being aware of their own limited life expectancy, even vigorous adults in their 80s and 90s can usually talk quite openly about death. It is remaining alive with major disabilities or being a burden to others that is a major source of concern. Chronic disabling diseases, such as stroke and Alzheimer's disease, are particularly feared.

MEMORY LOSS

Short-term memory loss is common in the elderly, and differentiating this "benign forgetfulness" from early dementia is often impossible. Formal mental status evaluation is indicated if there is any concern about cognitive impairment. Worrying about memory loss itself is a symptom of normal aging more than of Alzheimer's disease, in which the sufferer is generally unaware of any mental impairment.

Even exceptionally healthy older persons experience mental fatigue and memory lapses. As humorously related by B.F. Skinner, the noted Harvard psychologist, when he was in his mid-70s:

Forgetting is a classical problem. It is most conspicuous in forgetting names because names have so little going for them by way of context. I have convinced myself that names are very seldom wholly forgotten. When I have time—and I mean something on the order of half an hour—I can almost always recall a name if I have already recalled the occasion for using it. . . . But that will not work in introducing your wife to someone whose name you have forgotten. My wife and I use the following strategy: If there is any conceivable chance that she could have met the person, I simply say to her, "Of course, you remember. . . .?" and she grasps the outstretched hand and says, "Yes, of course. How are you?" The acquaintance may not remember meeting my wife, but is not sure of his or her memory, either.[12]

▼ *MARTHA HILLIARD ROBINSON (Part VI)*
Age 90

For her ninetieth birthday, Mrs. Robinson was interviewed for a feature by a reporter from the Durham Morning Star. An independently wealthy widow, Mrs. Robinson had donated an undisclosed sum of money to the Roth School of Nursing. At the interview, her white hair was pulled back into a thin, neat bun, her posture was stooped, and she walked with the assistance of a four-pronged cane. She wore a hearing aid and an eye bandage, having recently undergone laser surgery on her left eye. Nevertheless, she continued to live alone in her one-story home, receiving homemaker services 3 hours a day. Her daughter, 15 miles away, assisted with transportation and shopping. A visiting nurse was coming daily to check on her eye but would discontinue services soon.

The interviewer, a journalism graduate student from a local small college, had gone to considerable length to prepare for the interview. She had learned that Mrs. Robinson was somewhat hard of hearing and bothered by bright lights. She also knew that Mrs. Robinson preferred a morning interview, generally taking a nap and then visiting with friends in the afternoon.

"Based on your own experience," the interviewer asked, "is it better to let things go or to keep as active as possible?"

"A little of both, I guess," responded Mrs. Robinson. "I'm not as active as I used to be, but I still do as much as I feel able. I guess I'd say I pace myself. I'm an early riser, take my pills, do a few exercises, and have breakfast. Morning is my work time—for shopping, writing letters, paying bills, seeing the doctor, or being interviewed by you. Two mornings a week I go to the senior center, where I'm in a bridge group. We use large-print playing cards."

HEALTHY AGING

Gerontologists have developed several theories to explain psychological adaptation to aging. The *disengagement theory* suggests that healthy aging involves voluntary cutting back on work, social, and even family ties. The disengaged individual becomes more satisfied with vicarious activities and especially with reminiscence. Often, a review of his or her life allows the individual to come to terms with and to accept past failures. The prototypical disengaged person is an older adult, well known and loved by neighbors, who happily spends all day rocking on the front porch, offering a cheerful word to everyone who passes by.

A contrasting view is represented by the *activity theory*. This position, which is often more readily grasped by young, energetic professional students, suggests that healthy aging implies staying as active as possible. Thus the active older adult finds meaning in continued professional or volunteer work, social activities, family, hobbies, and interests. As Eric Pfeiffer said, "It struck me as though the successfully aging person was someone who somewhere along the way had decided to stay in training. He or she had decided to stay in training physically, intellectually, emotionally, and socially."[13]

The limitation of the activity theory is its inability to appreciate the extent to which even the most active and energetic older adults must continually adjust to diminished capabilities and to physical and role losses. A third theory of psychological adjustment to aging, the *continuity theory,* may serve as a bridge between the proponents of disengagement and those of activity. According to the continuity theory, successful psychological adaptation to aging involves allowing personal preferences from earlier years to manifest themselves as the individual responds to the stresses and challenges of older age. Thus some individuals will remain more active because it suits their personality, whereas others will become more disengaged. Great variation in responses is seen; the goal is that the older adult lives a personally satisfying and socially satisfactory life.

CASE DISCUSSION

Healthy aging, as exemplified by Martha Hilliard Robinson, involved preparation, adaptation, and good fortune. Mrs. Robinson prepared for a healthy old age by adopting good health habits early in life. She did not overeat, did not smoke, exercised regularly, got plenty of sleep, married, and raised a family. Her life-style during older years involved routines of exercise, eating, rest, productive work, and socializing. All of these factors have been linked to longevity. Furthermore, she managed to enter old age relatively well off economically; the well-to-do live longer and remain healthier than the impoverished.

In spite of entering old age with superior health habits and economic resources, Mrs. Robinson needed to adjust successfully to a variety of losses. She retired, her husband became ill and died, and she suffered from osteoarthritis, osteoporosis, and hearing impairment. In her case, successful adaptation involved being able to give up some activities and continue others. Thus she was able to continue to find meaning in life, in spite of limitations and losses. She maintained a strong faith in God and a close attachment to her family, drawing strength from these in difficult times.

STUDY QUESTION

- *Mrs. Robinson had many advantages that helped her age gracefully. Identify some of the problems that a less advantaged person might face and what physicians can do to provide assistance in addressing each.*

▼ *MARTHA HILLIARD ROBINSON (Part VII)*
Age 94

At age 92, Mrs. Robinson suffered a stroke, which left her aphasic and unable to use her right hand. After rehabilitation, she was able to walk with a cane. She moved in with her daughter, whose care was supplemented by home health nursing. She died of pneumonia at age 94.

CASE DISCUSSION

Death and dying are a normal part of aging. Those like Mrs. Robinson, who have led a long, full life, often face death unafraid. Nevertheless, the period of dependency and disability that often accompanies the final years is trying for the older person and his or her family. Mrs. Robinson was fortunate to have a supportive daughter and physician and to die in relative comfort at home.

POSTTEST

1. Which one of the following normal aging changes contributes to impaired night driving skills among 80-year-olds?
   a. Reduced dark adaptation
   b. 19% decrease in foot reaction time compared with young adults
   c. 70% reduction in light reaching the retina
   d. 70% decrease in pinprick sensation in the feet
   e. Reduced ability to hear approaching sirens
2. Which one of the following statements is false about individuals aged 65 to 70 years?
   a. Reported happiness is greater than at any other age.
   b. Percentage of body fat is greater than at age 20.
   c. They report less independence and more financial worries than younger adults.
   d. Sexual activity is correlated with physical health.
3. All of the following are true about normal aging except which one?
   a. Established routines often constitute a helpful adjustment to aging.

   b. Sensory impairments limit many older persons' ability to make friends.
   c. Major disability is uncommon among older persons.
   d. Worrying about memory loss is more often a symptom of normal aging than of Alzheimer's disease.
4. Mr. Carter, an 80-year-old retired engineer, is active in a bridge club, the local church, and a daily exercise class. His wife, on the other hand, spends the majority of her time either watching television (during cold days) or sitting on the front porch (during warm days). Which one of the following is false about this couple?
   a. Mrs. Carter exemplifies the disengagement theory of successful aging.
   b. Mr. Carter exemplifies the activity theory of successful aging.
   c. Mr. Carter is likely to live longer than Mrs. Carter.
   d. The continuity theory could apply to either spouse.

REFERENCES

1. Larrabee WF, Caro I: The aging face, *Postgrad Med* 76(7):37-46, 1984.
2. Karp DA: A decade of reminders: changing age consciousness between fifty and sixty years old, *Gerontologist* 28:727-738, 1988.
3. Perlman PE, Adams W: Physiologic changes as patients get older, *Postgrad Med* 85:213-217, 1989.
4. Beck JC, ed: *Geriatrics review syllabus: a core curriculum in geriatric medicine,* New York, 1989, American Geriatrics Society.
5. Williams ME: *The American Geriatrics Society's complete guide to aging and health,* New York, 1995, Harmony Books.
6. Sheehy G: The happiness report, *Redbook,* July 1979.
7. Kenney RA: *Physiology of aging: a synopsis,* Chicago, 1982, Year Book Medical Publishers, Inc.
8. Shock NW et al: *Normal human aging: the Baltimore Study of Aging,* NIH Publication No 84-2450, Washington, DC, US Government Printing Office.
9. Kokmen E et al: Neurological manifestations of aging, *J Gerontol* 32:411-419, 1977.
10. Carter TL: Age-related vision changes: a primary care guide, *Geriatrics* 49(9):37-45, 1994.
11. Dybkaer R: Relative reference values for clinical chemical and haematological quantities in "healthy" elderly people, *Acta Med Scand* 209:1-9, 1981.
12. Skinner BF: Intellectual self-management in old age, *Am Psychol* 38:239-244, 1983.
13. Pfeiffer E, ed: *Successful aging: a conference report,* Durham, NC, 1974, Center for the Study of Aging and Human Development.

PRETEST ANSWERS

1. b
2. b
3. d

POSTTEST ANSWERS

1. b
2. c
3. c
4. c

CHAPTER 4

Illness and Aging

RICHARD J. HAM

OBJECTIVES

Upon completion of this chapter, the reader will be able to:

1. Describe the typical ways acute illness is modified in its modes of presentation in older patients, including the significance of cognitive and functional change as presentations of acute illness.

2. Understand the factors that inhibit presentation of older individuals for health care.

3. Initiate methods to improve communication both with and about older individuals, especially at times of change in the site of care.

4. Reduce deconditioning, dysmobility, and immobility resulting from illness in old age, especially in the hospitalized or institutionalized patient.

5. Prioritize the management of multiple concurrent problems of differing types in elders.

6. Avoid the problems of multiple prescribers for one patient.

7. Integrate health promotion and maintenance of function into the management of acute and chronic illnesses.

8. Understand the roles, problems, and utility of the family and other surrogates in the care of elderly patients.

9. Utilize and manage the family, other caregivers, and community support systems effectively and efficiently in diagnosis and management.

10. Identify and relieve the factors increasing family and caregiver stress.

11. Describe the range of housing alternatives to be considered and the principles of organizing placement when an elder has to relocate.

12. Understand the influence of environment on presentation and management of illness in old age.

13. Understand the principles of decisions about intensity of treatment and the financial and ethical aspects of care.

14. Describe the rationale for physician involvement in the design of public policy.

15. Outline the principles and characteristics of good geriatric primary care.

PRETEST

1. Which one of the following is not a characteristic presentation of illness in old age?
   a. Depression without sadness
   b. Infectious disease without leukocytosis
   c. Fever without cause
   d. Apathetic thyrotoxicosis
   e. Myocardial infarction without chest pain
2. Which one of the following statements is false concerning ways in which physicians might "harm" older persons?
   a. The half-life of many medications is prolonged in healthy older people.
   b. Twenty percent of hospitalizations of older people are prolonged by a major adverse event.
   c. Follow-up to assess the effect of prescriptions is often lacking.
   d. Communication between physicians about patients often excludes consideration of their functional level.
   e. Longer hospital stays have been shown to improve recovery prior to discharge.
3. Which one of the following aspects of a dependent older person has not been demonstrated to be a major stressor of the caregiving family member?
   a. The patient's ingratitude
   b. The use of multiple medications
   c. The patient's being awake at night
   d. The physical dependency of the patient
4. Following brief office assessment of a 69-year-old black woman who lives with her daughter and works full time, four problems were defined. Which one problem takes most priority in the initial management?

   a. A blood pressure of 175/90
   b. Demonstrable stress incontinence, which restricts her from leaving the home
   c. Hearing difficulties: she keeps the television loud but can manage one-on-one conversation
   d. A brown nevus on her anterior chest, which has been unchanged for several years
5. A 75-year-old woman is taking amitriptyline, isophane insulin suspension, digoxin, and a thiazide diuretic, and has established diagnoses of congestive heart failure with left bundle branch block, diabetes mellitus, and depression. Which one of the following concerning the interactions between her diagnoses and treatments is false?
   a. The thiazide predisposes to digoxin toxicity.
   b. The amitriptyline may be the cause of the bundle branch block.
   c. The hyperglycemia may be worsened by the diuretic.
   d. The digoxin predisposes her to risk of hypoglycemia.
6. Which one of the following statements concerning family members and the care of elderly patients is false?
   a. The physician is obligated to carry out noninvasive investigations if demanded by the health care proxy.
   b. An individual named as health care proxy has the right to refuse treatment on behalf of the patient.
   c. If an older person is deemed competent, the family has no right to be involved in medical decisions on the patient's behalf.
   d. Disturbed nights head the list of patient characteristics stressing caregivers.

The changes that usually occur with increasing age, the way our society treats the old, and the way individuals view themselves as they age combine to modify the ways in which illnesses present and the methods required for their optimal management. People become more unique as they age, and each individual situation must be very carefully evaluated. Yet certain issues and characteristics are sufficiently frequent and recurrent in the elderly that they require special approaches. The primary care physician needs to be familiar with these issues and characteristics in order to appropriately plan his or her practice style in such a way that elderly people in need are optimally served. Rather than the traditional "investigate, diagnose, treat, and cure" sequence and a one-on-one re-

lationship with the patient, the physician to the older patient must consider the family members and others, who frequently have differing perceptions from the patient, and must take into account function and the long-term consequences of many concurrent factors, illnesses, treatments, and their interactions.

▼ THREE MODIFIED PRESENTATIONS

Virginia Tsadlick, an 82-year-old nursing home resident, falls twice during the day. She has previously been functioning well, with no problems with gait or balance. She eats less supper than usual but has normal vital signs both that evening and the following morning. The following afternoon, her blood pressure is found to be very low, and she is transferred to the emergency room, where abnormal bowel sounds and abdominal x-ray examination leads to a diagnosis of perforated diverticulum; she is in a state of sepsis and shock from peritonitis. At no time does she have abdominal tenderness or abdominal pain.

Harold Robinson *is a 76-year-old man who lives a comfortable retired life with his wife in a self-contained small house with a half-acre garden that is his major hobby and pastime. He complains of fatigue, saying he lacks energy to carry out his normal functions. His mood appears fine, and at a glance he looks quite well. However, on physical examination he has marked cardiomegaly, rales at both bases, and other signs suggestive of congestive heart failure. He denies any history of dyspnea, nocturnal coughing, or orthopnea.*

Donna Wilkinson *is an 83-year-old woman cared for by her disabled sister. Her main problem has been an ongoing, progressive dementia. Over a period of 24 hours, she develops respiratory symptoms and a cough that sounds productive, although no sputum is seen. An in-home chest x-ray examination is performed less than 24 hours after her symptoms start; it is reported as clear. Within another 24 hours, she has overt physical signs of right lower lobe consolidation, tachypnea, and a temperature of 103° F. She has to be hospitalized, at which time a diagnosis of right lower lobe pneumonia is made. After a stormy hospital course, she recovers.*

People become more unique as they age, so their symptoms and how they perceive them are inevitably "different."

NONSPECIFIC PRESENTATION

Severe, acute illness in older individuals will often present with vague, nonspecific, or seemingly trivial symptoms. Sometimes the illness manifests itself in an organ system remote from the one primarily affected. Typical signs and symptoms may be absent or delayed. The brain is especially vulnerable to the toxic effects of illness (and treatment). Typical nonspecific symptoms that may represent specific illnesses in old age include confusion, falling, incontinence, fatigue, anorexia, and self-neglect.

The onset of such symptoms, either abruptly or over a matter of days, should alert the physician to the possibility of a developing acute illness. "Premonitory falls" are falls occurring as a "prodrome" to a developing illness. An older individual presenting with a new onset of falling or confusion (or any of the other symptoms mentioned above and summarized in Box 4-1) should be observed for the development of acute illness. An abrupt change in functional status of any kind (e.g., ceasing to go shopping or withdrawing from other previous activi-

---

BOX 4-1
Nonspecific Symptoms That May Represent Specific Illness

Confusion	Apathy
Self-neglect	Anorexia
Falling	Dyspnea
Incontinence	Fatigue

---

ties) should similarly be regarded as a sign of potential illness, including depression.

In the elderly, an abrupt change in functional status is a cardinal sign of potential illness.

PRESENTATION IN A DIFFERENT ORGAN SYSTEM

The brain is an especially vulnerable organ, thus a change in mental status is one of the most frequent presenting symptoms of acute illness in older persons; but the limited reserve of several organ systems leads to certain illnesses frequently presenting in the "wrong" system. *Thyroid disease,* although it can present in typical fashion, often presents symptomatically with cardiac, gastrointestinal, or cerebral complications. *Cardiovascular* presentations, secondary to the lack of reserve in many older persons' cardiovascular systems, are often presentations or concurrent complications of other illnesses, especially if there is an increased hemodynamic state, as with hyperthyroidism or an acute infection. Sometimes congestive heart failure (CHF) treatment is continued for years or for life, when in fact the state of CHF was induced by intercurrent illness; once the underlying illness is resolved, the CHF may not need such vigorous continuing management.

TYPICAL ALTERED PRESENTATIONS

A number of altered presentations of disease in the elderly occur so frequently that they almost may be regarded as specific syndromes for which to be clinically alert (Box 4-2).

Depression Without Sadness

Major depression in an older individual may have very little overt dysphoria (sadness); often, apparent mental confusion dominates the clinical picture, demonstrating the vulnerability of the brain to an illness that is physical in nature. This phenomenon is generally referred to as the "dementia syndrome of depression." In other elders with major depression, somatic symptoms dominate the picture. Although masked, the sadness of the depression is often (but not always) present, if carefully sought.

Mass Without Symptoms

This describes the sometimes incidental finding of a malignant mass, especially gastrointestinal, which has produced remarkably little functional impairment, such as bowel disturbance. This is sometimes secondary to lesions located in clinically "silent" parts of the bowel (e.g., the ascending colon), but it may be secondary to reduced neuronal sensitivity in the gastrointestinal tract itself and/or reduced central awareness.

Silent Infectious Disease

Often, an older patient has sepsis but without leukocytosis, fever, or tachycardia. In pneumonia, chest x-ray examinations may be normal. Many clinicians believe that the radiological changes are delayed in old age. Possibly the pneumonic appearance manifests only when associated dehydration is corrected.

Silent Surgical Abdomen

The normal sequence of localized tenderness and pain leading to generalized tenderness and pain as local peritonitis spreads and generalizes is often greatly modified. The patient may present with tachypnea and pneumonia-like symptoms or with vague mental or urinary symptoms, without anything specifically pointing to the acute abdominal problem itself. Physicians must be familiar with the conditions likely to produce an abdominal catastrophe in old age. Ischemic colitis (mesenteric insufficiency) may produce only vague but persistent, nonspecific bowel disturbance, or even general symptoms like anorexia or fatigue, until completion of the thrombotic process or embolization to the bowel leads to ischemia and ultimately gangrene of the bowel, a life-threatening situation. Presentation of other major abdominal problems, including appendicitis and cholecystitis, the most common cause of acute abdominal conditions in old age, can be remarkably clinically silent.

Myocardial Infarction Without Chest Pain (Silent MI)

By most estimates, approximately one third of acute myocardial infarctions in older individuals are clinically silent, with no chest pain or other symptoms to identify them; they are found later on routine electrocardiography. Perhaps another one third have symptoms but not symptoms like chest pain that would necessarily identify the cardiac origin of the problem.[1] Again, the clinician should be alert to the elderly individual who has a history of several days of vague illness, perhaps with a little exercise intolerance, and should obtain an electrocardiogram or (if suspicions are raised early enough) cardiac enzyme studies which may be confirmatory.

Nondyspneic Pulmonary Edema

The frequent phenomenon is of a patient with definite signs of CHF who does not experience subjective dyspnea, paroxysmal nocturnal dyspnea, or coughing and instead has vague symptoms or none at all. Unfortunately, the ultimate morbidity and mortality, if uncorrected, is the same as in the symptomatic patient. This phenomenon may be partially explained by reduced sensation and partially by self-limitation of activity, keeping within insidiously reduced, and thus perhaps unnoticed, exercise tolerance limits.

Apathetic Thyrotoxicosis

Although much hyperthyroid disease (and most hypothyroid disease) presents the typical clinical picture, this well-recognized syndrome of tiredness and slowing down caused by hyperthyroidism is sufficiently well recognized for this to be one of the classic "altered presentations" of illness in old age.[2]

WHY PRESENTATION IS MODIFIED IN OLD AGE

There are several possible explanations for these delayed and modified presentations. *Altered central processing* may be present either because of reduced cognitive status as a result of the cerebral effect of the illness itself or because of preexisting, often previously unrecognized, dementia. Some individuals, because of *negativity* about what is likely to happen to them with increasing age, will tolerate or ignore symptoms, limiting their activities if necessary, and accepting the symptoms as "old age." Although the ease of developing tolerance to a very insidious onset of disability is understandable, this same negativity, surprisingly, is often seen when more acute changes strike. Some health professionals, lacking an adequate explanation of different phenomena, will attribute symptoms to "old age"; this encourages patients and their family members to do so as well. *Fear*, not only of illness but of its treatment (hospitalization or placement in an institution), is often a factor. These factors may lead to *denial*. Actual *ignorance* of the significance of bodily changes may be an issue. Neuronal degeneration causing reduction of *peripheral sensitivity* provides a physical explanation for reduced sensation and awareness. Many elders suffer unrecognized *depression;* this frequent and treatable illness will create negativity and reduce the individual's initiative to seek medical care. Many illnesses, especially chronically progressive ones, are associated with an increased prevalence of depression.

CASE DISCUSSIONS

Mrs. Tsadlick *has the characteristic presentation of a "silent acute abdomen" with vague, nonspecific symptoms and normal vital signs even just a few hours before impending collapse in a life-threatening situation.*

Mr. Robinson *exemplifies the classic insidious presentation of "nondyspneic pulmonary edema": a patient of clear mental status who lacks specific symptomatology and presents with a rather vague symptom for which the differential diagnosis is very wide. He could have been suffering a depression or any number of medical illnesses. Finding signs of CHF is not sufficient in a presentation such as this. The generic rule in geriatric medicine (see below) is that individual signs and symptoms often have multiple causes. Thus proper investigation of a previously well-functioning individual like Mr. Robinson must include attention to the many other potential causes of fatigue. Laboratory tests with organ-specific testing should be carried out (if any symptoms point to specific organ deficits). Depression should be seriously considered, even while initiating treatment for the CHF itself.*

Mrs. Wilkinson *shows classical delay in the development of objective radiological evidence, although she was clinically in clear need of medical attention. (The white blood cell count may have been normal, too, had it been obtained.) Her case emphasizes the importance of observation over time, the need to record changes in signs and symptoms, and the necessity to act on them and on clinical suspicions rather than merely relying on comprehensive exclusionary laboratory and radiological data at one point in time.*

NONPRESENTATION WHEN ILL

Physicians are trained to start the write-up of the patient's history with the abbreviation "c/o," meaning "complains of." Patients are expected to "complain" and thus attract medical attention. But many older individuals do not do that. As mentioned above, denial, ignorance, fear, or negativity about the aging process lead some people to tolerate problems which they may not have tolerated at a younger age. The psychological and cultural barriers to declaring mental symptoms, such as depression or memory loss, lead to the known underutilization of mental health services by the older population, given the known incidence of such illnesses. Certain conditions accepted by many as "normal" in old age, such as musculoskeletal stiffness, hearing loss, and even urinary incontinence are often not presented for medical attention; a review of symptoms, including very specific inquiry for the symptoms commonly not presented through embarrassment or negativity, is vital. To save time, this review can frequently be done at the time of the physical examination.

Studies in Scotland[3] decades ago demonstrated the extent of untreated illness among older individuals, even when access to health care is exemplary (in this case by the well-publicized development of the National Health Service after World War II). Illnesses that were tolerated, despite being treatable, included mental disturbance, depression, diabetes, anemia, and malnutrition, as well as lesser problems like earwax buildup producing deafness, and dental and podiatric problems. A number of such characteristic "hidden illnesses" are summarized in Box 4-3.

> *BOX 4-3*
> *"Hidden" Illnesses in the Elderly*
>
> | | |
> |---|---|
> | Depression | Hearing loss |
> | Incontinence | Dementia |
> | Musculoskeletal stiffness | Dental problems |
> | Falling | Poor nutrition |
> | Alcoholism | Sexual dysfunction |

▼ ROBERT OSBORNE

Robert Osborne is a 76-year-old man who lives on his own. He is brought to you by community social service workers who have been called to the house by neighbors because of the weight loss and self-neglect they have observed in this isolated elderly man as he putters around in his garden. On formal testing, his mental status is normal, but his limited mobility (secondary to degenerative joint disease), hearing loss, diminished visual acuity, and urinary incontinence are clinically obvious, with apparent weight loss, dehydration, and undernutrition.

CASE DISCUSSION

Mr. Osborne typifies the isolated older individual who tolerates slowly increasing difficulties, the functional effects of which will ultimately be quite difficult to correct even though the "treatment" is medically simple. Major efforts will need to be made in this case to institute appropriate therapy to try to improve Mr. Osborne's mobility, investigate and control his incontinence, and improve his nutrition. After what has probably been several years of silence, it is unlikely that efforts to get him to use a hearing aid will be successful. If he later needs care in a skilled nursing facility, his hearing loss will be very isolating.

COMMUNICATION PROBLEMS

Hearing loss is very common in old age. Many of us fail to take the time to allow for the lipreading which many older individuals rely on for full comprehension; this requires that the physician arranges to be in a lighted area and on the same level as the patient, looking full into the face. In old age, environmental noise (universally present in emergency rooms and in many medical offices) diminishes auditory acuity. Under the stress of a medical visit when ill, even without dementia, many older persons find their concentration reduced.

The preserved social facade of patients with dementia frequently misleads health professionals; the patient may appear to be (and may actually be) both registering and understanding information but failing to memorize it. For this reason, objective screening for impaired cognitive status should be carried out much more readily than it is. Individuals with unrecognized cognitive deficits are likely to be placed at unnecessary risk. Both the family and the physician must realize that in some cases the patient "can't" rather than "won't" comply. Even in younger, unimpaired individuals, remarkably little information is actually learned and retained by patients during their interactions with their physicians. Reinforcements, written reminders, and utilization of the family, if available, to increase compliance and understanding are essential adjuncts for effective management of many older patients.

This necessary involvement of family members and caregivers itself produces communication problems. These other concerned individuals will have their own anxieties to address and will often have more to say privately about their relatives than they would ever say in their presence. Family members are frequently the means of implementing the management plan. Good communication includes both time away from the patient for family members and other caregivers and sufficient time for the patient, too, whose autonomy and input must be respected. It is up to the patient, if competent, to decide what is to be done; some family members "take over" too soon; others deny problems and expose vulnerable individuals to unnecessary risk.

Once good communication with the family is in process, the primary care physician is in a much better position to address complex ethical issues, such as resuscitation, tube feeding, and other aspects of the intensity of treatment.

Communication between health professionals about elders is a special skill. The ability to work as a team, using and interacting with a wide range of health professionals—often by telephone and fax—is essential to good care. Physician-to-physician communication can be problematic; elderly patients often have several physicians involved in their care. Who is "in charge"? The primary care physician should be, but there is sometimes competition for this role. Many organ-specific specialists take on primary care roles for patients with whom they are involved. This is partly because of the shortage of primary care physicians. When several physicians are involved, it is important to have one of them be declared the primary care physician, or "personal physician," the others being relegated to specific roles.

Special communication is needed when a patient transfers from one setting to another; this often involves an entirely new set of health professionals. Communication must include the medications (including the reasons for prescription, the "target symptoms" or other purpose for each, suggested follow-up plans to assess their utility, and the plans to stop them); the current formal diagnoses and functional problems, with an impression of the speed of change; other therapeutic interventions that have been helpful; social and other health professional services already involved (including the names of the agencies and, if possible, the individuals involved); the patient's insight into their problems; and the patient's interests and ethnic, cultural, and religious backgrounds when significant. Objective measurements, numeric if possible, of mental status, activities of daily living (ADLs) and instrumental ADLs (IADLs), the range of movement in degrees, exercise tolerance by distance, etc. should be used whenever possible so that change can be appreciated and acted upon.

▼ WILLIAM HENRY

William Henry is an 80-year-old man, who has been led to believe that he has been brought to your office for a "routine physical." He describes himself as well, having a little difficulty moving around, but otherwise not needing attention. You have a pleasant conversation with him about his activities in World War II. After a physical examination, you find him to be a "delightful old man." You are then surprised to receive an emotionally charged phone call from the son, who had felt constrained from speaking in front of his father. The son gives a history of tolerating more than a year of multiple late-night phone calls from his father, who lives alone and gets confused and suffers hallucinations at night; the father has in fact been brought back by the police on more than one occasion after being found walking around, improperly attired, in the night.

CASE DISCUSSION

This case dramatically illustrates the difference between the patient's and the family's perceptions. Mental status screening in this case would have revealed considerably more impairment than the brief interview, which, by focusing not on current events but rather on events in the past, entirely missed the patient's deficits and needs. Better communication, with the son describing the problems by phone to the office staff, could have prevented the misunderstanding.

DECONDITIONING AND DYSMOBILITY

Hospitals and nursing homes are still characterized by the number of "beds." Marjorie Warren, a pioneer geriatrician in the 1940s in Britain, used to ask her junior physicians time and again, "Why is this patient in bed?" All health professionals still need to do the same.

Deconditioning refers to the loss of musculoskeletal strength and suppleness and the loss of coordinated balancing and righting reflexes familiar to anyone who has suddenly been immobilized for a few days by an intercurrent illness or surgery. Recovery from such deconditioning is prolonged in many older persons, and the consequences may be severe: falling and injury, loss of confidence, further prolonged immobility, and even a continuing downhill spiral of deterioration that can be difficult to stop. The primary physician must continually interfere in the management of his or her older patients, especially when they are temporarily immobilized by other conditions while under the care of others (e.g., perioperatively and while in intensive care). Efforts to maintain range of motion, to physically get the patient out of bed, to continue weight bearing exercise, and to keep the patient moving around must be vigorously maintained. This is one of the most vital functions for the generalist physician in the specialized or tertiary care setting.

Dysmobility is the current term for a range of problems: instability, gait disturbance with poor balance, falling and its consequences (including the loss of self-confidence that is so often consequent to falling), partial immobility (with assistance being needed for transfers), and being "bed-bound" or at least "chair-bound." This can be a progressively downward spiral over weeks to months for older individuals, in whom the consequences of immobility are many and severe and include life-threatening conditions, conditions that increase morbidity, and conditions that cause potentially permanent disability, such as flexion contractures. (See Box 4-4.)

Maintaining the patient's mobility in the hospital and elsewhere is a vital function of the primary care physician.

▼ WILLIAM WILKINSON

William Wilkinson is a 73-year-old patient of yours who was hospitalized for urosepsis while on vacation out of town. He had previously been independently mobile, although he had morning stiffness in his hips. Before hospitalization, he had regular bowel movements, and his morning habit of walking around the house both helped this and helped to move bronchial secretions that "sat on his chest" overnight. (He suffered chronic obstructive pulmonary disease.) Septic and unwell in a tertiary care hospital, he is initially given intravenous therapy and antibiotics but rapidly develops fecal impaction with fecal incontinence, becomes confused, and develops a persistent but nonproductive cough. His son, alarmed at this rapid deterioration, is personally instrumental in initiating respiratory and physical therapy. However, Mr. Wilkinson's bowel habits and the stiffness in his hips are still problems for him 2 months after hospitalization, which he describes to you as "the worst thing that has ever happened to me."

CASE DISCUSSION

This case demonstrates a relatively minor range of complications; at least he is on the road to recovery. The much more depressing scenario of patients suffering virtually all the consequences listed in the box above can be seen in any tertiary care hospital any day of the week.

MULTIPLICITY OF CONCURRENT PROBLEMS

Frequently an older individual's management is complicated by several ongoing chronic conditions and their medical treatment, together with acute superimposed illnesses. Added to these multiple diagnoses are the various unique psychosocial and environmental factors that influence function and management.

The primary care physician is ideally set to be the coordinator when multiple systems are impaired; this often involves coordinating the ongoing attention of several organ-specialists. The principle of restricting prescription of medications to only one coordinating physician could reduce polypharmacy, duplicate prescribing, and drug-drug or drug-disease interactions.[4] *Setting priorities* for treatment or management is a particular skill. Physicians are often tempted to treat the problem that is easiest to treat, which often means a prescription of a medication.

BOX 4-4
Consequences of Immobilization

Stiffness, contractures
Loss of muscle strength
Confusion, sensory loss, depression
Dependence, institutionalization
Instability, loss of confidence
Dehydration, electrolyte imbalance
Malnutrition
Osteoporosis
Thrombosis: arterial and venous, pulmonary embolism
Pneumonia, atelectasis
Hypothermia
Pressure sores
Urinary retention, urinary incontinence, urinary tract infection, calculi
Constipation, fecal impaction, fecal incontinence

However, this may not be the most important problem in functional terms (which is probably what matters most to the patient and family members) nor in terms of its consequences as an immediate threat to life or as an ongoing threat to full health. The initial comprehensive assessment recommended for most older persons includes the evolution of a comprehensive *problem list* including not only formal diagnoses but also broader symptom complexes that do not fall into traditional diagnostic categories (such as falling or instability) and that, although they may have identifiable contributory diagnoses, require a management plan in and of themselves. The problem list must also include contributory psychosocial features ("lives alone," "recent bereavement," etc.), in view of the impact of such psychosocial and environmental factors on the patient and on the illness(es) themselves. The problem list can then be consulted so that attention to even one individual problem will efficiently and appropriately take into account the other factors. A well organized, current problem list can ensure a coordinated approach. Such a problem list also aids communication at times of transition from one clinical site to another.

▼ KATHLEEN TRAVIS

Kathleen Travis is an 81-year-old patient who is brought by her grandson to initiate primary care with you. He is concerned about the number of medications she is on and her rather depressed state of mind. He and his wife give most of the history.

She has lived for years in the same ranch-style house with three of her sisters, the last of whom died several months ago. On an average day she is "bored," but she avoids going out. For 4 weeks her right arm has been aching, a constant and dull pain. She has previously suffered chronic low back and neck pain, and she currently has stiffness in multiple joints. She brings several medications with her that have been prescribed and that she takes sporadically. She uses eye drops and medication for glaucoma and sees an ophthalmologist; she cannot see well enough to watch the television or read. She has been having problems sleeping for several months, and 3 or 4 times a week she takes flurazepam (Dalmane) 30 mg to help her sleep. She wakes often, frequently experiencing pain in her back or arm, and she generally has to get up to urinate more than once in the night. She is constipated and gets very tired on the few occasions she visits with her family. Physical examination confirms her poor visual acuity and shows that her mental status is good, at least on screening. She is almost impacted with feces on the rectal examination; and she has signs suggestive of slight CHF with cardiomegaly, as well as kyphoscoliosis, restricted neck movements, and diminished range of motion of her shoulders and hips. Her muscle tone is poor. She walks with an unsteady gait and becomes dizzy on movement of her neck.

CASE DISCUSSION

Ms. Travis' problem list includes recent symptoms but is dominated by major ongoing problems and by several prescribed medications that she is taking intermittently. She has signs suggestive of depression, and must be investigated for osteoporosis as well as osteoarthritis, the former being a particular hazard since she lives alone, has an unsteady gait, and is at risk of falling and therefore fracture (which would probably be the beginning of the end). Since she did not choose to come, it is particularly important for you and the grandson to set priorities for her safety. The problem list will assist in this process. Her medications include a long-acting benzodiazepine, which may be impairing her in the day, or at least contributing to apathy and depression. Her ophthalmologist, who is the physician whom she has seen most frequently in the past few years, must be included in the planning. She may well need to continue several medications for some of the conditions already hinted at; they must be coordinated through you in order to avoid problems.

POLYPHARMACY AND OTHER MEDICATION PROBLEMS

Polypharmacy is a term generally used to imply the indiscriminate giving of multiple concurrent medications. Often the problem results from *reflex prescribing*, that is, responding with a medication prescription to each of many presented problems. Many chronic problems of old age benefit from medication, but nonmedication therapies should be considered first or at least concurrently. The risk of drug-drug and drug-disease interactions increases with the number of prescriptions. When more than one physician is prescribing, duplicate prescription can occur; confusion between generic and proprietary names can contribute to this (e.g., taking Lasix and furosemide together).

Another major factor in polypharmacy is *failure to follow-up* on the effectiveness, the potential side effects, and the continuing need for prescribed medications. Physicians are often hesitant to stop medications, fearing that an already fragile patient will come to further harm. This especially occurs when a physician takes over a patient's care (e.g., following nursing home or hospital transfer). The high incidence of iatrogenic illness[5,6] makes it good practice not to prescribe anything without a thorough review of existing medications and always to define and record clearly the intended effect of your prescription. If the target symptom or sign is defined, then follow-up can be specific and the medication's effectiveness can be judged. Using numeric, or at least objective, measurements could be practiced more often: measuring sadness on a validated scale, measuring range of motion in degrees, measuring joint circumference with a tape measure, and numerically scoring mental status using one of the recognized, scoreable tests.[7]

⚭ *"Start low, go slow," but ultimately give an adequate dose.*

Changing *pharmacodynamics* with increasing age make many older individuals either more susceptible to side effects at a given dose or responsive to lower doses than would be used in younger patients.[8] Many medications have an increased half-life in older individuals, exerting their effects, for good and ill, for longer. Knowing the patient's renal function (preferably by calculating the creatinine clearance) when renally excreted drugs are prescribed is a help. The traditional phrase is "start low, go slow"; but sometimes clinicians make the mistake of failing to raise the dose (slowly) to therapeutic levels. Quite often elderly patients are chronically underdosed, especially with antidepressants and pain relievers.

Psychotropic medications (i.e., those deliberately given for psychotropic effect) require special attention because of the widespread appreciation of their adverse potential. Family members sometimes totally oppose them, and advance directives and health care proxies may even include clauses forbidding their use. But they are vital in certain situations; some of the family issues are discussed later in this chapter.

⚭ *With psychotropics, the physician, the family, and the staff must all understand the target symptoms and how narrow the "therapeutic window" often is.*

To avoid the inevitable confusion of having several physicians prescribing for one patient, it is ideal if all prescriptions are routed through the primary physician. But patients establish links with organ-specific specialists, and routing all prescriptions through one office can lead to communication errors. If there must be several physicians, at least encourage the patient or family to use one pharmacist. Most pharmacists have more capability to be alert to potential interactions than most physicians.

⚭ *When prescribing for elders, the rule should be "one physician," or at least "one pharmacist," otherwise the result will be confusion.*

Make it a standard rule to review all medications, both prescribed and over-the-counter (OTC), when any change in prescription is anticipated. OTC medications are increasing in availability: patients can now directly access not only antihistamines, with their anticholinergic, sedative, orthostatic, and other effects, but also interactive medications like nonsteroidal antiinflammatory agents (NSAIDs) and H_2 blockers.

A useful geriatric medical technique is the "paper or plastic bag test," in which either a family member or a visiting health professional brings in *all* the medications found in the house, including the spouse's and other "borrowable" ones. This technique can be extraordinarily revealing and is particularly recommended in making the initial evaluation for patients new to your practice.

▼ WILLIAM POWERS

William Powers is a 72-year-old man who is a new patient of yours. He is a heavy smoker who has had symptomatic chronic obstructive lung disease (COPD) for nearly 10 years. After several hospitalizations for exacerbations, including at least one episode with complicating CHF, he is now taking many medications. He is on an antihypertensive and an antidepressant that was started 2 years ago for impotence. He has been sleeping badly, and he has been taking some phenobarbital that his late wife used to take to help her sleep when she was terminally ill with cancer. Last year on vacation, during some hot days in Florida, he became dizzy and faint and was started on cyclizine. He has continued using it because it calms him, and he feels it dries some of his chest secretions. He still gets a little dizzy on standing. His son comes with him to your office and brings a large bag of medications: chlorthalidone 100 mg every other day, potassium chloride 20 mEq 3 times a day, oxtriphylline 200 mg 4 times a day, docusate twice a day, digoxin 0.25 mg daily, methyldopa 250 mg 4 times a day, terbutaline 5 mg 3 times a day, amitriptyline hydrochloride 50 mg at night, cyclizine 3 times a day, phenobarbital 60 mg at bedtime, an over-the-counter sinus medication containing an antihistamine, a decongestant, and acetaminophen, and also some diphenhydramine hydrochloride for sinus congestion and to help him sleep.

CASE DISCUSSION

It is unlikely that most of these medications are really needed long term. It is not known if his COPD is responsive to the bronchodilators, and they may be contributing to his anorexia and insomnia. He could be depressed; he is taking several medications that could produce this effect, and his antidepressant dose is low. He takes several anticholinergics in any one day, which could be effecting his thinking, motivation, and balance. He is on the most highly anticholinergic antidepressant available (amitriptyline). He lacks current signs of CHF, yet he continues on CHF treatment. Chronically taken barbiturates interfere with sleep. Polypharmacy may be his number one problem.

IATROGENESIS

"First do no harm" is the beginning of the Hippocratic oath. Whereas the term *iatrogenesis* is usually equated with physicians harming patients by the prescribing of medication, the potential to "cause harm" goes beyond this.

Relocation of elderly individuals can cause great disruption, precipitating confusion and falling, anorexia, and even malnutrition. Primary care physicians must act as advocates for their patients to reduce to the minimum, and minimize the effects of, the often multiple relocations older individuals must frequently undergo, especially when ill.

Hospitalization is hazardous to an older person's health: around 20% of older individuals' hospitalizations are prolonged by major adverse events.[4-6,9] These events include nosocomial infections; falls, accidents, and other trauma; problems with pressure sores and other consequences of the relative immobility of hospitalization; and delirium, depression, and medication side effects. The primary care physician has a vital role in shortening and appropriately planning hospital stays and in assisting nursing and medical colleagues to respond behaviorally and environmentally to the needs of the individual elderly patient. All health professionals have a role in "reducing the harm."

MULTIPLE ETIOLOGIES

The rule in geriatric medicine is that each phenomenon (symptom, sign, syndrome, functional deficit) is usually the end result of many different factors, and optimal management involves identifying and correcting all of them. It is always a mistake to assume that the etiology found explains everything. Whereas it is exciting to find, for example, a recurrent cardiac dysrhythmia in a patient who is falling, it is unlikely to be the only factor. The patient with stress incontinence, even with obvious physical predisposition (e.g., marked prolapse), will probably have other factors influencing the continence; in the past, disappointment with surgical management frequently occurred because of failure to adequately investigate for other causes. This "multifactorial etiology" principle is important when planning management: careful attention to *all* the precipitating and predisposing factors will often reveal potential medication-free approaches.

> In geriatrics, always look for the multiple factors that are likely to have produced the patient's problem, even when one apparently clearcut explanation has been found.

▼ HAROLD STEINKAMPF

Harold Steinkampf is a 75-year-old patient of yours with mild cognitive impairment, who 1 week ago saw another physician in your group because of persistent agitation while staying temporarily with his daughter following lens implants for cataracts; haloperidol 0.5 mg tid was prescribed. You are called by the ER physician. Harold has been taken there following a fall in the night; he had been found on the floor in the dark between his bedroom and the bathroom. He has been found to have a subcapital fracture of the right femur, with displacement and an urgent need for internal fixation and pinning. He is known to have ischemic heart disease, and he is on hydrochlorothiazide 50 mg daily for hypertension. The ER physician has found that Mr. Steinkampf has a dysrhythmia, atrial fibrillation, which had not previously been recorded.

STUDY QUESTIONS

- *There are many factors to consider in the work-up for an apparent fall. What factors are already identified as predisposing in this case?*
- *What steps could have been taken to prevent this fall in the first place?*

CASE DISCUSSION

Like most falls in elders, Mr. Steinkampf's was caused by multiple factors interacting. His agitation, the unfamiliar place, possibly the nocturia that made him get up in the first place, potential orthostasis, the darkness, and the recent prescription of a tranquilizer, which may have reduced his attention as well as potentially added to orthostasis, are all contributors, along with variation in his visual acuity following the recent surgery. These are all much more likely precipitants than the dysrhythmia, and several of them could have been approached preventively in such a high-risk situation.

FUNCTION: ITS LOSS AND MAINTENANCE

> The loss, maintenance, and promotion of function is what geriatric care is mainly about.

In setting treatment priorities for the patient with multiple problems, the functional implications often matter most when deciding what to treat first and how to treat.[10]

It is often not fully appreciated that the already functionally impaired person is exquisitely sensitive to even a very slight change. For example, a seemingly minor podiatric problem developing in the person already barely able to make it to the bathroom will render them wholly dependent for essential functions. Recognizing that function is of such overriding importance affects all medical, environmental, and social decision making for older individuals.

The abilities to measure, record, and be aware of change in functional status are essential skills in geriatric care. A change in functional status may be a sign of developing illness. Functional status must be precisely known when plans are made for the provision of support services. If those caring for the hospitalized elderly person do not know the prior functional status, they will not be able to judge the potential for recovery. Health professionals now speak much more readily in terms of functional status, using the technical terms ADL for personal self-care skills and IADL for skills involving interaction with objects and the environment, or the practical daily skills needed for life like shopping, telephoning, and traveling. Health professionals are also using more or less standardized ways of recording these two sets of skills.

> The cardinal caregiving mistake is to "take over" too soon; there will be resentment as well as premature dependency.

Description and diagnosis of elderly patients should always be made in functional terms. It is truly "ageist" to describe an individual only in terms of their chronological years; to improve communication and to avoid assumptions made on the basis of the patient's age, all health professionals should become used to quickly defining a person's level of function. Anecdotal incidents of individuals being treated differently because of a typographical error on the record of their chronological age underscore such assumptions. Age in and of itself is *never* a criterion for medical decision making—function is.

MODIFIED SPEED OF RECOVERY

Some physiologically "young" older persons recover as quickly as younger individuals from acute illness and disability, but as a general rule, recovery from illness is prolonged by various factors in the frail. With today's emphasis on short hospitalization and the desirability of the most rapid recovery possible, a complacent attitude toward rehabilitation in old age is unforgivable. It may not be possible to rehabilitate to full independence, but rehabilitation to the previous level of function should normally be the aim. (This is why the previous level of function needs to be known and recorded before hospitalization.) Recording the overall functional status (ADLs and IADLs) at intervals ensures that very slow change over time can be appreciated as the individual shifts from one level and site of care and one set of professional caregivers to others.

ENVIRONMENTAL INFLUENCES

There are many examples of ways in which environment influences the symptoms, signs, and effects of illness in older persons. Noise reduces auditory acuity. Because the quantity of light reaching the retina is reduced, darkness profoundly reduces visual acuity. Mobility depends on the familiarity and convenience of the surroundings.

Poor cognition is less impairing in a familiar place, yet physicians are frequently asked to assess patients' capabilities in conditions very unlike those that they will be in from day to day. That is why the home must be accessed by someone in many cases, especially if there is long-term impairment of daily living skills or if it is anticipated that the problems will be progressive (e.g., Alzheimer's). Even an ideal office environment impairs elders to some extent. Physicians rarely exercise the influence they potentially could to change the environment in long-term care facilities, yet the environment clearly influences the behavior and disability of patients. Physicians should prescribe both psychotropics *and* environments.

INVOLVEMENT OF FAMILY

When or if an older patient presents for care is greatly influenced by family members or other caregivers. The increased dependency of many frail elders creates a parallel between the parent and child. Just as the manifestation and reaction to illness in a child are influenced by the parental response, so it often is with illness in the more dependent older person. Just as the implementation of management in a child generally depends on the parent, guardian, or some other caregiver, so too with an older person. In certain situations, the family member or caregiver must be trained to be therapeutically skilled, especially when behavioral techniques are required, as in the patient with dementia. (See Box 4-5.)

It is often necessary to work through surrogates or family members at times when "life or death" decisions about the intensity of treatment need to be made. This is in part secondary to the frequent impairment of the patient's cognition (either long-term from a dementing illness or short-term due to the effect of illness, relocation, or treatment). Even when the elderly patient is clearly competent, family members and other concerned carers, aware of the vulnerability of elderly people and of the problems they face, feel bound to be involved. Dealing with families, utilizing their energy, and training them to become part of the team are some of the most important skills of the health professional helping an older patient. It is up to the physician to set the tone for family involvement from the outset.

It is important to identify and agree upon which one family member is to be the family spokesperson. This can help, but not entirely prevent, the familiar syndrome of the "long distance" family member who often disagrees with the intensity of treatment endorsed by the local fam-

---

BOX 4-5
Principles of Family Involvement in Elderly Care

The physician sets the tone for family involvement at the outset.

Family observations are essential and must be valued.

The family should be part of the therapeutic team.

The family, or any member of it, is not "in charge of the case."*

The family must nominate one spokesperson for communication who will communicate with the others (especially if there are long-distance relatives).

The physician is not obligated to carry out unreasonable medical treatment.

The family cannot deny the patient helpful treatment (e.g., pain relief or antidepressants).

Physicians must be careful about psychotropics: family and societal prejudice makes their reasonable use difficult.

Good communication between physician and nursing home and hospital staff is the key; they may be the main link between physician and family.

---

*Even if a family member is the health care proxy or named in the durable power of attorney for health care; he or she is to act then as the patient not as the physician.

ily members. Recognition of the powerful caring feelings of such an individual and efficiently maintaining contact with them (perhaps mailing them a copy of your notes) can help.

▼ PETER LASALLE

Peter LaSalle is a patient of yours with known dementia of Alzheimer's type, who for several weeks has required intermittent doses of lorazepam for control of his tendency to be very "hyper" and agitated at times. You are called in the middle of the night by police who have been called to the house because Mr. LaSalle has become aggressive and violent. The local psychiatric emergency services will not help because this is not a "mental illness," so he is taken to the emergency room and admitted by you to a general medical ward. He is extremely restless and makes fists and gestures when attempts are made to redirect him or even to feed him. A progressive course of increasing tranquilization with haloperidol and intermittent lorazepam is initiated. On the first day an explanation of the intent to progressively increase the doses until he is calmed is given to his wife, and you express the hope that once calm he will return home to her care. Under considerable pressure to contain the situation because of his wife's understandable distress and the nursing administration's difficulty to "special" this restless individual who, if unsupervised, will walk into other patients rooms and tinker with IVs, you

sedate him over 3 to 4 days. Finally he falls into a deep sleep, exhausted, for a whole night and most of the rest of the next day. His son visits and complains to nursing staff that his father has been "drugged." The next day the family complains to the hospital administration that the patient is being oversedated to a nonacceptable degree and that they have been insufficiently involved in the treatment decisions.

STUDY QUESTIONS

- Given the inevitability of Mr. LaSalle's finally falling asleep in response to the titrated doses, what could have been done to increase the family's understanding of your therapeutic attempts?
- What input do family members have the right to in treatment decisions in such potentially dangerous situations?

CASE DISCUSSION

This case illustrates the dilemma of the clinician when an inappropriate environment is the only one available and psychotropic drugs are involved. Rather than risk the physician appearing to be for medication and the family against it, family (and professional staff) need to realize the objectives of treatment and the potential side effects. The family need to understand that their input is vital for the physician to make the right therapeutic decisions, especially when, as in this case, the patient cannot have input. If a family member is a health care proxy, then he or she has the right to act as the patient and refuse treatment; the physician's role is to explain fully to a designated family member, on behalf of the patient, an appropriate amount of information about the treatment plan. In this case an additional family member who disagreed with the plan contributed to the misunderstanding. Even though an explanation was given to the stressed caregiving spouse, it may be that the explanation was not "heard." The optimistic plan to return home may have lead to unrealistic expectations: "wait and see" would have been wiser advice.

A principle demonstrated throughout this book is to use the family and make them, if possible, into part of the therapeutic team. However, family members need to recognize that they are not directing the management of the case. An exception to this may occur when the patient has appointed a health care proxy or has a durable power of attorney for health care; in this situation the family member or other surrogate is really acting as the patient and therefore has the same right to refuse treatment as any competent patient. However, even in such instances, the health care team may have reached consensus about a certain direction of management, and a family member may disagree. Although every effort should be made to understand the family member's point of view, health care professionals are not obligated (and ethically should not) carry out medically inappropriate investigations or treatments, especially treatments that may harm or distress the patient; nor are they obligated to deny the patient the potential benefit of medications, such as antidepressants or analgesics.

> *Patients should not be denied the opportunity for treatment merely because of the fear of side effects.*

Medications, especially psychotropics, are a problem for some families. Negative images of older patients "drugged" and incapable are widespread, and physicians may frequently find themselves in opposition to family members who would prefer to see the patient alert and frightened, rather than calm yet sometimes less attentive. Whereas one must bring every possible skill (including family observations of the patient as well as those of other staff) to bear in assessing the effect of each medication or dose change, the "therapeutic window" for drugs in many older patients is extremely narrow. It is best to prepare the family by mentioning the possibility of oversedating during the dose titration of sedatives, for example. Often, family members' fears are meaningless, based on anecdotes from friends or alarming reports in the press that have no application to the situation at hand.

> *When using tranquilizers, the alternatives are not alert versus "drugged," but frightened versus calm.*

Families and health care professionals alike often do not realize that unless there is a legal authority (health care proxy or durable power of attorney), the rights and obligations of family members are quite limited. Whereas it is clearly undesirable to have to act against family members' wishes, that may at times be necessary. Before such issues become contentious, one would be wise to involve colleagues, other health professionals, ethics committees, hospital administration, and even legal counsel. Especially in nursing home and hospital sites, such disagreements sometimes reach a crisis before it is realized that no one has actually spent time with the family member to find out what is creating the misdirected advocacy.

In the nursing home and sometimes in the hospital, the physician may not have a long prior history of knowing the family and patient. In both sites, the "bonding" between a health professional and a family member may have occurred with a nurse or social worker, rather than the physician. Good communication between these professionals and the physician is then essential.

> *In the case of a health care proxy or durable power of attorney, the family member or surrogate acts as the patient but does not act as the physician.*

▼ GEORGE HEILENKAMPF (Part I)

George is a long-term nursing home patient of yours who is kyphotic, dependent, and immobilized. For several weeks he has been overtly depressed, disinterested, weeping, refusing food, even refusing his medications and pulling off his oxygen. Thinking he might be depressed you initiate sertraline (Zoloft), with strikingly good effect, and virtually all the target symptoms respond. His niece, whom you have never met, sees him 4 weeks later. She is shocked to find him on a psychotropic medication and insists that it be stopped. She feels that her uncle is "different" than he used to be and that the medication is interfering with his mind.

STUDY QUESTIONS

- *How would you justify the medication to the niece?*
- *Does she actually have the right to insist on the medication being stopped?*

▼ GEORGE HEILENKAMPF (Part II)

Despite explanations of the treatment and the lack of an official proxy, Mr. Heilenkampf's niece insists on the medication being withdrawn. Following discussion with the nursing home administration, it is decided to temporarily discontinue the medication; but you insist that it will be restarted should his symptoms break through again. The trial period without the medication commences and all the symptoms return. When you call to describe this to the niece, she mentions that he was previously on an antidepressant following a suicide attempt and that she had suppressed both facts in giving the history when he was first admitted to the facility, since she feared that he would be treated differently if they thought he was "mentally ill" or a suicide risk.

STUDY QUESTIONS

- *What common misapprehensions and prejudices are here revealed?*
- *Was it right to withdraw his medication even though everyone on the team knew that it had been effective?*

CASE DISCUSSION

It was convincingly demonstrated to the niece that the medication was a necessity, and she did not have the right to interfere. The withdrawal of a potential medication when there was adequate record that the patient had responded well to it and was not suffering side effects was inappropriate. Further discussion would have revealed the niece's unreasonable, though common, prejudices and embarrassment about a "mental" history in her uncle. The stigma of mental illness is an issue for many family members, and it can interfere profoundly with treatment and contribute to misunderstandings.

FAMILY AND CAREGIVER STRESSES

The role of the family or other caregiver can be extremely stressful; situations often continue over years, with increasing dependency. The primary care physician's role in enhancing the caregiver's coping and behavioral skills must be balanced by an active approach to preventing and relieving these stresses.[11,12]

Characteristics of the dependent patient that are especially stressful include: disturbed nights, aggressive or abusive behavior by the patient, physical dependence on the caregiver for ADLs, incontinence, and "ingratitude." The latter incorporates a range of behaviors that are not necessarily under the patient's conscious control.

Factors in the caregiver that increase the caregiver's stress include: the caregiver's own frailty, alcoholism or other emotional problems in the caregiver, other stressful responsibilities of the caregiver, and poor health of the caregiver.

Caregiving frequently falls to one individual, even when there are multiple family members; the primary caregiver is often a woman who generally has many other responsibilities, including job and family.

The primary care physician must be familiar with and recommend (and even initiate locally if such services are not available) the vital services known to improve the patient's quality of life and to provide respite for the caregiver: day care programs (both "social" and "medical," as appropriate to the intensity of the patient's needs), senior centers, nutrition programs, transportation, legal and management services, in-home respite ("grannysitting," home aides, volunteers, etc.), and short-stay respite programs (short admissions up to 2 weeks to long-term care facilities).

PLACEMENT AND HOUSING ALTERNATIVES

As an individual becomes more and more frail, the potential need for *long-term institutional placement* increases. This is an important factor in the presentation of illness to the physician and to the system. After prolonged care of a dependent relative, a "burned-out" family member may find a small additional complication is more than they can cope with. Fear of institutionalization underlies nonpresentation by some older persons when ill or abused. Exceptional skill is required by the primary care physician in carefully balancing the patient's needs against the caregiver's and family members' potential, anticipating and advising so that the move to a facility, if it becomes necessary, is made in a less precipi-

tate and emotionally fraught manner than usual. Societal prejudice regarding long-term care facilities, the actual dourness of some institutional environments, and the long delays in placement because of waiting lists in some areas, all make smooth integration of long-term institutional care into the continuum of an increasingly dependent and frail person quite challenging and sometimes unachievable.

> *The physician must help to skillfully balance the patient's needs against the caregiving family members' potential.*

As the patient becomes more dependent, a number of services should be brought into action to relieve caregiver burden and to postpone institutionalization where dependency is developing insidiously. It is usually appropriate to consider *other housing alternatives* prior to full skilled nursing home care: supervised housing, apartment complexes with resident management, home-sharing with others, other community or group home arrangements, and licensed adult homes are some examples of the spectrum of housing that may respond to the continuum of need as the patient deteriorates. In such situations, the physician clearly has a role in matching the prognosis and the speed of deterioration with such placement plans; it is inappropriate to relocate a person several times over a short interval, but also inappropriate to consign them to too high a level of care too soon, which has often been the fault of management in the past.

NEED FOR MULTIDISCIPLINARY MANAGEMENT

The concept of using a multidisciplinary/interdisciplinary team is well established in geriatrics, but many physicians are not comfortable with team management. It is widely believed that many physicians do not understand the availability and scope of available services, such as in-home aides, occupational and physical therapists, or, for example, the range of a social worker's skills in integrating the limitations, capabilities, and financial aspects of the system with the family's and the individual's autonomy and function. There is better understanding of disciplines like dentistry, podiatry, and nursing; but integration could still be improved. Whereas this "team" of several health professionals will frequently be working on one patient, it is unrealistic to think of them coming together in "team meetings," except in exceptional crises and circumstances. Good communication between the disciplines (phone, fax, letter) can encourage each to understand the full range and potential of the others.

FINANCIAL CONCERNS/PUBLIC POLICY

Although the health care of older persons consumes a large proportion of public spending on health care, at least half of health care costs are still direct expenses to the elderly themselves or their families. Older persons may avoid health care or at least not fill prescriptions, fearing their own impoverishment or the impoverishment of their family after they have gone.

Since health care for older persons is publicly financed, changing policies regarding payment for services and limitations on these payments are issues for everyone. All health professionals can and must provide strong input into policy development.[13,14]

> *Health professionals must provide strong input into policy development: these are issues for everyone.*

The cost of good, comprehensive health care is high: as a person becomes more dependent, increasing professional time from a variety of disciplines is justified; this might postpone the period of maximal dependency, including long-term institutional care, which still forms the closing chapter of many older persons' lives (at considerable public expense). It is of course impossible to prove in any individual case that earlier provision of extra services (at extra expense) actually saves money later on. This impossibility and the generally short-term nature of many policy decisions (often annual, sometimes longer—e.g., the length of an electoral term), in addition to the real difficulties inherent in the type of long-term epidemiological/financial research that would be involved to obtain solid data, are some of the bases for the present difficulties. In this context, the clinician needs to bring his or her advocacy and case examples (as unscientific and emotive as this seems) to some aspects of the political process, especially at local and state levels.

Geriatric care is thus carried out with due consideration of the issues of the cost of care and its potential limitations. Physicians must always act as advocates for their patients to receive optimal medical management; physicians must also be advocates for change in the health care system, encouraging payment for and development of health care services that will fit the characteristics of older persons when ill and the patterns of illnesses and disabilities that can be anticipated.

ETHICAL ISSUES

Humanitarian and financial concerns, issues of intensity of treatment and of resuscitative efforts, and how much, how invasively, and how expensively to investigate and manage medical problems in older persons are among the core ethical issues in geriatric medical care.

The central principle of the patient's autonomy as the prime decision maker in his or her health care must always be maintained and acknowledged. Yet in older persons, the cognitive impairment so frequently accompanying illness makes it necessary for substituted judgments, leading to the necessity for legal steps such as power of attorney, health care proxy, and different types of advance directives. Much of this effort is directed at preventing unnecessary, sometimes inappropriate, life-prolonging modes of care for the individual. However, the issue is not as simple as merely omitting expensive aspects of care. Often, an expensive intervention, one that would appear to be "high tech," may in fact be palliative and reduce the person's dependency on others for some considerable time.

Every decision in an older person's medical management must be coordinated with the patient's known wishes, the physician's knowledge of how medically worthwhile the procedure or intervention is (information which is often difficult to obtain accurately), and other factors. It must be remembered that competence is task-specific (i.e., the patient may be competent to take part in some decisions yet not able to take part in others that are more complex). For the physician to make a positive contribution to this process, he or she must have full knowledge of the patient and family, based on a comprehensive assessment.

> *Everyone has the right to refuse treatment, but many older persons lack the ability to be assertive enough to get the care they need.*

UNMET PREVENTIVE AND PROMOTIVE NEEDS

The health care system, its financing, and a societal attitude that favors illness care over prevention has led to a system that, at least until the past few years, responds to crisis but does little to prevent dependency and illness in the long term. In addition to the specific screening and preventive measures that have become somewhat established for younger persons but that are often entirely omitted in older persons (cancer screening, immunizations, etc.), many other preventive efforts could be effective in older persons. Efforts must be directed to prevent long-term dependency. The primary physician must look ahead to foresee the next few years and beyond in a patient's life in order to help plan. When an older person is already ill and dependent, a preventive, active, forward-looking approach is vital—always look for the ways in which even a small degree of dependency can be reduced.

SUMMARY: PRINCIPLES OF GERIATRIC PRIMARY CARE

The principles of geriatric primary medical care flow naturally from the characteristics of older persons and the incidence of the major chronic and acute diseases. Older individuals lacking a family member or other advocate require the advocacy of professionals: community social services, the primary care physician, volunteers, and others. Yet elders have the right to refuse "help," and skill is required to properly comprehend an individual's competence. For example, living alone is not without risk, although it may be what the patient wants. If so, it is up to the professionals involved to do everything possible to make things safe, even if there is risk. The following principles of geriatric primary care should be observed. Practicing physicians using this text may wish to compare these principles with their own practice.

1. *Accessibility:* This includes the physical ability of the patient to get in to see the health care professional, with home visitation available as an alternative. Good telephone access is also necessary.
2. *Comprehensiveness:* All involved health professionals must be comfortable handling not only physical and social but also sexual, psychological, fiscal, and ethical problems; they must be familiar with the range and roles of other professional services.
3. *Coordination:* This extends to the coordination of not only other health professional disciplines but also nonhealth professionals, such as those concerned with housing, legal issues, and tax liability.
4. *Continuity:* This is often challenging. Ideally, the same primary care physician and health care team cares for the patient in the differing clinical sites. Especially during some hospitalizations or with long-term care facility placement, the primary physician may have to take a secondary role in medical care of the patient; continuity must then be achieved by good communication.
5. *Accountability:* This vital principle implies that since the frailty of many older persons may lead to inability to be assertive in obtaining care, health professionals must take responsibility (while never overlooking the autonomy of the patient) in following up on prescriptions and plans. One may need to actively follow up an unwilling or noncompliant patient if harm or dependency can be predicted.

The characteristics of old people when ill mandate the following principles of geriatric care:

6. *Clinical alertness:* Look for subtle changes in mental status and function so that an anticipatory approach is achieved and emergent acute illness is identified early.
7. *Advocacy:* The physician's role sometimes extends beyond accountability since the patient often needs a health care professional to act as advocate through the complexity of the system. This may involve the physician in shared control of decision making, including sharing such control with fiscal managers.
8. *Integrating the family's and other caregivers' roles:* The family is part of the team, but they must often be trained and can sometimes be adversarial.
9. *Emphasis on function:* The principle is to maintain physical and psychosocial function if at all possible, including during hospitalization. Health professionals must be aware of their patient's functional level, objectively measure and record it, and always work to maintain or regain it.
10. *Accurate diagnosis:* Recognize that several diagnoses may contribute to one symptom or problem, making it necessary to hunt for contributory medical illnesses and other problems (environmental, behavioral, familial, psychological) in all cases.
11. *Serial observation:* Use *time* to assess diagnosis and function rather than relying on the acute care technique of comprehensive tests at a specific point in time. This involves tolerating ambiguity on occasion: "watchful waiting" is too low key for many professionals and families, but it is often the best approach.
12. *Recognition that even a good intervention may produce harm:* Older persons should not be denied the many benefits of modern medical management simply in order to avoid potential side effects. Careful follow-up is the safety net to discover unexpected problems.
13. *Setting clear goals, identifying target symptoms, and organizing good follow-up:* Everyone (especially the physician) needs to know what the intervention (prescription, relocation, procedure) is intended to do, and the follow-up process should establish whether these objectives were achieved or not.
14. *Allowing sufficient time:* When detailed observation is necessary, allow sufficient time for it and for addressing the many concerns of the patient and family. Also, allow enough time for recovery of function: it is appropriate to hurry patients out of hospital before *full* recovery, but the primary care physician and community services then have to ensure that further recovery is facilitated.
15. *Postponing dependency:* A central principle of geriatric medicine, postponing dependency also makes postponing institutionalization possible. A multidisciplinary effort must be made to maintain

individuals in the familiarity and dignity of their home surroundings for as long as possible. This must not be done at too high a cost to the functioning and financial status of the caregivers and their families.

16. *Communication:* Ongoing clear communication with the patient, the family, and all others involved, especially at times of transfer from one level of care to another, is vital. It must be done in "functional" language.

CONCLUSION

The special characteristics of many older patients and of their responses to treatment and other interventions mandate significantly different approaches to their care than have become the standard for younger adults. In particular, the physician and family have a much greater role in ensuring safety and good health care because older patients frequently cannot advocate for themselves.

POSTTEST

1. Which one of the following is not a typical nonspecific presentation of illness in old age?
   a. Self-neglect
   b. Headache
   c. Falling
   d. Anorexia
   e. Fatigue

2. Even when access to health care is good, symptoms that have been shown to be disproportionately not presented to physicians include all except which one of the following?
   a. Falling
   b. Depression
   c. Deafness
   d. Nocturia
   e. Incontinence

3. Which one of the following has not been demonstrated to be a consequence of immobilization?
   a. Osteoporosis
   b. Venous thrombosis
   c. Insomnia
   d. Pressure sores
   e. Instability

4. Which one of the following statements concerning illness in old age is false?
   a. Depression can be diagnosed in the absence of sadness.
   b. Peritonitis often fails to localize in acute appendicitis.
   c. Congestive heart failure, once established, rarely resolves.
   d. One third of myocardial infarctions in old age are asymptomatic.
   e. Peripheral sensitivity is reduced.

5. A 75-year-old man has diagnoses of prostatism, constipation, depression, CHF, and allergic rhinitis. He regularly takes furosemide, amitriptyline, dioctyl, and an over-the-counter hay fever medication. Which one of the following is false?
   a. Three of his four medications will increase the need for the dioctyl.
   b. The over-the-counter preparation may worsen three of his five diagnoses.
   c. Only two of his medications increase the risk of acute retention of urine.
   d. He is at risk of orthostasis from three of the medications.

Questions 6 and 7 relate to the following patient:

A 79-year-old lady who lives in the country with her retired farmer husband, age 92, comes to your office for the first time. She has not been seen by any physician for 3 years, but has remained on the following long-term medications, generally renewed by telephone. She brings them in a paper sack at your request: furosemide, 40 to 80 mg per day (the dose varying depending upon how much ankle swelling she has); potassium chloride (Slow-K), 3 times a day; hydrochlorothiazide/triamterene (Dyazide), 50 mg daily; cyclizine (Antivert), 25 mg 3 times a day; oxybutynin (Ditropan), 5 mg 3 times a day; doxepin, 50 mg at night; phenobarbital, 30 to 60 mg at night as needed for sleep; digoxin, 0.25 mg daily.

Her husband asks for her to be seen because she has been dizzy on standing for over a year, and she has fallen 3 times in the past 2 weeks, though without injury. She is chronically short of breath on exertion and has some stress incontinence. He describes her as very nervous, often "down" in mood, and tired; she wakes frequently in the night.

On examination, she is a little confused. Her pulse is regular and there are no signs of CHF. However, her blood pressure is 125/80 sitting and 90/60, with dizziness, on standing.

6. Which one of the following statements relating to the above patient is false?
   a. Four of her existing medications could be contributing to her feelings of depression.
   b. Phenobarbital is probably making her sleep worse.
   c. Digoxin should not be discontinued since her CHF is not controlled.
   d. Ankle swelling is an unreliable indicator of diuretic need.

7. Which one of the following plans of action, in addition to having her seen by the visiting nurse at her home in 2 days and by the physician in the office in 2 weeks, represents the best course of action in the above patient?
   a. Obtain an electrocardiogram, a serum potassium, and immediately stop all potentially hypotensive medications.
   b. Stop *all* the medications and prescribe elastic support hose to increase the venous return and reduce orthostasis.
   c. Stop the diuretics and doxepin, but retain the cyclizine and oxybutynin since she still has symptoms that they may be relieving.
   d. Stop all the medications and photograph the contents of her paper bag of medications in anticipation of a formal complaint about her prior physician.

REFERENCES

1. Barsky AJ et al: Silent myocardial ischemia: is the person or the event silent? *JAMA* 264:1132-1135, 1990.
2. Nordyke RA, Gilbert FI, Harada ASM: Graves' disease: influence of age on clinical findings, *Arch Intern Med* 184:626-631, 1988.
3. Williamson J et al: Old people at home: their unreported needs, *Lancet* 1117-1120, 1965.
4. Steel K: Iatrogenic illness on a general medical service at a university hospital, *N Engl J Med* 304(11):638-642, 1981.
5. Jahnigen D et al: Iatrogenic disease in hospitalized elderly veterans, *J Am Geriatr Soc* 30(6):387-390, 1982.
6. Gillick MR, Serrell NA, Gillick LS: Adverse consequences of hospitalization in the elderly, *Soc Sci Med* 16(10):1033-1038, 1982.
7. Gallo JJ, Reichel W, Anderson LM: *Handbook of geriatric assessment,* ed 2, Rockville, Md, 1995, Aspen.
8. Lamy PP: The elderly and drug interactions, *J Am Geriatr Soc* 34(8):586-592, 1986.
9. Reichel W: Complications in the care of five-hundred elderly hospitalized patients, *J Am Geriatr Soc* 13(11):973-981, 1965.
10. Ham RJ: Functional assessment of the elderly patient. In Reichel W, ed: *Clinical aspects of aging,* ed 3, Baltimore, 1989, Williams & Wilkins.
11. Gwyther LP, Matteson MA: Care for the caregivers, *J Gerontol Nurs* 9(2):93-116, 1983.
12. Rabins PV, Mace NL, Lucas MJ: The impact of dementia on the family, *JAMA* 248:333-335, 1982.
13. Ball RM: Public-private solutions to protection against the cost of long-term care, *J Am Geriatr Soc* 38:156-163, 1990.
14. Schneider EL, Guralnik JN: The aging of America: impact on health care costs, *JAMA* 263:2335-2340, 1990.

PRETEST ANSWERS

1. c
2. e
3. b
4. b
5. d
6. a

POSTTEST ANSWERS

1. b
2. d
3. c
4. c
5. c
6. c
7. a

CHAPTER 5

Assessment

RICHARD J. HAM

OBJECTIVES

On completion of this chapter, the reader will be able to:

1. Describe the role of home visitation in the assessment and ongoing care of older patients.

2. Describe the techniques for assessing cognitive status.

3. Describe the importance of overall function and of the objective assessment of activities of daily living (ADLs) and instrumental activities of daily living (IADLs).

4. Outline the "review of symptoms," including those that generally require specific inquiry.

5. Understand the importance of nutrition in the comprehensive assessment.

6. Describe how to plan the initial interview when family members are present and/or the patient has cognitive impairment.

7. Describe the ways in which an office-based physical examination should be modified for many older patients.

8. Understand the principles of the comprehensive problem list and its utilization in office-based and home-based care.

9. List the range of contents of a comprehensive, functional geriatric assessment.

10. Understand the role of other health professionals in such assessment.

PRETEST

1. Which of the following is an instrumental activity of daily living (IADL) rather than an activity of daily living (ADL)?
   a. Bathing
   b. Dressing
   c. Toileting
   d. Shopping
2. Which one of the following statements regarding physical examination in older persons is false?
   a. The "silent gap" phenomenon can result in falsely elevated readings of systolic blood pressure.
   b. A split second heart sound, with inspiration increasing the gap, is generally not significant.
   c. Patients with undiagnosed cardiac murmurs generally should be "covered" by antibiotics for elective dental surgery.
   d. A pulsatile abdominal swelling smaller than 2 cm with no bruit is not likely to be an aneurysm.
   e. The left lateral position for pelvic examination is especially indicated in osteoarthritic individuals.
3. Which of the following tests should not be considered as a baseline investigation to be carried out in the majority of older individuals?
   a. Hemoglobin and hematocrit levels
   b. Creatinine level
   c. Electrocardiogram
   d. Purified protein derivative (PPD) (tuberculin) skin test
   e. Vitamin B_{12} level

Many older patients have multiple concurrent problems that interact with their environment and circumstances. There is a need to plan continually for the long-term future care of older persons and to help them maintain their function. Thus it is vital that the primary care physician to the older individual obtains comprehensive and accurate information and clearly records this in the patient's records for other health professionals to access so that appropriate decisions can be made both in emergency and in more chronic or elective situations. A comprehensive assessment, which incorporates the traditional history and physical, may evolve over time over many visits and must be achieved economically, not wasting the time of the health professional, the patient, or the family. It should result in screening, preventive and health-promoting plans, and practical plans for implementing comprehensive and continuing future care.

This chapter will detail special modifications that can be made in history-taking technique and in the physical examination, including assessment of mental status and function, and other aspects of assessment that can be realistically achieved in primary care settings.

▼ GEORGE ANDERSON (Part I)

George Anderson is an 81-year-old widower who is brought to the attention of the county's social service department by concerned neighbors. They are requesting that you help him and become his physician. He lives alone and is increasingly confused and self-neglected. He and his wife had always been somewhat reclusive, and she died 5 years ago. He apparently continues to care for himself, driving out to local shops and maintaining himself with some supplies delivered. He is well known in his small community. A social worker calls your office and describes her home visit. The house is neglected and dirty; and because there is much uneaten food and debris, she is concerned about his nutritional and hydration status and fears for his safety. During her visit, he walked slowly around the house and did not appear to have been out of the house in weeks. She found him a little confused, but he mentioned that he does not speak to his son, who lives in town. He is somewhat short of breath, and he smells of urine. His only "complaint" is continual lower back pain. He does not wish to see a doctor.

STUDY QUESTIONS

- *How should you proceed?*
- *What common diagnoses and problems are likely to need consideration in this case?*
- *This individual is not seeking care (and therefore is not really a "patient" yet); how should you gain access to him?*

GOALS OF GERIATRIC ASSESSMENT

Comprehensive assessment of an older person should result in the following information being obtained and recorded. The information is derived from a comprehensive history and physical examination incorporating functional, cognitive, and screening examinations.

1. Current symptoms and their functional impact
2. Current illnesses and syndromes and their functional impact

3. All current medications, their indications, and effects
4. Current health professionals involved
5. Relevant past illnesses
6. Recent and planned life changes
7. Current and future living environment
8. Objective measure of overall functionality
9. Appropriateness of environment to function and prognosis
10. Family situation and availability
11. Current caregiving network, its problems and potential
12. Objective measurement of cognitive status
13. Objective assessment of mobility and balance
14. Rehabilitative status or prognosis if disabled or ill
15. Emotional health (mood and motivation)
16. Nutritional status and needs
17. Preventive, screening, and health maintenance status
18. Overall social functioning
19. Health-promoting activities
20. Services received and required
21. Problem-oriented plan for future care

The overall result of a comprehensive assessment will be that a problem list can be produced and recorded, outlining all problems, medical illnesses, risk factors, and other issues of which the primary physician (or other physicians or health professionals who might subsequently become involved) should be aware whenever further medical or social decision making is implemented (Box 5-1).[1,2]

THE HOME VISIT

Assessment of an older person must include information about the home.[3,4] In many cases, a health professional should visit the home and make direct observations and recommendations. Such a visit should be focused and will often be done by a nurse or other health professional, perhaps working with a certified home health agency or in public health. Clearly the results of the assessment must be well communicated to the primary care physician. The physician will personally gain much from making a home visit; such a visit will often quickly clarify complex issues of environment, family relationships, compliance, and planning. Although the financial return remains distressingly low, the presence of the physician in the home considerably reinforces the commitment of the health care team to maintaining the individual in their chosen environment, and it can be very personally satisfying to the physician in giving a complete and vivid view of a patient's situation.

Indications for a home visit[5] are summarized in Box 5-2. In the case of an unwilling or unable patient, the home visit may be the entire assessment, with the history, physical examination, and labs completed in that setting.

Although the home visit may be the entire assessment, it should generally be used to complement information obtained in the office. Certain aspects of the assessment that are especially difficult to achieve in the office, such as nutrition, alcoholism, actual function, and the suitability and safety of the environment, can be quickly clarified. To assess home safety and to plan for the home care of a disabled person, it is best for an occupational therapist to visit to make recommendations for mobility and safety aids. Even for relatively independent elders, an appreciation of the difficulties involved in food preparation, heating or cooling the house, accessing and using the bathroom, showering, etc., can be vividly obtained by a home visit. Outside the home itself, the environment, the accessibility of transportation, the availability and cooperativeness of neighbors (or their hostility), and the crime rate can all be directly observed. The range of information that can be obtained on a home visit[5] is summarized in Box 5-3.

▼ GEORGE ANDERSON (Part II)

Your office nurse practitioner makes an assessment of the home and of the patient. The previous impression of neglect of self and home is confirmed, and in addition to the evidence of un-

---

> **BOX 5-1**
> *Outline of Comprehensive Geriatric Assessment*
>
> A functional
> physical, social, and mental
> assessment of patient
> and caregivers
> and assessment of environment
> in order to plan care
> and prevent problems

> **BOX 5-2**
> *Indications for a Home Visit*
>
> Living alone, especially if recently bereaved or separated
> Mental impairment
> Major mobility problems
> Several risk factors for dependency
> History of falling or accidents
> Imminent institutionalization
> Recent hospital discharge, especially if recovery was incomplete

From Ham RJ: Geriatrics: I. Monograph ed 89, Home Study Self-Assessment Program, Kansas City, Mo, Oct 1986 American Academy of Family Physicians.

BOX 5-3
Information Obtained from a Home Visit

Suitability and safety of home for patient's functional
   level
Attitudes and presence of other persons at home
Proximity and helpfulness of neighbors and relatives
Emergency assistance arrangements
Nutritional and alcohol habits
Actual and required daily living skills
Hygiene habits
Safety and convenience modifications needed
Problems in getting to local stores and services

From Ham RJ: Geriatrics. I. Monograph ed 89, Home Study Self-Assessment Program, Kansas City, Mo, Oct 1986 American Academy of Family Physicians.

eaten food, it is evident that alcohol has been delivered to the house on many occasions, as the empty bottles and cans confirm. The home is in a neighborhood that formerly was quietly residential but now is sadly run down with uneven sidewalks and sporadic commercial and industrial development. The adjacent buildings are no longer homes: on one side is a warehouse and on the other, an open parking lot. A gang of youths runs away from the lot when the nurse practitioner parks there.

The house itself is old, and uneven steps without railings lead up to both of the outside doors. Mr. Anderson has evidently adapted to living mostly on one floor, but the only toilet, tub, and shower are up a long flight of poorly lit stairs. The tub is high and deep. He has started sleeping downstairs in the living room. There is a step down to the kitchen and heating supplies outside. He relies on a wood-fired stove which heats the downstairs and heats his water. It does not provide heat upstairs.

Mr. Anderson is suspicious and does not welcome the visitor. After she gains his confidence, he says his only problem is "back pain." He is unwilling to discuss his son, merely implying that they do not now speak to one another. He describes his wife as dying "last year." (She died 5 years ago.) He is somewhat short of breath, and on the limited physical examination that he will permit, it is noted he has extensive rales at both lung bases, with occasional rhonchi in the rest of the lung fields. His blood pressure is 140/95, standing. His mouth is dry and his teeth neglected. He appears to hear quite well.

STUDY QUESTIONS

▪ *What other specifics might be sought on the limited physical examination allowed?*

▪ *How should the hints of some mental confusion be further evaluated in this setting?*

▪ *What immediate steps can be taken to improve the situation?*

CASE DISCUSSION

It is urgent to assess Mr. Anderson's mental status, and it can be done in this setting. The visitor must confirm which medications are being taken. A "plastic bag test" could be done with the patient's consent. It is important to establish other family contacts for his future care, but clearly some in-home services ("meals on wheels" at least) might be started with benefit if he will consent to receive them. The nurse practitioner could also observe his gait and how safely he negotiates his home environment. How does he get supplies? Is he still driving? What would happen if he fell to the floor and could not get up?

ASSESSING MENTAL STATUS

 Preserved social skills, even in patients with marked cognitive impairment, can mislead family and physician alike.

The characteristic retention of social grace and skill long after memory, judgment, abstract thought, and orientation have become severely impaired can easily mislead both the family and the physician unless objective measurement of mental status testing is used in cases where there is any suspicion of a decrement in cognitive function. It is recommended that brief, validated mental status tests with numeric scores, as used in formal geriatric assessments and research, be used much more often in primary care physicians' offices. Two of the most frequently used mental status questionnaires are the Mini–Mental State Examination[6] (Fig. 5-1) and the Short Portable Mental Status Questionnaire[7] (Box 5-4), both of which are validated screening tests for several areas of cognitive function.

Such assessments do not require a physician and have validity when measured by different observers in different situations, although the interviewer must be properly trained and reasonable efforts must be made to ensure the patient is making a maximal effort. The latter point is particularly important if the patient is depressed or unwilling.

Incorporating such an assessment into the office-, home-, or hospital-based assessment makes some health professionals uncomfortable, as they are unused to asking formal questions and are used to their own free-flowing style of interaction between patient and professional, professional and family. In order to avoid the discomfort of a patient feeling that they are being "tested" while conversing with their physician, it is better to clearly distinguish testing from history taking. The mental status examination should be performed and recorded as part of the physical examination. When the history is obtained in one setting and the physical examination done in a separate room, it is helpful to complete the

Mini–Mental State Examination

I.   Orientation (Maximum score:10)
Ask "What is today's date?" Then ask specifically for parts omitted, such as "Can you also tell me what season it is?"

Ask "Can you tell me the name of this hospital?"
"What floor are we on?"
"What town (or city) are we in?"
"What county are we in?"
"What state are we in?"

Date (e.g., January 21)	1	____
Year	2	____
Month	3	____
Day (e.g., Monday)	4	____
Season	5	____
Hospital	6	____
Floor	7	____
Town/City	8	____
County	9	____
State	10	____

II.   Registration (Maximum score: 3)
Ask the patient if you may test his memory. Then say "ball," "flag," "tree" clearly and slowly, allowing about one second for each. After you have said all three words, ask the patient to repeat them. This first repetition determines the score (0–3), but continue to say them (up to six trials) until the patient can repeat all three words. If he does not eventually learn all three, recall cannot be meaningfully tested.

"ball"	11	____
"flag"	12	____
"tree"	13	____

Number of trials: _____

III.   Attention and calculation (Maximum score: 5)
Ask the patient to begin at 100 and count backward by 7. Stop after five subtractions (93, 86, 79, 72, 65). Score one point for each correct number.

If the subject cannot or will not perform this task, ask him to spell the word "world" backward (D, L, R, O, W). Score one point for each correctly placed letter, e.g. DLROW = 5, DLORW = 3.
Record how the patient spelled "world" backward: _____
                                                                              D   L   R   O   W

"93"	14	____
"86"	15	____
"79"	16	____
"72"	17	____
"65"	18	____

or

Number of correctly
placed letters .... 19 ____

IV.   Recall (Maximum score: 3)
Ask the patient to recall the three words you previously asked him to remember (learned in Registration).

"ball"	20	____
"flag"	21	____
"tree"	22	____

V.   Language (Maximum score:9)
Naming: Show the patient a wristwatch and ask "What is this?"
Repeat for a pencil. Score one point for each item named correctly.

Watch	23	____
Pencil	24	____

Repetition: Ask the patient to repeat "No if's, and's or but's. "Score one point for correct repetition.

Repetition .... 25 ____

Three–stage command: Give the patient a piece of blank paper and say "Take the paper in your right hand, fold it in half and put it on the floor." Score one point for each action performed correctly.

Takes in right hand	26	____
Folds in half	27	____
Puts on the floor	28	____

Reading: On a blank piece of paper, print the sentence "Close your eyes" in letters large enough for the patient to see clearly. Ask the patient to read it and do what it says. Score correct only if he actually closes his eyes.

Closes eyes .... 29 ____

Writing: Give the patient a blank piece of paper and ask him to write a sentence. It is to be written spontaneously. It must contain a subject and verb and make sense. Correct grammar and punctuation are not necessary.

Writes sentence................ 30 ____

Copying: On a clean piece of paper, draw intersecting pentagons as illustrated, each side measuring about 1 inch, and ask the patient to copy it exactly as it is. All 10 angles must be present and two must intersect to score 1 point. Tremor and rotation are ignored.

Draws pentagons .... 31 ____

Score: Add number of correct responses. In Section III, include items 14 through 18 or item 19, not both. (Maximum total score: 30).

Total Score: _____

Level of consciousness: ____coma ____stupor ____drowsy ____alert

FIG. 5-1   From Folstein MF, Folstein SE, McHugh PR: Mini–mental state: a practical method for grading the cognitive state of patients for the clinician, *J Psychiatr Res* 12:189-198, 1975.

BOX 5-4
Short Portable Mental Status Questionnaire

1. What is the date today (month/day/year)? (All three correct needed to score.)
2. What day of the week is it?
3. What is the name of this place? (Any correct description needed to score.)
4. What is your telephone number? If you do not have a telephone, what is your street address?
5. How old are you?
6. When were you born (month/day/year)? (All three correct needed to score.)
7. Who is President of the United States now?
8. Who was the President just before him?
9. What was your mother's maiden name?
10. Subtract 3 from 20 and keep subtracting 3 from each new number all the way down. (Whole series correct needed to score.)

Error score (out of 10): Add one if patient is educated beyond high school; subtract one if patient is not educated beyond grade school.

Scoring: 0 to 2 errors—intact intellectual function
       3 to 4 errors—mild intellectual impairment
       5 to 7 errors—moderate intellectual impairment
       8 to 10 errors—severe intellectual impairment

From Pfeiffer E: *J Am Geriatr Soc* 23:433-441, 1975.

mental status examination along with the physical examination. After engaging the patient in some discussion about memory, the physician should properly inform the patient: "I am now going to test your memory," or some such phrase. Use of such formal questionnaires is more likely to produce useful, objective information than it is to cause embarrassment for the physician or patient. Because of the reproducibility of the test and its numeric score, it can be used as a measure of change of mental status over time.

FUNCTION AND ITS ASSESSMENT

Maintaining optimal function, with the patient doing as much as possible physically, intellectually, and socially, and being as independent as possible, is the overriding objective of good geriatric care.[8] Since the loss, maintenance, and promotion of function is the basis of geriatric medical interventions, it is important that function be assessed as objectively and accurately as possible. It is vital for professionals to be able to communicate effectively about function in order to assist continuity and transfers. Measuring functional status objectively as it changes over time helps everyone involved to appreciate both deterioration and improvement. Improvement may be very slow following an acute episode and may not be fully appreciated unless measured at intervals.

 Preserving, nurturing, measuring, recording, and communicating function is the core of good geriatric medicine.

Changed functional status is an important *presenting symptom:* medical illness will often present, for example, as "failure to go shopping" or "taking to bed" without other typical symptoms. Knowing the existing functional status enables change to be appreciated and thus facilitates earlier diagnosis of emerging illness presenting as functional change.

Function helps in *prioritizing individual problems* and thus helps in prioritizing management when there are multiple problems; the issue that most impacts the person's daily life and function may be more significant even than some potentially life-threatening factor.

In deciding on *intensity of treatment* and overall *effectiveness of treatment,* the functional impact of an individual problem and its treatment must be understood in order for the risk-benefit ratio of each intervention to be properly appreciated. For example, treating the complaint of a disturbed night's sleep at the expense of producing postural instability with its attendant risks may be reasonable in one situation but quite unreasonable for someone already having gait problems. A marginal increase in respiratory function as a result of an additional medication may seem hardly worth it until the functional impact of that improvement is seen: perhaps the patient can now independently access the bathroom whereas previously help was needed. On the other hand, if an improvement does not result and the individual suffers anorexia or agitation as a result of the new medication, then the functional impact of the treatment is not worthwhile. Each diagnosis and intervention in an older person must include an assessment of its functional impact.

Baseline functional information helps to *manage acute illness.* If the prior functional status is not known, reasonable decisions cannot be made about the target for recovery of function following a major catastrophe such as a hip fracture or cerebrovascular accident. The primary care physician must be able to intervene effectively in secondary- and tertiary-level situations, bringing organized and specific knowledge of the person's previous level of function in order to assist in setting reasonable targets for recovery.

Functional assessment should be recorded objectively so that the *degree of change over time* and the *speed of functional change* can be fully grasped. In this manner, the potential functional impairment of a new medication or of an institutional placement, for example, can be objectively known.

ACTIVITIES OF DAILY LIVING

Activities of daily living (ADLs) is the term now generally used to describe basic self-care skills. The six basic ADLs, as measured on the scale developed by Katz, include: bathing, dressing, toileting, transferring, continence, and feeding.[9] The Katz Index records loss of independence in these six skills in the order stated, since this is generally the order in which such skills are lost. They are regained in the reverse order during rehabilitation in the majority of patients. Many other ADL instruments have been validated[10-13] and give not only a quantitative indication of the skill level, but have been shown to be sensitive to change over time in clinical use and to have reliability when recorded by different interviewers (inter-rater reliability). Other ADLs include communication, grooming, visual capability, walking, and use of the upper extremities.

The Katz Index,[9] one of the more widely used measures of ADL capability, is reproduced in Box 5-5. Formal measurement of ADL status is increasingly being incorporated into assessments by social service agencies, although there is unfortunately no standardization from state to state. Physicians should remember that objective information about certain of these functions (which can be difficult to establish with accuracy in the office) may already have been recorded by trained professional workers in the community, often by visiting the home. Many states utilize such assessments to assess more fairly a person's need for services and to objectively assess the "level of care" need when long-term care institutional placement is anticipated.

Unlike the issue of mental status assessment, where the numeric score is much more useful than an unscored set of questions, for ADLs (and IADLs—see below) it is

---

BOX 5-5
Katz Index of Independence in Activities of Daily Living

The index of Independence in Activities of Daily Living is based on an evaluation of the functional independence or dependence of patients in bathing, dressing, going to the toilet, transferring, continence, and feeding. Specific definitions of functional independence and dependence are provided.

A. Independent in feeding, continence, transferring, going to the toilet, dressing, and bathing
B. Independent in all but one of these functions
C. Independent in all but bathing and one additional function
D. Independent in all but bathing, dressing, and one additional function
E. Independent in all but bathing, dressing, going to the toilet, and one additional function
F. Independent in all but bathing, dressing, going to the toilet, transferring, and one additional function
G. Dependent in all six functions
Other: dependent in at least two functions not classifiable as C, D, E, or F

Independence refers to the ability to function without supervision, direction, or active personal assistance except as specifically noted in the definitions. This is based on actual status and not ability. Patients who refuse to perform a function are considered not able to perform the function even though they are deemed able.

Bathing (sponge, shower, or tub)
Independent: assistance only in bathing a single part (such as the back or a disabled extremity) or bathes self completely
Dependent: assistance in bathing more than one part of the body; assistance in getting in or out of the tub or does not bathe self

Dressing
Independent: gets clothes from closets and drawers; puts on clothes, outer garments; manages fasteners; act of tying shoes is excluded
Dependent: does not dress self or remains partly undressed

Toileting
Independent: gets to the toilet; gets on and off the toilet; arranges clothes, cleans organs of excretion (may manage own bedpan used only at night and may use mechanical supports)
Dependent: uses bedpan or commode or receives assistance in getting to the toilet and using it

Transferring
Independent: moves in and out of the bed independently; moves in and out of the chair independently (may use mechanical supports)
Dependent: assistance in moving in or out of the bed and/or chair; does not perform one or more transfers

Continence
Independent: urination and defecation entirely self-controlled
Dependent: partial or total incontinence in urination or defecation; partial or total control by enemas or catheters or regulated use of urinals and/or bedpans

Feeding
Independent: gets food from the plate or its equivalent into the mouth (precutting of meat and preparation of food, such as buttering bread, are excluded from evaluation)
Dependent: assistance needed in act of feeding; does not eat at all or uses parenteral feeding

From Katz S et al: *Gerontologist* 10(1):20-30, 1970.

generally recommended that physicians simply incorporate information regarding dependence or independence in each of these activities into their interviews and start to record them and discuss them as "ADLs."

INSTRUMENTAL ACTIVITIES OF DAILY LIVING

Instrumental activities of daily living (IADLs) is the term used to describe the more complex activities an individual needs for independent living. They convey perhaps more vividly a sense of the older individual's dependence or independence in daily life, but they are slightly less objective since they involve the interaction of the individual (often with an "instrument") and the environment. IADLs include the ability to go shopping, manage transportation, prepare food, climb stairs, manage finances, do housework, use the telephone, do the laundry, manage medications, walk outdoors, drive, hold down a paying job, and prepare meals (a separate activity, for example, from eating them, which would be a self-care skill and one of the ADLs). IADLs thus include learned skills, and the individual's capability to carry them out depends on the environment itself as well as the individual's characteristics. IADL capability, especially if it can be directly observed, has clear implications

for future management. A brief IADL measure has been developed by Fillenbaum[14] (Box 5-6), and several other IADL questionnaires are available.[12,13] As with ADLs, it is probably more important for most office- and home-based assessments that physicians routinely incorporate such information into their accounts of an individual, rather than using and scoring formal instruments.

▼ GEORGE ANDERSON (Part III)

The nurse practitioner tests Mr. Anderson's mental status using the Mini–Mental State Examination and he scores 23/30, consistent with mild dementia. The deficits are in orientation to time and place, short-term memory, and visuospatial skills. He allows physical examination of his lower spine since it is giving him trouble; loss of normal lumbar lordosis and some tenderness over the L2-3 region is noted. His gait, observed while he is showing the nurse practitioner his home, is the stiff gait of a person with osteoarthritis. While walking around his familiar living room, he knocks against the chairs and does not seem to notice items near the floor. The nurse practitioner has him accompany her upstairs, and he is markedly dyspneic by the time he reaches the top. It is difficult to visualize him being able to get into the tub to bathe. Dressing and undressing for the limited physical examination shows

---

BOX 5-6
Five Instrumental Activities of Daily Living

1. Can you get to places out of walking distance?
   - 1   Without help (can travel alone on buses or taxis or drive your own car)
   - 0   With some help (need someone to help you or go with you when traveling), or are you unable to travel unless emergency arrangements are made for a specialized vehicle like an ambulance?
   - —   Not answered
2. Can you go shopping for groceries or clothes (assuming the patient has transportation)?
   - 1   Without help (take care of all shopping needs yourself, assuming you had transportation)
   - 0   With some help (need someone to go with you on all shopping trips), or are you completely unable to do any shopping?
   - —   Not answered
3. Can you prepare your own meals?
   - 1   Without help (plan and cook full meals yourself)
   - 0   With some help (can prepare some things but are unable to cook full meals yourself), or are you completely unable to prepare any meals?
   - —   Not answered
4. Can you do your housework?
   - 1   Without help (can scrub floors, etc.)
   - 0   With some help (can do light housework but need help with heavy work), or are you completely unable to do any housework?
   - —   Not answered
5. Can you handle your own money?
   - 1   Without help (write checks, pay bills, etc.)
   - 0   With some help (manage day-to-day buying but need help with managing your checkbook and paying your bills), or are you completely unable to handle money?
   - —   Not answered

From Fillenbaum GG: Screening the elderly: *J Am Geriatr Soc* 33(10):698-706, 1985.

his difficulties with fine hand movements, and he agrees that his fingers have "gotten stiff" and that he cannot see small things well. He used to read but does not bother any longer. He resists any intimate examination (the nurse practitioner is female), but a uriniferous odor is noted. He denies having problems with urination. He cannot remember seeing a physician for years, but he can remember where he keeps his medications. In the cupboard are old expired bottles of prescription medications, including sublingual nitroglycerin, digoxin 0.25 mg, hydrochlorothiazide 25 mg, and phenobarbital 15 mg (prescribed as needed for sleep, 1 to 2 hours before bedtime). Other bottles of aspirin, acetaminophen, and antacids contain medications mixed together. His pulse is 96 beats per minute and irregularly irregular.

STUDY QUESTIONS

- How should the patient's changed mental status be investigated?
- Construct a problem list on this patient at this time.
- What should be the focus of an office-based assessment if Mr. Anderson can be persuaded to come to the office?
- Which ADLs and IADLs are impaired or potentially a source of concern?

▼ GINA GOHRENBERGER (Part I)

Gina Gohrenberger's daughter calls you because she is concerned that her mother, who "hates doctors," has had no health checkup for over 5 years. The daughter has observed that her mother is having increasing problems with urinary incontinence, and she has mentioned that she has felt a lump in her left breast. Her mother has been increasingly forgetful and has not been sleeping well lately. She is 73 years old and lives with her husband George, who is 17 years her senior but has no apparent health problems. Gina's daughter wants to bring her mother in for a thorough checkup but is concerned that her mother will not be open about her symptoms when she attends your office.

STUDY QUESTIONS

- This may be a unique opportunity for a comprehensive checkup; on what areas should you focus to gain as much information as possible?
- A gynecological examination is indicated, especially in view of the symptoms; are there any special considerations in an older patient when planning a pelvic examination?
- How should the interview be set up to give the daughter private access to you to express her concerns about her mother?

PLANNING THE INITIAL INTERVIEW

Though it is usual for the relationship between a primary care physician and his or her patient to be built up over multiple visits and other contacts over time, it is sometimes necessary to attempt a comprehensive interview in one visit in the office setting. This occurs especially when a patient has not been seen for a considerable time or when a patient is brought in by relatives (a common occurrence) and is actually unmotivated to attend.

If the first visit is to be in the office, a relaxed and efficient atmosphere for the interview with good acoustic conditions and no interruptions is important. An efficient appointment system, a pleasant and well-lighted waiting area, and an office in which an older person with some mobility problems (or a wheelchair) can move without difficulty all help to put the patient at ease.

Always arrange to have eye contact, full face if at all possible, with you on the same level as the patient while interviewing. Sit on the "good hearing" side if necessary.

For optimal communication the physician must be prepared for hearing impairment. Assume a face-to-face position that enhances eye contact with the patient. The physician's chair should be on the same level as the patient, and the lighting should be good on both the physician's face and the patient's. If a hearing aid has been recommended, instruct the patient to wear it to the interview. If the patient has impaired hearing but no hearing aid, the physician should ideally have a communication device available. (A simple amplifier and a straightforward microphone will improve communication. Such devices are available from many radio stores.) With the physician thus prepared, rarely would a patient's poor hearing preclude the necessary questions or, for example, assessment of mental status.

Frequently, others accompanying the patient have things to tell the physician. It is inappropriate to talk about patients in their presence unless this is clearly with their consent and unless they can take part actively in the conversation. Too often, health professionals display outrageous behavior, whispering to the family members in front of the patient, which will add to suspiciousness and unrest. Unless it is specifically set up, family members will not have an opportunity to speak freely about their concerns, which are often markedly different or even at odds with the patient's own concerns. Planned utilization of office staff, who, for example, can take the patient away to weigh them and undress them for the physical examination, can allow sufficient time for a brief private interview with the family member or other caregiver. If this will not work, it may be necessary to set a separate appointment or to encourage telephone contact before or after for confidential and private communication.

The "paper or plastic bag test" is the only way to be reasonably certain about which medications are available to the patient on a daily basis.

For all new assessments, the "paper or plastic bag test" should be applied. Ask the family member or someone else to gather all the medications in the house, including over-the-counter, borrowed, and out-of-date prescriptions, so that a true picture of the patient's medication habits can be obtained. Also, before the appointment ask the patient or caregiver to organize a list of the names and telephone numbers of previous physicians and past hospitalizations and to bring copies of available medical records, prior radiological reports, and electrocardiograms.

Many physicians use *preappointment questionnaires,* generally one they design themselves to fit their particular practice style, covering a range of issues. This is highly recommended for elderly patients, as it saves time in the office. The questionnaire can be sent to patients and/or family caregivers before the initial interview to be filled out at home (Box 5-7). This gives an opportunity to gather full background information and prior historical data so that the first appointment can review and priori-

---

BOX 5-7
Suggested Items for Preappointment Questionnaire

Patient name, address, and date of birth
Current physician(s) and pharmacy
Current medical problems
Past medical problems
Past psychiatric history
Past hospitalizations
Past operations/surgeries
Past fractures or other accidents
A review of systems, to include questions about sexuality, continence, falling, mood, memory loss, as well as dyspnea, chest pain, pain, and mobility problems
Recent health maintenance or screening procedures
Describe the meals and drinks on a typical day
Describe the exercise taken on a typical day
Specifics about immunizations
Specifics about cancer screening
What services are already provided in the home?
Are special arrangements for emergency contact such as "life line" made?
Does the patient wear some identification or emergency bracelet?

---

tize the current problems. Such a questionnaire can clarify to the patient and caregiver the physician's range of interests: for example, that he or she is prepared to deal with issues of sexuality, continence, falling, mood, memory loss, etc., as well as the more "traditional" areas that people expect physicians to address. Such a questionnaire will also clarify that the physician is interested in screening, prevention, and health promotion, with questions concerning nutrition and exercise, for example, as well as immunization and cancer screening. Especially in the more frail, specific information about ADLs and IADLs should be included. Emergency contact arrangements such as a "life line" or identity bracelets should be inquired after. The questionnaire can ensure that details of the home circumstances and the services already provided there (this is vital information in the more fragile patient), as well as phone numbers of family, pharmacy, etc., are all available in your office record since the questionnaire can be simply incorporated physically into it. The questionnaire can be resubmitted and updated at the time of annual reviews or after major events, such as hospitalizations.

OFFICE-BASED ASSESSMENT OVER TIME

In the following account, the history, physical, and other aspects of the assessment are described such that they could all be done at one long appointment, but often such information is obtained at many short appointments over time. A number of aspects of the comprehensive assessment can be postponed until a later visit.

Generally a very long initial visit is undesirable, unless the patient is really unlikely to return. Certain embarrassing procedures that need to be done but not urgently, such as screening pelvic and rectal examinations, should be postponed to a subsequent visit, but these procedures must not be postponed indefinitely. Often the initial visit will raise many questions, some that cannot be resolved quickly, and will require the obtaining of medical records and also perhaps laboratory tests, a home visit, or information from existing community services.

The primary care setting gives the physician the ability to observe the situation over time, with the certainty of being able to "look again" and follow up the patient. In geriatrics, the sometimes inevitably long periods of diagnostic ambiguity and the observation and adjustment of treatment make the continuity of primary care essential, safer, and less costly.

MODIFYING TECHNIQUE IN THE ACUTE HOSPITAL AND THE NURSING HOME

The primary care physician-patient relationship will sometimes have to begin in the hospital or nursing home. Try to adapt the same techniques as above to maximize communication. Obtain information not only from the patient but also from others who objectively observed the patient's functionality before the acute illness and who can predict problems after recovery. The distracting atmosphere of the emergency room is particularly challenging, but the physician who makes a conscious effort to pull up a chair or who, in a hospital, sits down on the hospital bed has immediately improved communication and contact. It is in the acute situation that the experience and skill of the physician is particularly exposed. Geriatric medicine does not consist solely of slow and detailed history taking and examination: the very difficulties that make some geriatric work slow make it even more important to *ask the right direct questions* and to lead the interview toward focusing on the relevant systems and on problems that must be discovered. A few direct questions, often regarding pieces of information that are not traditionally communicated, can be vitally helpful: *who* lives at home with the patient, *where* does the patient live, what is the previous level of *function*, and is the patient *aware* of where he or she is and what is happening, as well as some general observations about frailty are typical examples. The art of the geriatrician is to be quick and efficient despite the complexity of the situations and the frequently unfocused nature of the patient, family members available, and presenting situation. Of course, in an acute situation it is often appropriate to examine only the immediately relevant areas, but the tendency for systems other than the clinically obvious one to be involved, even in acute situations, is well recognized; so a reasonably broad assessment should be attempted, whatever the setting. Seeing the patient on a stretcher or already in bed encourages the physician to look at only one side of the patient; and although it is often physically time consuming and difficult to get the patient up to assess gait, mobility, and skill with transfers, this must be done unless the acuity or morbidity of the patient obviously precludes this. Many hospitals and nursing homes are poorly organized even for a private interview, which may be essential to obtain caregiver information or to do objective mental status testing effectively. The setting may make a comprehensive physical examination difficult, especially discouraging rectal and pelvic examinations; but these things can be achieved in suboptimal circumstances with adaptation and flexibility. The lateral position for the pelvic and rectal examinations (described later) is one such adaptation. Frequently, much of the physical examination must be made with the patient sitting in a chair. Parts of the examination may need to be deferred.

> *In geriatric medicine, it is less a matter of taking a considerable amount of time and more a matter of asking the right questions: Does the patient live alone? Is this patient eating or drinking enough? Who does the shopping? The answers to questions such as these are the "vital signs" of geriatrics.*

THE ASSESSMENT TEAM

In the nursing home setting, the physician works as a member of a multidisciplinary team. Many physicians are uncomfortable with the "team concept" and avoid multidisciplinary settings.[15] However, other disciplines (such as dietitians, physical and occupational therapists, and social workers) bring information and advice outside of most medical training, and nursing colleagues are with the patients, observing their functionality and problems, for a far greater proportion of the time than physicians ever are and have specific disciplinary input about many aspects of patient care. Team work goes well beyond delegation and sharing of the medical tasks, although this must be done as well. Physician assistants and nurse practitioners can obtain much assessment information appropriately and economically and are skilled in the management of many of the details of care that frequently can be overlooked, especially if somewhat acute problems are dominating; PAs and NPs are increasingly available in nursing home and hospital settings, and their role as colleagues and professional partners in primary care practice is valuable and increasing. Regulations for PAs and NPs vary in different states but can effectively relegate the individual to being a "physician extender" (for example, some regulations require that the physician be physically present at the office when NPs or PAs are working with patients). Fortunately, increasing recognition of the autonomy of many health professionals is decreasing the phenomenon of the "physician sign-off"; however, skilled interprofessional communication and teamwork becomes more important as each discipline carries out its tasks more independently and with less supervision.

> *Geriatric medicine is a team effort: physicians must be open to working with colleagues in several disciplines and to accepting these colleagues' specialized input.*

Outside of the hospital and institutional setting the team may be more loosely organized and rarely, if ever, come together as a group. Many frail elderly persons with multiple problems benefit from several health professionals from different services and backgrounds working together. Many aspects of the comprehensive assessment implied here should be covered by professionals other than physicians. Implementing plans based on the evolving problem list requires the physician to be thoroughly knowledgeable about the range and capabilities of the other team members (and they need to know the physician's interests and abilities). Although the primary care physician will often be the central team member and will predominate when the patient is medically unstable or when new therapeutic modalities are being considered, other involved professionals will take the lead at other times: the social worker takes charge of placement, ongoing community, family, or supportive therapy, and the integration of fiscal arrangements; the community nurse oversees the ongoing professional handling of the patient's behaviors and functions and the home care services for dependent patients; the occupational therapist guides patients who need to relearn specific daily living skills or who need home safety improvements and special home adaptations; the physical therapist is of primary importance when handling major mobility problems; the activity aide assists patients who are socially withdrawn by guiding them to enjoyable activities; and a case manager guides the management of and access to multiple services, emphasizing efficient fiscal management and promoting cost containment.

A wide range of health professionals exists in most urban communities and elements are often available in more rural settings. However, rarely are their activities well coordinated. The logical place for their coordination is through the primary care physician's office, with notes kept in the primary care physician's record. Currently, much communication between physicians and home care agencies is by means of the physician "signing off" on generally rather dense, triplicated patient management protocols. More personal communication, especially communicating both ways in less bureaucratic language than many care protocols allow, will considerably enhance mutual understanding of the differing professional roles and improve the specificity and individualization of patient management.

ASSESSING THE CAREGIVER

It is essential that family members and other caregivers provide their input about the patient's history, symptoms, and function. As the caregiver contributes to the assessment, so too is the caregiver being assessed. For example, in the common situation of progressive dementia, the quality, skills, and knowledge of the caregiver are essential determinants of the standard of future care. The

good caregiver can be the therapeutic tool to maintain optimal function despite disability. Failure of caregiver skill and capacity often precipitates hospital or institutional placement or even abuse.[16] The challenge is to ensure that the caregiver is operating optimally so that the more dependent phase can be postponed as long as possible.

A number of questionnaires exist to quantify caregiver stress.[17] Aspects of caregivers that make them especially vulnerable to stress include their own frailty (often the spouse is the caregiver, or a person in their 70s is caregiver to a parent in their 90s), alcoholism, depression, and the presence of other caregiving demands (e.g., the caregiver's own spouse or the typical "sandwich-generation" dilemma of the caregiver caring for the generation above and below, often while holding down a job and career as well). The caregiver's approach to the patient is an important determinant. Some will attempt to "do everything" in order to expiate guilt or a prior poor relationship with the patient, whereas others, more appropriately, encourage independence. Overzealous care can easily induce dependence.

Aspects of patient care that caregivers find especially stressful include disturbed nights, uncontrolled aggression, wandering, falling, uncontrolled incontinence, and the inability to walk without assistance. As might be predicted, increasing physical dependency for ADL functions is particularly stressful, especially in a parent of the opposite sex.

HISTORY

The majority of the diagnosis, assessment, and planning for any patient derives from a comprehensive history. The data will be obtained not only from the patient but from other witnesses, including caregivers and family members. The opportunity must be provided for the patient's and caregiver's own concerns to be expressed. Because of the phenomenon of "hidden" illnesses and the tendency not to realize the significance of certain symptoms (due to negativity or other biases), the physician needs to adopt a direct questioning technique for the sake of efficiency. But health professionals often tend to be too sickness-oriented in their direct questioning. A preappointment questionnaire, individually designed by the physician to reflect his particular skills and interests but emphasizing those areas especially important in older persons, should be completed by the patient, if possible, and at least one outside observer in most cases; this will greatly facilitate and direct the process (see Box 5-7).

The traditional approach of defining a "chief complaint" is not appropriate to the assessment of most older persons unless it is clearly realized that these words are a medical code for "the reason why the patient is being seen today." The content of the history is summarized in Box 5-8. Experienced clinicians reading this text may

BOX 5-8
Content of the History of the Elderly Patient

Patient profile, social history
History of current problems
Review of symptoms and systems
Medical history
Medication history
Caregiver's status
Family history
Functional history, abilities in activities of daily living
Community services currently provided

BOX 5-9
Minimal Social Assessment

Content of average day for the patient
Abilities in activities of daily living
Suitability and safety of home
Availability, attitude, and health of caregivers and
   neighbors
Availability of emergency help
Services received and/or needed
Transportation needs
Financial status
Occupational history and interests

From Ham RJ: Geriatrics. I. Monograph ed 89, Home Study Self-Assessment Program, Kansas City, Mo, Oct 1986, American Academy of Family Physicians.

balk at breaking down the assessment in such formal terms, but it enables a clinician to analyze the process and make recommendations that are essentially practical by focusing the time available on the areas most relevant to the elderly patient.

The interview should be carried out with the patient fully clothed and comfortably seated in a reasonably well-lit and quiet environment. Direct questions must be put to the patient first, and then to the caregiver, to clarify the priority the physician gives to the patient's own input. Many older persons do not appreciate being addressed by their first names. An open, non–sickness-oriented question such as, "How can I help you today?" is preferable to somewhat patronizing openers such as, "What seems to be the problem?" With an unwilling patient, a suggested approach is, "Your daughter has been concerned about you recently. Could *you* tell me about it?"

The content of the history begins with the *patient profile and social history.* This is essential general background information about the patient's current or previous occupation, hobbies, and interests and provides a basis for determining how detailed an assessment of mental status is required. Detailing the *average patient day* is a speedy technique of assessing the degree of dysfunction and disability and its influence on the patient's life-style. This naturally leads to an assessment of *activities of daily living,* details of the measurement and assessment of which are given above. For those who want to divide the history conceptually into its different elements, Box 5-9 summarizes a suggested "minimal social assessment" that should be incorporated into this aspect of the history. The patient profile and social assessment thus give a functional picture of the patient and family, the patient's daily life, the available support, and the social environment.

The *history of current problems* (the "chief complaint" and more) is a listing of the patient's and caregiver's major concerns and will be the core of the problem list. In assessing the timing and duration of symptoms, it is often useful to relate symptoms to their functional effect

and to major events such as Thanksgiving, Christmas, and Hanukkah ("Were you having trouble walking up the stairs last Christmas?").

The *review of systems and symptoms* goes beyond the presented problems and consists of responses to direct questions by the clinician looking for "hidden illnesses"—those many symptoms which, through a combination of ignorance, fear, or negativity, are often not mentioned to the physician at all. The preappointment questionnaire, although setting the basis for much of this, does not completely substitute. Box 5-10 summarizes information often forgotten in the "review of systems and symptoms."

It is always useful to obtain old medical records for verification of the *past medical history.* Prior electrocardiograms and other cardiovascular investigations, previous assessments of mental status, precise details of prior surgeries, histologies, and discharge summaries are particularly useful. Technological advances (computers, fax machines) have greatly improved the dissemination of such past records, but it will sometimes be necessary to be in contact with several different physicians' offices; it is generally advised that a physician should not send out another physician's opinions and reports, although this is reasonably accepted practice when a primary care physician is in effect handing over the complete record and care of a case. In sharing records with a colleague when transferring a patient for whatever reason, it is considerate to be selective and to send only (legible) information that is likely to be relevant.

The *family history,* while vital in younger persons to assess future risk of familial illness, has different significance in older persons; personal family experience will greatly influence the patient's attitude to the development of comparable symptoms and can often lead to negativity or nonpresentation. Certain familial illnesses are particularly significant as "risk factors": alcoholism,

---

BOX 5-10
Items Often Forgotten in the Review of Systems and Symptoms

General	Locomotor	Genitourinary
Appetite	Stiffness or pain	Incontinence
Fatigue	Range of movement	Frequency
Weight change		Nocturia
Falling	**Cardiorespiratory**	
Balance	Cough	**Cerebral**
Sleep	Dyspnea	Memory loss
Depression		Confusion
Hearing loss	**Gastrointestinal**	Headache
Visual change	Constipation	Transient weakness or visual symp-
Alcoholism		toms (transient ischemic attacks)

From Ham RJ: Geriatrics. I. Monograph ed 89, Home Study Self-Assessment Program, Kansas City, Mo, Oct 1986, American Academy of Family Physicians.

---

osteoporosis, premature cardiovascular mortality, depression, and Alzheimer's disease.

The *medication history* is crucial. The "paper (or plastic) bag test" should be performed, and thorough details of prior responses and idiosyncrasies to medications (as well as actual allergies) plus a list of current medications (prescribed, over-the-counter, and borrowed, including eye preparations) should be obtained.

▼ *GINA GOHRENBERGER (Part II)*

You instruct your receptionist to schedule Mrs. Gohrenberger so that there is time for an individual interview with her daughter. You arrange for the visit to take place at a relatively quiet time at the office, when staff will be available to accompany, occupy, and assess the patient during your interview of the daughter.

Mrs. Gohrenberger is relieved to see you because a lesion in her left breast has been worrying her. She allows examination, and a hard mass is found in the upper outer quadrant of the left breast, tethered to the skin, with some skin puckering but no associated lymph nodes. You ask several questions about other aspects of bodily function, and the answers are generally negative. She initially denies incontinence, but when pressed she says she would "prefer to leave well enough alone." Interviewing her daughter, you find that the incontinence is a major problem, with much of Ms. Gohrenberger's clothing and furniture stained from urine. Her daughter believes that Mrs. Gohrenberger is extremely embarrassed about this and would not allow a male physician to examine her "private parts." During the examination, Mrs. Gohrenberger had given an upbeat account of her life at home, describing looking after her husband, cooking meals, and visiting with friends. Her daughter, however, says that neither her mother or father have been out of the house for months. She knows that at times her mother has entirely forgotten to cook meals and has had a number of near-accidents in the kitchen; so her father, who is nearly 90 but physically quite fit, sometimes has to fill in and cook meals at short notice. He seems to tacitly accept all this and will not discuss his wife's apparent memory problems, even with his daughter.

STUDY QUESTIONS

- How should you now proceed?
- Since this patient does not wish her incontinence to be dealt with, do you have a right or obligation to intervene anyway?
- How should the problems with cooking and memory loss be followed up?

PHYSICAL EXAMINATION

Conducting a good physical examination of an elderly individual requires an appropriate setup: an examining table which can be lowered closer to the floor so that the patient can get on it, privacy for dressing and undressing, and physical assistance when necessary. If your office is not set up to make, for example, pelvic and rectal examinations convenient in frail elderly people, such examinations will inevitably be "deferred" permanently; this is often the case for such examinations. Whereas cardiac and chest examinations can sometimes be effectively achieved with the patient sitting in a chair, a comprehensive examination requires a good table with a 45-degree tilt for the upper body to properly assess the possibility of congestive heart failure. An adequate, soft pillow to go under the patient's neck is an important piece of equipment, since many older persons have a degree of kyphosis and will not be able to relax the abdominal wall when lying supine unless the neck is properly supported.

In addition, there must be enough space to observe the patient's ability to walk, balance, and turn. Many clinicians partially achieve this by escorting their patients from the waiting area, or they complete this part of the assessment in the interview room with the patient fully dressed, which is appropriate. The formal examination must also include direct examination of the range of movement of the joints and the assessment of musculoskeletal mobility, stability, and strength. Dividing these examination tasks and interview time between the physician and the office nurse, nurse practitioner, or physician assistant can be very efficient. A nurse can complete many of these observations and thus facilitate private time for the physician, nurse practitioner, or physician assistant with the caregiver.

A suggested sequence for the physical examination in the office setting follows (Box 5-11): First assess the gait and mobility before the patient undresses. The patient, in a robe (not paper but toweling, if possible), can then sit upright on the end of the examining table for examination of vital signs, ears, eyes, mouth, neck, chest, cardiovascular system, cranial nerves if indicated, and the musculoskeletal and neurological examination of the upper extremities, including range of movement. Then tilt the top of the table and extend the leg support and have the patient sit back at a 45-degree angle in order to examine the neck veins (jugular venous pressure, JVP). Then the patient can lie flat to complete the abdominal examination and, for men, the genital examination. With the patient flat, the examination of the lower extremities can be completed, including range of movement at the hips and knees, neurological assessment, and careful examination of the feet. In some patients, the neurological examination is more easily achieved when the patient is still sitting upright with the legs dangling over the end of the table, which encourages relaxation for the elicitation of tendon jerks. The patient is turned onto the left side for the rectal examination and, in women, a lateral-position pelvic examination, as described later. While in this lateral position, the back can be observed for flexibility or tenderness and pressure areas checked. The pelvic examination can be completed on returning the patient to the supine position if the patient prefers this. While the patient is lying flat and while they are moving around on the table, observations regarding orthopnea and physical capability are made. At the end of the supine part of the examination, the patient should sit up slowly in case of orthostatic hypotension, and certain parts of the neurological examination may be left until the end, thus filling in a short period of time while the patient sits up before he or she is helped down from the table. Always look at the feet after they have been dangling down for a while. The patient can then be assisted to stand down, and further assessment of balance and the lumbosacral spine can be made. If the pelvic examination or history indicate it, an upright examination of the female genital tract can be done, especially to check for prolapse and urinary stress incontinence. By dividing up the physical examination in this manner, there is mini-

---

BOX 5-11
Suggested Sequence for Full Physical Exam of Older Persons in the Office Setting

Patient Fully Clothed in Walking Shoes:

Observation of gait and balance, rising unassisted from chair, etc.

Patient Sitting Upright on End of Table, Legs Down:

Vitals/ears/eyes/mouth/neck/chest/heart/cranial nerves/upper extremity, neurological and range of movement

Patient Lying Back at 45 Degrees, Legs Extended:

JVP/abdomen, if patient orthopneic

Patient Lying Flat, Head and Neck on Pillow:

Abdomen/male genitals/lower extremities range of movement/lower extremities, neurological (may complete later, see below)/feet

Patient on Left Side, Knees Drawn up Symmetrically:

Rectal/lumbosacral mobility and tenderness/pressure areas

Patient on Left Side, Upper Limb Flexed More Than Lower Limb, Upper Shoulder Rolled Away from Clinician:

Lateral-position pelvic examination if indicated (Patient slowly returns to next position in case of dizziness)

Patient Sitting on End of Table, Legs Down:

Lower extremities neurological completed/can see feet while dependent

Patient Assisted to Stand Down from Table:

Demonstrates depth perception, mobility

Patient Standing:

Gait/balance/stress incontinence, uterovaginal prolapse exam if indicated/lumbosacral mobility and tenderness if indicated

---

mal repositioning of the patient, minimal exposure of the patient's nude body by judicious use of paper sheets, and all parts are adequately examined.

The *lateral-position pelvic examination* is rarely taught in U.S. medical schools. It is essentially the same position as would be adopted for a rectal examination in the lateral position, but it is different from the lumbar puncture position, although the patient is lying on the left side. The lateral position for pelvic examination is sometimes necessary because of the frequently limited range of movement of the hip and knees in older women. To be placed in stirrups or in the dorsal position for a pelvic examination requires flexion and external rotation of the hips, which is often impossible or uncomfortable if osteoarthritis is present. In addition, especially if there is little prior experience of pelvic examinations, the traditional supine position exposes the genitalia in a way which many older persons find embarrassing. The lateral position is also very useful if the examination must be made in an ordinary soft low bed, as in the patient's home or in many nursing home settings. The positioning of the patient is crucial. The patient lies on her left side, with a soft pillow under the head and neck and with her knees flexed up towards her chest, the upper hip more flexed than the lower, and the superior (right) shoulder rolled forward so that she is comfortable and slightly rolled over away from the examiner. It may be desirable to have an assistant support the patient's upper leg. Then a bimanual technique can be used to palpate the pelvic organs: with the physician's right hand in the vagina and left hand reaching over onto the abdominal wall, adequate exclusion of pathological enlargement of the uterus (which should be virtually impalpable) and of the ovaries (which should be impalpable) can be made except in the case of urinary retention or an exceptionally obese or tense patient. Especially if compact lightweight disposable pelvic speculae are used, the cervix and vagina can be well visualized in this position, a Pap smear can be obtained, and an assessment of any uterovaginal descent can be made.

Weight and Height

It is useful to ask what height the patient believes himself or herself to be, since loss of height may be an early indicator of osteoporosis; this also better approximates the patient's "real" height for purposes of figuring the desirable body weight (DBW). However, it must be borne in mind that accurate figures for the "desirable" (or even the "average") weight are not universally agreed upon in this age group. But the significance of *change* in weight is considerable as an indicator of disease and poor nutrition; thus not only the scales must be accurate, but the quantity of clothing worn must be consistent and recorded. The scales must at least have a steadying bar for the patient to hold on to (physically attached to the platform of the scale so that the weight is accurate). Tables are available to assess the patient's effective height if they cannot stand; they are based on upper arm length, which it is always possible to measure, even in the chairbound.

Temperature

This is only required in acute assessments. It is now recognized that high fever is associated with very severe and overwhelming sepsis in older persons, even if the patient appears otherwise relatively "well," and should not be attributed to a viral infection (e.g., in the flu season) as readily as it might be in a younger adult. In addition, there should be a low-reading thermometer available for situations in which hypothermia needs to be a consideration.

Blood Pressure

Blood pressure recording requires special techniques in the elderly. Not only is there disagreement about what should be regarded as normal and what should be treated, but inadequacies in recording the pressure abound. The cuff must be large enough to cover at least two thirds of the arm's circumference, and this may be a consideration in the obese. Cachectic patients may need a pediatric cuff. The "silent gap" auscultatory phenomenon, in which the Korotkoff sounds are absent for an interval between the true systolic and true diastolic pressures, can easily lead to serious underestimation of the systolic pressure (which is the more significant risk factor). Thus it is desirable to palpate the radial artery and inflate the cuff to above the point where the radial pulse is obliterated; then the systolic pressure (the point at which the pulse returns as the cuff is deflated) can be recorded manually. In addition, nonelastic atherosclerotic arteries may require excess cuff pressure to constrict the blood vessels, giving an inaccurately high reading to which the term "pseudohypertension" has been given. The Osler maneuver is designed to elucidate this and is indicated in individuals in whom there is apparent hypertension but no fundal or other peripheral or end organ evidence of hypertension.[18] The cuff is inflated to above the systolic pressure: if the nonelastic atherosclerotic radial artery remains palpable, a firm "cord," then pseudohypertension may be present.

Eyes

Ophthalmological examination, especially of the fundi, and assessment of visual acuity is crucial in all (unless the person already receives regular eye care). Papilledema occurs less readily in older persons even in the presence of raised intracranial pressure. Direct observation for macular changes, lens opacities, and atherosclerotic or hypertensive changes is vital.

Ears

Hearing must be considered, ear wax must be checked for, and at the very least a whisper test should be carried out since hearing loss is so often unreported but is functionally significant. An otoscope with a built-in high-tone screening device can be a useful screen.

Mouth

The mouth must be examined and the dentures taken out, if present, so that the whole oral mucosa can be inspected for problems such as dryness, presence of oral cancers, and dental and periodontal problems.

Neck

The neck examination, which includes examination of the thyroid and observation of the range of movement of the cervical vertebrae, should also include auscultation for carotid bruits.

Heart

The cardiac examination is carried out as in any other patient. A split second heart sound, with inspiration increasing the gap between the aortic and pulmonary components, is a relatively normal finding in older individuals. However, as in younger patients, narrowing of such a gap during inspiration does imply left ventricular strain or reduced left ventricular function, often from a recent myocardial infarction. Another special issue in examining the elderly patient is the high frequency of systolic murmurs present in probably more than 60% of older patients; this finding is often not as significant as in younger adults. Most authorities believe that a patient with a cardiac murmur, whether known to be significant or not, should have antibiotic coverage to prevent bacterial endocarditis when facing elective bowel or dental surgery. Aside from this consideration, a "normal systolic murmur" requiring no further intervention would have the following characteristics: an ejection type of murmur heard loudest at the base, possibly audible at the apex, but still soft (grade 2/6 at most). Such normal murmurs are probably representative of turbulence over sclerosed aortic valves. Some such patients may merit echocardiography, which also remains the most reliable test for assessing left ventricular size. Since left ventricular enlargement is of such prognostic significance, especially in the hypertensive patient, careful examination for cardiac size using percussion as well as indirect methods such as chest x-ray examination and ECG is recommended. But it should be recognized that echocardiography provides the best documentation of this important phenomenon. The phenomenon of "nondyspneic pulmonary edema" has been described previously, and it requires careful examination for signs of congestive heart failure (CHF) even if the patient is not dyspneic or orthopneic. CHF is sometimes overdiagnosed, and the assumption that CHF is the cause for peripheral edema is a mistake. Most cases of peripheral edema are caused by poor venous return, which is often subsequently overtreated with diuretics. Also, many older persons have moist sounds at the lung bases, and most such sounds do not represent CHF. The liver edge may be palpable below the right costal margin, especially in emphysematous persons, and thus percussion can be helpful in making a diagnosis of hepatomegaly (although overlying lung, which will be resonant, may disguise this).

Chest

The chest can be difficult to examine in an older person since the rib cage is often quite fixed and the deformities of kyphosis or scoliosis may produce general hyperresonance with little chest movement and breath sounds that are sometimes difficult to hear. Use of simple in-office respiratory function tests, such as a peak flow meter, can be a useful adjunct and will assist in judging reversibility of obstructive lung disease and avoiding unnecessary use of bronchodilators.

Upper Extremities

The examination of the upper extremities should include assessment of fine finger movement and examination for tremor (Table 5-1).

Abdomen

Often the colon and its contents can be palpated; sometimes it is useful to reexamine after fecal masses that could mimic a malignancy have had time to pass. The classical geriatric "mass without symptoms," which is usually a gastrointestinal tract mass with few functional symptoms, can occur. Therefore relaxation of the abdominal wall is important in this examination. The patient must be comfortably flat, which generally requires a proper pillow underneath the head. Suprapubic percussion to check for urinary retention, which is often asymptomatic, is also vital. If there is any suspicion at all or if symptoms such as incontinence suggest this, the abdominal examination should be extended by a straight catheterization to measure postvoid residual urine (or, if available, use the less invasive procedure of ultrasound). Often, aortic pulsation will be easily felt; if a pulsatile swelling is less than 3 cm and there is no bruit, an aneurysm is unlikely. The hernial orifices should be palpated. Inguinal hernias are frequently tolerated but probably

Table 5-1   Types of Tremor in Elderly Patients

Type	Description
Anxiety/ hyperthyroidism	Fine, rapid, increased by activity, reduced by relaxation
Parkinsonism	Regular, fine, at rest, inhibited by movement
Cerebellar	Variable rate, only with movement, shows dysmetria (rapid patting movements are of unequal force and hit different places)
Senile/essential	Rate as in parkinsonism, may be familial, disappears with relaxation, especially after drinking alcohol
Metabolic	Flapping, patient obviously ill (respiratory or hepatic failure)

From Ham RJ: Geriatrics. I. Monograph ed 89, Home Study Self-Assessment Program, Kansas City, Mo, Oct 1986, American Academy of Family Physicians.

should be repaired, and femoral hernias must be repaired, in view of the high likelihood of strangulation. Where the possibility exists of an acute abdominal condition, the recognized tendency to have no generalized or localized peritoneal signs frequently makes it necessary to extend the examination to abdominal x-ray examinations and to recheck the physical examination in hours or the next day, as well as to obtain serial white blood cell counts. Examination of a potentially acute abdomen is incomplete until rectal and pelvic examinations have been carried out.

Lower Extremities and Feet

The lower extremities are an area of dermal vulnerability that must be checked, and signs of peripheral vascular disease and poor venous return should be sought. Cyanotic, cold feet and unhealthy, dry, or erythematous skin constitute risks and require attention. The feet must be checked for hygiene, peripheral pulses, the condition of toenails and other indicators for podiatric care, deformity, and skin condition, especially in diabetics.

Range of Movement

The range of movement (ROM) of all joints of both extremities should be assessed. Any limitation should be recorded and the amount of limitation measured in degrees, as an angle from the horizontal or straight position. Rotation at the hip should be attempted bilaterally (a common and easily elicited early sign of osteoarthritis).

Central Nervous System

An examination of the CNS consisting of an assessment of tone, power, and coordination and functional testing of balance and gait, with the physician looking especially for lateralizing differences, may often be sufficient. However, a more thorough neurological examination must be made in many circumstances, such as when the patient has an abnormal gait, when there is a history suggesting a dementing illness, or when flatness of affect suggests Parkinson's disease or other problems. A number of neurological changes occur that may be "normal" in older persons (Box 5-12).

Skin

Examination of the entire skin (remember to turn the patient over and see the pressure areas) will generally produce findings of a combination of "normal" and "pathological" lesions in most older persons.

Gait and Balance

This assessment should include having the patient perform the following: rising from a sitting position to a standing position without assistance, bending forward at

---

BOX 5-12
Frequent Neurological Changes in Elderly Patients

Eye signs
  Small, irregular pupils
  Diminished reaction to light and near reflex
  Diminished range of movement on convergence and upward gaze
  Slowed pursuit movements with cogwheel-like motion
Motor signs
  Flexion posture
  Tendency to tremor (>69 yr: 43% have hand tremor, 7% have head tremor [titubation])
  Gait: short-stepped or broad-based with diminished associated movements
  Dysmetria (in all >65 yr)
  Dysdiadochokinesia*
  Atrophy of interossei muscles (thenar wasting in 66%, anterior tibial wasting in 25%)
  Increased muscle tone (legs more than arms, proximal more than distal)
  Diminished muscle strength (legs more than arms, proximal more than distal)
Sensory signs
  Diminished vibratory sense distally, legs much more than arms
  Possible change in proprioception
  Mildly increased threshold for light touch, pain, and temperature
  Impaired double simultaneous stimulation
Reflex signs
  Diminished or absent ankle jerks
  Some reduction in knee, biceps, and triceps reflexes
  Abdominal reflex sometimes lost
  Babinski's sign may not occur (when it would in younger patients)
  Primitive reflexes occur in 20% to 25% (palmomental, snout, and nuchocephalic [doll's eyes])

From Caranosos G, unpublished materials.
*Dysdiadochokinesia is the impaired ability to arrest a motor function and substitute the opposite motor function.

---

the waist, squatting down (or bending down if squatting is not possible) and picking up an object from the floor, standing upright and rotating the head slowly from left to right through its whole range of movement, and walking to one side of the room, turning, walking back, and sitting down again in the chair. All of this should be done without a sense of imbalance or dizziness. More formal versions of this test have been described.[19,20] Some such test must be done in virtually all older persons. Normal and pathological gaits are summarized in Box 5-13 and Table 5-2.

Table 5-2   Pathological Gaits in Older Persons

Gait	Cause	Characteristics
Apraxic	Frontal lobe disease	Patient leans backward and has slowed initiation of movement
Hyperkinetic-hypotonic	Extrapyramidal dysfunction	Slow, short deliberate steps with muscular rigidity
Marche à petits pas	Arterial degeneration	Short uncertain steps that do not adapt to the walking surface
Parkinsonian	Parkinson's disease	Shuffling movement and walking at running pace

---

BOX 5-13
Normal Gait Changes in Older Persons

Women	Men
Waddling gait	Small-stepped gait
Narrow walking and standing base	Wide walking and standing base

---

▼ *GINA GOHRENBERGER (Part III)*

Mrs. Gohrenberger is persuaded to allow a physical examination by the nurse practitioner who is female. She says that this is a "woman's problem." The nurse practitioner is able to complete a lateral pelvic examination, and even in that position she can demonstrate stress incontinence and marked anterior wall prolapse. On standing, there is almost a procidentia; and on slightly bearing down, urine leaks to the floor. The nurse practitioner immediately and vigorously reinforces that something can be done about this situation and that it is not necessary for her to tolerate this condition.

The physician is able to complete a mental status screening examination, on which Mrs. Gohrenberger scores 15/30; this is consistent with moderate dementia. She has poor short-term memory, poor orientation to time (although not to place), and problems with language and the three-stage command. Whereas she gives a good account of her present life, it is evidently optimistic and inaccurate; and her memory for the duration of symptoms is grossly impaired.

STUDY QUESTIONS

- *What should the problem list now consist of?*
- *What should be done next?*

CASE DISCUSSION

This case demonstrates the combination of embarrassment and denial that characterizes the presentation of many symptoms in older persons. There is urgent need to deal with the probable malignant breast neoplasm. In case metastatic disease from this is the cause of the patient's recent memory loss, there is an urgent need for brain imaging. Addressing future preventive and health maintenance activities clearly takes second place to these urgent medical considerations. A "dementia workup" needs to be completed in view of the impaired cognitive status; this should include special attention to potentially

malignant influences (e.g., liver function and calcium level). The urinary incontinence does not appear related to the malignancy or the dementia since it is classically of the stress type, and it appears to have a physical cause (the marked uterovaginal prolapse). Attention must be given to this, but it should probably be postponed until after dealing with the breast lesion and investigating the memory loss. Meanwhile, proper diapering techniques are to be used, and urinary tract infection should be ruled out as a (treatable) contributory factor. Urodynamic investigation of the incontinence during Mrs. Gohrenberger's upcoming hospitalization for the lumpectomy is a possibility, although the lumpectomy will probably be performed on an outpatient basis.

PROBLEM LIST: ORGANIZING AND SUMMARIZING THE ASSESSMENT

The comprehensive set of data, obtained from either a few or many patient visits to the office and perhaps a physician visit to the home, results in a large amount of information that must be organized into one problem list if it is to be useful in the subsequent care of the patient. The problem list should be designed in such a way that it can be modified easily as the situation and diagnoses change and refine over time.

The problem list should include both long-term and short-term problems (some physicians prefer to divide it into the two categories), all medical diagnoses, all of the special risk factors for dependency, functional symptoms (even where there is not a specific diagnosis), and any relevant aspects of the social situation and past history that either require active intervention or that will be important in future decision making (e.g., lives alone, prior suicide attempt, etc.). The problem list should clearly go beyond "formal" diagnoses and traditional medical illnesses.

 The problem list should cumulatively include all items that either require an active intervention or will be important in future situations.

In writing up each problem, an initial plan should be evolved for each. The specific follow-up plan, the target result desired from any intervention, and the ways in which that result will be assessed must be clarified. Too often, different treatments and investigations are all started at once, and it becomes impossible after only a short time to know what has worked and what has not worked. The principle is to simplify the situation into a list of action plans. This should be given to the caregiving family member (and the patient, if competent) to involve them directly in the management; often patient and caregiver should have a copy of the whole record for the same reason.

▼ GINA GOHRENBERGER (Part IV)

Mrs. Gohrenberger's initial problem list is as follows:

1. Impaired cognitive status. Plan: investigate with a computed tomography (CT) scan; perform blood work for both thyroid and liver function, calcium, electrolytes, CBC, VDRL, B$_{12}$, folate, and plasma proteins.

2. Probable carcinoma left breast. Plan: surgical referral for probable lumpectomy and consideration of staging, if malignant, depending upon the histology.

3. Urinary stress incontinence with marked uterovaginal prolapse. Plan: extensive diapering while problems 1 and 2 are investigated and treated. Check for UTI. Following that, probable referral for uterovaginal surgery, with consideration of urodynamic testing and investigation to assess other potential causes before considering surgery.

BASELINE INVESTIGATIONS AND TESTS

It is debatable how much baseline investigation should be carried out in an older person. Because these investigations may reveal otherwise occult problems, the initial investigations listed in Box 5-14 include some that should probably be performed in all older persons and repeated at intervals (which may not be as frequently as annually) and others that are useful in many cases. Since clinical examination for anemia can miss even the markedly anemic, hemoglobin and hematocrit tests are probably useful. Before prescribing any renally excreted drug, the physician should obtain blood urea nitrogen (BUN) and creatinine values to rule out severe renal impairment. (Ideally, a creatinine clearance should be calculated if renally excreted drugs are to be given.) The urinalysis is an economical screen for glycosuria, urinary infection (although some chronic bacteriuria patients will be found and should not be treated unless symptomatic), and proteinuria. The baseline ECG is probably useful, although one witty authority is reputed to have said, "Obtain the baseline ECG, but do not look at it!" This statement rightly implies that the major utility of an "interval" ECG is to enable the physician to assess change in it in the event of a potential cardiac episode. Purified protein derivative (PPD), or tuberculin, status should be known on all patients, and it is often a requirement prior to institutional placement, as is a chest x-ray examination. The other investigations listed in Box 5-14 could probably be justified in many ill older patients: thyroid disorders are frequently missed, electrolyte upsets may be occult (and are always a consideration in patients taking medications that may modify their electrolytes), liver function tests may pick up malignancy and alcohol-induced cirrhosis when it is not suspected (the test could be restricted to an aspartate transaminase [AST] in screening for alcoholism), and venereal disease screening (although it may produce information that is sometimes difficult to interpret) is inexpensive and will reveal the occasional case of previously unrecognized syphilis. HIV testing is a consideration in any older person at risk. Routine screening for calcium, magnesium, and B$_{12}$ is not recommended but should be considered, and folate and albumin measurement, again not a routine consideration, may help to confirm suspicions of poor nutritional status.

STUDY QUESTIONS

- *Based on the above information, review Parts 1, 2, and 3 of George Anderson's case. What tests might be useful in this case?*

- *Construct a problem list and plans for this immobilized, unwilling, dyspneic, self-neglected, and possibly demented, isolated elderly man.*

BOX 5-14
Initial Investigations in Older Persons

Most Patients:
  Hemoglobin and hematocrit
  Creatinine and BUN
  Urinalysis with microscopy
  Chest x-ray examination
  ECG
  PPD

Many Patients:
  Thyroid-stimulating hormone (TSH)—with or without T$_4$
  Rapid plasma reagin (RPR) or venereal disease research laboratory (VDRL)

Selected Patients:
  Complete blood count (CBC)
  Electrolytes
  Hepatic function
  Calcium
  Magnesium
  B$_{12}$
  Folate
  Albumin

CASE RESOLUTION AND DISCUSSION

George Anderson's case demonstrates the challenge of the unwilling but high-risk individual; as he challenges the physician's sense of advocacy, he also displays independence and autonomy. He is an individual who does not seek help but who is in danger. The approach of winter, the increasingly crime-ridden area in which Mr. Anderson lives, his unsuitable house, his poor gait and nutrition, his probably persistent alcoholism, his access to some potentially dangerous medications, and the lack of available family do not allow the same type of ordered approach that was possible with Mrs. Gohrenberger. Yet Mr. Anderson is equally, if not more urgently, in need of help and medical and social intervention. A "comprehensive geriatric assessment" for this case is obtained sporadically over a period of time and mostly in the home setting; the information is slowly accumulated in the ongoing problem list. Mr. Anderson is able to remain in his home for 2 more years, and his nutrition is improved. He also becomes socially involved in his local church community, which gets him out of the house and improves his physical mobility. He never consents to come to the office, but after the 2 further years at home, he is hospitalized with a hip fracture following a fall. He recovers sufficiently to be placed in an adult home rather than at a skilled level of care. It could be reasoned that he was in much better shape physically at the time of his fracture and that this contributed to his relatively good rehabilitation from the incident. He lives for 5 more years in the adult home, stops drinking, and is for some time a mainstay of many of the social activities in the facility, being one of the few men available in the pleasant home setting in which he is able to spend his remaining days.

SUMMARY

The techniques for obtaining comprehensive geriatric assessment information in a variety of settings, centered around the home and office, have been outlined. In obtaining this information, emergent medical problems often dominate. Direct and basic questions about function and situation must be asked; geriatric assessment should be efficient and not waste the time of the patient, family, or physician. Plans for health maintenance and health promotion must also be incorporated into the problem list and plan that the primary care physician develops for each patient.

POSTTEST

1. Which one of the following statements concerning physical examination in the elderly is false?
   a. A split second heart sound with narrowing of the gap during inspiration is generally an insignificant finding in older persons.
   b. A "normal" systolic murmur requiring no further intervention is an ejection type of murmur heard loudest at the base but still soft.
   c. High fever is more often associated with extreme sepsis in older individuals than it is in younger adults.
   d. The Osler maneuver indicates that firm blood vessels may give a falsely elevated blood pressure reading.
2. Which one of the following statements concerning laboratory screening in older persons is false?
   a. A PPD is generally required prior to nursing home admission.
   b. Creatinine and/or BUN values must be known prior to the prescription of a renally excreted drug.
   c. Annual CBC, BUN/creatinine, and electrolyte tests are recommended in frail elders.
   d. Bacteriuria found on routine urinalysis should only be treated if symptomatic.
3. Which one of the following statements is false concerning ADLs and IADLs?
   a. Independence of feeding is generally lost before independence in bathing.
   b. Feeding is an ADL; cooking is an IADL.
   c. Many states screen for long-term care services by assessing ADLs and IADLs.
   d. ADLs are the skills required for self-care.
4. Which one of the following statements is false concerning tremor in older patients?
   a. Cerebellar tremor shows dysmetria.
   b. A parkinsonian tremor is inhibited by movement.
   c. Alcohol generally worsens an essential (senile) tremor.
   d. The rate of cerebellar tremor is variable.
5. Which one of the following statements concerning neurological changes common in older persons is false?
   a. There is increased muscle tone—more in the legs than in the arms.
   b. There is reduced muscle strength—more in the arms than in the legs.
   c. There is diminished vibratory sense—more in the legs than in the arms.
   d. There is a diminished range of eye movement on convergence.
6. Which one of the following statements concerning gaits in older persons is false?
   a. The gait of frontal lobe disease involves the patient leaning backward.
   b. Walking at running pace is characteristic of Parkinson's disease.
   c. In extrapyramidal dysfunction, there are short steps that do not adapt to the walking surface.
   d. In osteoarthritis, the gait is wide-based, waddling, and swaying.
   e. Normal gait changes in older men include a wide walking and standing base.
7. Which one of the following items is not a component of the Folstein Mini–Mental State Examination?
   a. Spelling WORLD backwards
   b. Proverb interpretation
   c. Drawing intersecting pentagons
   d. Remembering three words for a time
   e. Carrying out a three-stage command

REFERENCES

1. Solomon DH: National Institutes of Health Consensus Development Conference Statement: geriatric assessment methods for clinical decision-making, *J Am Geriatr Soc* 36:342-347, 1988.
2. Rubenstein LZ, Wieland D: Comprehensive geriatric assessment, *Annu Rev Geriatr Gerontol* 9:145-192, 1989.
3. Ham RJ: Home and nursing home care of the dependent elderly patient, *Am Fam Phys* 31:163-169, 1985.
4. Keenan JM et al: A review of federal home-care legislation, *J Am Geriatr Soc* 38:1041-1048, 1990.
5. Ham RJ: Geriatrics: I. Monograph ed 89, Home Study Self-Assessment Program, Kansas City, Mo, Oct 1986, American Academy of Family Physicians.
6. Folstein MF, Folstein SE, McHugh PR: Mini-mental state: a practical method for grading the cognitive state of patients for the clinician, *J Psychiatr Res* 12(3):186-198, 1975.
7. Pfeiffer E: A short portable mental status questionnaire for assessment of organic brain deficit in elderly patients, *J Am Geriatr Soc* 23:433-441, 1975.
8. Ham RJ: Functional assessment of the elderly patient. In Reichel W, ed: *Clinical Aspects of Aging,* ed 3, Baltimore, 1989, Williams & Wilkins.
9. Katz S et al: Progress in development of the index of ADLs, *Gerontologist* 10:20-30, 1970.
10. The Older Americans' Resources and Services (OARS) Methodology: *Multidimensional Functional Assessment Questionnaire,* ed 2, Durham, NC, 1978, Duke University Center for the Study of Aging and Human Development.
11. Mahoney FI, Barthel DW: Functional evaluation: the Barthel index, *Md State Med J* 14:61-65, 1965.
12. Kane RA, Kane RL: *Assessing the elderly: a practical guide to measurement,* Lexington, Mass, 1981, DC Heath.

13. Gallo JJ, Reichel W, Andersen LM: *Handbook of geriatric assessment,* ed 2, Rockville, Md, 1995, Aspen.

14. Fillenbaum GG: Screening the elderly: a brief instrumental activities of daily living measure, *J Am Geriatr Soc* 33:698-706, 1985.

15. Goldstein MK: Physicians and teams. In Ham RJ, ed: *Geriatric medicine annual 1989,* Oradell, NJ, 1989, Medical Economics Books.

16. Kosberg JI, ed: *Abuse and maltreatment of the elderly: causes and interventions,* Boston, 1983, John Wright-PSG.

17. Zarit SH: Relatives of the impaired elderly: correlates of feelings of burden, *Gerontologist* 20:649-655, 1980.

18. Messerli FH, Ventura HO, Amodeo C: Osler's maneuver and pseudohypertension, *N Engl J Med* 312:1548-1551, 1985.

19. Tinetti ME, Williams TF, Mayesski R: Fall risk index for elderly patients based on number of chronic disabilities, *Am J Med* 80(3):429-434, 1986.

20. Mathias S, Nayak USL, Isaacs B: The "Get Up and Go" test: a simple clinical test of balance in old people, *Arch Phys Med Rehabil* 67(6):387-389, 1986.

PRETEST ANSWERS

1. d
2. a
3. e

POSTTEST ANSWERS

1. a
2. c
3. a
4. c
5. b
6. c
7. b

CHAPTER 6

The Health Care System

L. GREGORY PAWLSON, DONNA LIND INFELD, and DEBORAH M. LASTINGER

OBJECTIVES

Upon completion of this chapter, the reader will be able to:

1. Describe the nature, source, potential, and restrictions of the five major areas of federal funding that support health services for the older population: Medicare, Medicaid, Title XX of the Social Security Act, the Older Americans Act, and the Veterans Administration.

2. Describe and define current aspects of the implementation of these programs, including Medicare Part A and Part B, diagnosis-related groups (DRGs), and Medigap.

3. Describe the range, limitations, and proportions of nursing home care costs from the three principal sources: patient's and family's personal funds, long-term care insurance, and Medicaid.

4. Describe the range of support available for home and community-based care and the emerging role of case management.

5. Describe the nature and purpose of currently available community support programs: nutritional support services, respite, adult day care, continuing care resident facilities, "social" HMOs, and transportation.

6. Describe the generally expected and desirable trends in the direction of organization and payment for health care services for the elderly in the next one to two decades.

7. Apply the preceding information to typical, brief case scenarios concerning older individuals at risk of needing increasing resources for their health care.

PRETEST

1. Which one of the following statements concerning payment sources for Medicare services is correct?
   a. Hospital care and nursing home care are paid for mainly by Medicare and Medicaid, whereas physicians' services are paid for mainly by individuals and private insurance.
   b. Hospital and physician care is paid for by Medicare and private insurance, whereas nursing home care is paid for by individuals and Medicaid.
   c. Hospital care and physician care are paid for mainly by individuals and Medicare, whereas nursing home care is paid for by private insurance and Medicaid.
2. Which one of the following statements concerning aspects of payment for health care is false?
   a. The resource utilization groups (RUGs) system is designed to encourage nursing homes to accept complex, dependent patients.
   b. Nearly half of Medicaid funding is spent on long-term care.
   c. Medicare pays for less than 10% of all nursing home days.
   d. Title XX funds are exclusively for the elderly and the mentally ill.
3. Which one of the following sets of figures correctly describes the 1994 annual deductible and copayments due from patients for hospital care if they are fully eligible for Medicare?
   a. Annual deductible $403, copayment $174 a day from day 91
   b. Annual deductible $796, copayment $148 a day from day 61
   c. Annual deductible $696, copayment $174 a day from day 61
   d. Annual deductible $403, copayment $198 a day from day 31
   e. Annual deductible $592, copayment $198 a day from day 61

Clinicians can no longer separate themselves from public policy and the financing of health care. This is particularly evident in the care of the older person because the vast majority of funding is controlled federally or by the state. Care of the elderly consumes a disproportionate portion of the health care budget, a trend that is expected to continue far into the next century. The common illnesses and syndromes afflicting older individuals interact with the aging process to produce functional decline and dependency. The aggregate costs and benefits of medical interventions in the high-risk older patient presents a special challenge for clinicians. Physicians are intimately involved in the decision making that affects the lives of both older persons and those who pay for public programs like Medicare and Medicaid. It is especially critical for clinicians who care for older persons to be fully aware of how the health care system for older persons is structured and paid for in order to assist both their patients and society in achieving optimal value from health care now and in the future.

▼ RITA SALTER

Mrs. Salter is an 85-year-old widow with osteoarthritis, diabetes mellitus, cataracts, macular degeneration, and hypertension. Over a 2-year period she experiences gradually increasing problems with shopping, food preparation, bathing, and dressing. Her income consists of $450 per month in Social Security and $200 per month in interest from a bank savings account left by her deceased husband. She pays $400 per month in rent for her one-bedroom apartment on the second floor of a building in a high-crime section of a large city. Her medications cost $50 per month, and Medicare premiums, deductible, and copayments average another $70 per month.

Mrs. Salter then begins to lose weight, in part because of her inability to shop and prepare food. Her diabetes and hypertension are in poor control largely as a result of difficulty paying for medication and poor vision, which hampers her use of insulin. She becomes increasingly reclusive because of embarrassment at being unable to bathe and dress herself appropriately. A social work consultant recommends a minimum of 10 hours per week (at $10 an hour) of home health aide time, and a visiting nurse one time per week (at $60 per visit). Her income and assets are too high to qualify for Medicaid assistance, and since she is not homebound, she is not eligible for the Medicare home care benefit.

After 6 months of largely futile attempts to improve her situation, she suffers a severe stroke. Following this she spends 1 week on an acute hospital service and 2 weeks in a rehabilitation unit at a total cost of $15,475 to Medicare and $696 to the patient. She is then discharged to a nursing home where the cost is $120 per day. Medicare pays the full amount for 20 days; then she has to pay $87 per day. After 60 days of skilled nursing care, she is denied further Medicare coverage because her rehabilitation potential is limited. She spends her life savings ($10,000) over the next 3 months paying for nursing home care, after which she becomes eligible for Medicaid.

She remains in the nursing home, except for four hospital admissions, until her death 3 years later. The cost to her is all but $360 per year of her income; the remainder of her nursing home expenses are paid by Medicaid, and her hospital and physician expenses are paid by Medicare and Medicaid. The total costs of care in the last 5 years of her life exceed $130,000 for medication, physicians, and hospitals and over $120,000 for nursing home care.

STUDY QUESTIONS

- How could the impact of her nutritional status and preexisting chronic illnesses have been reduced by increased home support earlier in her illness?
- What are the most important factors in the failure to prevent the actual outcomes?
- What policy changes might have created a higher quality of life before her death?
- What other payment sources are available to certain categories of individuals in similar economic circumstances?

Until recently, few health care providers felt they needed to understand the details of access and provision of services for older persons. Now, however, providing high-quality primary care includes knowing about types of insurance, benefits, or eligibility, issues related to financing of care (including expenditures and source of financing), and available services. This chapter explores the issues and problems related to access and financing of care for older individuals that affect the provision of care for these individuals.

> *Unless clinicians understand the system, neither patients nor society will receive good value for health care.*

The relationship of access and financing to the provision of care is of special interest in older persons for several reasons. First, persons 65 years and older, because of their high burden of chronic illness, consume a disproportionate share of health care services. Although they make up approximately 12% of the population, they utilize nearly 20% of all physician services, 40% of all hospital days, and over 90% of all nursing home days. Furthermore, those 85 years and over use substantially more services than those 65 to 69 years old. This high utilization results in substantially higher per capita expenditures for medical care (nearly $10,000 per person per year) in those over 65 as compared to those under 65 ($2,500).

Second, the financing of much of the care of older persons is through publicly financed programs, principally Medicare and Medicaid. Federal and state governments, faced with stable or falling revenues and, in the case of

the federal government, increasing debt, have been increasingly active in their attempts to control costs. Changes in eligibility, benefits, and reimbursement have become very evident to older persons and to the institutions and individuals providing health care services to them.

In the past three decades, demographic changes caused by declining age-specific death rates have accounted for less than 10% of the growth in medical care expenditures. However, beginning in 2010 the increase in the number of elderly because of the aging of the "baby-boom" cohort will have a profound impact on medical practice. To illustrate this effect, consider the following: in 1994, the 12% of our population over 65 accounted for 36% of total health care expenditures—$300 billion out of a total of over $800 billion; if 20% of our population is over 65 (as we are likely to have in 2040), expenditures for those over 65 will be over $500 billion out of total expenditures of $1.1 trillion. Most of the $200 billion in additional expenditures will come from the Medicare and Medicaid programs.

Finally, while a substantial proportion of the care of older persons is concerned with long-term care for chronic illness, our health care system is organized and financed largely around acute care. Thus the care of older persons with chronic illness is often made more difficult and less efficacious because of the problems of coordinating, managing, and paying for long-term care.

CASE DISCUSSION

Ms. Salter's functional deterioration when she first presented to her physician was already quite marked: she had problems with shopping, food preparation, bathing, and dressing. Her poor vision interfered with these functions and with control of the diabetes mellitus. Her preoccupation with providing these care services to herself and anxiety related to living in a high-crime area undoubtedly contributed to her reclusiveness and to her noncompliance with antihypertensive treatment, increasing her risk of stroke. With less than $150 of expendable income, she could not afford the simple activities of daily living (ADL) assistance she needed. Ultimately, she cost the system more than she might have, had the acute stroke and her subsequent dependency been postponed or prevented.

PUBLIC PROGRAMS

In the United States in 1994, over $300 billion was spent for health services provided to persons over 65 years. The largest portion of these expenditures was for hospital care (about 35%), followed by physicians (25%), and nursing homes (20%). The source of payment for care is dramatically different between acute and long-term care: hospital and physician services are paid for largely by Medicare and private insurance while payment for nursing home care comes from individuals and Medicaid (Fig. 6-1).

There are five major areas of federal funding that support health services for the older population: Medicare, Medicaid, Title XX of the Social Security Act (Block Grants), the Older Americans Act, and the Veterans Administration. Each program has different funding sources, different eligibility requirements, and a different set of services that are paid for by by different mechanisms (Table 6-1).

Medicare

Acute care services for nearly all persons over 65 years are covered by Medicare but with substantial gaps in coverage (Tables 6-2 and 6-3). Thus while access to hospital care is not usually a problem for persons over 65 years, paying for long stays can be a major problem. Medicare is administered and paid for through the federal government, with services delivered by the private sector. There are two parts of Medicare coverage.

Medicare Part A, Hospital Insurance. Medicare Part A, hospital insurance, is made up of revenues derived from Social Security taxes paid by employers and employees and credited to the Medicare Hospital Insurance Trust Fund. Part A provides reimbursement for hospital and hospice care and for some posthospital skilled care provided by nursing homes and home care agencies. All older persons who receive Social Security are enrolled in Medicare Part A. Most services covered by Part A require that beneficiaries pay substantial copayments and deductibles (see Table 6-2). Those persons with long hospital stays can face copayments in the thousands of dollars.

For providing this care, hospitals receive a predetermined payment based on the diagnosis-related group (DRG) to which the case is assigned at discharge. The assignment is based on the diagnosis that resulted in the admission or on a surgical procedure. The payment is based on the relative weight (complexity) of the DRG to which the case is assigned and a geographic modifier (primarily based on relative labor costs). Hospitals are not paid directly by Medicare but rather by Medicare intermediaries (generally insurance companies), and they

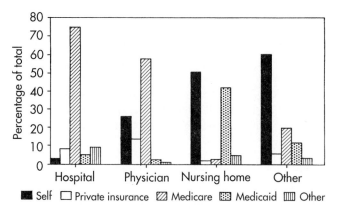

FIG. 6-1   Source of payment for health care services for persons 65 and older.

Table 6-1   Funding Sources for Care Services Commonly Used by Older Persons

Setting	Medicare	Medicaid	Block Grants	Older Americans Act	Veterans Administration
Eligibility based on:	Age	Income + assets	Income + other	Age	Vet status
Institutional					
Acute care	Yes	Yes	No	No	Yes
Rehab facility	Yes	Optional*	No	No	Yes
Skilled nursing	Limited	Optional*	No	No	Yes
Mental hospital	No	No	No	No	No
Community-based					
Physician services	Yes	Yes	No	No	Yes
Adult day care	No	Waiver	Some†	Yes	Yes
Congregate meals	No	No	Some†	Yes	No
Respite care	No	Waiver	No	No	Yes
In home					
Case management	No	Waiver	Some†	No	Yes
Information/referral	No	No	Some†	Yes	Yes
Chore/repair	No	Waiver	Some†	Yes	Yes
Homemaker	No	Waiver	Some†	Yes	Yes
Home meals	No	No	Some†	Yes	No
Transportation	No	No	Some†	Yes	No
Home health aide	Yes	Waiver	Some†	Yes	Yes
Home health	Yes	Yes	No	No	Yes
Respite	No	Waiver	Some†	No	No

*Optional means states have the choice whether to include as a covered service.

†Some means that some states cover for the service for the elderly while others do not.

Table 6-2   Services Available Under Medicare Part A (1994)

Medicare Part A 1994	Services Included	Conditions That Must Be Met—Care Must Be:	Deductible (d), Copayment (c)	Reimbursement
Inpatient hospital care	Semiprivate room, special units, lab, x-ray, medication, supplies, blood (except for first 3 U), meals, nursing (not private duty)	Ordered by physician, care that can only be provided in hospital for stay approved by peer review organization	d: $696 for each benefit period* c: $174, day 61-90; $348, day 90-150; no coverage beyond day 150	Prospective payment per case modified by DRG
Skilled nursing facility (SNF)	Semiprivate room, rehabilitation services, meals, nursing, medications, use of appliances	For skilled nursing or rehabilitative services on daily basis after a 3-day hospital stay for related condition within 30 days before SNF admission ordered by physician; approved by Medicare intermediary	d: none c: $87 for days 21-100; no coverage beyond day 100	Cost based on each facility's approved cost
Home health care	Skilled nursing, physical therapy (PT) or speech therapy (ST), occupational therapy, part-time home health aide and medical equipment also covered if skilled nursing, PT, ST needed	For intermittent (up to 8 hr per day for up to 21 days) skilled nursing, PT, ST, ordered by physician approved by Medicare intermediary; patient must be confined to home	d: none c: 20% only for durable medical equipment	Cost based on but limited by maximal approved costs
Hospice	Inpatient and outpatient nursing, physician, drugs, PT, OT, ST, homemaker, counseling, inpatient respite (5 days), medical social services	For care of patient certified by a physician as terminally ill, patient chooses hospice over standard Medicare benefits for terminal illness	d: none c: none except $5 copayment for drugs and 5% of inpatient respite care; limited to 210 days, but extension possible	Daily fixed rate per case for up to 210 days (patient may be billed for additional days but care must be provided if patient cannot pay)

*Benefit period: begins with day of admission and ends after patient has been out of a hospital or skilled nursing facility for 60 consecutive days.

must accept Medicare payment as full payment (except for specified copayments and deductibles).

Medicare Part B. Physician services are supported by an optional program in which Social Security retirees do not have to participate, the Supplementary Medical Insurance program (SMI; Medicare Part B), which is funded by general tax revenues (75%) and a premium paid by those eligible for Social Security benefits who elect to enroll in Medicare Part B (25%). Over 98% of those eligible for Part B choose to enroll. Persons not eligible for Social Security can also enroll in Part B by paying the full cost (which is usually still less than other insurance available to them). Part B also pays for some medical devices, hospital outpatient visits, and some outpatient rehabilitation services. As of 1994, participation in Part B requires a monthly premium of $41.10, an annual deductible ($100), and a coinsurance payment (20%

for allowed physician charges and certain other services and 50% for mental health services; Table 6-3).

Reimbursement to physicians under Medicare Part B has undergone a fundamental change from allowed charges (the lesser of what the physician charges, what the physician has historically charged, or the average of what other physicians have charged for the same service) to a Medicare fee schedule. The fee schedule is based on the relative work required for different services, modified by geographic differences for labor costs.

At present, physicians, unlike hospitals and other providers, can decide on a case-by-case basis whether to accept the Medicare fee schedule as full payment for services (referred to as "accepting assignment"). Physicians who do not accept assignment may bill the patient no more than 15% more than the fee schedule.

Medicare payment for care in a long-term care facility

Table 6-3   Services Available Under Medicare Part B (1994)

Medicare Part B (Premium = $28.60/mo)	Services Included	Conditions That Must Be Met—Care Must Be:	Deductible (d); Copayment (c)	Reimbursement
Physician services	Medical and surgical services, diagnostic procedures, radiology, pathology, drugs, and biologicals that can't be self-administered	Medically necessary for diagnosis and management of acute or chronic illness and approved by Medicare carrier	d: one $100 deductible for all Part B services; c: 20% (50% for mental health, recipient pays all charges in excess of allowable by nonparticipating physicians)	Allowable charge (lesser of actual charge, the physician usual charge or 75% of the area prevailing charge with annual increase limited by Medicare Economic Index)
Hospital outpatient services	Ambulatory surgery services incident to services of physician, diagnostic tests (lab/x-ray), emergency room, hospital-based medical supplies	Medically necessary, approved by Medicare carrier	d: same as physician services; c: same as physician services	Varies by service: outpatient surgery in transition from hospital cost to average cost, lab, and x-ray on fee schedule, emergency room on hospital-specific costs
Independent lab services	Clinical diagnostic laboratory	Ordered by physician	d: none; c: none	Approved standard fee—all labs must take assignment
Durable medical equipment (not oxygen)	Wheelchairs, oxygen equipment for use in home to serve a medical purpose	Ordered by physician	d: same as physician services; c: same as physician services	Usually on approved amount for rental fee

or in one's own home is very restricted. Medicare coverage of home health care is limited to patients who need skilled nursing or physical or speech therapies, whose needs are intermittent (not chronic), and who are confined to their homes. Medicare payments for nursing home care are even more limited and account for less than 2% of annual nursing home care costs. Further details of this are in this chapter's section on payment for nursing home care.

Older individuals concerned about paying for their Medicare copayments and deductibles for hospital and physician services often purchase private health insurance known as a Medigap policy. Approximately 70% of older persons have purchased such private insurance, and another 12% percent have their deductibles and copayments covered by Medicaid. Because of the misunderstandings about private insurance coverage, many older individuals think they are buying insurance to cover other costs, such as long-term care, and some purchase more than one policy that essentially cover the same Medicare copayments and deductibles. The premiums for many Medigap policies exceed $100 per month.

Medicaid

Medicaid (Title XIX of the Social Security Act) is a means-tested, joint federal and state program for certain categories of indigent persons. Persons over 65 years old

qualify provided that they meet the income and asset criteria set by the state in which they live. Many states use the federally determined income and asset level for supplemental security income (SSI) to determine Medicaid eligibility for the aged (over 65 years), the blind, and the disabled, but others set both higher and lower limits. In 1994, the federal limits were an income of less than $634 per month for an individual and $841 per month for a couple and countable assets of less than $4,000 for an individual and $6,000 for a couple. A home that is owned by an individual or a couple and is the primary residence is not a countable asset. Forty-three states and the District of Columbia have higher limits than those set federally. A majority of states (38) also permit the aged, blind, and disabled to receive Medicaid benefits if their medical expenses reduce their income to a level below that required for Medicaid (the assets test must still be met). These beneficiaries are often referred to as medically needy Medicaid recipients. Many older persons who end up requiring nursing home care either spend down their income and assets on medical expenses before needing nursing home care or do so shortly after entering the nursing home. Medicaid funding comes primarily from general tax revenues at both the state and the federal level. The proportion of total Medicaid costs that are paid by the federal government ranges from 50% to 77.5% (depending on the relative income of the state), with poorer states receiving a higher proportion of federal funds.

The federal government has established a set of minimum services for Medicaid-eligible persons that each state is required to cover. These services include hospital inpatient care, hospital outpatient services, laboratory and x-ray services, skilled nursing care, skilled home health care, physician services, family planning, rural health clinic services, and care for children under 21 years of age. States have the option of including additional services such as drugs, eyeglasses, prosthetics, private duty nursing, intermediate nursing home care, inpatient psychiatric care, physical therapy, dental care, personal care and home health services, and medical transportation. Even though it is considered optional, all states (except Arizona, which does not participate in Medicaid) include intermediate-level nursing home care.

Medicaid is a direct-vendor payment program, which means payments are made directly to providers of care including nursing homes, hospitals, and physicians. Medicaid reimbursement levels are generally lower than those for private insurance or Medicare and must be accepted as payment in full by participating providers. States have considerable flexibility to determine eligibility, benefits, payment mechanisms, and rates, and as a result there is little consistency of coverage across states and a wide range of expenditures (from under $90 to over $200 per capita per year). While Medicaid is designed to cover a variety of health services for poor people of all ages, its largest program by far is long-term care. Payments for long-term care services account for nearly 50% of total federal and state Medicaid vendor payments. Nearly 70% of the long-term care expenditures are for institutional care.

Medicaid programs are required to pay Medicare premiums, copayments, and deductibles for persons covered under both programs (known as dual eligibility). About 12% of Medicare enrollees are covered by state Medicaid programs. The actual levels and methods of nursing home reimbursement vary widely from state to state.

Many states have attempted to control overall spending for Medicaid long-term care benefits by setting maximum reimbursement rates and limiting the number of nursing home beds covered by the program. More recently, some states have begun to use various forms of case mix reimbursement systems. Case mix payments are based on patient characteristics that influence the amount of care needed. One goal of case mix reimbursement is to encourage nursing homes to admit more dependent, heavy-care patients. Several methods, using measures of functional levels of ADL, have been developed for use in nursing homes.

The resource utilization groups system (RUGs) is a case mix reimbursement system that is used in several states. This system categorizes patients as heavy rehabilitation, special care, clinically complex, severe behavioral problem, or reduced physical functioning. In a case mix system, patients must be reassessed periodically. There is concern that case mix systems could provide an incentive to keep patients at lower levels of functioning; therefore quality assurance mechanisms are critical to be sure that appropriate services are being delivered.

Older Americans Act

Coverage for care management and nonskilled services is also provided in some communities through the Older Americans Act (OAA). OAA funds can be used to support a variety of community-based social services. These federal funds are channeled through a designated agency in each state to a local area agency on aging. Area agencies are housed in governmental offices (city, county, or multicounty units), or quasigovernmental agencies (e.g., councils of governments). They have authority to conduct community needs assessments, provide information and referral (developing directories of elderly services in most communities), and can contract for gap-filling services to meet specific community needs. Under this provision, some area agencies on aging support care management. In 1993, total OAA expenditures for programs and activities were $754.3 million.

Title XX Programs

The final program that covers some case management and/or nonskilled services for older persons is Title XX of the Social Security Act, social services block grants. Social services block grant funds are distributed to states, each of which can determine eligibility and services to be provided. Title XX funds can be spent for a range of target groups such as the mentally ill, mentally retarded, pregnant teenagers, and the elderly. As a result, the proportion of state funds that go to elderly services in general, and to case management in particular, tends to be limited. In addition, there is minimal reporting required of how Title XX funds are spent, so it is difficult to determine how many older persons receive services under this program.

Veterans Administration Programs

Veterans have additional service options. In 1994, the total U.S. Veterans Administration health care expenditures exceeded $15 billion, much of which was spent on care for the increasing proportion of veterans over the age of 65. Some veterans hospitals offer a full range of long-term care services including geriatric assessment, case management, skilled and unskilled in-home services, and nursing home care. Unfortunately, the severe limits on funds available for long-term care (about 7% of the total) for the growing number of aged veterans means that in most localities, only veterans who have service-connected disabilities or who are indigent can receive VA-based long-term care.

NURSING HOME CARE

Nursing home placement for maintenance of functioning and assistance with ADL can be paid for in three ways: a patient's own funds, private long-term care insurance, and Medicaid.

In 1994, approximately 40% of nursing home care was paid for by private funds.[1] This expenditure represented more than 30% of total health care out-of-pocket expenditures for persons over age 65. For the large majority of elderly, nursing home costs far exceed monthly income. As a result, they must spend savings and sometimes liquidate other assets.

The second way is an option only for the few older persons (approximately 4% in 1990) who have purchased private long-term care insurance.[2] In 1994, only 2.5% of nursing home costs were paid by private insurance, including both Medigap and true long-term care policies.[1] While there are a growing number of long-term care insurance policies available on the market, most offer nursing home coverage that is limited in duration or absolute amount. Many have restrictions on prior conditions or have waiting periods for the benefit to begin; some even require a prior hospital stay. The policies are quite expensive (over $3,000 per year) for those most likely to need nursing home care (women over 80 years) and relatively expensive (over $1,400 per year) for those over 65 years old.[3] The typical policy covers 5 years of nursing home care and pays $69 per day in benefits. It has been estimated that between 6% and 20% of Americans over 65 years old can afford private long-term care insurance.[4]

For the rest of the older population, those who do not have private funds or insurance to cover nursing home costs, Medicaid is the program of last resort. In the absence of a national strategy for long-term care, and because of the exclusion of long-term services from Medicare coverage, Medicaid, by default, constitutes our national long-term care program, financing almost half (47% in 1987) of national nursing home expenditures.[1]

> *Medicaid, by default, has become our national long-term care program.*

Medicare pays for skilled nursing care provided in a facility with substantial restrictions. To be eligible for nursing home coverage, the patient must need skilled rehabilitation following a 3-day or longer stay in a hospital for a condition related to the need for rehabilitation. While a maximum of 100 nursing home days can be covered per year, most patients lose their eligibility sooner because their condition no longer requires skilled level care or because they have a poor rehabilitation potential. As a result, Medicare payments account for only 2% of annual nursing home care costs.[1] Skilled nursing home stays require a copayment of $87 per day (1994) for days 21 through 100. While most private Medigap insurance policies cover the Medicare skilled nursing care copayment, they are limited to the same requirements and eligibility that hold for Medicare skilled care coverage.

In addition to these problems with funding, elderly patients face serious concerns about access to and quality of nursing home care. Nursing homes in the United States operate at near full capacity (94.5% occupancy rate, 1992) and therefore access is limited.[5] While local referral agencies review applicants for appropriate placement, many must wait for care. As a result of concerns over quality, Congress passed sweeping nursing home reforms in the Omnibus Budget Reconciliation Act of 1987 (OBRA 87). New regulations stress residents' rights and ensure a care planning process that responds to residents' needs and preferences. These regulations have resulted in increased minimum staffing levels, more individualized care, and reductions of restraint use in nursing homes.

These changes, coupled with early discharge from hospitals, have increased the level of medical care provided in nursing homes. While subacute care is a growing trend, patients who need less care are more likely to move to an assisted living facility, which provides help with activities of daily living but no nursing care, or to remain in their own homes.

▼ *JAMES FREEMAN*

Mr. Freeman is a 74-year-old man who has a history of intermittent depression, occasionally complicated by psychotic symptoms. He has rarely been able to hold a steady job and qualifies for only a minimal Social Security benefit. His current income is $515 per month, all from Social Security. His Medicare Part B premium costs $41.10 per month and his rent another $200. During the past year, he has become increasingly withdrawn and has lost 20 lb. He has not paid his utility bills for 2 months, and his telephone and gas have been disconnected. He is brought in by a neighbor to see you and you diagnose recurrent depression and possible dementia. You refer him to a psychiatrist (no community mental health center is available nearby) for further evaluation of the depression, but he fails to return to either you or the psychiatrist because of concern that he cannot afford the 50% copayment for Medicare-covered mental health services (the psychiatrist charges $100 per visit). He becomes more withdrawn and several weeks later is taken to the emergency room suffering from pneumonia and dehydration. He is diagnosed during the hospitalization as having dementia and is discharged to a nursing home, where he dies 2 months later.

- *Could the compliance and follow-up of this dependent, psychiatrically ill individual have been improved by more accessible primary care services?*
- *Would the system have responded better and/or could there have been cost saving if there had been more active interventions before his terminal illness?*
- *Critique the way in which cost influenced his nontreatment.*

MENTAL HEALTH SERVICES

There are very few resources available in most communities for mental health care of older persons. Most communities have community mental health centers, although they serve disproportionately few older persons. The Medicare benefit for outpatient mental health services requires a 50% copayment.

Inpatient care for older persons with severe mental health problems is even more of a problem. Medicare pays only for acute treatment. State mental hospitals are generally understaffed and underfunded and resist taking cognitively impaired patients. In fact, regulations at the federal level now distinguish between "mental illness" and the dementias, regarding the latter as a nonpsychiatric illness. Whatever the manifestation and care need might be, if dementia alone is the cause of the patient's behavior or emotional problems, care will not be forthcoming or reimbursed through mental health services or resources. This contrasts with the policies of many other Western countries where it is recognized that psychiatric expertise and expert mental health services have an important, although limited, place in the overall management of individuals with dementia. Nursing homes are therefore often the only resort for such persons, but entry by persons with mental health disorders has been restricted by a mandatory screening for mental illness given before nursing home placement. A person judged to need active treatment of a mental disorder is not usually allowed to be admitted into most nursing homes.

HOME AND COMMUNITY-BASED CARE

Services for the elderly are complex and overlapping. Older persons often have difficulty understanding how to gain access to community services. Case management helps with this process. A case manager is typically a nurse or a social worker trained to conduct an in-depth assessment of the patient's needs and resources. In an ideal situation the case manager coordinates assessments by several members of an interdisciplinary team. The review includes areas such as ability to perform ADLs (e.g., need for assistance with meal preparation and dressing), environmental barriers to independent functioning (e.g., second floor apartment), financial resources, mental functioning, and availability of family or friends to provide support. After determining the client's needs, the case manager arranges for the delivery of services from available community sources. Finally, the case manager monitors the services to make sure that they are delivered and to arrange for changes in services if a client's condition changes.

Many older persons also need nonskilled services such as homemaker and home chore services. Homemakers can provide help around the house making beds, preparing meals, and giving general assistance. Home chore services include house cleaning and grocery shopping, for example.

Unfortunately, neither case management nor nonskilled services are covered by Medicare unless the patient qualifies for skilled nursing home care and other criteria are met (Table 6-2). These services are available on a fee-for-service basis in some communities, but patients are rarely able or willing to pay for them. Other sources of funds that are occasionally available for such programs include Medicaid, Older Americans Act funds, or Title XX of the Social Security Act (Social Services Block Grant).

Homemaker and chore aides are supported by Medicaid programs in general, but case management services are not. However, many states have established Medicaid waiver programs, which allow the utilization of Medicaid funds for additional services to a defined target population. Some states also spend general revenues to support these services.

Patients' access to such services depends, to a large extent, on where they live. In some communities, area agencies on aging have contracted for delivery of these services to targeted high-risk groups. In other locations, these services are available under the provisions of a Medicaid waiver or other demonstration program. Unfortunately, limited funding, limited geographic availability, and lack of knowledge about these programs result in many older persons going without such services.

Another set of available community programs are nutritional support services. The largest support for these programs comes from the Older Americans Act (OAA), which in 1992 provided $246.2 million for congregate meals and $122.6 million for home-delivered meals. Home-delivered meals are provided to homebound elderly in many communities, and congregate meal programs, often in churches or senior centers, provide both meals and social interaction. Approximately 10% of older persons living alone receive home-delivered meals and another 10% participate in congregate meal programs.

Respite refers to care given to provide relief to family or other caregivers. Respite services can be provided in the home for a few hours or a few days, in a community setting such as an adult day-care center, or in an institutional setting such as a hospital or a nursing home.

Adult day care is provided in community settings

where older persons go for daytime hours and receive a range of social and/or health services. Most often adult day care is used by persons living with family members who need a break from the demands of constant care. However, people living alone may also benefit from the social interaction and health services available in these settings. Most adult day care is funded by out-of-pocket payments by the older people or their family members. Limited OAA or Title XX funds are available, and Medicaid may support this care in states with waiver programs.

To be able to use adult day care, participate in congregate meals, or visit their physician, patients often need to use special transportation services. In some cases, service providers have special vans and provide transportation. In other cases, senior transportation services provide access to a range of services and locations. Approximately 5% of older persons use specialized transportation services.

Most recent initiatives in the area of long-term care services are aimed at improving the integration among and access to a complete continuum of services. Social HMO demonstration programs in four cities are attempting to integrate acute and long-term care services. In addition, several hospital systems active on this front have formed the National Chronic Care Consortium to encourage further development. However, different funding sources and requirements for health and social services create substantial barriers to effective integration.

In summary, the major funding sources for case management and community-based services are the Older Americans Act funds, Title XX of the Social Security Act (Block Grants), and Medicaid waivers. Table 6-1 shows a summary of the services supported by each of the five major federal programs that help the elderly with health and long-term care needs.

THE FUTURE

There are significant problems with the current patchwork system of financing health care for the elderly in the United States. Services funded by more than one program, eligibility restrictions, and copayments and deductibles result in a system almost impossible to use effectively.

The demographic and health parameters of the elderly population have provoked and will continue to engender major public policy debates because older persons have a relatively high need for medical care services and often use public funds as payment. This situation creates a number of policy issues ranging from limits on benefits included in public programs to the relative proportion of health care costs of older individuals that should be paid by the older persons themselves rather than by those still employed.[6]

The old are medically needy, and public money pays for much of their care; so geriatric medicine is a matter of public policy, and vulnerable to political change.

Financing health care for the elderly will increase as a societal concern. A problem looming large with the aging of the baby-boom generation is a decrease in the ratio of persons 18 to 65 years (i.e., those of working age) to those over 65 years (presumed to be retirees) from 3:1 in 1987 to 2:1 in 2040. The impact of this change will be exacerbated by the trends toward earlier retirement, smaller families, and middle-aged caregivers entering the work place. These changes and others will have a profound impact on our ability to maintain the current system of Social Security and health benefits financing for the elderly. Any discussion of financing care for older individuals must be placed in the context of the continued increase in total health care expenditures, the substantial likelihood of recessions in the future, and the expanding federal debt.[7]

Demographics alone suggest a need to focus on better ways to manage chronic illness and on prevention and management of disability. Some of this effort must be directed at basic research that might lead to the prevention of chronic, dependency-producing conditions such as Alzheimer's disease or osteoporosis. In addition, efforts will have to be directed toward developing and financing a health care system that is more effective in managing chronic illness by providing comprehensive, continuing primary and community-based care (as has been achieved in other countries).[8]

Innovations in and expansion of in-home and community-based services must be developed at an accelerated rate to have a substantial impact. Devices such as motorized wheelchairs, self-actuated emergency alarms, environmental control systems, and services such as chore aides, friendly visitors, and respite care have already made significant contributions to chronic illness care.

Demonstration projects involving case assessment and management, whether with a medical, nursing, social, or combined focus or combined with financing mechanisms (as with the channeling or the social HMO projects) have provided some promise in the area of service coordination. However, no single approach has emerged as superior when costs are considered.

Linkage of housing for older persons with provision of chronic home care services is one strategy to address long-term care services. Some approaches, such as lifecare at home or nursing home without walls, have served individuals with substantial deficits in function, offering a relatively broad range of coordinated services. Others, such as life-care communities or continuing care retirement communities (CCRCs), have linked older person–oriented housing facilities with a gradation of home care and, in some cases, nursing home services. Such settings are expensive: most CCRCs require an entry fee over $100,000 plus a monthly payment covering some, but often not all, long-term care services. Relatively high costs, reluctance of many older persons to move from their family home, and financial problems experienced by some of the early facilities are all of concern.

The 1983 Social Security law reforms have increased the stability of Medicare financing, but the current level of income of the Hospital Trust Fund (which is the source of Part A Medicare payments) is insufficient to prevent a large deficit just after the year 2005. The shortfall could reach nearly $1 trillion by the year 2020, just when the baby-boom generation will be generating a high demand for medical care services.

Medicare provides less than 2% of the funding for nursing home care. Unless major changes occur in the system, the burden of increased nursing home care funding will continue to fall on Medicaid and individuals in that segment of the older population with the highest risk of nursing home placement and the least ability to pay (women over 85 years old). In recent years the proportion of long-term care expenses paid by Medicaid has steadily increased. Given the large numbers of poor people under 65 years with neither health insurance nor Medicaid coverage, the pressures on Medicaid will be substantial. As a result, concerns about the quality, financing, and organization of long-term care in our society will continue.[9]

A variety of factors have led to current efforts to move more Medicare and Medicaid recipients into managed care plans. Clearly, the most compelling of these factors is the apparent success of HMOs in reducing employer health care costs, as contrasted with repeated failures to control costs in the Medicare and Medicaid programs. Also, the proportion of new Medicare enrollees who have received their prior health care in HMO settings is steadily increasing. In addition to pressure from federal and state governments, the saturation of employer-based markets with managed care is causing HMOs to see the Medicare and Medicaid markets as more attractive.

This trend will have a profound effect on the care of older persons in the next decade, but a large number of critical policy issues remain unclear, including the fundamental question of whether HMOs in their current mode of practice actually do reduce costs of care in older persons. In the past, most apparent cost savings have been due to selection of a relatively low risk population by the HMOs. On the positive side, the use of capitation as a reimbursement mechanism creates a substantial opportunity for expanding the use of comprehensive geriatric assessment and case management. It also provides opportunities for a creative blending of acute, subacute and long-term care if, for example, an HMO is able to create a program for persons with dual Medicare and Medicaid eligibility. In the final analysis, whether lower payments to providers, better case management, or other elements of managed care will really enable Medicare and Medicaid to maintain quality, while substantially decreasing the long-term rate of increase in expenditures, could truly be termed the "trillion dollar" question.

To ensure access to a reasonable level of health care for all persons, including the old, additional methods of organizing and financing that care must be developed and must address critical issues, including demographic-driven increases in demand, rising prices for health care, increasing but highly skewed relative wealth in the older population, and decreasing ratio of workers to the over-65-year-old population. Recent proposals (in addition to national health insurance) include increases in the age at which persons become eligible for Social Security and Medicare, indexing Medicare premiums to income, further reductions in Medicare reimbursement to hospitals and physicians, the use of the equity in homes of older people (currently estimated at over $500 billion) to pay for insurance or care, medical savings accounts (medical IRAs), and private long-term care insurance.

Given the ever-increasing proportion of the gross national product going for medical care of older persons, our failure to find an equitable solution could result in intensification of our current implicit rationing of medical care by income or by type of care (acute vs. long-term care). It is ironic that our dilemma in providing and financing health care to older persons is largely a result of the success of health care, especially public health, in increasing life expectancy. The challenge to the health care system, and indeed to our whole society, is to adapt successfully to this new reality.

POSTTEST

1. Which one of the following statements concerning health care expenses is false?
   a. Of the $150 billion spent on health services in 1989 on persons over 65 years, the largest proportion was on hospital care.
   b. Medicare Part B is an optional insurance to cover excess hospital care.
   c. Medigap policies are private insurances to pay Medicare copayments and deductibles.
   d. Twenty percent of the payment for health services in this country in 1989 was spent on nursing home care.

2. Which one of the following statements concerning Medicaid is false?
   a. Medicaid covers Medicare deductibles and copayments.
   b. Most states have higher income limits for Medicaid eligibility than are federally determined.
   c. Federal rules for Medicaid require states to ensure that it covers physical therapy when medically indicated.
   d. Not all states allow the medically needy (in whom medical expenses have dropped their income below Medicaid eligibility requirement lines) to receive Medicaid.

3. Which set of figures expresses the federal Medicaid eligibility levels for 1994?
   a. Income $857 per month per individual, $1243 per month per couple
   b. Income $634 per month per individual, $841 per month per couple
   c. Income $450 per month per individual, $648 per month per couple

4. Which one of the following statements is false concerning Medicare?
   a. Medicare Part B covers 80% of the Medicare-approved physician charge.
   b. Medicare Part B covers 70% of approved mental health services.
   c. Accepting assignment means that the physician accepts Medicare's approved amount as full payment.
   d. Medicare pays for less than 3% of nursing home costs.

5. Which one of the following sets of figures correctly describes the 1994 annual deductible and copayments due from patients for hospital care in patients fully eligible for Medicare?
   a. Annual deductible $696, copayment $210 a day from day 91
   b. Annual deductible $856, copayment $245 a day from day 61
   c. Annual deductible $756, copayment $174 a day from day 91
   d. Annual deductible $596, copayment $148 a day from day 31
   e. Annual deductible $696, copayment $174 a day from day 61

REFERENCES

1. Short P, Feinleib S, Cunningham P: *Expenditures and sources of payment of persons in nursing and personal care homes,* AHCPR Pub No 94-0032, Rockville, Md, April 1994, Agency for Health Care Policy and Research, Public Health Service.
2. Cohen MA, Kumar N, Wallack SS: New perspectives on the affordability of long-term care insurance and potential market size, *Gerontologist* 33(1), 1993.
3. Consumers Union: *Consumer Reports* 56(6):425-442, 1991.
4. Cohen M et al: Long-term care financing proposals: their costs, benefits, and impact on private insurance, *Research Bulletin,* Washington, DC, Health Insurance Association of America.
5. *Managed care digest,* Long term care edition, Kansas City, 1993, Marion Merrell Dow.
6. Fuchs VL: *The future of health policy,* Cambridge, Mass, 1993, Harvard University Press.
7. Mendelson D, Schwartz W: The effects of aging and population growth on health care costs, *Health Affairs* 12:119-124, 1993.
8. Schneider EL, Guralnik JM: The aging of America: impact on health care costs, *JAMA* 263:2335-2340, 1990.
9. Wiener J, Rivlin A: *Caring for the disabled elderly: who will pay?* Washington, DC, 1988, Brookings Institute.

PRETEST ANSWERS
1. b
2. d
3. c

POSTTEST ANSWERS
1. b
2. c
3. b
4. b
5. e

CHAPTER 7

Minorities

SHARON A. BRANGMAN

OBJECTIVES

On completion of this chapter, the reader will be able to:

1. Understand the significance of the increasing number of minority elders in the United States and their impact on the health care system.

2. Understand the health status of minority elders and factors that contribute to their health.

3. Better appreciate the influences race, culture, and ethnicity have on health status.

4. Appreciate the diversity that exists within each minority group and the challenges of providing culturally sensitive care.

5. Be familiar with the correct methods of incorporating an interpreter into the clinical setting.

Select the single best answer:

1. Which of the following statements is false?
   a. The number of minority elders is increasing rapidly, and this growth is expected to continue into the next century.
   b. Minority elders, in general, are a homogenous group with similar health concerns and needs.
   c. Minority elders are similar to white elders in that they develop the same chronic diseases.
   d. Illiteracy and poor language skills can be considered barriers to receiving good health care.

2. All of the following may be considered barriers to accessing health care except:
   a. Lack of health insurance
   b. Low personal income
   c. Services located outside of patient's neighborhood
   d. Fluency in English

3. Which one of the following statements is true?
   a. Older African-American women do not usually live longer than men.
   b. Large, extended American Indian families eliminate the need for nursing home placement for their elders.
   c. Most minority elders develop the same diseases as older whites, but at younger ages.
   d. The idiomatic use of Spanish by Mexicans is identical to that used by Puerto Ricans.

▼ BESSIE MAE JOHNSON (Part I)

Mary, a temporary clerical worker in your office, comes to you to discuss her aunt, Bessie Mae Johnson, because of concern about her health care. Mrs. Johnson is a 73-year-old African-American woman and a diabetic with a history of hypertension, obesity, and osteoarthritis. Yesterday she told Mary that she was giving up going to her doctors, the young physicians in training who staff the public health clinic where she obtains her primary care. She says she feels sick and has become tired of "all those young doctors practicing" on her; they don't seem to know what they are doing. She is tired of sitting in the waiting room for hours before she can see someone, and the doctors change all the time. All of them call her "Bessie" and talk to her in a loud voice using fancy words. They told her to change her diet, but all the foods are expensive and none of them are things that she likes. She has said that she is not going to live forever and that God will call her when He is ready.

STUDY QUESTIONS

- *What barriers can you already see to effective health care for Mrs. Johnson?*
- *What could be done to improve her management and her compliance?*
- *Are these problems characteristic of issues facing minority elders in America today?*

▼ NHAN QUOC HO (Part I)

Mr. Ho, an 80-year-old Laotian man who has been in the United States for 15 years, is referred to your office by Adult Protective Services. Neighbors had become concerned because of his reclusiveness and Mrs. Ho's frightened demeanor. Mrs.

Ho is 45 years old, and she and her husband live with their 10-year-old son in a small apartment. Both are illiterate and speak only Hmong and a little French, but no English. Mr. Ho has had no regular medical care. He is neglecting himself and is threatening his wife, who, he has said to the agency worker, is trying to poison him so that she can marry a younger man. As a result, he will not eat anything that she prepares for him.

STUDY QUESTIONS

- *How can the language barriers be overcome to allow assessment of this man's mental status?*
- *Does the stigma of "mental illness" mean more in minority cultures?*
- *What problems will arise, should institutional care become required?*

Traditionally, minority elders in America have included African-American, Latino, Asian/Pacific Island American, and American Indian/Alaska Natives. There are also other ethnic groups not traditionally included in the definition of minority elders. These elders represent a large, diverse group of Americans that cannot be narrowly defined. The challenge in understanding older minority group members is to understand the group in context, while avoiding stereotypes and appreciating individual similarities and differences.

Within any one minority group there is considerable variation. African-American elders may live in rural areas of the South or urban areas in the North and have a variety of backgrounds and experiences. American Indians represent many tribes, languages, and traditions that define their attitudes on aging and health. Latinos may have origins in countries as distinct as Mexico, Cuba, or Guatemala and speak Spanish in varied forms. Asians may be recent immigrants or the third generation in the United States.

Although there has been an increase in data on minority aging in recent years, there is still much that needs to be examined. Much of the data on minority elders offers cohort comparisons to whites. This type of comparison can limit data interpretation, since it obscures intragroup characteristics. Similarly, data that compare "whites" to "nonwhites" are difficult to examine, since these designations obscure the individual characteristics of specific groups. At this time, we have little information on how health status, health perception, or health-seeking behavior may be influenced by such factors as socioeconomic status, gender, culture, and race.

DEMOGRAPHICS

The number of minority elders is increasing at an even faster rate than the rest of the elderly population, and this increase is projected to continue well into the next century (Figs. 7-1 and 7-2). According to census data, the number of elderly whites should increase by 16% by the year 2001 and 45% by 2015. African-American elders, in contrast, should increase by 21% by 2001, and 72% by 2015. As with white elders, minority women generally live longer than men.[1]

> By 2030, one in four elders will be a minority.

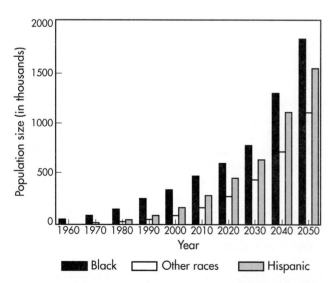

FIG. 7-1   Growth in minority population 85 years and older. (Data from Current Population Reports Series P-25, No 1018, table 4, 1989; No 995, table 2, 1986; and Angel JL and Hogan DP: The demography of minority aging populations. In *Minority elders: longevity, economics, and health,* Washington, DC, 1991, Gerontological Society of America.)

Poverty

Minority elders are more likely to be living in poverty than older whites. In urban areas, 32% of older African-Americans live in poverty compared with 11% of white elders; the poverty rates are similar for Latino, American Indian, and Asian/Pacific Island elders (Tables 7-1 and 7-2). Minority elders are more likely than white elders to work past traditional retirement age. Lifetime employment histories are those of low-paying, menial jobs with little or no pension or other benefits. Minority elders are more likely to depend on income derived from Social Security and supplemental security income rather than on dividends from stocks or other investments. Many lack private insurance and therefore have higher out of pocket expenses for medical care than white elders.

Education

White elders are more likely to have completed high school than similar minority elders. According to 1980 census data, only 17% of African-American elders completed high school compared with 41% of whites. Many African-American elders had no formal education or were educated in segregated schools. Among Latinos, older Cubans are more likely to have completed high school than older Mexicans. As many as half of older Latinos

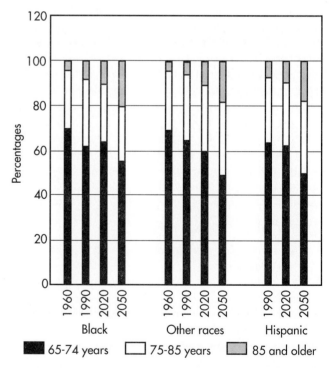

FIG. 7-2   Increasing percentage of elders by racial group. (Data from Current Population Reports Series P-25, No 519, 1974; No 917, 1982; No 995, 1986; No 1018, 1989; No 1045, 1990; and Angel JL and Hogan DP: The demography of minority aging populations. In *Minority elders: longevity, economics, and health,* Washington, DC, 1991, Gerontological Society of America.)

may be functionally illiterate in both English and Spanish.

As a group, minority elders are poorer and less educated than their white counterparts, and they are likely to have spent their adult lives working in low-skilled, low-paying jobs. Most have not achieved the same standard of living as similar elderly whites. All of these factors have a significant role in increasing the risk for many indicators of poor health, including reduced life expectancy, multiple chronic diseases, functional impairment, and reduced access to high-quality health care.

Life Expectancy

The average life expectancy for minority elders, with the exception of Asians, is lower than that of white elders (Table 7-3). Asians have the longest life expectancy of all groups, followed by whites, Latinos, African-Americans, and American Indians. There are many explanations for this disparity. Double jeopardy, or the cumulative negative effects of race and age, has been offered as one explanation; however, this does not fully account for the differences. It is likely that a variety of factors, including poorer health over a lifetime, limited access to health services, and lower socioeconomic status, are also critical. Research is needed to differentiate the factors related to race from those associated with socioeconomics.

> *Minority elders are in general poorer and less educated, and, except for Asians, their life expectancy is reduced.*

The racial mortality crossover effect occurs when an older minority group member reaches an age at which his or her remaining years of life are longer than those of similar whites. For example, this crossover occurs approximately at age 75 for African-Americans, but no crossover is observed for Chinese or Japanese elders. Latinos, in some cases, show a much smaller crossover effect, and American Indians demonstrate a crossover at about age 55. This crossover effect suggests that the aging process might occur at different rates for some minority group members. Minority elders who have survived to advanced ages may be more hardy or fit than others. However, they often still have multiple chronic illnesses and disabilities. This variation in life expectancy suggests that health service needs, particularly long-term care, will remain prominent issues for minority elders, even at advanced ages. More research is needed to better understand why life expectancies vary by age among various populations.

Health Status

Race and ethnicity are important determinants of health and disease, yet most of the statistical data on older Americans do not evaluate these variables as they relate to age, socioeconomic status, or social and behavioral determinants of health. Despite this lack of information on specific factors that determine health status, it is clear that the health of minority elders lags far behind that of whites. There has been a general improvement in the health status of seniors in this country that minority elders do not enjoy. In general, minorities have poorer health at all ages. Impaired health and disability during midlife directly affect health in late life. More information is needed so that effective health promotion and disease prevention programs can be developed, especially those that are sensitive to the cultural needs of these elders.

Data on possible genetic determinants of health and disease are likewise limited, and no conclusions can be drawn at this time. Health is directly influenced by poverty, educational level, work history, and other socioeconomic factors. It is possible that these factors have a

Table 7-1 Percent of Aged Persons in Poverty, 1990

	Percent
All races	12.2
Whites	10.1
African-American	33.8
Latino origin*	22.5
White, not of Latino origin†	9.6
Mexican†	23.1
Puerto Rican	31.7
Asian or Pacific Islander	12.1

From US Bureau of the Census, published and unpublished data.
*Latino may be of any race.
†Unpublished Census Bureau data courtesy of Eleanor F. Baugher.

Table 7-2 Percent of All Persons 65 or More Years Old and Below the Poverty Level

	African-American	Latino*	White
1985	31.5	23.9	11.0
1991	33.8	20.8	10.3

From US Bureau of the Census: *Statistical abstract of the United States,* 1993.
*Latino may be of any race.

Table 7-3 Life Expectancy at Birth in 1990 (yr)

	African-American		White		All Races*
	Male	Female	Male	Female	Both Sexes
At birth in 1990	64.5	73.6	72.7	79.4	75.4

Modified from Current Population Reports, Series P-20, No 444, Table 1, 1990, and Horner LL, ed: *Black Americans: a statistical sourcebook,* Palo Alto, Calif, 1994, Information Publications.
*All races includes other races not shown separately.

greater role in determining health or life expectancy than race.[2]

Minority elders develop the same diseases as older whites; however, the diseases often begin at earlier ages and result in a greater degree of disability and functional impairment for a greater portion of life. Functional status is an important means of assessing overall health and well being. The ability of an individual to complete daily living tasks and remain independent in the community setting is expressed as functional status. Elders with impaired functional status are at higher risk for dependency and institutionalization. Despite this, minority elders have lower rates of admission to long-term care facilities than white elders.

Acculturation, or the acquisition of the norms and values of the majority society, can influence many aspects of the health status of a minority group member. Thus there may be differences in the rates of cancer or heart disease between foreign and native-born Chinese elders. The health status of an American Indian who resides in a large city may be very different from one living on a reservation. These variations within a given group emphasize the importance of appreciating individual differences while simultaneously gaining an understanding of the larger group.

Current data indicate higher rates of several diseases, including diabetes, hypertension, cancer, and cerebrovascular disease, in minority elders when compared with majority elders. African-American, Latino, and American Indian elders have significantly higher rates of diabetes than older white Americans. Japanese elders have higher rates of diabetes compared with elderly whites, and these rates vary significantly between Japanese elders born in the United States and those born in Japan.

There is a considerable stigma associated with mental illness in many cultures, including the minority groups discussed in this chapter. Most elders are reluctant to discuss mental illness or related symptoms, and there is a low utilization rate of mental health services. Depression is the most common mental illness in minority elders and is underdiagnosed and undertreated as it is in all elderly patients. Since it is more acceptable to discuss somatic symptoms, minority elders may present with multiple somatic complaints when the actual problem is psychiatric in nature. Further, the diagnosis of depression or other psychiatric illnesses may be complicated by the lack of normative standards for minority elders; objective tests frequently have inherent cultural biases.

Barriers to Care

Even though current data suggest that minority elders have poorer health and more disabilities than white elders, many are not able to access appropriate health care services. Health care may be sought only at late stages of disease or disability when a successful outcome is much less likely to be achieved. Both physical and psychological barriers affect the manner in which minority elders access care.

The financial burden of health care, large out of pocket expenses, and lack of affordable services or health insurance are barriers to accessing care for low-income minority elders. Language barriers exist for those who do not speak English. Services may not be bilingual or bicultural, thus increasing communication difficulties. Services may be located outside of a minority community, limiting access for those without transportation.

Patients and families may perceive services to be culturally incompatible with their needs. They may have encountered discrimination in the past or be unable to wade through the bureaucracy that is often required to secure care. Immigrants may fear jeopardizing their immigration status or being deported when they seek care. Patients and families may not understand eligibility requirements for programs or services. Ineffective outreach programs developed by health agencies may lack the scope or focus to reach minority communities, limiting awareness of programs.

> *Culture, finances, and language contribute to the low use of long-term care services by minority elders.*

Compared with the rate of use for elderly whites, the rate of long-term care use is significantly lower for minority elders. This may be due to cost, discrimination, personal choice, or social and cultural differences.[3] The location of long-term care facilities outside of minority communities may also be a factor. The relative importance of these factors varies with each minority group. Cost and discrimination were considered the primary barriers to African-Americans. Mexican-American elders indicated discrimination, cost, language, and cultural differences, while American Indians cited social and cultural factors as barriers. Asian Americans and Pacific Islanders listed language, social, and cultural differences that isolated them from other residents and staff.[4]

Some providers, aware of the strong sense of family responsibility in many minority communities, may feel that minority elders are best cared for by their own families. They may then neglect to make appropriate referrals to services such as home care, long-term care, or rehabilitation for their minority patients.

With an understanding of these barriers, providers and agencies must begin to address the issues that keep minority elders from the care that is available. Programs and services must be structured to be affordable, conveniently located, and culturally sensitive to the needs of those they serve.

▼ BESSIE MAE JOHNSON (Part II)

Mrs. Johnson says that her medications make her feel sick and don't seem to bring her blood pressure down. She has told her niece that she stopped taking them after her last visit. She is planning to go back to drinking her garlic tea and lemon juice for her blood pressure and just take it easy for a while. She feels this should be enough to bring her pressure down. She says that there is no way she is going to eat the foods the dietician suggested to lose weight, especially since fish costs $7.99 per pound in her neighborhood store. She will just watch her sweets and cut back on rich foods. Mrs. Johnson's young doctor warned her on the last visit that she would have to be switched to insulin injections if her glucose remained elevated. She is terrified of needles and can't imagine injecting herself.

Mrs. Johnson's husband has been dead for 23 years. She has eight children, but her niece Mary usually takes her to her appointments. Mary has been helping her regularly, especially since the arthritis in her knees made it difficult for her to walk. It is getting harder for Mrs. Johnson to do things around her apartment like get in and out of the tub, make the bed, and stand at the stove to cook. She still does occasional domestic work for which she is paid in cash but she has no pension and is receiving Medicaid, Medicare, and food stamps.

Her physicians are medical residents doing a rotation in ambulatory care. She has to take two buses to get to the appointments. She sometimes sees the same physician more than once but usually has a new physician every few months. Most of the resident physicians are at least 35 years younger than Mrs. Johnson and have had little substantive exposure to someone with her background. Each resident has medical clinic once a week for 4 hours, with nine patients scheduled each session. It is not unusual for her physician to get paged during clinic sessions about new admissions or inpatient consults, which distracts from the task at hand. On average, each clinic visit takes her more than 4 hours.

She has been gaining several pounds each visit, and her blood pressure and glucose are never under control. She has recently begun having low back pain. On the last visit, she was put on a strict 1500 calorie diet in an effort to encourage weight loss and better glucose control. She was sent to a dietician in the clinic who gave her a list of foods describing what she was allowed to eat and what she should avoid. The list of acceptable foods included many that she does not usually eat. Specifically, she was instructed to eat fresh fish at least three times a week, along with a variety of raw fruits and vegetables. She was to avoid fried foods, pork, and beef. The dietician gave Mrs. Johnson a small scale to weigh her food portions to help measure exactly how much she should eat.

A previous medical resident gave Mrs. Johnson several pamphlets on the etiology and management of essential hypertension and diabetes. Both pamphlets were in small print and written in a style that she could not understand, but she was too embarrassed to tell the doctor.

Mrs. Johnson's medications include metoprolol tartrate (Lopressor), hydrochlorothiazide, potassium, glyburide (DiaBeta), and ibuprofen (Motrin). She recently has been taking Anacin and Doan's Pills for her back pain, but her physician never asked, and she did not volunteer this information.

STUDY QUESTIONS

- What is most crucial to be done medically to improve Mrs. Johnson's health care?
- What are the barriers to her receiving good care and complying with the recommended management?
- What could be done to improve her overall situation and the risks to her future health?

AFRICAN-AMERICAN ELDERS

African-American elders are a heterogeneous group representing a vast array of histories and experiences. According to 1980 census data, almost one third of older African-Americans live in New York, Texas, Georgia, North Carolina, and California.[5] The majority live in urban areas of large cities. Like other minority group members, they were more likely to receive substandard health care in their younger years, directly impacting their current health status.

Older African-Americans develop the same diseases as their white counterparts, including cardiovascular disease, cerebrovascular disease, and cancer. However, diagnosis is often made at advanced stages of disease when there is more disability and functional impairment.

> *Survival rates for breast cancer in women and for prostate, lung, and pancreas cancer in men are reduced in African-Americans.*

African-American men die twice as often from strokes as other men. They are more likely to develop carcinomas of the prostate, lung, and pancreas and have lower rates of survival. African-American women are less likely to develop breast cancer than white women but have more aggressive disease with lower survival rates.[6] However, when African-Americans are compared with whites of similar socioeconomic backgrounds, the differences in cancer incidence disappear.[6]

> *Hip fracture morbidity, stroke mortality (doubled in men), and prevalence of diabetes (three times as common) are all increased in African-Americans.*

Hip fracture as a result of osteoporosis is less common in African-Americans, but morbidity is higher. After a hip fracture, African-Americans are more likely to have longer hospital stays, with discharge back to the community rather than to a rehabilitation facility.[7] Diabetes is three times more common in African-Americans than whites. Older African-American females have a higher risk for diabetes, partly related to higher rates of obesity.

STUDY QUESTIONS

- *What are the special health risks for Mrs. Johnson?*
- *If she can be persuaded to continue medical care, what specific issues should be focused upon in health maintenance plans?*

LATINO ELDERS

Latinos are the second largest minority group in the United States. The largest subgroup of Latinos are Mexican-American, followed by Cuban-Americans. Other subgroups include Puerto Ricans and South and Central Americans (Table 7-4). Each subgroup has a distinct and varied experience in the United States, along with diverse cultural backgrounds, socioeconomic status, educational level, and use of language. Latinos, as a group, are younger, with elders representing only 5% of the total Latino population. Cuban-Americans, however, are an exception with approximately 15% over the age of 65. The number of Latino elders will have increased significantly by the year 2000, and in fact this group is the fastest growing segment of all older Americans.

Latinos can be of any race, yet in much of the available data they are grouped together with no distinction made between race or ethnicity. This has complicated the data interpretation, making it difficult to make comparisons or draw conclusions about the health status of Latino elders.

Major health concerns include diabetes, cardiovascular disease, cerebrovascular disease, and cancer. Older migrants from Mexico, Puerto Rico, and Cuba have relatively lower death rates from heart disease and cancer. This may be partly related to self-selection with stronger, healthier elders more likely to immigrate.

Mexican-Americans and Puerto Ricans have a significantly higher prevalence of diabetes compared with whites. Cuban-Americans, however, have a lower prevalence of diabetes, only slightly higher than whites.[8] Spanish-surname men and women have higher morbidity and mortality from cerebrovascular disease at younger ages than similar whites. Mexican-born elders have the highest rates of mortality from cerebrovascular disease in comparison with Puerto Ricans or Cubans.

There is little data on cancer rates and mortality in older Latinos. In general, Mexican-Americans have cancer rates below the national average, with the exception of Mexican-born women, who have higher rates of cervical cancer. Within the Latino subgroups, Cuban-Americans have higher cancer rates than Puerto Ricans or Mexican-Americans. Immigrant women with Spanish surnames in Los Angeles County have lower incidence rates for breast cancer than non-Latino whites but are more likely to have high numbers of positive axillary nodes at the time of treatment.[8,9]

The rate of dysphoria and depression in one study of older Latinos in Los Angeles County was 26% and correlated with medical disability. Affective disorders were also associated with certain factors such as being female, the inability to speak English, low income, and loneliness, even if not living alone.[8,10] The diagnosis and management of depression may be complicated by language limitations of both patient and provider.

AMERICAN INDIAN AND ALASKA NATIVE ELDERLY

There are over 400 federally recognized tribal groups representing more than 250 different languages designated as American Indian in the United States.[11] Elderly American Indians are concentrated on reservations in the western part of the country, many of which are located in isolated rural areas.

As with the other groups discussed, there is great diversity among American Indians and Alaska Natives, making generalizations difficult. The Indian Health Service (IHS) is the primary provider of care to those Indians who are members of federally recognized tribes and living on reservations. IHS services are generally not available to Indians living in urban areas. Historically, the focus of the IHS has been on acute care issues with particular attention given to child and family services. Geriatric issues have not been a primary focus partly because few Indians lived to old age. Now, with the number of older American Indians rapidly increasing, policy changes will be required to incorporate the needs of older Indians into health planning and policy.

Although life expectancy is improving for American Indians, it is still significantly lower than that of elderly whites. Mortality rates are significantly higher for Indians below the age of 65, but there is lower mortality after age 65. Overall, the number of Indians over the age

Table 7-4   Latino Elderly Population by Nation of Origin, 1989

	Percent
Mexican American	47.6
Cuban American	18.1
Other Hispanic	15.0
Puerto Rican	10.9
Central/South American	8.4

Modified from *Current Population Reports,* Series P-20, No 444, Table 1, 1990, and *Minority elders: longevity, economics, and health,* Washington, DC, 1991, The Gerontological Society of America.

of 65 is small when compared with whites. Disabilities and functional impairment begin at younger ages for Indians, suggesting that chronologically they may be considered "old" at ages as young as 45.[12]

Of all U.S. elders, American Indians have the lowest socioeconomic status: more than one third live in poverty.

Data are limited on health status, but American Indian elders have the lowest socioeconomic status of all elders in this country. This has a direct impact on health status and utilization of services. More than a third live below the poverty level compared with only 10% for whites. As with other elders, leading causes of mortality include heart disease, cancer, and cerebrovascular disease, but these illnesses occur at lower rates in Indians than in other races.[13] Diabetes and diabetes-related disorders are significant causes of morbidity and mortality in Indians of all ages. Non–insulin-dependent diabetes is approximately 10 times more common in Indians than in whites.[14] Other major health concerns are arthritis, tuberculosis, malnutrition, injuries related to accidents, hearing and visual impairment, and alcohol abuse and its complications.

Access to adequate health care is affected by low income, limited availability of IHS centers, and lack of transportation for those living in isolated rural areas. Many older American Indians prefer traditional medical treatments and healers and are suspicious of American health care and practices.

▼ *NHAN QUOC HO (Part II)*

Mr. Ho stays in his room with the door locked all day and comes out only at night to eat a light meal he prepares. He sleeps with a large knife and threatens to use it if his wife disturbs him. He has had several episodes of incontinence of both bowel and bladder, and he no longer bathes. He does not change his clothes regularly and refuses to let his wife assist him with any activities of daily living. He is having more difficulty walking and is at high risk of falling. The agency worker relates that Mr. Ho's concerns have no truthful basis and that his wife is very supportive and concerned; the worker suspects dementia and asks you to evaluate.

STUDY QUESTIONS

- *What are the primary issues in Mr. Ho's care?*
- *How will you overcome the language barriers effectively?*
- *How would you organize the evaluation of his potential dementia?*
- *How can health care be organized for this couple?*

ASIAN AND PACIFIC ISLAND AMERICAN ELDERS

Asian Americans and Pacific Islanders represent more than 20 different ethnic groups and over 30 languages, with origins in East Asia, Southeast Asia, the Indian subcontinent, Hawaii, Polynesia, Melanesia, and Micronesia. Asian Americans and Pacific Islanders demonstrate vast diversity of ancestry, culture, and language, with only vague geographic similarities.[15,16] As with other minority groups, data on the health status of Asian Americans and Pacific Islanders have been grouped together, making it difficult to evaluate the health status of specific ethnic groups. The Chinese, Filipinos, and Japanese represent more than 75% of all older Asians (Table 7-5).

About 65% of the Asian and Pacific Island American population are refugees or immigrants, with a wide variety of patterns of immigration to the United States. Typical immigration patterns have included younger Asians coming to the United States, leaving older family members in their native countries. Consequently, as a group, Asians are younger, with elders representing only 6% of the total Asian and Pacific Island American population, and less than 1% of all elders in this country.[15]

Rates of morbidity and mortality are different for each Asian subgroup. The life expectancy for elderly Chinese, Japanese, and Filipinos is higher than the life expectancy for older whites. Differences in rates of disease may vary between American-born and foreign-born elders. The prevalence of coronary heart disease in China and Hong Kong is significantly lower than in the United States. As Chinese Americans become Westernized, their rates of heart disease increase. Older Chinese have a higher incidence of carcinomas of the liver, pancreas, and esophagus. Japanese Americans have a higher prevalence of diabetes and impaired glucose tolerance than both the native population in Japan and whites in the United States.[17]

Asian heritage is considered a risk factor for osteoporosis. Both Japanese and Chinese elders are at higher risk for osteoporosis than whites. This may be due to lower bone density, as well as other contributing factors such

Table 7-5   Asian Elderly Population by Nation of Origin, 1980

	Percent
Filipino	26.7
Chinese	26.6
Japanese	24.7
Asian Indian	14.6
Korean	4.2
Vietnamese	2.2
Other Asian	1.0

From US Bureau of the Census, PC-80, Vol I, 1988.

as body size, physical activity, or dietary habits.[16,18] Major health issues for elderly Southeast Asians are related to infectious diseases, malnutrition, and depression.[16] Despite a high prevalence of depression, cultural stigmas may reduce the use of mental health services. Pacific Islanders have high rates of obesity and are at high risk for hypertension, heart disease, and diabetes.

APPROACH TO THE PATIENT: ESTABLISHING CULTURALLY SENSITIVE CARE

Many factors shape an individual's health beliefs, response to illness, and health-seeking behaviors. These characteristics are determined in part by race, cultural background, and economic status. When these differences are contrary to the model taught in medical schools, conflicts can arise. Illnesses may not be brought to medical attention until advanced stages, or care may be sought only on an urgent basis. Health care may be delayed because of perceived poor or culturally insensitive care, financial limitations, or lack of transportation.

An open physician-patient relationship is crucial to providing and receiving high-quality care. Poor communication by both the patient and physician is damaging. What the physician may perceive as indifference, or lack of concern, may be a sign of respect for authority. For example, an American Indian elder would avoid direct eye contact when speaking to an authority figure, such as a physician; many Americans ordinarily interpret lack of eye contact as a sign of dishonesty or rudeness. Unawareness of this and other cultural nuances might compromise care.

Generalizations regarding establishing a relationship with the older minority patient are inappropriate. A good relationship begins with genuine concern. An understanding of the patient's cultural system is vital, since each will have unique values from his or her heritage and beliefs. Stereotypes must be avoided, and care individualized.

In general, establishing a successful relationship with any elderly patient requires time and effort. More time must be spent listening and allowing the patient to provide information in his or her own way. This can be difficult with heavy patient loads and busy schedules. Such relationships develop over months or years; instant rapport should not be anticipated.

Many clinical training programs encourage a degree of distance with patients in order to minimize emotional involvement and maintain objectivity. However, health professionals willing to more informally discuss themselves outside of their medical role will thereby foster honesty and openness and set the tone for an open relationship, overcoming inadvertent cultural errors.

Be respectful and open with patients from different cultures. Be somewhat informal; step outside the medical role, and overcome inevitable, inadvertent cultural errors.

Minority elders must be addressed respectfully, using appropriate titles and names. Clinicians should learn to pronounce names correctly. It is often considered disrespectful to address an elder by the first name; this should be avoided unless the patient directs otherwise. Clinicians should respect their patients' values and beliefs and avoid the imposition of personal values. Illnesses and treatments should be explained using simple, nonmedical terms, avoiding medical terms and jargon. In addition, clinicians should ask for explanations of words or terms the patient uses that are unfamiliar. Pamphlets and other patient education materials that have become standard methods of medical communication may not be the best way to inform a minority elder about an illness, given the low rates of literacy many have attained.

It should not be assumed that a minority elder has no level of knowledge or understanding about an illness or has not sought other means of treatment or care. Nonjudgmental inquiries into the use of traditional healers or home or folk remedies should be made and incorporated into care plans where appropriate. Some professionals wisely incorporate traditional practices into their medical care.

Direct eye contact or staring may be considered rude or overly familiar with some elders, particularly American Indians. Some older African-Americans may avoid eye contact, especially when answering questions. Other elders may withhold information or avoid the problems that cause most concern if the relationship with the provider is not yet established. American Indians and Latinos may be reluctant to discuss a subject such as cancer or other diseases for fear that simply discussing it will cause it to happen.

Some cultures may have different boundaries for privacy than those in American culture. For example, the Chinese consider discussions of sex, emotion, or personal feelings to be very private and not discussed outside of the immediate family. Physical boundaries may differ, as well. American Indians shake hands using a light touch of the fingers and thumb, not the palm.[14]

CASE DISCUSSION

There are a number of factors directly affecting Mrs. Johnson's health status. Her medical care is provided in a busy, impersonal public hospital where there is limited time to become familiar with her personal characteristics, background, or values. Her physicians are young, busy residents with histories and backgrounds very different from Mrs. Johnson's. Be-

cause of the frequent turnover of staff, there has been inadequate opportunity to develop a strong physician-patient relationship. Mrs. Johnson perceives her physicians as young and disrespectful, and she feels she is there only to enhance their educational experience. Her obesity and diabetes are serious, and referral to a dietician was appropriate. However, the dietician made several assumptions that reduced her likelihood of compliance. The suggested foods were not a usual part of her diet and required her to purchase expensive foods, weigh her portions, and then prepare them in a manner to which she was not accustomed. The diet might have been more successful if time had been taken to review Mrs. Johnson's budget for food and her customary methods of food preparation, and then incorporate these if possible into the recommended diet.

Patient education materials were not presented in a manner that would increase Mrs. Johnson's knowledge. Although more time consuming, a one-on-one discussion using simple terms adapted to Mrs. Johnson's life-style and individual characteristics would have been more effective in encouraging compliance and increasing her understanding.

More frequent, brief (but punctual and efficient) appointments would probably help Mrs. Johnson's understanding. Involving her niece Mary in this process would also be efficient and help compliance. Mrs. Johnson's physicians failed to learn about her personal understanding of her health and home treatments she may have tried; patent medicines and nontraditional treatments often play a large role in self-medication, particularly when prescribed medications result in side effects or are perceived to be ineffective.

▼ BESSIE MAE JOHNSON (Part III)

You naturally offer to take over Mrs. Johnson's care. Recognizing that her situation is symptomatic of the fragmented and episodic care she received from the residents in the local residency program, you communicate your concerns to the director of the program and offer to become involved in teaching them how to overcome cultural and ethnic barriers to care.

▼ NHAN QUOC HO (Part III)

Before Mr. Ho is brought to your office, you make arrangements to have an interpreter accompany him. He refuses to allow his wife to come along. The interpreter turns out to be a 16-year-old boy who has provided interpretation in the past for the Laotian community. He can't stay long because he has to rush back to school to avoid missing an exam.

You begin asking questions with the young boy translating. Mr. Ho's responses are long and animated, but the interpreter gives all replies in monosyllables without elaborating. After 20 minutes the interpreter announces he has to leave for school and the visit ends.

STUDY QUESTION

- What different preparations should have been made to ensure a more successful outcome for this visit?

USE OF TRANSLATORS IN THE MEDICAL SETTING

Frequently, non–English-speaking patients, or patients who do not speak English fluently, require an interpreter to assist with communication in the medical setting. It is often a unique challenge to provide medical care to a patient whose primary language is not English. The provider may also be foreign born and not fluent in the patient's language. Unfortunately, an interpreter may contribute to the confusion of the encounter and inhibit the development of a good relationship.

A professional interpreter, who is both bilingual and bicultural, should be used whenever possible. Professionals are trained in the complexities of extracting pertinent information while clarifying concepts and ideas between different cultures, individuals, and languages. The interpreter should also be familiar with medical terminology and procedures. Untrained interpreters such as family members or ancillary staff can complicate the transfer of information. They may inappropriately omit or add information or inaccurately condense or substitute words or phrases that can completely alter the message. An untrained interpreter may also exchange roles with the interviewer, replacing the interviewer's questions with his or her own. The interpreter also can improperly impose his or her own values, obscuring the patient's values and beliefs.

There is the potential to breach confidentiality when family or ancillary staff are used. Patients may be reluctant to discuss certain topics in the presence of family members. Even in instances in which adult children translate for parents, role reversal and shifts in familial control and power can impede the transfer of information.

> Always use a professional interpreter if possible: when interpreting, family members inevitably impose their own values.

The provider should speak slowly, using simple words and phrases and avoiding jargon, idioms, and metaphors. Medical terms or procedures must be specific, clear, and concise. Periodically during the interpretation, thoughts should be summarized and repeated so that any miscommunications can be promptly corrected. Even when speaking through an interpreter, it is important for the provider to maintain visual contact with the patient so that indirect or nonverbal cues are not missed or ignored.

▼ NHAN QUOC HO (Part IV)

On the next visit, you have arranged for another interpreter. This time it is a middle-aged man who works full-time as a medical interpreter for the Laotian community. Before the visit, you review the case with the interpreter. The interpreter is able to reveal that Mr. Ho is paranoid and confuses events from his boyhood in Laos with recent events. Mr. Ho feels that he can no longer take care of himself, and he no longer trusts his wife. You make a rough attempt at traditional Western mental status testing and find that Mr. Ho demonstrates poor short-term memory and disorientation to time. Through the agency you attempt to involve Mrs. Ho, but she will not come to your office, so you are unable to involve her in any decision making. Blood is obtained at this visit to rule out contributory or causative factors that can be detected on blood tests, but brain imaging is deemed impractical. Home care is arranged to assist Mr. Ho in daily care and nutrition, but this is limited by the lack of aides and nurses fluent in Hmong.

On a subsequent visit, Mr. Ho's functional and mental status shows continued evidence of decline. A tentative diagnosis of dementia of Alzheimer's type is made. Mr. Ho becomes agitated at the prospect of returning to his home. He is admitted into a respite program until long-term care arrangements can be made. Nursing facilities are reluctant to accept him, since they have no staff members who speak Hmong and there is concern about his being able to communicate his needs. The interpreter assists in organizing members of the Laotian community to visit Mr. Ho and is able to find a nursing aide fluent in Hmong to work on Mr. Ho's floor at the nursing facility where he is eventually transferred. Mr. Ho's wife remains distant and uninvolved in her husband's care.

CASE DISCUSSION

The complexities of a dementia evaluation across cultures and languages are evident in this case. An appropriate bilingual and bicultural interpreter is essential. Standard mental status tests are not useful in this situation, since most have biases against those who are illiterate or whose primary language is not English. The clinical history becomes crucial in making an accurate diagnosis. It is important to involve family members whenever possible, since they may be able to contribute critical information.

Medical interpretation is a complex task, and it requires interest and commitment from both the provider and interpreter. The interpreter must assist in the communication of ideas and thoughts across cultural and language barriers and should have experience in the medical setting. Responses and questions should not be condensed, since this could alter the meaning or understanding of the concepts. In this case the first interpreter was young, inexperienced, and too distracted by school to provide meaningful interpretation.

Home care and long-term care placement can be particularly challenging when the patient is not fluent in English. Most agencies and facilities lack cultural diversity or do not offer services in languages other than English. There may be a reluctance to accept patients like Mr. Ho if there are no staff to support their admission. In some states, nursing home regulators require that the facility have someone on each shift who can communicate with the resident. Although it is important that patients be able to communicate and make their needs known, there should also be programs and activities that meet the cultural needs of the residents and their families.

As the number of ethnic elders increases, agencies and facilities will have to meet the challenge of providing culturally and linguistically appropriate services and staff to all elders.

SUMMARY

The dramatic increase in older Americans is already making a significant impact on the health care system in this country. Minority elders, whose numbers are anticipated to increase well into the next century, have specific health care issues and needs that are defined in part by their unique blends of culture, race, gender, and socioeconomic status. Most geriatricians and related health care professionals can expect to care for members of these groups, so it is important that all providers develop an understanding of the health care needs of minority elders and become familiar with the components of culturally sensitive health care.

POSTTEST

1. Which of the following statements about medical interpretation is true?
   a. Family members are the ideal interpreters.
   b. Fluency in the required language is the only criterion.
   c. Nonverbal communication plays a small role in interpretation.
   d. Knowledge of the patient's cultural context is important for good interpretation.

2. All of the following statements about current data on minority elders are true except:
   a. Data are frequently lumped together, obscuring intragroup characteristics.
   b. Data about African-Americans can be easily applied to American Indians.
   c. Most of the research has been performed using small sample sizes.
   d. Latino subgroups have ethnic distinctions that may affect attitudes about health.

3. Which of the following statements is false regarding life expectancy?
   a. A racial mortality crossover effect occurs in all minority groups.
   b. Life expectancy has improved for all groups since the beginning of the century.
   c. Japanese-American men have the longest life expectancy of all minority elders.
   d. Life expectancy is influenced by socioeconomic factors.

REFERENCES

1. US Bureau of the Census: Estimates of the population of the United States, by age, sex, and race, Series P-25, No 985, Washington, DC, 1986, US Government Printing Office.
2. Guralnik JM et al: Educational status in active life expectancy in blacks and whites, *N Engl J Med* 329(2):110-116, 1993.
3. Moss FE, Halamandaris VJ: *Too old, too sick, too bad,* Germantown, Md, 1977, Aspen Systems.
4. Yeo G: Ethnicity and nursing homes: factors affecting use and successful components for culturally sensitive care. In Barresi CM, ed: *Ethnic elderly and long-term care,* New York, 1993, Springer Publishing.
5. Manuel RC. In Jackson JS et al, eds: *The Black American elderly: research on physical and psychosocial health,* New York, 1988, Springer Publishing.
6. Baquet CR et al: Socioeconomic factors and cancer incidence among blacks and whites, *J Natl Cancer Inst* 83:551-557, 1991.
7. Furstenberg A, Merzey MD: Differences in outcome between black and white elderly hip fracture patients, *J Chron Dis* 40(10):931-938, 1987.
8. Cuellar J: Aging and health: Hispanic American elders, *SGEC Working Paper Series,* No 5, Stanford, Calif, 1990, Stanford Geriatric Education Center.
9. Lee YT: Surgical treatment of carcinoma of the breast: changes in patient population and therapeutic modalities at a metropolitan hospital, *J Surg Oncol* 29(3):147-153, 1985.
10. Kemp BJ et al: Epidemiology of depression and dysphoria in our elderly Hispanic population: prevalence and correlates, *J Am Geriatr Soc* 35(10):920-926, 1987.
11. Edwards E: Native-American elders: current issues and social policy implications. In McNeeley RL, Colen JN, eds: *Aging in minority groups,* Beverly Hills, Calif, 1983, Sage Publications.
12. Weibel-Orlando J: Elders and elderlies: well-being in Indian old age, *Am Indian Culture Res J* 13:149-170, 1989.
13. US Department of Health and Human Services: Health status of minorities and low-income groups, ed 3, Rockville, Md, 1991, US Government Printing Office.
14. Rhoades ER: Profile of American Indians and Alaska Natives. In Minority aging: essential curricular content for selected health and allied health professions, DHHS Publication No HRS(P-DV-90-4), Washington, DC, 1990, US Department of Health & Human Services.
15. Liu WT, Yu E: Asian/Pacific American elderly: mortality differentials, health status, and use of health services, *J Appl Gerontol* 4:35-64, 1985.
16. Morioka-Douglas N, Yeo G: Aging and health: Asian/Pacific Island American elders, *SGEC Working Paper Series,* Stanford, Calif, 1990, Stanford Geriatric Education Center.
17. Fujimoto WY et al: Prevalence of complications among second generation Japanese American men with diabetes, impaired glucose tolerance, or normal glucose tolerance, *Diabetes* 36:730-739, 1987.
18. Yano K et al: Bone mineral measurements among middle aged and elderly Japanese residents in Hawaii, *Am J Epidemiol* 119(5):751-764, 1984.

PRETEST ANSWERS

1. b
2. d
3. c

POSTTEST ANSWERS

1. d
2. b
3. a

CHAPTER 8

Health Maintenance and Promotion

NEIL K. HALL

OBJECTIVES

On completion of this chapter, the reader will be able to:

1. Discuss the potential value of preventive health screening.

2. Understand the principles of screening and apply them to evaluate specific screening modalities.

3. Locate references to help decide which techniques to apply in practice.

4. Discuss specific prevention and screening procedures appropriate for the elderly.

5. Discuss the role of health education in prevention.

PRETEST

1. Which one of the following statements is false?
   a. Primary prevention attempts to prevent a condition from occurring at all.
   b. Screening for hypertension is secondary prevention.
   c. Detecting unreported angina is secondary prevention.
   d. Stopping smoking can result in longer life for the elderly.
2. Which one of the following statements concerning cancer prevention is false?
   a. Mammography is recommended every 1 to 2 years at least to age 75.
   b. Pap smears are not necessary for elderly patients who have had regular, normal smears until age 65.
   c. Routine chest x-ray examinations are an effective preventive technique for lung cancer.
   d. Testing the stool for occult blood is of uncertain value as a preventive technique for colon cancer.
3. The most common causes of mortality in the elderly are:
   a. Heart disease, cancer, and accidents
   b. Heart disease, strokes, and cancer
   c. Heart disease, strokes, and infections
   d. Strokes, cancer, and infections

Maintaining and promoting health is the overall goal of any health professional. The incidence and severity of most major causes of death and disability can be reduced by prevention, early recognition, and treatment. Screening for common conditions is more likely to be positive in the older patient, and there is extensive evidence that interventions, both to prevent illnesses from occurring and to reduce their impact, are much more effective than is frequently recognized by professionals or the public. An active approach, incorporating screening, health maintenance, prevention, and health promotion should be incorporated into the daily practice of the primary care physician.

 It's never too late: exercise and other good health habits improve well-being even in the very old.

▼ JAMES CREIGHTON (Part I)

Mr. Creighton is a 70-year-old retired construction worker in for a routine checkup. He has been relatively healthy and currently has no complaints, but he is having an examination because his wife wanted him to.

▼ VIOLA SCHULTZ (Part I)

Mrs. Schultz is an 85-year-old woman with hypertension and diabetes mellitus. She comes to your office for her yearly physical.

STUDY QUESTIONS

- What are the goals of a routine health maintenance examination?

- What actions help achieve these goals, and how frequently should these examinations be done?

GOALS OF HEALTH MAINTENANCE

Aging is characterized by a general and gradual decline of physical and physiological capacity. Much of this decline is related to unhealthy habits, such as smoking, excess alcohol consumption, inappropriate diet, and sedentary lifestyle. Environmental factors, including infectious and toxic agents, and physical hazards, such as motor vehicles, uneven flooring, and poor lighting, may also contribute. These factors often combine to lead to physical, cognitive, or emotional problems that cause a functional decline. The loss of independence and the feeling of being a burden to others is often more feared by the elderly than death itself.

The goal of health maintenance in the elderly is to maximize both the quality and quantity of life. This includes maintaining independence and limiting physical and emotional pain. Although preventive techniques are best begun at an early age, they can still have major impact later in life.

Exercise and nutrition are the two factors that, if vigorously addressed, will lead to improved health in old age.

ROLE OF THE PRIMARY CARE PHYSICIAN

Changing people's health behavior is paramount in preventive medicine. Whether starting an exercise program, obtaining a mammogram, or coming in for a physical and immunizations, people must overcome their inertia. Be-

Table 8-1   The Ten Leading Causes of Death Among Persons Aged 65 or Older in 1990

Cause of Death	Number of Deaths	Death Rate (per 100,000 population)	Percentage of All Deaths in Those ≥ 65 yr
All Causes	**1,542,493**	**4,963.2**	**100.0**
1. Heart disease	594,858	1,914.0	38.6
2. Malignant neoplasms, including neoplasms of lymphatic and hematopoietic tissues	345,387	1,111.3	22.4
3. Cerebrovascular diseases	125,409	403.5	8.1
4. Chronic obstructive pulmonary disease and associated conditions	72,755	234.1	4.7
5. Pneumonia and influenza	70,485	226.8	4.6
6. Diabetes mellitus	35,523	114.3	2.3
7. Accidents and adverse effects	26,213	84.3	1.7
Motor vehicle accidents	7,210	23.2	0.5
All other accidents and adverse effects	19,003	61.1	1.2
8. Nephritis, nephrotic syndrome, and nephrosis	17,306	55.7	1.1
9. Atherosclerosis	17,158	55.2	1.1
10. Septicemia	15,351	49.4	1.0
All other causes, residual	222,048	2,045.9	14.4

From National Center for Health Statistics: Advanced report of final mortality statistics, 1990, Monthly Vital Statistics Report Vol 41, No 7(Suppl) Hyattsville, Md, 1993, Public Health Service.

cause of repeated interaction with patients and trust developed over tie, the primary care physician has the potential to teach and motivate patients. The physician must actively promote health.

TYPES OF PREVENTION

Primary prevention attempts to keep a condition from occurring (e.g., immunization and health education).

Secondary prevention is the detection of disease at an asymptomatic stage (e.g., screening for hypertension, cancer, or elevated cholesterol).

Tertiary prevention is the detection of symptomatic but unreported conditions or their complications, and it includes the management of these conditions (e.g., detection of [unreported] transient ischemic attacks, angina pectoris, and falls). Management includes medical treatments and health education for patients and families.

Screening is the application of procedures to detect risk factors, asymptomatic disease, and unreported conditions. It is the first step in a preventive program.

SCREENING AND HEALTH PROMOTION FOR SPECIFIC CONDITIONS

There are little data concerning which preventive approaches could influence the impact of the leading causes of death and major causes of disability in the elderly (Tables 8-1 and 8-2).[1,2]

Criteria to help decide which screening measures should be used in a population are listed in Box 8-1.

Table 8-2   Principal Causes of Severe, Chronic Disability Among Disabled Persons Aged 85 and Older

Condition	Percent
Dementia	19.43
Arthritis	16.75
Peripheral vascular disease	14.88
Cerebrovascular disease	12.86
Hip and other fractures	8.81
Ischemic heart disease	1.88
Hypertension	1.38
Diabetes	1.01
Cancer	0.91
Emphysema and bronchitis	0.26

There is conclusive evidence for the effectiveness of screening in only a few conditions (Box 8-2). Several groups have made recommendations based on the available research literature and on the opinions of experienced clinicians and epidemiologists.[3-9]

The text that follows describes the screening and health promotion methods primary care physicians can use with their older patients. There is insufficient evidence that most elements of the traditional history and physical and most laboratory tests are effective in screening. Mass laboratory screenings do not contribute enough to offset their cost and often cause unnecessary further evaluation because of false-positive results.

BOX 8-1
Six Criteria for Evaluating Preventive Services in the Elderly

1. The condition must have a significant effect on health.
2. Acceptable methods of preventive intervention or treatment must be available for the condition.
3. For *primary* preventive services (counseling, chemoprevention, immunizations), the intervention must be effective in preserving health.
4. For *other* preventive services or interventions:
   (a) There must be period before the individual (or his or her caregiver) is aware of the condition, or of its seriousness or implications, during which it can reliably be detected by providers;
   (b) Tests used to identify the condition must be able to reliably discriminate between cases and noncases of the condition;
   and
   (c) Preventive services or treatment during this "preawareness" period must have greater effectiveness than care or treatment delayed until the individual or caregiver brings it to a provider's attention.
5. For individuals cared for by caregivers, the benefit offered by the preventive service must outweigh any negative effects on the quality of life of caregivers.
6. The relative value of the preventive service or intervention must be determined by a comparison of its costs with its expected health benefits.

From Klinkman MS et al: *J Fam Pract* 34:205-224, 1992.

▼ *JAMES CREIGHTON (Part II)*
Mr. Creighton requests an exercise electrocardiogram. He has no symptoms of heart disease, but his wife has read that this should be done.

▼ *VIOLA SCHULTZ (Part II)*
Mrs. Schultz, having read about the dangers of hypercholesterolemia, asks you to check her cholesterol.

STUDY QUESTION

■ *What should you do to evaluate your patients' risk of cardiovascular disease?*

CARDIOVASCULAR DISEASE

Major modifiable risk factors for cardiovascular disease are hypertension, cigarette smoking, and hypercholesterolemia. Inactivity, obesity, and diabetes mellitus are lesser risk factors. Screening questions about smoking, exercise habits, dietary fats and cholesterol, and symptoms suggestive of transient ischemic attacks should be considered. Blood pressure should be measured yearly: systolic values above 160 mm Hg and diastolic values above 90 mm Hg need further evaluation. The dramatic decrease in cerebrovascular accidents in the past two decades is thought to have been in part due to the detection and reduction of hypertension. Treatment of diastolic hypertension in the elderly is as effective as in younger persons in reducing morbidity and mortality, and reducing systolic hypertension in elders significantly reduces the risk of stroke.[10,11]

Serum cholesterol screening in the elderly is controversial. The effectiveness of cholesterol reduction in lowering cardiovascular morbidity and mortality in the elderly is questionable,[12,13] and it is not cost effective.[14] Stress electrocardiograms are not productive screening tests for the asymptomatic. In smokers or those with hypertension, diabetes mellitus, or peripheral vascular disease, auscultation for carotid bruits and regular electrocardiograms may be appropriate.

Health education and promotion include discussing smoking, weight control, restriction of fat intake to no more than 30% of total daily calories, and aerobic exercise.

Regular physical exercise is associated with reduced cardiovascular mortality in elderly men (and presumably women also). Positive cardiovascular effects include reduced blood pressure, favorable modification in blood lipids, and reduced incidence and severity of obesity and diabetes mellitus. Not only vigorous physical exercise but also less intense activity has benefits. There is general consensus that physicians should recommend regular physical exercise.

Smoking is responsible for up to 30% of myocardial infarctions and is a major contributor to stroke. The vast majority of lung cancers and chronic pulmonary disease are tobacco induced, and oral, pharyngeal, laryngeal, and esophageal cancers are mostly caused by tobacco use. Counseling by physicians can influence patients to quit smoking. Most patients already know the health hazards and have already attempted to quit. The urging of their personal physician, particularly if given repeatedly and coupled with self-help materials and nicotine prescription, can be the difference that helps them succeed. Stop-

BOX 8-2
Appropriateness of Various Preventive Screening Techniques In Elderly Persons

Widely Accepted

Blood pressure measurement
Mammogram
Breast examination
Pap smear unless previously normal
Tetanus/diphtheria immunization
Infuenza immunization
Pneumococcal immunization
Hearing tests
Vision screens
Dental examinations
Smoking history and education
Weight measurement and education
Diet history and education
Physical exercise education

Controversial

Cholesterol measurement
Digital rectal examination
Prostate specific antigen
Routine estrogen use
Stool for occult blood
Thyroid function tests
Blood/urine sugar

High Risk Only

Colon/sigmoid endoscopy
Skin cancer examination
Oral cancer examination

Not Appropriate for Well Elders

Complete physical examination
Extensive history
Screening blood tests
Cancer screening of
   Lung
   Ovary
   Uterus
Auscultation of carotid arteries
Tuberculosis screen

Uncertain Value, Often Used in Elders

Mobility/fall risk
Cognitive decline assessment
Incontinence test
Depression test
Accident evaluation
Nutrition evaluation
Osteoporosis examination
Social situation evaluation
Activities of daily living history

ping smoking does result in longer life for some elderly.[15] Reduced cardiovascular mortality occurs within 1 year of cessation.

Use of estrogen in postmenopausal women has been repeatedly shown to be associated with decreased coronary artery disease and around a 50% reduction in the risk of death. This is probably secondary to its effect on raising HDL cholesterol levels. Although estrogen use is associated with increased gallbladder disease and possibly with a slightly increased risk of breast cancer, the beneficial cardiovascular effect and the protection from osteoporosis outweigh the risks.[16] Women with an intact uterus should also have progesterone to prevent the increased risk of endometrial cancer from unopposed estrogen. The withdrawal bleeding of cyclical estrogen and progesterone use and the spotting with combined daily regimens make hormone replacement unacceptable to many.

> *Daily aspirin is probably reasonable for all elders if there are no contraindications.*

Prospective studies show aspirin's association with decreased myocardial infarction in both men[17] and women[18] over age 50; it also protects against recurrent infarction. It prevents strokes in those with transient ischemic attacks or previous stroke. Opinion is not uniform about routine prophylactic aspirin. Patients at high risk of cardiovascular disease, or perhaps all elderly patients, are advised to take 325 mg daily if there is no contraindication. An added benefit is the decreased incidence of colon cancer in aspirin users.[19]

Reduced fat intake can slow the development of atherosclerosis by reducing cholesterol; it helps obesity and diabetes and thus affects cardiovascular risk. Limiting alcohol consumption may prevent hypertension. Many studies demonstrate reduced coronary events in persons who drink in moderation, but the risks of precipitating alcohol excess prevent this from being a routine recommendation. Reduced sodium intake (from the typical 4 to 6 g per day in Americans) may decrease blood pressure, perhaps more in the elderly; increased potassium, calcium, and magnesium may lower blood pressure, but there is no clear consensus.[20]

▼ JAMES CREIGHTON (Part III)

Mr. Creighton's blood pressure is 160/100 mm Hg. He is approximately 40 lb over his desired weight and has no regular exercise regimen. You advise him to return for follow-up blood pressure evaluation and give him information about weight control and a walking exercise program. He asks you if he should have the prostate cancer test.

▼ *VIOLA SCHULTZ (Part III)*

Mrs. Schultz is normotensive, has a satisfactory weight, and tells you she exercises regularly. During the breast examination, she mentions that her sister recently died of breast cancer and asks if she should have a mammogram.

STUDY QUESTION

▪ *What cancer screening should be applied to your patients?*

CANCER

Cancer is the second leading cause of death in the elderly. The incidence of cancer death increases dramatically with age. Lung, breast, prostate, and colorectal tumors are the most common causes of mortality. Cancers of the breast and cervix are the most accessible to screening. Health education may reduce the risk of others. Recommendations about cancer screening differ substantially. Knowledge of the effectiveness of such efforts is limited.

Breast cancer mortality is reduced by screening; this applies to the elderly as well.[21,22] The incidence of breast cancer increases with age, so the likelihood of a lump or mammographic abnormality being a malignancy is much higher. There are fewer false-positive results. Obtaining the history of a lump or of risk factors is not recommended as part of the screening. Yearly physical examination is recommended by all experts. Evidence of its effectiveness is limited, however, to studies that combine such examination with mammography. Routine screening mammograms have been shown in several studies to reduce mortality from breast cancer; they are appropriate every 1 to 2 years, through age 75.[23] Medicare now pays for them. Teaching breast self-examination is recommended, although the evidence is slight to support this.

Cervical cancer is comparatively rare in old age, and older women with previously normal Pap smears rarely develop it. Those who have not received screening are more likely than younger women to have abnormal smears and invasive disease,[24,25] so obtaining the history of previous smears and performing smears on unscreened women is mandatory. Women with a record of normal Pap smears do not need screening beyond age 70. Those with previously abnormal results should have continued Pap smears at regular intervals, probably yearly. Those who have not had regular previous screening should have at least two annual Pap smears.

Colon cancer is a disease for which there is no clear consensus on screening.[26] Digital rectal examinations are not effective as a screen. Stool guaiac tests produce frequent false-positive results and therefore further unnecessary evaluations. False-negative results are also common. However, this test can detect both early malignancies and premalignant lesions. It is inexpensive (if done

in isolation), and many groups recommend it every 1 to 2 years for those over 40. Sigmoidoscopy is expensive and often unacceptable to patients; it is probably best reserved for persons at high risk, such as those with a history of colon cancer in first-degree relatives or of familial polyposis. Health education should include encouraging decreased fat and increased fiber in the diet and seeking medical attention promptly for rectal bleeding. Regular use of aspirin is associated with a lower risk of colon cancer.[19]

Oral cancer treatment at an early stage improves outcome, and most expert groups recommend regular oral examination. Tobacco and alcohol increase the risk, and individuals who use these substances might be especially targeted for examination. However, evidence is lacking about the effectiveness of routine oral examination. Health education includes recommending reductions in tobacco and alcohol use.

Prostate cancer is very common in older men and is often asymptomatic. There is no good study to show that prostate cancer screening reduces morbidity and mortality compared with waiting until symptoms develop.[27] Digital examination of the prostate, while generally recommended, has not been shown to affect outcome. Yearly prostate-specific antigen (PSA) screening is recommended by the American Cancer Society, but a high false-positive rate makes this test a costly screen.[27] Ultrasound of the prostate is expensive and not recommended. Health education includes informing the patient that decreased fat intake may reduce risk.

Skin cancers, both basal cell and squamous cell, are common and treatable. Malignant melanoma, much rarer, is responsible for the majority of skin cancer deaths. The effectiveness of screening is unknown, but a routine skin examination is recommended, particularly in those with prolonged exposure to sunlight. Health education includes recommended use of sunscreens.

Lung cancer is a major killer of the elderly, but routine screening including x-ray examination and sputum cytology is ineffective and not recommended. Health education includes recommending smoking cessation (associated with reduced cancer risk even in long-term smokers).

There is insufficient evidence of effectiveness to lead to recommendations for screening asymptomatic persons for other cancers (pancreatic, uterine, testicular, etc.). Health education includes advising medical attention for postmenopausal bleeding.

▼ *JAMES CREIGHTON (Part IV)*

During Mr. Creighton's skin examination, actinic keratoses are found on his face and hands. The remainder of the examination is negative. He is advised to return to the office for further evaluation and treatment of these premalignant skin lesions.

▼ *VIOLA SCHULTZ (Part IV)*

Mrs. Schultz's breast and skin examinations are negative. Because she had regular and normal Pap smears through age 70, you do not obtain a Pap smear. You advise a screening mammogram and stress its importance because of her family history of breast cancer.

INFECTIOUS DISEASES

Infections are the fifth leading cause of death in the elderly, becoming increasingly common as immunity and general resistance wane. Frail nursing home residents are at greatest risk, in part because of their exposure to many people in the institutional setting. Pneumonia and influenza are the primary causes, so virtually all experts recommend yearly influenza immunization for individuals 65 and older, particularly if institutionalized. Although the immune response is decreased in the elderly, the vaccine has been shown to reduce the incidence of influenza and its complications.[28] It is remarkably cost effective,[29] the cost of the vaccine is reimbursed by Medicare, and a sore arm is its only significant side effect.[30] Patients at highest risk of influenza complications should receive prophylaxis with amantadine (100 mg per day) or rimantadine during influenza A outbreaks.

Pneumococcal vaccine is also recommended for those over age 65, and its effectiveness has been documented in the elderly.[31] It is given only once, although some experts suggest repeating for high-risk individuals after 6 years or more. Repeat vaccination with the newer 22-valent vaccine is *not* routinely recommended if the patient previously had received the 14-valent one.

Tetanus and diphtheria immunizations should be every 10 years in a combined vaccine, although a single revaccination at age 65 may be sufficient.[32] The effectiveness is high, complications minimal, and the diseases, although rare, are often fatal. If the patient has never had a primary vaccination, a series of three injections should be given, the second approximately 4 to 8 weeks after the first and the third 6 to 12 months later.

The elderly have often not received vaccinations and are frequently reluctant to accept them. The physician should always obtain the immunization history and vigorously promote patient compliance.

Tuberculosis (TB) screening is not advised for the general elderly population because of the low frequency of active disease. TB has a much higher incidence and prevalence in the nursing home, so annual intradermal purified protein derivative (PPD) is often recommended and may be required by the state health department. Because of the decreased immune response of the elderly, a repeat PPD is recommended 1 to 2 weeks after an initial negative test, using the immunological booster phenomenon to improve sensitivity. Chest x-ray examinations are reserved for further evaluation of those with positive PPDs.

FUNCTION

While it is clear that functional evaluation can detect previously unrecognized problems, it is not known what, if any, difference in outcome results from mass application of functional screening in primary care. Many geriatricians believe that periodic evaluation of function is worthwhile.

Both activities of daily living (bathing, dressing, toileting, mobility, urine and stool continence, and feeding) and instrumental activities of daily living (using the telephone and transportation, preparing food, managing finances, etc.) can be assessed by history from the patient, family member, or other caregiver. Inquiry can be made about memory difficulty, emotional symptoms (particularly depression), social contacts, and support and financial difficulties. Brief rating scales and questionnaires are available to assist in this process.[33]

SENSORY LOSS

Hearing and vision losses have dramatic effects on social, physical, and emotional life and can often be treated. A Snellen chart or near card visual screen and a whisper test[34] or simple audiogram are sufficient. The hand-held audioscope (Welch Allyn, Skaneateles, New York) is an effective tool. Hearing aids improve communication and overall function of persons with hearing loss.[35] Persons found to have hearing loss that interferes with communication should be referred to an audiologist if they are willing to consider a hearing aid. Periodic eye examinations by an optometrist or ophthalmologist are recommended, particularly to screen for glaucoma, although there is no evidence that glaucoma screening, even by ophthalmologists, results in improved vision outcomes. The primary care physician's glaucoma screen is to evaluate the optic cup size, with cups greater than 0.5 disk diameter being suspect for glaucoma. Schiøtz tonometry is not accurate enough to use in screening.

MOBILITY

Ambulation can be assessed with a simple gait and balance evaluation: have the patient arise from a chair without using the arms, walk a short distance, and turn around; check for Romberg's sign, assess postural stability and resistance to a push on the chest with the patient's eyes closed, then have the patient pick up an object from the floor and sit back down. (Be sure to guard against falling with these last two maneuvers.) If there is difficulty with any of these, the patient is at risk for falling and further history and assessment are vital; physical therapy referral should be considered.

COGNITIVE DECLINE

Routine screening for cognitive function has not been well studied. Dementia is common and can be devastating; it can cause considerable familial disruption before it is recognized as an illness. Even though most dementias are not curable, early diagnosis may assist patients and families to plan and to take positive approaches to future management. Brief dementia screens are available,[36,37] although their sensitivity is questioned.[38] Screening for dementia has been either not discussed or advised against by the major groups evaluating prevention practices. Primary care physicians should suspect dementia often and seek to confirm it when suspicions are present, but they should not feel compelled to screen for it.

INCONTINENCE

Urinary incontinence is one of the most common hidden problems in the old. Occurring in 15% or more of the community dwelling elderly, it can interfere with social and physical function, cause emotional discomfort, and result in substantial expense. Despite these effects, patients (mostly women) rarely ask their physicians for assistance. Inquiring about incontinence at the time of the routine examination often confirms this embarrassing problem, allowing further evaluation. Usually these patients can be helped, sometimes dramatically. Although the cost-effectiveness of this screening is undetermined, geriatricians usually include this brief question as part of their routine.

SOCIAL SUPPORT

Because the social support system is crucial, knowledge of family and friends available for assistance and emotional support for any functionally impaired elder must be known. A questionnaire requesting such information can be economically given to patients and family members and can include a simple screen for financial difficulties, potential abuse, and emotional and cognitive problems.

DEPRESSION

Depression is common in the elderly and may lead to suicide, particularly in men living alone. Treatment with medications or psychotherapy is effective. Short, simply administered depression screens are available,[39] but the efficacy of these in primary care is unknown. Primary care physicians should remain alert to the possibility of depression, especially in patients at highest risk, such as those with recent bereavement, excessive alcohol consumption, Alzheimer's disease, and Parkinson's disease. Those who are caregivers of the chronically ill are also at high risk. When detected, depression should be treated vigorously.

ACCIDENTS

Injury is a major cause of morbidity and mortality. Falls and their complications are most significant, causing about half the injury deaths, with motor vehicle accidents and burns from fire and hot water also important. The effectiveness of physician intervention to prevent accidental death is unknown, but risk screening and health education are often advised. Fall risk can be assessed by asking about a history of falls (since many are unreported), checking for use of medications associated with falls (e.g., antidepressants, major tranquilizers, sedatives), and by screening for the level of function in skills such as vision and ambulation. In addition to encouraging exercise and other techniques that improve these functions, health education to modify environmental factors, such as poor lighting and inadequate stair rails, may help. Promoting the use of seat belts, the avoidance of smoking in bed, and the use of smoke alarms and advising the elderly to lower the hot water temperature to 120° F have also been suggested as having the potential to reduce accidental injury and death.

OSTEOPOROSIS

Osteoporosis causes morbidity and mortality from vertebral, hip, and other fractures, particularly in elderly white women. Screening can include the family and personal history of osteoporotic fractures. More expensive radiological tests to assess bone density are not generally recommended. Health promotion includes weight-bearing exercise and adequate calcium intake, probably best achieved by supplementation with oral calcium, possibly combined with vitamin D. The most important preventive technique, use of estrogen, should be instituted long before old age to be most effective, but it may be helpful even in the elderly.

CHRONIC OBSTRUCTIVE PULMONARY DISEASE

Chronic obstructive pulmonary disease (COPD) is one of the major killers of the elderly, but it is not generally modifiable by screening, except for asking about cigarette use; persons with this disease should be strongly encouraged to give up smoking and to have immunizations. Promotion of regular exercise and good nutrition, possibly including nutritional supplements, may help maintain functional status.

NUTRITION

Screening for nutrition is best accomplished by comparing patients' weights with expected weight for height and by observation of interval weight loss. The diet history may be helpful. However, the value of nutritional screening, education, and promotion by physicians is unproven. The Nutrition Screening Initiative has validated a brief nutritional screening questionnaire to detect those at risk for poor nutrition.[40] The role of dietary modification in reducing cardiovascular and cancer risk has been mentioned elsewhere. Eating items from each of the standard food groups is strongly advised for all. Vitamin and mineral supplements (other than calcium) are not needed for people with an adequate, varied diet, although there is some evidence to support their use in the frail.[41]

DIABETES MELLITUS

Early detection and treatment of diabetes mellitus in the elderly have not been shown to improve outcome compared with treatment only after symptoms develop. However, some experts think that a simple urine dipstick test for glucose and protein is reasonable. This may detect urinary tract malignancy, too.

HYPOTHYROIDISM

Patients with a history of neck irradiation may benefit from thyroid screening; elderly women, in general, who are most at risk of hypothyroidism, may also benefit. However, screening for hypothyroidism is not routinely recommended.

DENTAL

Dental evaluation should be advised by the primary care physician and should be performed by a dentist on an annual basis. Even persons with dentures can benefit from the examination, which also helps detect oral carcinomas.

MEDICATIONS

Medication complications, both side effects and drug-drug interactions, are more common in the elderly, mainly because of the high number of drugs used. Physicians may help prevent such complications by reviewing drug use at routine visits. It is reasonable to discuss potential problems, particularly the risks associated with using drugs from multiple physicians, using over-the-counter medications, and combining drugs with alcohol.

ALCOHOL

Alcohol can be a major problem in the elderly, who are more affected by "a dose" of alcohol than when younger. Approximately one third of elderly alcoholics begin their problem drinking after age 65. It often goes unrecognized by the physician. Questionnaires such as CAGE can be used as a brief screen. Preventive techniques should also be used; these include asking the patient about alcohol use and counseling about moderation of alcohol, the risks of driving after drinking, and the alcohol-drug interaction.

▼ *JAMES CREIGHTON (Part V)*
Further questioning of Mr. Creighton reveals that he drinks 8 or more ounces of whiskey a day, along with occasional wine and beer. He is still driving his car but does not wear seat belts and occasionally drives after drinking. You talk about the possible negative consequences of alcohol, including its possible effect on his blood pressure and strongly encourage him to not drive after drinking and to always wear seat belts.

▼ *VIOLA SCHULTZ (Part V)*
On being asked, Viola Schultz relates that she frequently loses small amounts of urine when she coughs or sneezes. Because of this, she must wear an incontinence pad, at a cost of $5 to $10 a week. She has limited some of her activities because of this problem, but she has never discussed this with a doctor. You tell her this problem is quite common and frequently can be helped; you schedule a urinalysis and urine culture and give her an appointment to return for further evaluation.

PREVENTION IN PRIMARY CARE

Primary care physicians have great freedom in making decisions about which interventions they will use and how often. Certain screens and procedures are standard (mammograms, breast examinations, Pap smears, and immunizations), although there is variation in recommended frequency and the age at which to stop. Box 8-3 shows the chart developed by the U.S. Preventive Services Task Force.[5] However, preventive practice must be individualized to the patient. Extremely frail incapacitated individuals often have differing priorities (for care rather than screening); the discomfort and inconvenience may outweigh the benefits, especially if life expectancy is short.

Use every patient interaction as an opportunity for prevention and health promotion.

Every visit is an opportunity for prevention. Each time the follow-up plan should include the next preventive examination. Some procedures (e.g., pneumococcal immunization and mammograms) can easily be updated during hospitalizations. A practice orientation toward prevention can be heightened by having your staff audit charts for the preventive procedures you selected.[9]

Office staff can check when the last examination was done and remind both physician and patient (or family if appropriate) when it is due again; this may include mailing reminders. Computer-generated reminders can assist. Staff can obtain and review much of the history and can complete social and personal data updates. Blood pressure, hearing, and vision screens should be done by the office nurse, who can also assist in patient education (although the physician should emphasize this, too). A nurse practitioner in the primary care setting will often specially emphasize patient education. Instead of asking patients all the questions directly, a self-administered questionnaire can be sent before the visit. This should include the activities of daily living (ADLs), instrumental activities of daily living (IADLs), and depression scales mentioned previously, as well as questions about nutrition, physical activity, and other habits. The physician should review these answers at the time of the visit to emphasize their importance to the patient.

A form in the patient's records should be individually developed by the physician to record preventive data, health maintenance, and screening activities on one page, preferably in a different color.

▼ *JAMES CREIGHTON (Part VI)*
You treat Mr. Creighton's skin lesions with topical 5-fluorouracil. On your advice, he cuts back on his drinking. His diastolic blood pressure remains elevated and is treated successfully with 25 mg of hydrochlorothiazide daily. He is compliant taking his medication and with his follow-up visits, but he returns to his previous drinking habits. Three years later he is killed in an auto accident. Had he been wearing his seat belt, he probably would have survived.

▼ *VIOLA SCHULTZ (Part VI)*
Mrs. Schultz' mammogram is negative. She continues under your care and remains very active. Two years later a mam-

---

BOX 8-3
Interventions Considered and Recommended for the Periodic Health Examination of Those Age 65 and Older

Leading Causes of Death
Heart diseases
Malignant neoplasms (lung, colorectal, breast)
Cerebrovascular disease
Chronic obstructive pulmonary disease
Pneumonia and influenza

Interventions for the General Population

SCREENING
Blood pressure
Height and weight
Fecal occult blood test[1] or sigmoidoscopy or both
Mammogram ± clinical breast exam[2] (women ≤69 yr)
Papanicolaou (Pap) test (women)[3]
Vision screening
Assess for hearing impairment
Assess for problem drinking
COUNSELING
Substance use
Tobacco cessation
Avoid alcohol or drug use while driving, swimming, boating, etc.*
Diet and exercise
Limit fat and cholesterol; maintain caloric balance; emphasize grains, fruits, vegetables
Adequate calcium intake (women)
Regular physical activity

Injury prevention
Lap or shoulder belts
Motorcycle and bicycle helmets*
Fall prevention*
Safe storage or removal of firearms*
Smoke detector*
Set hot water heater to <120-130° F*
CPR training for household members
Dental health
Regular visits to dental care provider*
Floss, brush with fluoride toothpaste daily*
Sexual behavior
STD prevention: avoid high-risk sexual behavior; use condoms
IMMUNIZATIONS
Pneumococcal vaccine
Influenza[1]
Tetanus-diphtheria (Td) boosters
CHEMOPROPHYLAXIS
Discuss hormone prophylaxis (perimenopausal and postmenopausal women)

From US Preventive Services Task Force: Guide to clinical preventive service, ed 2, Baltimore, 1996, Williams & Wilkins.
[1]Annually. [2] Mammogram q1-2 yr, or mammogram q1-2 yr with annual clinical breast exam. [3]All women who are or have been sexually active and who have a cervix. Consider discontinuation of testing after age 65 yr if previous regular screening with consistently normal results.
*The ability of clinician counseling to influence this behavior is unproven.

Continued.

BOX 8-3
Interventions Considered and Recommended for the Periodic Health Examination of Those Age 65 and Older—cont'd

Interventions for High-Risk Populations

POPULATION	POTENTIAL INTERVENTIONS (See detailed high-risk definitions)
Institutionalized persons	PPD (HR1); hepatitis A vaccine (HR2); amantadine/rimantadine (HR4)
Chronic medical conditions; TB contacts; low income; immigrants; alcoholics	PPD (HR1)
Persons ≥75 yr or ≥70 yr with risk factors for falls	Fall prevention intervention (HR5)
Cardiovascular disease risk factors	Consider cholesterol screening (HR6)
Family history of skin cancer; nevi; fair skin, eyes, hair	Avoid excess and midday sun, use protective clothing (HR7)
Native Americans/Alaska Natives	PPD (HR1); hepatitis A vaccine (HR2)
Travelers to developing countries	Hepatitis A vaccine (HR2); hepatitis B vaccine (HR8)
Blood product recipients	HIV screen (HR3); hepatitis B vaccine (HR8)
High-risk sexual behavior	Hepatitis A vaccine (HR2); HIV screen (HR3); hepatitis B vaccine (HR8); RPR/VDRL (HR9)
Injection or street drug use	PPD (HR1); hepatitis A vaccine (HR2); HIV screen (HR3); hepatitis B vaccine (HR8); RPR/VDRL (HR9); advice to reduce infection risk (HR10)
Health care/lab workers	PPD (HR1); hepatitis A vaccine (HR2); amantadine/rimantadine (HR4); hepatitis B vaccine (HR8)
Persons susceptible to varicella	Varicella vaccine (HR11)

HR1 = HIV positive, close contacts of persons with known or suspected TB, health care workers, persons with medical risk factors associated with TB, immigrants from countries with high TB prevalence, medically underserved low-income populations (including homeless), alcoholics, injection drug users, and residents of long-term care facilities.

HR2 = Persons living in, traveling to, or working in areas where the disease is endemic and where periodic outbreaks occur (e.g., countries with high or intermediate endemicity; certain Alaska Native, Pacific Island, Native American, and religious communities); men who have sex with men; injection or street drug users. Consider for institutionalized persons and workers in these institutions, and day-care, hospital, and laboratory workers. Clinicians should also consider local epidemiology.

HR3 = Men who had sex with men after 1975; past or present injection drug use; persons who exchange sex for money or drugs, and their sex partners; injection drug-using, bisexual, or HIV-positive sex partner currently or in the past; blood transfusion during 1978-1985; persons seeking treatment for STDs. Clinicians should also consider local epidemiology.

HR4 = Consider for persons who have not received influenza vaccine or are vaccinated late; when the vaccine may be ineffective due to major antigenic changes in the virus; for unvaccinated persons who provide home care for high-risk persons; to supplement protection provided by vaccine in persons who are expected to have a poor antibody response; and for high-risk persons in whom the vaccine is contraindicated.

HR5 = Persons aged 75 years and older; or aged 70-74 with one or more additional risk factors including: use of certain psychoactive and cardiac medications (e.g., benzodiazepines, antihypertensives); use of ≥4 prescription medications; impaired cognition, strength, balance, or gait. Intensive individualized home-based multifactorial fall prevention intervention is recommended in settings where adequate resources are available to deliver such services.

HR6 = Although evidence is insufficient to recommend routine screening in elderly persons, clinicians should consider cholesterol screening on a case-by-case basis for persons ages 65-75 with additional risk factors (e.g., smoking, diabetes, or hypertension).

HR7 = Persons with a family or personal history of skin cancer, a large number of moles, atypical moles, poor tanning ability, or light skin, hair, and eye color.

HR8 = Blood product recipients (including hemodialysis patients), persons with frequent occupational exposure to blood or blood products, men who have sex with men, injection drug users and their sex partners, persons with multiple recent sex partners, persons with other STDs (including HIV), travelers to countries with endemic hepatitis B.

HR9 = Persons who exchange sex for money or drugs and their sex partners; persons with other STDs (including HIV); and sexual contacts of persons with active syphilis. Clinicians should also consider local epidemiology.

HR10 = Persons who continue to inject drugs.

HR11 = Healthy adults without a history of chickenpox or previous immunization. Consider serologic testing for presumed susceptible adults.

mogram reveals a suspicious lesion. This is removed by lumpectomy and found to be a carcinoma. She does well on tamoxifen and has no further problems until age 90, when she falls and fractures her right femur. After hip surgery she dies from a pulmonary embolism.

EXERCISE IN OLD AGE

Many adults enjoy an increased sense of well-being as a result of regular exercise. Clinical experience indicates that osteoporosis, arterial and venous insufficiency, gastrointestinal stasis, postural instability, and musculoskeletal stiffness are all increased in the immobilized. Many geriatricians recommend the initiation of exercise in old age as a means of improving well-being, helping other parameters, and postponing morbidity.[42-44] Exercise has the greatest impact on the sedentary. There are many studies confirming beneficial effects of exercise training in relatively healthy older individuals: cardiovascular function can be improved, bone loss reduced, lean body mass and muscle strength can be increased, flexibility can be increased, and glucose tolerance and cholesterol levels can be improved.[45] In more vulnerable, frail elders, further studies are needed regarding the benefits of exercise, but short-term benefits on cardiovascular function, flexibility, balance, and strength have been shown in some studies in such individuals.[46-48] A recent prospective study confirms lower mortality rates in higher fitness categories, with all-cause mortality reduced because of lowered rates of cardiovascular disease and cancer.[49] (See Box 8-4.)

> *Encouraging exercise has most effect on the sedentary.*

There are enough experience and data to conclude that it is clinically wise for the primary care physician to attempt to increase the level of exercise of all older patients. The right amount of exercise in old age is "more exercise than yesterday." For the sedentary older person the recommendation should be for slow reacquisition of regular, low-impact, unstressed but progressively increasing exercise. Walking, swimming, stationary cross-country skiing, and bicycling are the most useful. Walking has the disadvantage of involving impact, so footwear and the surface walked upon are crucial. Bicycling and walking may be bad for the knees. Swimming and the indoor cross-country ski track are best for many elders.

> *The best exercise for elders? Walking, swimming, stationary skiing, and bicycling.*

BOX 8-4
Potential Benefits of Exercise in the Elderly

Decreased overall mortality
Decreased cardiovascular disease
Decreased blood pressure
Decreased obesity
Decreased stroke
Decreased osteoporosis
Improved glucose tolerance
Improved cardiorespiratory fitness
Improved strength, agility, flexibility
Improved balance
Improved osteoarthritic pain and function
Improved sleep
Improved mood
Improved cognition

Since many of the phenomena associated with growing old are the very changes that regular exercise can potentially reverse or prevent, primary care physicians must actively encourage their older patients to exercise. The prescription must be unique for the individual but should be followed up at any later interaction with the patient to assist in continuing compliance. Remember "we don't wear out, we rust out."[43]

> *Many of the phenomena associated with growing old can be partially reversed and largely prevented by exercise.*

SUMMARY

Applied preventive health techniques can be beneficial to older patients. The goal is to maximize quality of life by minimizing suffering, loss of function, and development of dependence. Although the efficacy of many screening and prevention procedures remains unproven, the opinion of experienced clinicians and epidemiologists allows logical recommendations when proof is lacking. A complete history and physical are not necessary, but a brief examination focusing on specific areas relative to common conditions that affect the elderly is appropriate. By using the advantage of a long-standing, trusting relationship with the patient and integrating screening history, examinations and procedures, health education, and health promotion into regular office and hospital care, the primary care physician has a potentially major impact. Planning and organization, making use of the office support staff, and incorporating questionnaires, checkoff lists, and patient education materials can facilitate efficient and effective implementation even in the busiest primary care setting.

POSTTEST

1. Which one of the following statements is false?
   a. Most skin cancer deaths in old people are caused by malignant melanoma.
   b. Annual digital rectal examination has not been shown to be of value in detecting colorectal cancer.
   c. Prostate-specific antigen, if combined with rectal digital examination, has been shown to improve the outcome of prostatic cancer.
   d. Women over 70 years with previously abnormal Pap smears should continue to have regular smears.

2. Which one of the following statements concerning infectious disease prevention is false?
   a. High-risk patients can be protected from influenza A by the use of amantadine.
   b. Individuals immunized with the 14-valent pneumococcal vaccine should be reimmunized with the 22-valent vaccine.
   c. Tetanus-diphtheria immunization is important in the elderly, since both illnesses are frequently fatal.
   d. An initial PPD test, if negative, should be repeated 1 to 2 weeks later.

3. The best statement about cholesterol screening in the elderly is:
   a. Screening should be done on all elderly because lowering cholesterol has a dramatic result in reducing cardiac death.
   b. Screening is unlikely to be effective because lowering cholesterol levels in the elderly has a small effect on reducing cardiac death.
   c. Cholesterol screening should be done yearly until age 75 years, then stopped.

   d. The value of cholesterol screening in the elderly is controversial and uncertain at this time.

4. Select the one statement that includes the physical examination components most appropriate for preventive health care in the elderly:
   a. Breast examination, blood pressure determination, and visual acuity
   b. Breast examination, rectal examination, and visualization of the cervix
   c. Breast examination, blood pressure determination, and auscultation of the heart
   d. Blood pressure determination, auscultation of the heart, and rectal examination

5. Of the following, the most important health education items for the elderly patient are:
   a. Smoking cessation, cholesterol reduction, accident prevention
   b. Smoking cessation, regular exercise, accident prevention
   c. Regular exercise, accident prevention, breast self-examination
   d. Accident prevention, breast self-examination, dietary fiber intake

6. Which of the following procedures would be most appropriate for an asymptomatic, apparently healthy woman between age 65 and 75 years who had never had any screening procedures done in the past:
   a. Mammography, Pap smear, chemistry screen
   b. Mammography, sigmoidoscopy, thyroid screen
   c. Mammography, Pap smear, stool for blood
   d. Pap smear, thyroid screen, chemistry screen

REFERENCES

1. National Center for Health Statistics: Advanced report of final mortality statistics, 1990, Monthly Vital Statistics Report Vol 41, No 7 (Suppl), Hyattsville, Md, 1993, Public Health Service.
2. Williams TF, Cooney LM: Principles of rehabiliitation in older persons. In *Principles of geriatric medicine and gerontology,* New York, 1994, McGraw-Hill.
3. Klinkman MS et al: A criterion-based review of preventive health care in the elderly, Part 1, *J Fam Pract* 34:205-224, 1992.
4. Omenn GS: Health promotion and disease prevention, *Clin Geriatr Med* 8(1):1-233, 1992.
5. US Preventive Services Task Force: *Guide to clinical preventive service,* ed 2, Baltimore, 1996, Williams & Wilkins.
6. Institute of Medicine: *The second fifty years: promoting health and preventing disability,* Washington, DC, 1990, National Academy Press.
7. Kennie DC: *Preventive care for elderly people,* Cambridge, 1993, Cambridge University Press.
8. Zazove P et al: A criterion-based review of preventive health care in the elderly, Part 2, *J Fam Pract* 34:320-347, 1992.
9. US Department of Health and Human Services Office of Disease Prevention and Health Promotion: *Clinician's handbook of preventive services,* Washington, DC, 1994, US Government Printing Office. (Available as "Put Prevention into Family Practice," from the AAFP at 1-800-994-0000.)
10. The fifth report of the Joint National Committee on Detection, Evaluation, and Treatment of High Blood Pressure, NIH Pub No 93-1088, Bethesda, Md, 1993, National Institutes of Health.
11. Applegate WB: Hypertension in elderly patients, *Ann Intern Med* 110:901-915, 1989.
12. Taylor WC et al: Cholesterol reduction and life expectancy: a model incorporating multiple risk factors, *Ann Intern Med* 106:605-614, 1987.
13. Grover SA, Palmer CS, Coupal L: Serum lipid screening to iden-

The self-assessment questionnaire referred to on pp. 117 and 119 is mistakenly cited as Fig. 9-2. The citation should read Fig. 9-4, which is reproduced below.

Determine Your Nutritional Health

The warning signs of poor nutritional health are often overlooked. Use this checklist to find out if you or someone you know is at risk.

Read the statements below. Circle the number in the yes column for those that apply to you or someone you know. For each yes answer, score the number in the box. Total your nutritional score.

	YES
I have an illness or condition that made me change the kind and/or amount of food I eat.	2
I eat fewer than 2 meals per day.	3
I eat few fruits or vegetables, or milk products.	2
I have 3 or more drinks of beer, liquor, or wine almost every day.	2
I have tooth or mouth problems that make it hard for me to eat.	2
I don't always have enough money to buy the food I need.	4
I eat alone most of the time.	1
I take 3 or more different prescribed or over-the-counter drugs a day.	1
Without wanting to, I have lost or gained 10 pounds in the last 6 months.	2
I am not always physically able to shop, cook, and/or feed myself.	2
TOTAL	

Total Your Nutritional Score. If it's –

0-2 **Good!** Recheck your nutritional score in 6 months.

3-5 **You are at moderate nutritional risk.**
See what can be done to improve your eating habits and lifestyle. Your office on aging, senior nutrition program, senior citizens center, or health department can help. Recheck your nutritional score in 3 months.

6 or more **You are at high nutritional risk.**
Bring this checklist the next time you see your doctor, dietitian, or other qualified health or social service professional. Talk with them about any problems you may have. Ask for help to improve your nutritional health.

NOTE: Remember that warning signs suggest risk, but do not represent diagnosis of any condition.

FIG. 9-4 Self-assessment checklist for determining nutritional health. (From materials developed and distributed by the Nutrition Screening Initiative, a project of the American Academy of Family Physicians, the American Dietetic Association, and the National Council on Aging, Inc., and sponsored in part through a grant from Ross Products Division, Abbott Laboratories.)

tify high-risk individuals for coronary death, *Arch Intern Med* 154:679-684, 1994.

14. Toronto Working Group: Efficiency considerations: the cost-effectiveness of treating asymptomatic hypercholesterolemia, *J Clin Epidemiol* 43:1093-1101, 1990.

15. Hermanson B et al: Beneficial six-year outcome of smoking cessation in older men and women with coronary artery disease: results from the CASS registry, *N Engl J Med* 319:1365-1369, 1988.

16. Marshburn PB, Carr BR: The menopause and hormone replacement therapy. In *Principles of geriatric medicine and gerontology*, New York, 1994, McGraw-Hill.

17. Hennekens CH et al: An overview of the British and American aspirin studies (letter), *N Engl J Med* 318:923-924, 1988.

18. Manson JE et al: A prospective study of aspirin use and primary prevention of cardiovascular disease in women, *JAMA* 266:521-527, 1991.

19. Giavannucci E et al: Aspirin use and the risk for colorectal cancer and adenoma in male health professionals, *Ann Intern Med* 121:241-246, 1994.

20. National High Blood Pressure Education Program Working Group: Report on primary prevention of hypertension, *Arch Intern Med* 153:186-208, 1993.

21. Eddy DM: Screening for breast cancer, *Ann Intern Med* 111:389-399, 1989.

22. Mandelblatt JS et al: Breast cancer screening for elderly women with and without comorbid conditions, *Ann Intern Med* 116:722-730, 1992.

23. American Geriatrics Society Clinical Practice Committee: Screening for breast cancer in elderly women, *J Am Geriatr Soc* 37:883-884, 1989.

24. American Geriatrics Society Clinical Practice Committee: Screening for cervical carcinoma in elderly women, *J Am Geriatr Soc* 37:885-887, 1989.

25. Fletcher A: Screening for cancer of the cervix in elderly women, *Lancet* 335:97-99, 1990.

26. Toribara NW, Sleisenger MH: Screening for colorectal cancer, *N Engl J Med* 332:861-867, 1995.

27. Krahn MD et al: Screening for prostate cancer: a decision analytic view, *JAMA* 272:773-780, 1994.

28. Patriarca PA et al: Efficacy of influenza vaccine in nursing homes: reduction in illness and complications during an influenza A epidemic, *JAMA* 253:1136-1139, 1985.

29. Final results: Medicare influenza vaccine demonstration—selected states, 1988-1992, *MMWR* 42:601-604, 1993.

30. Margolis KL et al: Frequency of adverse reactions to influenza vaccine in the elderly: a randomized, placebo-controlled trial, *JAMA* 264:1139-1141, 1990.

31. American College of Physicians Task Force on Adult Immunization and Infectious Disease Society of America: *Guide to adult immunization*, Philadelphia, 1994, American College of Physicians.

32. Balestra DJ, Littenberg B: Should adult tetanus immunization be given as a single vaccination at age 65? A cost-effectiveness analysis, *J Gen Intern Med* 8:405-412, 1993.

33. Gallo JJ, Reichel W, Anderson LM: *Handbook of geriatric assessment*, ed 2, Rockville, Md, 1995, Aspen.

34. Uhlmann RF et al: Validity and reliability of auditory screening tests in demented and non-demented older adults, *J Gen Intern Med* 4:90-96, 1989.

35. Mulrow CD et al: Quality of life changes and hearing impairment: results of a randomized trial, *Ann Intern Med* 113:188-194, 1990.

36. Gallo JJ, Reichel W, Andersen L: Mental status testing. In *Handbook of geriatric assessment*, ed 2, Rockville, Md, 1995, Aspen.

37. Katzman R et al: Validation of a short orientation-memory-concentration test of cognitive impairment, *Am J Psychiatry* 140:734-739, 1983.

38. Jones TV, Williams ME: Mental status questionnaires: an opposing view, *J Fam Pract* 189:197-200, 1990.

39. Yesavage JA: The use of self-rating depression scales in the elderly. In Poon LW, ed: *Clinical memory assessment of older adults*, Washington, DC, 1986, American Psychological Association.

40. *Nutrition screening manual for professionals caring for older Americans*, Washington, DC, 1991, The Nutrition Screening Initiative.

41. Chandra RK: Effect of vitamin and trace-element supplementation on immune responses and infection in elderly subjects, *Lancet* 340:1124-1127, 1992.

42. Shephard RJ: The scientific basis of exercise prescribing for the very old, *J Am Geriatr Soc* 38:62-70, 1990.

43. Elward K, Larson EB: Benefits of exercise for older adults: a review of existing evidence and current recommendations for the general population, *Clin Geriatr Med* 8(1):35-50, 1992.

44. Fries JF: Aging, natural death and the compression of morbidity, *N Engl J Med* 303:130-135, 1980.

45. Rubenstein LZ: Geriatric medicine, *JAMA* 263:2644-2646, 1990.

46. Morey MC et al: Evaluation of a supervised exercise program in a geriatric population, *J Am Geriatr Soc* 37:348-354, 1989.

47. Foster VL et al: Endurance training for elderly women: moderate versus low intensity, *J Gerontol* 44:184-188, 1989.

48. Posner JD et al: Effects of exercise training in the elderly on the occurrence and time to onset of cardiovascular diagnoses, *J Am Geriatr Soc* 38:205-210, 1990.

49. Blair SN et al: Physical fitness and all-cause mortality: a prospective study of healthy men and women, *JAMA* 262:2395-2401, 1989.

PRETEST ANSWERS

1. c
2. c
3. b

POSTTEST ANSWERS

1. c
2. b
3. d
4. a
5. b
6. c

CHAPTER 9

Nutrition

JANE V. WHITE and RICHARD J. HAM

OBJECTIVES

Upon completion of this chapter, the reader will be able to:

1. Describe the outcomes of poor nutritional status in older persons.

2. List the risk factors for poor nutritional status in older Americans.

3. State the general dietary recommendations for older adults and cite examples of situations in which these recommendations may require modification.

4. Identify a system for assessing nutritional risk in older Americans.

5. List the indicators of poor nutritional status in older Americans.

6. Describe the diagnostic criteria for kwashiorkor and marasmus (the syndromes of protein energy malnutrition, or PEM).

7. Describe a methodology for the detection and diagnosis of malnutrition in primary care in older persons.

8. List and give examples of the range of nutrition interventions available to older persons in poor nutritional health.

9. Describe the general principles involved in the implementation of nutritional support.

PRETEST

1. When assessing food intake in older persons, evaluation of which one of the following parameters is essential?
   a. Serum albumin and cholesterol levels
   b. Body mass index (BMI)
   c. The frequency, type, and amount of food eaten
   d. Past medical history
2. Which one of the following represents a frequently unrecognized set of contributory factors to involuntary weight loss in older persons?
   a. Lack of sleep, restlessness, and irritability
   b. Oral health problems and depression
   c. Constipation with laxative abuse
   d. Caffeinated beverages and herbal teas
3. Which one of the following is not an indicator of poor nutritional status in an older person?
   a. Albumin of 3 g/dl
   b. Body mass index (BMI) of 23
   c. Cholesterol of 150 mg/dl
   d. Loss of 10% of body weight in 1 year

Many older Americans are undernourished, and this important aspect of their health is frequently unrecognized. Undernutrition places individuals at increased risk, especially if they become ill or need surgery. Chronic undernutrition contributes to long-term effects on health and well-being, energy, healing capacity, resistance to infection, and bowel function, to name but a few examples.

Older adults display a greater variance in nutritional needs and concerns than younger people do.[1] After middle age, adjustments to food intake must be made as metabolic needs decline and activity levels change. There is great heterogeneity: careful assessment of nutritional status in each individual and a nutrition prescription based on the unique and specific needs, culture, and education are essential.[2] Dietary enhancement with the least restrictive regimen possible is the aim.

> *Poor nutrition in old age is frequently unrecognized and neglected; it makes people more ill and more dependent than they need to be. Preventing it, recognizing it, and doing something active about it is everyone's responsibility.*

▼ BENJAMIN SMITH (Part I)

Benjamin Smith is a 75-year-old white man, never married, who was recently hospitalized for pneumonia with malnutrition. He returns to your office for follow-up, 2 weeks post hospitalization. His height is 72 inches; his weight at discharge was 148 lb (up from 132 lb on admission). His current weight is 145 lb. He completes a nutritional self-assessment questionnaire, which confirms that he lives alone; his closest neighbor lives 3 miles away on an adjacent piece of lakefront property. Although he worked as a chief loan officer for the bank for almost 30 years, he developed and maintained few close friendships, living with his widowed, chronically ill mother. As her only child, he had assumed total responsibility for her well-being for much of his adult life. She had refused domestic help and performed most of the household chores herself. You had forgotten that Mr. Smith's mother died about 6 months ago. Since that time, he has been feeling increasingly abandoned, tearful, and depressed. The questionnaire also reveals that he has limited food preparation skills, keeps little food in the house, and eats only one meal a day.

STUDY QUESTIONS
- *What factors place Mr. Smith at increased risk of poor nutritional status?*
- *What additional parameters could be used to further assess his nutritional health?*

RISK FACTORS FOR POOR NUTRITIONAL STATUS

Nutrition is vital to health promotion, disease prevention, chronic disease management, and illness and injury treatment. The outcome of chronically poor nutritional status and unrecognized or untreated malnutrition is frequently considerable dysfunction and disability,[3] reduced quality of life,[4-7] premature or increased morbidity and mortality,[8] and increased health care cost.[9-11]

A *risk factor* for poor nutritional status is defined as a characteristic or occurrence that increases the likelihood that an individual has, or will have, problems with nutrition.[12] Risk factors are typically cumulative and interrelated. As an individual's number of risk factors increases, the prevalence and the degree of impaired nutrition also increase.

Risk factors for poor nutritional status have been identified in older populations in a number of countries and are quite similar in nature, despite the ethnic, racial, and cultural differences of the populations reported.[12] Nutritional risk factors identified for U.S. elderly and the criteria by which they are assessed are summarized in Box 9-1.

Inappropriate Food Intake

It is critical to accurately estimate the food and fluid intake. Physicians should routinely evaluate the type,

---

BOX 9-1
Risk Factors for Poor Nutritional Status in Older Americans: Including Elements by which Risk is Assessed

Inappropriate Food Intake

Meal/snack frequency
Quality/quantity food
 consumed
 Milk/milk products
 Meat/meat alternates
 Fruit
 Vegetables
 Grain products
 Fats/sweets
Dietary modifications
 Self-imposed
 Prescribed
 Compliance
 Impact
Nutritional supplements
 used
 Type
 Amount

Poverty

Income
 Source
 Adequacy
Food expenditures/
 resources
Reliance on economic
 assistance program

Isolation

Support systems
 Availability
 Utilization
Living arrangements
 Cooking/food stor-
  age facilities
 Transportation
 Other

Dependence/Disability

Functional status
 ADLs
 IADLs
Disabling conditions
 Lack of manual dex-
  terity
 Use of assistive de-
  vices
Inactivity/immobility

Acute/Chronic Diseases or Conditions

Abnormalities of body
 weight
Alcohol abuse
Cognitive/emotional
 impairment
 Depression
 Dementia
Oral health problems
Pressure sores
Sensory impairment
Diet-related diseases
Others

Chronic Medication Use

Prescribed/self-
 administered
Polypharmacy
Quackery

Advanced Age

From White JV: Risk factors for poor nutritional status in older Americans, Washington, DC, 1991, Nutrition Screening Initiative, a project of the American Academy of Family Physicians, the American Dietetic Association, and the National Council on Aging, Inc. and funded in part by a grant from Ross Products Division, Abbott Laboratories.

---

amount, and frequency of food and fluid consumption in older patients. Recent food frequency surveys in U.S. adults document habitually poor intakes of vegetables, fruit, and dairy products by the majority of adults.[13,14] Other factors contributing to deficient or excessive food and nutrient intakes include mistaken health beliefs; distorted attitudes regarding food or body image; excessively restrictive dietary prescriptions; excessive or inadequate use of nutritional supplements; inability to shop for or to prepare food; and the need to adjust food consistency, flavor, or temperature. These factors must also be regularly assessed. Minorities and the educationally or economically deprived tend to have the poorest food and nutrient intakes. The declines in total body water and the ability to concentrate urine and the diminished sensation of thirst that all occur with aging place the elderly at increased risk of dehydration. Because of this possibility, attention must focus on fluid management as well as food intake.

Published guidelines regarding recommended nutrient intakes[1] and healthful diets[15,16] for older persons are somewhat limited by a lack of reference data specific to the needs of the older population. However, such guidelines offer a reasonable starting point for nutrition education and counseling (Fig. 9-1). Table 9-1 summarizes the basic food intake recommendations for older adults. These include increased consumption of complex carbohydrates (grains, fruits, and vegetables), moderate protein intakes, and limitation of dietary fat to 30% or less of the total daily calories. Moderation in salt, sugar, and alcohol consumption is stressed. Of course, dietary guidance must always be individualized.

A variety of formulas for estimating caloric needs are available. Two that are frequently used are shown in Box 9-2. Both are based on the utilization of either actual weight (if appropriate) or desirable body weight (DBW). Although in ambulatory populations a less complex formula can be used to estimate caloric needs reliably, in metabolically stressed individuals (such as in acute or long-term care settings), estimates of caloric needs must be more precise. The caloric need is the starting point in providing individualized dietary guidance or nutritional support.

Poverty

Whereas the poverty rate for older persons is about the same as for younger adults (over 12%), another 8% of the elderly are "near poor" (their income is between the poverty level and 125% of it). Older women have a 15% poverty rate, compared with a poverty rate of only 8% in men in 1993, and older persons living alone or with nonrelatives were much more likely to be poor (24%) than if they lived in families (6%). Forty-four percent of older black women living alone lived in poverty in 1993. This means that approximately 31% of males and 61% of fe-

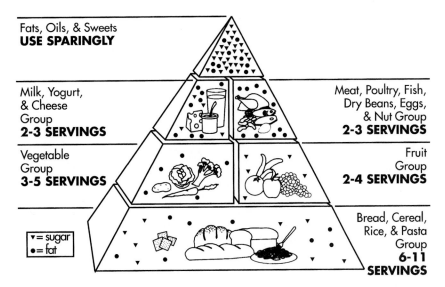

FIG. 9-1   Food Guide Pyramid. (From U.S. Department of Agriculture/U.S. Department of Health and Human Services.)

males aged 65 years and over subsist on annual incomes of $10,000 or less.[17] Clearly this reduces access to food and limits food choices. Basic needs such as utilities, phone, medication, and transportation compete for food dollars and are often perceived as more pressing. Anything indicative of limited economic resources, such as reliance on economic assistance programs, is a warning sign of nutritional risk.

Isolation

As individuals age, loss of family members, friends, income, independence, and self-esteem is virtually inevitable. In the United States, approximately 16% of males and 42% of females aged 65 years and older live alone.[17] Living alone contributes to nutritional risk through apathy, depression, and a lack of motivation to self-care.[18] There may be self-neglect or even suicidal tendencies.

Preparing and eating meals alone is difficult, even when an individual is in the prime of life and in perfect health. Thus questions regarding living arrangements and frequency of family member or other social contact should be routinely asked. Community resources to facilitate social life and interpersonal skills will enhance access to food.

Limited Literacy

Another factor that isolates and reduces compliance, leading to poor health outcomes, is limited literacy.[19] The average reading level of U.S. adults is fourth- to sixth-grade. However, much of physicians' patient education material and many of their instructions are written at a high school or college level.[20] Individuals who are unable to read may have difficulty grasping concepts such as one-to-one correspondence, sets (i.e., food

groups), time of day, and so forth. Information about medication schedules, appointment times, dietary guidance, and social services access may not be understood. Brief assessment of reading and comprehension level and learning style is necessary in patients who are noncompliant, require multiple medications, or are habitually late for, or chronically miss, appointments.[21] Simple language, pictures, videos, and other devices may improve comprehension.

Dependence and Disability

Progressive illnesses such as Alzheimer's, catastrophic events such as stroke with persistent disability, and age-associated, gradual, progressive decline are common causes of functional impairment.[22] But whether the cause is cognitive, emotional, or physical, functional impairment in older persons decreases independence, reduces self-esteem, impedes the maintenance of interpersonal relationships, and hampers the performance of customary activities, including self-care.[18,22,23] Functional assessment, especially the ability to procure, prepare, and consume adequate food and nutrients, must be routinely and recurrently reviewed. Should a problem be identified, a more focused evaluation of the many skills related to food acquisition, preparation, and eating should be implemented so that interventions can be appropriately targeted.[24]

Acute and Chronic Diseases or Conditions

Recent surgery, significant trauma or infection, recent hospitalization, or the initiation or withdrawal of nutrition support plus any acute or chronic illness, are elements of the medical history that should serve as warning signs of increased nutritional risk. Clinicians should

Table 9-1   Basic Meal Pattern for Older Adults

Food Group	Servings/Day	Serving Equivalents
Breads and cereals	6-11	1 slice whole grain or enriched bread
		1 dinner roll, muffin, tortilla
		½ English muffin, hamburger bun
		1 oz ready-to-eat cereal
		½ cup pasta, rice, cooked cereal
		3-4 small plain crackers
Vegetables	3-5	1 cup raw leafy vegetables
		½ cup cooked or chopped raw vegetable
		¾ cup juice
		Include dark green, leafy, or yellow/orange varieties at least 3-4 times per week.
Fruit	2-4	1 medium piece fresh fruit
		½ cup cooked or canned fruit
		¾ cup juice
		¼ cup dried fruit
		Include citrus fruit or juice, berries, melon, or other rich sources of vitamin C daily.
Dairy products	2-4	1 cup fluid milk or yogurt
		1 ½ oz natural cheese
		2 oz processed cheese
		½ cup cottage cheese, ice cream, frozen yogurt, pudding, or custard
		1 cup soup made with milk
		Cottage cheese, frozen desserts, pudding, and custard have ¼ to ⅓ the calcium per serving of milk, yogurt, or cheese.
Meat and meat alternates	2-3 (6-7 oz total)	2-3 oz cooked lean meat, fish, poultry
		The following equal 1 oz of meat:
		1 egg
		½ cup cooked dried beans or peas
		2 tbs peanut butter
		¼ cup seeds or nuts
Fats and sweets	As needed for calories	
Alcohol	In moderation	Do not exceed any one of:
		1-2 mixed drinks
		1-2 beers (12 oz cans)
		1-2 glasses wine (4-8 oz)

Modified from USDA Food Guide Pyramid, Washington, DC, 1992, Government Printing Office.

routinely inquire for signs or symptoms of nutritional deficiency or toxicity. They should also look for poor control of diet-related diseases, self-initiated supplements, "health food" consumption, and self-modification of the diet.[12]

Sensory changes that occur with age increase the risks, too. Hearing and visual losses have an impact upon one in three persons over age 65.[25] They contribute to social isolation, depression, and declines in mobility and functional status, leading to difficulty in obtaining, preparing, and consuming an adequate diet. Age-related declines in the senses of taste and smell are poorly understood but often impair food intake and dining pleasure.[26] A recent study suggests that the addition of flavor enhancers to food provided to older nursing home residents may significantly increase food intake and nutritional health.[27]

Poor oral hygiene contributes to dental caries, plaque accumulation, periodontal disease and, when unattended, to multiple missing or decayed teeth.[28-30] Many older adults also report changes in the type or texture of foods that they eat, changes in food taste, taking longer to eat, hesitation about eating with others, and discomfort in a variety of dining and social settings, all of which may be due to compromised oral health. As the number and type of dental problems increase in each individual, nutritional status declines.[29]

Significant changes in renal structure and function occur with age. Disease states such as atherosclerosis, sepsis, hypertension, diabetes mellitus, and heart failure make older persons more susceptible to acute and chronic renal failure, as do polypharmacy, the increased occurrence of obstructive uropathies (particularly in older males), and prerenal hemodynamic compromise.[31]

BOX 9-2
Formulas for Estimating Caloric Needs

Office Method:

1. Measure the patient's actual height and weight, obtain age.
2. Compare to established norms to determine whether the patient needs to change his or her caloric consumption.
3. Multiply the appropriate number of calories (listed below) by the patient's actual or ideal weight (in pounds) to derive an estimate of daily caloric needs:

Activity level	*Calories/lb*
Overweight:	
Sedentary	8-12
Moderate	14
Strenuous	16
Normal Weight:	
Sedentary	14
Moderate	16
Strenuous	18
Underweight:	
Sedentary	16
Moderate	18
Strenuous	20-23

1. Subtract 100 calories per decade from the above figure for individuals 35 years of age and older.
2. Add or subtract 500 to 1000 calories per day to or from the above figure, in order to gain or lose 1 to 2 pounds per week.

Hospital/Long Term Care Facility Method:
Harris-Benedict Equation:

Men: $66.47 + (13.75w) + (5h) - (6.76a) \times$ activity factor $\times$ injury factor

Women: $655.10 + (9.56w) + (1.85h) - (4.86a) \times$ activity factor $\times$ injury factor

w = weight in kg, h = height in cm, a = age in years

Activity Factor:	*Injury Factor:*	
Bed rest 1.2	Starvation	0.7
Ambulatory 1.3	Minor surgery	1.00-1.20
	Peritonitis	1.20-1.50
	Soft tissue trauma	1.14-1.37
	Skeletal trauma	1.35
	Major sepsis	1.40-1.80
	Fever (per degree F above 98.6° F)	1.07

---

nutrition education, creativity, and support are required to enhance patient acceptance and use. Products containing essential amino acids or their analogues are sometimes used to augment dietary efforts. Hemodialysis, peritoneal dialysis, and renal transplantation are of course the treatments of choice when conservative management is not effective.

The elements of a comprehensive nutrition history and physical exam are listed in Table 9-2. Leading diet-related causes of death in U.S. adults ages 65 years and older are heart disease (ischemic and hypertensive), cancer, stroke, and diabetes mellitus; these disease processes account for approximately 71% of deaths in those over 65.[17]

▼ ROSA WHITE (Part I)

Rosa White is an obese, hypertensive, diabetic, 67-year-old white female patient of yours with a history of congestive heart failure, esophageal reflux, hypothyroidism, diabetic neuropathy, and recent onset of mild renal failure. She is extremely independent and often cantankerous, with limited tolerance of her children's involvement in her personal life. She is 62 inches tall and her weight today is 162 lb, a decrease of 7 lb over the last month. Her blood pressure is 160/70 sitting and standing. Her son brings her to your office for follow-up and is concerned about her increasing confusion, decreased appetite, and recurrent urinary tract complaints. She has been a very difficult and frustrating patient to manage over the years because of her failure to keep appointments and her poor compliance. When you ask her to complete a nutrition self-assessment form, you discover that she is unable to read. Her son states that she has a very limited understanding of her medical condition and its implications. He indicates willingness to assist his mother in the management of her medical conditions, but he states that his reading ability is "not very good." He does understand how to tell time and count. He is able to assist his mother to complete a nutrition self-assessment questionnaire. Urinalysis shows 2 to 6 RBCs, WBCs too numerous to count, and a large quantity of bacteria. A urine culture is ordered.

STUDY QUESTIONS

- Which factors, if any, suggest that Ms. White is at increased nutritional risk?
- What additional aspects of nutritional status should be assessed?

Conservative management of renal disease properly includes regulation of the protein, sodium, potassium, phosphorus, and fluid content of the diet. Such diets are often poorly understood and marginally implemented, and they can be monotonous and tasteless. Considerable

Medication Use

The use of prescribed or self-selected medications, particularly on a chronic basis, has great potential to reduce nutritional status. Inappropriate prescription, misuse of prescribed or over-the-counter medications, concurrent or intermittent use of multiple drugs, and the interac-

Table 9-2   Components of the History and Physical That Assess Nutritional Status

History	
Identifying data	Age, sex, ethnic origin, religious preference, marital status
Medical component	Chief complaint (especially if diet-related)
	Presence of chronic disease or allergy
	Recent major illness or surgery
	Family history (diet-related disease)
	Usual weight and recent involuntary weight change
	Dental history
	Cognitive/emotional status
	Medications
	Exercise and sleep patterns
Psychosocial component	Occupation, income level
	Participation in economic assistance programs
	Living arrangements
	Transportation
	Shopping patterns
	Educational and reading level and learning style
	Motivation and compliance
Nutrition component	Changes in sensory perception
	Appetite
	Current meal and snack pattern
	Food intake over the last 24 hours
	Food preferences and tolerances
	Major food group intake
	Current and previous dietary modifications (duration, compliance, results)
	Use of supplements (purpose, content, frequency)
Physical	General appearance
	Measured height, weight, vital signs
	Other anthropometric parameters as indicated
	Physical signs and symptoms of nutrient deficiency or toxicity
	Oral cavity examination
	Vision and hearing status
Laboratory	Serum albumin (especially if hospitalized or institutionalized)
	Serum cholesterol (periodic monitoring: modify diet if elevated; check additional parameters if low)
	Blood glucose (especially postprandial)
	Hemoglobin/hematocrit, CBC
	Vitamin B_{12} (especially vegan diets or GI pathology)
	Individual nutrients: e.g., K, Mg, Na (signs, symptoms, or chronic drug use dictates choice)

tion of drugs with food, nutrients, or alcohol are all areas of concern.

Prescription drugs are estimated to be used by 82% of all older persons in the United States.[32] Three out of four office visits to primary care physicians are related to the initiation or continuance of medications. Many older individuals, particularly those living in institutional settings, consume multiple different drugs daily.[12,33,34] Table 9-3 lists the categories of drugs frequently consumed by older people that have the potential to influence nutritional status negatively. Drug use must be reviewed frequently. Ask about prescribed and over-the-counter medications, nutritional supplements, "health foods," and alcohol. Make patients aware of dietary precautions or special dietary instructions related to drug use.[35]

▼ ROSA WHITE (Part II)

A review of Rosa White's medical records reveals the following list of medications: insulin (Novolin) 70/30 U AM and 5 U PM; glyburide (DiaBeta) 5 mg tid; ciprofloxacin (Cipro) 750 mg bid; bumetanide (Bumex) 1 mg daily; captopril (Capoten) 6.25 mg bid; nizatidine (Axid) 300 mg hs; metoclopramide (Reglan) 10 mg bid; metolazone (Zaroxolyn) 2.5 mg daily, Niferex (iron/vitamins) bid; Maalox (aluminum hydrox-

Table 9-3   Common Drugs in the Elderly That Can Negatively Influence Nutrition

Drug	Nutrition-Related Side Effects
Alcohol	Anorexia, altered consciousness, amnesia, dizziness, headache, lethargy, paresthesias, vitamin/mineral deficiencies, weakness
Analgesics	
Aspirin	Anemia, GI hemorrhage
Antibiotics	Anorexia, diarrhea, nausea, vomiting
Antiinflammatory Agents	
Corticosteroids	Anorexia, appetite stimulation, edema, hyperglycemia, osteoporosis, weight gain
Nonsteroidal antiinflammatory agents (NSAIDs)	Anemia, GI hemorrhage, edema, weight gain
Cardiovascular Agents	
Antiarrhythmics	Anorexia, nausea, vomiting
ACE-inhibitors	Anorexia, dry mouth, gastritis, hypoalbuminemia, hyperkalemia, loss of taste, nausea, weight loss
β-Blockers (lipid soluble)	Constipation, cramping, diarrhea, epigastric distress, nausea, vomiting, worsening of diabetic glucose control
Calcium channel blockers	Anorexia, constipation, diarrhea, dry mouth, dysgeusia, edema, nausea, vomiting
Diuretics	Anorexia, constipation, cramping, dehydration, diarrhea, fluid/electrolyte imbalance, gastric irritation, hyperglycemia, hyperlipidemia, hyperuricemia, nausea, vomiting
Cardiac glycosides	Anorexia, drug interactions, nausea, loss of taste, weight loss
Potassium supplements	Anorexia, gastric irritation, hyperkalemia
CNS Agents	
Anticonvulsants	Anemia, antivitamin effects, hyperglycemia, oral health problems, nausea, osteoporosis, vomiting
Antidepressants	Anorexia, appetite stimulation, constipation, drowsiness, dry mouth, weight gain
Antipsychotics	Appetite stimulation, constipation, dry mouth, fluid retention, weight gain
Endocrine/Metabolic Agents	
Oral hypoglycemic agents	Appetite stimulation, dizziness, hypoglycemia
Gastrointestinal Agents	
Antacids	Drug/nutrient binding, malabsorption, reduced iron absorption
Laxatives	Dehydration, diarrhea, malabsorption, weight loss
H$_2$-receptor antagonists	Confusion, diarrhea, dizziness, somnolence

Modified from White JV: Risk factors associated with poor nutritional status in older Americans, Washington, DC, 1991, Nutrition Screening Initiative, a project of the American Academy of Family Physicians, the American Dietetic Association, and the National Council on Aging, Inc. and funded in part by a grant from Ross Products Division, Abbott Laboratories.

ide–magnesium carbonate gel) 30 ml at bedtime; K-Dur (potassium chloride) 40 mEq daily; levothyroxine sodium (Synthroid) 0.2 mg daily. She can take these medicines throughout the day, except for the insulin, glyburide, captopril, metolazone, and ciprofloxacin, all of which she takes as prescribed. She avoids "sweets" and salty foods. Her favorite foods are beef, pork, and cheese, which she eats daily. She is afraid to eat too many fruits, vegetables, or grain products, because she's heard they "run your sugar up." A random blood sugar measurement, approximately 2 hours after lunch, is 65 mg/dl.

STUDY QUESTIONS

- *Identify any additional contributors to Ms. White's poor nutritional status.*
- *Identify any revisions to Ms. White's diet and medication regimen that you feel are indicated, and outline an approach to their implementation.*

Summary

A self-assessment questionnaire designed for persons 65 years of age and older by which older persons themselves

Complete the following screen by interviewing the patient directly and/or by referring to the patient chart. If you do not routinely perform all of the described tests or ask all of the listed questions, please consider including them but do not be concerned if the entire screen is not completed. Please try to conduct a minimal screen on as many older patients as possible, and please try to collect serial measurements, which are extremely valuable in monitoring nutritional status. Please refer to the manual for additional information.

Anthropometrics

Measure height to the nearest inch and weight to the nearest pound. Record the values below and mark them on a Body Mass Index (BMI) scale.* Then use a straight edge (paper, ruler) to connect the two points and circle the spot where this straight line crosses the center line (body mass index). Record the number below; healthy older adults should have a BMI between 22 and 27; check the appropriate box to flag an abnormally high or low value.

Height (in): _____
Weight (lbs): _____
Body Mass Index
(weight/height^2): _____

Please place a check by any statement regarding BMI and recent weight loss that is true for the patient.

□ Body mass index <22

□ Body mass index >27

□ Has lost or gained 10 pounds (or more) of body weight in the past 6 months

Record the measurement of mid-arm circumference to the nearest 0.1 centimeter and of triceps skinfold to the nearest 2 millimeters.

Mid-Arm Circumference (cm): _____
Triceps Skinfold (mm): _____
Mid-Arm Muscle Circumference (cm): _____

Refer to the table and check any abnormal values:

□ Mid-arm muscle circumference <10th percentile

□ Triceps skinfold <10th percentile

□ Triceps skinfold >95th percentile

*A nomogram can be used if desired.

NOTE: Mid-arm circumference (cm)−[0.314 × triceps skinfold (mm)]=mid-arm *muscle* circumference (cm)

Percentile	Men		Women	
	55-65 yr	65-75 yr	55-65 yr	65-75 yr
Arm circumference (cm)				
10th	27.3	26.3	25.7	25.2
50th	31.7	30.7	30.3	29.9
95th	36.9	35.5	38.5	37.3
Arm muscle circumference (cm)				
10th	24.5	23.5	19.6	19.5
50th	27.8	26.8	22.5	22.5
95th	32.0	30.6	28.0	27.9
Triceps skinfold (mm)				
10th	6	6	16	14
50th	11	11	25	24
95th	22	22	38	36

From Frisancho AR: *Am J Clin Nutr* 34:2540-2545, 1981.

For the remaining sections, please place a check by any statements that are true for the patient.

Laboratory Data

□ Serum albumin below 3.5 g/dl

□ Serum cholesterol below 160 mg/dl

□ Serum cholesterol above 240 mg/dl

Drug Use

□ Three or more prescription drugs, OTC medications, and/or vitamin/mineral supplements daily.

Clinical Features

Presence of (check each that apply):

□ Problems with mouth, teeth, or gums

□ Difficulty chewing

□ Difficulty swallowing

□ Angular stomatitis

□ Glossitis

□ History of bone pain

□ History of bone fractures

□ Skin changes (dry, loose, nonspecific lesions, edema)

Eating Habits

□ Does not have enough food to eat each day

□ Usually eats alone

FIG. 9-2   Level II Screen (including mental status and functional assessment). (From materials developed by the Nutrition Screening Initiative.)

□ Does not eat anything on one or more days each month

□ Has poor appetite

□ Is on a special diet

□ Eats vegetables two or fewer times daily

□ Eats milk or milk products once or not at all daily

□ Eats fruit or drinks fruit juice once or not at all daily

□ Eats breads, cereals, pasta, rice, or other grains five or fewer times daily

□ Has more than one alcoholic drink per day (if woman); more than two drinks per day (if man)

Living Environment

□ Lives on an income of less than $6000 per year (per individual in the household)

□ Lives alone

□ Is housebound

□ Is concerned about home security

□ Lives in a home with inadequate heating or cooling

□ Does not have a stove and/or refrigerator

□ Is unable or prefers not to spend money on food (<$25-$30 per person spent on food each week)

Functional Status

Usually or always needs assistance with (check each that apply):

□ Bathing

□ Dressing

□ Grooming

□ Toileting

□ Eating

□ Walking or moving about

□ Traveling (outside the home)

□ Preparing food

□ Shopping for food or other necessities

Mental/Cognitive Status

□ Clinical evidence of impairment (e.g., Folstein<26)

□ Clinical evidence of depressive illness (e.g., Beck Depression Inventory>15, Geriatric Depression Scale>5)

Patients in whom you have identified one or more major indicator of poor nutritional status require immediate medical attention; if minor indicators are found, ensure that they are known to a health professional or to the patient's own physician. Patients who display risk factors of poor nutritional status should be referred to the appropriate health care or social service professional (dietitian, nurse, dentist, case manager, etc.).

FIG. 9-2, cont'd.

or a caregiver or family member can assess the risk of poor nutritional status has been developed (Fig. 9-2). This serves as an initial screen and as a general educational device. It is often a useful starting point for the initiation of nutrition assessment, diet and lifestyle education, and when necessary, the implementation of nutrition counseling and support for elders vulnerable to the ravages of malnutrition.

INDICATORS OF POOR NUTRITIONAL STATUS

If an individual is at increased risk of poor nutritional status, the physician must look for the signs and symptoms of it. Serial observation of such indicators can be done effectively in the primary care office to pick up insidious development of trends. Such an assessment may be needed as a matter of urgency if an individual becomes seriously ill (e.g., with sepsis) or is facing acute surgery, situations in which even slight nutritional compromise will rapidly deteriorate into a situation of acute undernourishment. Indicators of poor nutritional status are observable and recordable signs and symptoms that can be sought.[36] Box 9-3 lists the major indicators that were agreed on by expert consensus and are widely recognized as useful in the recognition and treatment of malnutrition in people of any age.[37] The importance of monitoring change over time in the majority of these indicators cannot be overemphasized; they can be used to assess the impact of intervention as well as the downward spiral of worsening malnutrition. Prompt recognition and early, appropriate intervention can reduce the misery, suffering, and expense of the sequelae of malnutrition.

Abnormalities of Body Weight

Height and weight are the most commonly used and most easily obtained measures of body composition. Weight should be measured each time an individual presents for care. It should be measured using a carefully calibrated scale, with the person dressed in indoor clothing and with shoes off. Height is generally measured by a sliding bar attached to the scale. Height should be measured with the individual's shoes removed and with the person's back to the measuring bar. It should be measured at least annually since it is subject to change. When actual measurement of height and weight is impossible because of disability or infirmity, an estimate of height and weight through alternative anthropometric techniques can be calculated and is reasonably accurate.[36-39]

Significantly low or high weight for height or a body mass index (BMI) less than 22 or greater than 27 indicate poor nutritional status. (BMI is the body weight in kg divided by the square of the height in meters.) Women with a waist/hip ratio indicative of significant abdominal fat accumulation show an increased risk of adverse health outcomes, a pattern observed in both smokers and nonsmokers.[39,40]

Serum Albumin

A low serum albumin (<3.5 g/dl) is a sensitive indicator of undernutrition, but many other factors including CHF, hypoxia, trauma, sepsis, renal failure, dehydration, hepatic insufficiency, major surgery, and bed rest can also modify it.[36,41,42] Low serum albumin levels are negatively associated with length of stay and outcome disposition.[41,42] Other laboratory investigations, all of which may be normal in an individual who is in fact nutritionally compromised but which may sometimes provide a clinical hint, include the *CBC* (look for macrocytosis from vitamin B_{12} or folate deficiency or for reduced lymphocyte count, which measures immune status), *folate* (serum or red cell, which if reduced indicates consumption of a limited variety and quantity of foods), *vitamin C* and B_{12} levels, *cholesterol* (levels below 160 mg/dl in

---

BOX 9-3
Major Indicators of Poor Nutritional Status in Older Americans

Significant Weight Loss Over Time
≥5.0% body weight in 1 month
≥7.5% body weight in 3 months
≥10.0% body weight in 6 months
Involuntary weight loss of ≥10 pounds in 6 months

Significantly Low or High Weight for Height
20% below or above desirable body weight for the individual (includes consideration of loss of height due to vertebral collapse, kyphosis, deformity)
BMI <22 or >27

Significant Reduction in Serum Albumin
<3.5 g/dl

Significant Decline in Functional Status
Change from "independent" to "dependent" in two of the ADLs or one of the nutrition-related IADLs

Significant Inappropriate Food Intake
Failure to consume the U.S. Dietary Guidelines recommended minimum from one or more basic food groups, with insufficient variety of foods
Failure to observe moderation in salt and sugar intakes or to observe saturated fat limitations (when indicated)
Alcohol consumption >1 oz/day (women) or >2 oz/day (men)

Significant Reduction in Midarm Circumference
<10th percentile NHANES standards

Significant Decrease or Increase in Skinfold Measurements
<10th percentile or >95th percentile NHANES standards

Selected Nutrition-Related Disorders
Osteoporosis
Osteomalacia
Folate deficiency
Vitamin B_{12} deficiency
Pressure sores

Modified from Ham RJ: Indicators of poor nutritional status in older Americans, Washington, DC, 1991, Nutrition Screening Initiative, a project of the American Academy of Family Physicians, the American Dietetic Association, and the National Council on Aging, Inc. and funded in part by a grant from Ross Products Division, Abbott Laboratories.

the elderly are consistent with poor nutritional status), and *BUN* (nonspecific, but elevated in dehydrated persons). Some physicians would add *zinc* and *vitamin A* as laboratory values to consider.

Physical Signs and Symptoms

Lists of the physical signs and symptoms of vitamin or mineral deficiency or toxicity have been developed and are readily available in most standard nutrition texts.[36] It is important to remember that a single physical finding (e.g., angular stomatitis) may have a variety of etiologies (e.g., malnutrition, candidiasis, poorly fitting dentures). A nutritional etiology for a physical finding is more probable when a series of related physical signs and symptoms occurs in more than one body part (e.g., skin, eyes, lips, hair).

PROTEIN-ENERGY MALNUTRITION

Primary care physicians must be familiar with protein-energy malnutrition (PEM; also known as protein-calorie malnutrition, or PCM), including the current nomenclature, in view of its increasing recognition in many vulnerable populations, especially in the nursing home. It is a syndrome characterized by a person's having too little lean body mass, secondary to too little energy or protein being supplied. Several of the general signs and symptoms of undernutrition already mentioned are often present in this syndrome, but there are two clinical patterns to be clinically distinguished: marasmus and kwashiorkor (hypoalbuminemic malnutrition). Increased risk of PEM occurs in those with dementia, the homebound or bedridden, the poor, those discharged after long hospital stays, those with hip fracture, those in long-term institutional care (especially if they have pressure sores), and persons with any long-term chronic illness.

Using the presence of just two indicators as the criteria for PEM, the prevalence in long-term care facilities ranges from 19% to 27% and from 33% to 58% in acute care hospitals on general medical and surgical units.[43,44] Data regarding the homebound are lacking.[45] The number of homebound, nutritionally vulnerable elders can be expected to increase, in view of the high cost of institutional care and increasing incentives to maintain patients at home. The documentation of an abnormally low body weight, recent significant weight loss, a BMI less than 22, or a low serum albumin level suggests that PEM is present and should be addressed. Frequent infections and pressure sore development are the common consequences and often the presenting symptoms of PEM.[46] Criteria are summarized in Table 9-4.

Marasmus is the PEM syndrome that develops gradually over time when energy intake is insufficient. It is the acute status in which many elders enter the hospital. In response to starvation, fat stores are mobilized. Decreased insulin secretion causes fatty acid release. Hepatic glucose is released and skeletal muscle is broken down. The basal metabolic rate (BMR) and proteolysis are both decreased in an attempt to conserve body mass, and fatty acids and ketones are used for energy. Since skeletal muscle, rather than plasma proteins or visceral protein, is metabolized, there are general wasting and prominent weight loss, but there is generally a normal serum albumin level. The clinical course is over months or years.

Kwashiorkor is the more acute or subacute type of PEM and is frequently superimposed on marasmus, the precipitant being the stress of acute illness; it may develop over weeks but is often more acute. Hormonal changes mediate a combination of stress and low intake, leading to an increase in the BMR. There is increased sympathetic output to maintain the blood pressure. Antidiuretic hormone and aldosterone secretion are increased, and there is retention of sodium and water. Skeletal muscle and fat are broken down, and several hormonal processes lead to hyperglycemia. Monokines and tumor necrosis factor are released, both tending to cause anorexia; tumor necrosis factor also decreases albumin production and accelerates skeletal muscle breakdown. Thus the appetite is lost, compounding the problem. Serum proteins are depleted, with consequent edema, so there is frequently no weight loss. Once developed, this PEM syndrome has a high mortality rate.

It must be emphasized that the symptoms and signs of PEM are nonspecific, and other conditions, such as underlying malignancy, malabsorption, hyperthyroidism, peptic ulcer, and liver disease, need to be ruled out. PEM frequently coincides and complicates other conditions, and it can easily be neglected while the clinician focuses elsewhere on the medical treatment.

NUTRITION SCREENING AND ASSESSMENT TOOLS

A simple, systematic approach to the screening and assessment of the nutritional status of individual older persons has been developed by consensus of the Nutrition Screening Initiative.[47] Key considerations in the development, design, and use of these tools are their ease of administration, acceptance, relevance, and cost-effectiveness. Not all aspects of each tool are needed in all settings. They are designed to be adapted to various sites of service delivery, ranging from senior centers to the primary care office. These protocols facilitate the collection of diverse elements of the history and physical examination, cognitive examination, and laboratory studies into one quickly reviewable database. Most elements do not require physician time to input.

Self-Assessment/Enhanced Awareness

The self-assessment tool shown in Fig. 9-2 is designed to heighten public awareness of nutrition in older persons.[47] It uses a checklist format and is written at a

Table 9-4 Classification of Protein-Energy Malnutrition (PEM)

ICD9-CM Code	Diagnosis	Anthropometrics	Weight as % of standard weight for height	Albumin	Cause	Characteristics
260.0	*Kwashiorkor:* nutritional edema with dyspigmentation of skin and hair	Normal	More than 90%	Less 3.0 g/dl	Acute energy and protein deficiency or metabolic response to injury	Edema, muscle catabolism, weakness, neurological change, loss of vigor, secondary infection, changes in hair
261.0	*Marasmus:* nutritional atrophy and severe malnutrition	Depressed	Less than 80% (or loss of more than 10% of usual in 6 months, with muscle wasting)	Over 3.0 g/dl	Chronic deficiency of intake	Catabolism of fat and muscle, generalized weakness, weight loss
262.0	*3rd-degree PEM:* edema without dyspigmentation of skin and hair	Depressed	Weight less than 60%	Less than 3.0 g/dl	Marasmic patient exposed to stress	Combination of marasmus and kwashiorkor, high infection risk, poor wound healing
263.0	*2nd-degree PEM:* moderate malnutrition	Depressed	60%-80%	3.0-3.3 g/dl		
263.1	*1st-degree PEM:* mild malnutrition	Depressed	75%-90%	Over 3.4 g/dl		

Modified from International Classification of Diseases, ninth revision (ICD-9).

fourth- to sixth-grade reading level. Simple language and concepts are used. The checklist is not a definitive diagnostic device. Overidentification of individuals at risk is intended so that those in greatest need of nutritional guidance or support will not be overlooked.

Community Assessment/Nutrition and Social Services Outreach

A simple, systematic approach to the recognition and quantification of nutritional risk in community dwelling elderly is offered by the Level I Screen.[47] It is designed to be used by a broad range of health or social services personnel in a variety of community settings, from health departments to senior centers to public assistance office. Assessment elements include a brief review of body weight, eating habits, living environment, and functional status. Neither a physician nor laboratory studies are required.

The Level I Screen helps to target those individuals who are at increased nutritional risk and who may need assistance in accessing a range of nutrition and social services to facilitate the selection, procurement, prepa-

ration, and consumption of a healthful diet. It offers a mechanism for identifying individuals with a significant involuntary change in weight or those whose weight falls outside of recommended norms. It prompts referral of such high-risk elders to a primary health care provider for assessment and intervention. Because the elements contained in the Level I Screen are repeated and expanded in the Level II Screen, the Level I Screen is not separately reproduced here. Copies of this screen are available from the Nutrition Screening Initiative.[47,48]

Professional Assessment/Definitive Diagnosis

Because the Level II Screen contains more sophisticated and targeted physical examination, laboratory, mental status, and functional assessment elements (Fig. 9-2), it is designed to be generally performed with involvement of a physician.[47] It is a structured approach to the diagnosis of nutritional problems common in U.S. elderly; it facilitates selection and implementation of diagnostic and therapeutic measures. An approach to the office implementation of such a protocol is outlined in Box 9-4.

Receptionist

Routes phone calls
Performs triage
Schedules appointments
Distributes self-assessment checklist

Nurse

Collects, reviews, and scores checklist
Performs anthropometric measurements (height, weight, others)
Alerts physician to individuals at risk
Facilitates access to interventions
Initiates patient education

Physician

Reviews checklist
Implements Level II Screen
Determines diagnosis
Writes prescription
Makes referral (Registered Dietitian, dentist, social worker, etc.)
Performs follow-up

Insurance Clerk

Does coding (ICD-9/CPT must match)
Manages billing and reimbursement

Modified from *Incorporating nutrition screening and interventions into medical practice: a monograph for physicians,* Washington, DC, 1994, Nutrition Screening Initiative, a project of the American Academy of Family Physicians, the American Dietetic Association, and the National Council on Aging, Inc. and funded in part by a grant from Ross Products Division, Abbott Laboratories.

Summary

The commitment to screen and assess the nutritional status of older individuals routinely is a low-cost, low-tech strategy that can be easily and efficiently implemented in a variety of health care settings. This provides an excellent opportunity to improve health and well-being and to limit health care costs for the nutritionally vulnerable segment of our society.

▼ BENJAMIN SMITH (Part II)

Completion of a Level II Screen shows that Mr. Smith is unwilling to spend money for food that he is not willing to prepare. He purchases and eats a sandwich and chips at the local deli, 6 days a week. On Sundays, he accompanies church members to the local cafeteria where he eats a large, fairly well-balanced meal. His intake of alcoholic beverages has in-creased to 4 to 6 drinks per day in the months since his mother's death. He has been actively trying to lose weight by eating no more than one meal a day since he read somewhere that "thin people live longer." His score is 8/15 on the Geriatric Depression Scale.

STUDY QUESTIONS
- *List additional contributors to Mr. Smith's increased nutritional risk.*
- *Identify appropriate nutrition interventions.*

NUTRITION INTERVENTIONS

Once a nutritional problem has been identified, persistent, often recurrent, action must be taken. The causes of poor nutritional status are multifactorial. Useful strategies can be implemented in many settings by many different types of health and social services professionals as well as by family members, caregivers, and the older individuals themselves. There are six general categories: social services, oral health, mental health, medication use, nutrition education and counseling, and nutrition support. A complete guide to nutrition interventions has been published by the Nutrition Screening Initiative.[48]

Social Services

Nutrition-related social services can address problems related to poverty, isolation, dependency, or disability. They are implemented in cooperation with public and private community-based organizations and are designed to facilitate retention of functional status and maintenance of an independent life-style. The majority of social services interventions mentioned here are accessible nationwide.

Programs such as Food Stamps, food banks, food kitchens or pantries, Social Security, Supplemental Security Income, Medicare, Medicaid, and Federally Assisted Housing programs are designed to address poverty while ensuring access to food. Interventions such as congregate nutrition and home-delivered meals programs, senior centers, transportation services, and adult day care enhance access to food, especially when economic resources are limited. They also assist older persons in the maintenance of social outlooks and interpersonal skills. Case management services, in-home health or personal care aides, and homemaker and chore services increase the availability of food because they enable older persons to manage additional needs that arise from increased dependency and disability. Information regarding access to these and other services is available in most communities through the County Welfare Office, Area Agency (or Office) on Aging, or Public Health Department.[49]

▼ *BENJAMIN SMITH (Part III)*

You refer Mr. Smith for dietary counseling to a Registered Dietitian who discusses the importance of maintaining a reasonable weight for height. His mistaken beliefs regarding the benefits of thinness are dispelled. Guidance regarding appropriate calorie and nutrient intakes is provided. He agrees to limit his alcoholic intake to 1 to 2 drinks per day. He agrees to work with social services providers in his community to ensure that his nutritional needs are met. He is to return to your office for weekly weight checks for the next 6 weeks.

Homemaker services are provided three times per week with cold breakfast foods and evening meals. These foods are acceptable to him; they can be reheated in the microwave and left in the refrigerator on the days he is without an aide. Senior center contact is made and he begins to eat at the center once or twice a week. He begins to participate socially. His alcohol intake declines. His weight at the 6-week check-up is 155 lb and continues to increase steadily.

CASE DISCUSSION

Mr. Smith's case is an ideal, but realistic, scenario. Early intervention had to be proactive, but the satisfactory results included improved quality of life and health for a patient who could easily have dwindled and become more dependent had he not been noticed early and assisted.

Oral Health

Often overlooked, oral health significantly influences nutrition. Poor oral health results in decreased food intake and is a significant cause of involuntary weight loss in the elderly.[29] Wholly or potentially edentulous individuals may restrict food intake and compromise nutrition. Modifications in food texture (chopping, grinding, or pureeing) may facilitate chewing and the resumption of eating.

Soft tissue lesions, temporomandibular joint dysfunction, candidiasis, sore tongue or lips, diminished salivation, or an inflamed oral cavity may cause pain or discomfort that prohibits eating. Treatment may include meticulous cleaning of the teeth or dentures, use of a dental prosthesis, antifungal agents, vitamin or mineral supplements when a deficiency is identified, artificial saliva, sugarless gum, discontinuance when possible of contributory medications (e.g., anticholinergic drugs),[28,30] and modifications in diet consistency and temperature. Timely dental referral or consultation is important.

Mental Health

Progression of chronic diseases, sensory impairment, loss of family and friends, and changes in job status or economic expectations all may impair mental well-being, appetite, and dining pleasure and thus impair the desire or ability to eat. Cognitive or emotional dysfunction, which affects over 25% of older people, is frequently unrecognized or is mistakenly categorized as a normal part of aging.[50] Depression is increasingly being identified as a common but previously unrecognized cause of involuntary weight loss in older persons, regardless of the setting.[51,52]

The nutritional problems that often accompany Alzheimer's disease and other dementias, depressive disorders, anxiety disorders, alcohol abuse, psychoses, suspiciousness, and paranoia frequently respond to specific nutritional interventions, once identified. Vitamin deficiency states resulting from poor food intake, alcohol abuse, or chronic drug use (i.e., antitubercular drugs, anticonvulsants, antineoplastic regimens) may be associated with a nutritionally correctable deterioration in mental status.[36] Eating dependency is often a major problem for patients with psychiatric conditions or disorders, particularly as their mental health deteriorates. The special nutritional problems of dementia patients are increasingly recognized; family members can benefit from advice about providing fewer choices, smaller servings, and nutritious snacks throughout the day early in dementia and about reducing stimulation and distraction at mealtime. They should also receive advice on handling the social aspects of eating in restaurants and at family occasions in the early phases of the disease. Oral feeding should be maintained as dementia progresses, with the deliberate intent of postponing the necessity for nutritional supplementation and in particular nutritional replacement (nasogastric feeding, gastrostomy (percutaneous endoscopic gastrostomy, or PEG tube) feeding, and parenteral feeding), for as long as possible. The use of an eating difficulties inventory[48] may help family members and other caregivers to define the problems so that specific strategies can be recommended.[24,48]

> *Managing oral feeding for as long as possible is the vital principle of nutrition in the frail.*

Medications

Many of the adverse drug reactions that are associated with multiple concurrent drugs involve nutritional risk (Table 9-3). Medications that limit mobility, contribute to disorientation or confusion, restrict or enhance appetite, alter sensory perception, decrease salivation, or induce constipation influence nutrition.

The timing of medications and their ingestion relative to food and beverage intake should be addressed. Questions regarding the use of nutritional supplements, salt or salt substitutes, caffeine, alcohol, and tobacco should be asked. The use of alternative forms of medicine, particularly herbal mixtures, vitamin compounds, teas, and enemas or colonics should be explored. Whenever possible, drug dosages and the number of substances that an individual is taking should be reduced. Drug-nutrient interaction screens that can be self-administered or professionally implemented have been developed.[48]

▼ ROSA WHITE (Part III)

Laboratory work on Mrs. White reveals: glycosylated Hgb 6.0%, down from 12.9% 6 months ago; BUN 5.1 mg/dl, creatinine 3.1 mg/dl; Na 128 mEq/L; K 5.3 mEq/L; and Mg 1.4 mg/dl. Mrs. White's urine culture is negative. A review of her laboratory values and medications leads to the reduction of the Novolin insulin 70/30 to 20 U q AM; the glyburide, ciprofloxacin, captopril, metolazone, nizatidine, and potassium chloride are all stopped. Continuing the levothyroxine, bumetanide, and metoclopramide is emphasized. Magnesium supplementation (L-lactate dihydrate [Magtab SR]) 84 mg tid is added. More aggressive dietary management of protein, potassium, sodium, and fluid intake is offered. Dietary education and hands-on learning experiences are offered to her son through a Registered Dietitian. Biweekly, in-home medication management and reinforcement of dietary and food purchasing principles are provided through the local Health Department's visiting nurse and shopping services programs. Compliance with diet and medication regimens modestly improves. Her confusion gradually diminishes and her appetite improves. Her glycosylated Hgb remains in the 6% to 9% range. Her BUN decreases to 38 mg/dl and creatinine to 2.5 mg/dl. Electrolyte values return to normal limits. Her weight stabilizes at 142 lb. Hemodialysis is delayed for 2 years.

CASE DISCUSSION

This was a complicated situation, with several illnesses and medications out of control. Aggressive dietary management postponed the need for expensive and dependency-producing treatment (hemodialysis) and involved a significant contribution from family members, who required and received appropriate education.

Nutrition Education and Counseling

Nutrition education provides general information regarding foods and nutrients, life-style factors, and community resources and services to individuals and their families.[47] The needs of individuals who are unsure of how to access food programs or resources, who skip meals, who consume poor-quality diets, or who experience difficulty with food selection, purchase, or preparation can often be adequately addressed this way. A wide range of individuals can provide such education. Family members, caregivers, community and social services professionals, the physician's office staff, nurses, and other health care professionals can both access and provide reliable information.

The current "basics" of nutrition education are the Dietary Guidelines for Americans and the Food Guide Pyramid. Although many older Americans would benefit from following this general advice (Table 9-1), recommendations must be individualized. For example, elderly individuals who maintain a reasonable weight and have only mild or modest lipid elevations may not benefit from extreme fat limitation (it lessens flavor and caloric content); individuals with normal blood sugars and reasonable weights may not need to be concerned with the sugar content of their diet; a limited salt intake should only be promoted for those whom it will specifically benefit (again, it lessens flavor and thus appetite). The overriding point is that such restrictions may make the diet so unattractive that the person's overall nutrition suffers, and this may be more hazardous than modest lipid, glucose, or sodium elevations. Nutrition education in this age group should promote the least restrictive regimen that is consistent with good health.

> *Restricting cholesterol, sugar, or salt makes food less attractive and less tasty, leading to the greater hazard of undernutrition.*

Dietary counseling offers individualized guidance about appropriate food and nutrient intake for those with complex or poorly managed chronic disease, those who self-impose or require considerable modification of diet or nutrient intake, or those with complex feeding difficulties or special needs.[47] The patient's unique cultural, socioeconomic, functional, and psychological status is considered. Such counseling may include increases or decreases in food, fluid, or nutrient intake; changes in the size, timing, or composition of meals; modification of the texture or consistency; or considerations about nutritional support. Dietary counseling is best provided by a Registered Dietitian (RD) or a qualified, licensed nutritionist who is skilled with old people and families and understands elders' proneness to undernutrition.

▼ MARTHA SHANKS (Part I)

Martha Shanks is an 87-year-old black woman who has lived alone for the last 35 years in apparently good health. You have seen her regularly over the last 15 years for checkups or minor health complaints. You have always been impressed with her independence and zest for life. From your office records you know that her height is 62 inches. Her weight at her last regularly scheduled office visit, 1 week ago, was 112 lb. She is brought to the ER today by her daughter-in-law because of severe abdominal pain. She has a temperature of 100° F and is jaundiced and mildly confused. Acute cholelithiasis with biliary obstruction is diagnosed, and the patient is treated surgically. Twelve days postoperatively, Ms. Shanks' weight has dropped to 95 lb, her appetite is poor, and she leaves most of the food on her tray. Her serum albumin level is 2.3 mg/dl. She has become increasingly confused in the acute care setting, and an area of erythema has developed in her sacral region. She wants to go home. You feel that she would perhaps be less confused at home and possibly eat better, but you are reluctant to discharge her because of her increasing frailty.

STUDY QUESTIONS

- *What, if any, are the indicators of malnutrition in Ms. Shanks?*
- *What types of interventions might be employed to improve her general health?*

Many physicians doubt the wisdom of embarking on long-term tube feeding when there is no chance of recovery of oral feeding.

Nutrition Support

Nutrition support is needed if an individual cannot eat a nutritionally adequate diet using regular food. Such support includes modifying nutrient content, density, consistency, and form. Oral feeding is best, and considerable efforts must be made to maintain it. Training professionals, volunteers, or family members in the proper techniques of spoon feeding is a low-tech method that has been widely and successfully implemented in many hospitals and other settings. However, if the caloric needs clearly cannot be met by the oral route despite improvements in nutrient density, enteral or intravenous routes must be considered (Fig. 9-3).[48] Whereas nasogastric tube feeding is essentially a temporary measure for resolvable situations (e.g., dysphagia following stroke), it is necessary at times to consider long-term tube feeding through a gastrostomy (PEG) tube. Whereas implementing this is not a difficult ethical consideration when there is a reasonable chance of the patient's recovering sufficient strength and motivation to restart oral feeding

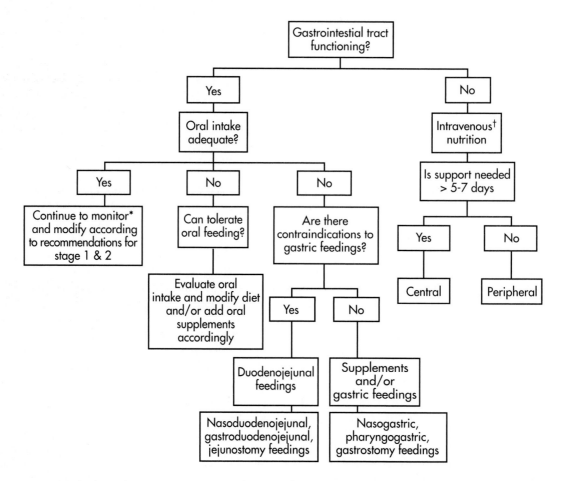

*Periodic "calorie counts" (protein, calories, and micronutrients/24 hr).
†Intravenous nutrition may be adjunctive or combined with partial gastrointestinal feedings.

FIG. 9-3   An algorithm for the provision of nutrition support. (Data from Barrocas A et al: Enteral and parenteral nutrition, *Probl Crit Care* 5[3]:442, 1991.)

eventually, the decision to move to long-term tube feeding when there is no chance of recovery of such function is a complicated ethical one. Many clinicians doubt the wisdom of embarking on such treatment, especially in chronically progressive illnesses such as Alzheimer's disease. When there is no advance directive or family and other input in an incompetent patient, an ethics committee, where available, is to be used. This is in part because legally it is difficult to withdraw such feeding once initiated. Long-term intravenous feeding (total parenteral nutrition) is rarely indicated in older individuals. The techniques, formulas, and protocols surrounding tube feeding are to be found in standard nutritional and medicine texts[36] and the diet manuals of acute or long-term care facilities, so they are not part of the content of this book. Assistance with a specific feeding regimen is obtained from RD consultation or through the institutional or home health agency nutrition support team.

> *It is not necessary to be well nourished, nor even well hydrated, to die comfortably and with dignity.*

▼ MARTHA SHANKS (Part II)

Ms. Shanks has no one to care for her at home. A functional assessment with a Level II Screen shows that she is having increasing difficulty with the ADL and IADL functional status parameters. Enteral nutrition support is instituted in the hospital and the patient is transferred to a long-term care facility. On your advice, the family transfers some familiar furniture, pictures, and other objects from her home to her room at the facility. The less intensive but more structured routine, with more consistent personnel than in the acute care setting, produces a gradual improvement in her attitude. As mobility improves and appetite increases, oral supplements and table foods gradually replace enteral nutrition support. The erythematous area in her sacral region resolves. Her weight stabilizes at 110 lb. Functional and mental status indicators return to prehospitalization levels. She is discharged to her home 6 months postoperatively. Biweekly home health care monitoring continues to be provided.

SUMMARY

Using widely accepted criteria and low-tech, cost-effective interventions, many of the nutrition-related problems that plague older persons can be reduced or eliminated. Compression of the morbidity associated with aging into a shorter time span, improved quality of life, and reduced health care costs are among the benefits to be accrued.

POSTTEST

1. Which one of the following statements regarding nutritional screening is false?
   a. Economic resources should be evaluated.
   b. Medications usage should be reviewed.
   c. Frequency of social contact should be determined.
   d. A functional status assessment is unnecessary.
2. Which one of the following does not indicate a significant weight concern in the elderly?
   a. A decrease of 6% in 1 month
   b. Being 20% below desirable body weight (DBW)
   c. A loss of 7 pounds in 6 months
   d. A decrease of 11% in 6 months
3. Which one of the following statements is false regarding nutrition-related social services interventions?
   a. They may be accessed through the Area Agency (or Office) on Aging.
   b. They include food stamps and meals delivery.
   c. They exclude housing and day care programs.
   d. They may be accessed without physician referral.
4. Dietary guidelines for older Americans include all but which one of the following recommendations?
   a. Increased consumption of cereals and grain products
   b. Moderation in sugar and salt consumption
   c. Avoidance of animal products
   d. Increased consumption of vegetables and fruit
5. The outcomes of unrecognized or untreated malnutrition in older people include all but which one of the following?
   a. Reduced health care costs
   b. Reduced quality of life
   c. Increased dysfunction and disability
   d. Premature morbidity and mortality

REFERENCES

1. National Research Council, Food and Nutrition Board: *Recommended Dietary Allowances,* ed 10, Washington DC, 1989, National Academy Press.
2. Berg RL and Cassells JS, eds and the Committee on Health Promotion and Disability Prevention for the Second Fifty Years, Institute of Medicine: *The second fifty years: promoting health and preventing disability,* Washington DC, 1990, National Academy Press.
3. Galanos AN et al: Nutrition and function: is there a relationship between body mass index and the functional capabilities of community dwelling elderly? *J Am Geriatr Soc* 42:368-373, 1994.
4. Brodeur JM et al: Nutrient intake and gastrointestinal disorders related to masticatory performance in the edentulous elderly, *J Prosthet Dent* 70:468-473, 1993.
5. Coe RM et al: Nutritional risk and survival of elderly veterans: a five-year follow-up, *J Comm Health* 19:327-334, 1993.
6. Zahler LP et al: Nutritional care of ambulatory residents in special care units for Alzheimer's patients, *J Nutr Elder* 12(4):5-19, 1993.
7. McEllstrum MC, Collins JC, Powers JS: Admission serum albumin level as a predictor of outcome among geriatric patients, *South Med J* 86:1360-1361, 1993.
8. Mowe M, Bohmer T: The prevalence of undiagnosed protein-calorie undernutrition in a population of hospitalized elderly patients, *J Am Geriatr Soc* 39:1089-1092, 1991.
9. Mowe M, Bohmer T, Kindt E: Reduced nutritional status in an elderly population (>70 y) is probably before disease and possibly contributes to the development of disease, *Am J Clin Nutr* 59:317-324, 1994.
10. Delmi M et al: Dietary supplementation in elderly patients with fractured neck of the femur, *Lancet* 335:1013-1016, 1990.
11. Veterans Affairs Total Parenteral Nutrition Cooperative Study Group: Perioperative total parenteral nutrition in surgical patients, *N Engl J Med* 325:525-532, 1991.
12. White JV: Risk factors for poor nutritional status, *Prim Care Clin* 21:19-32, 1994.
13. Patterson BH et al: Fruit and vegetables in the American diet: data from the NHANES II survey, *Am J Pub Health* 80:1443-1449, 1990.
14. Kant AK et al: Food group intake patterns and associated nutrient profiles of the US population, *J Am Diet Assoc* 91:1532-1541, 1991.
15. US Department of Agriculture/US Department of Health and Human Services: *Nutrition and your health: dietary guidelines for Americans,* ed 3, Washington, DC, 1990, US Government Printing Office.
16. US Department of Agriculture: *Food Guide Pyramid,* Washington, DC, 1992, US Government Printing Office.
17. US Bureau of the Census: *Statistical abstract of the United States: 1993,* ed 113, Washington, DC, 1993, US Government Printing Office.
18. Walker D, Beauchene RE: The relationship of loneliness, social isolation and physical health to dietary adequacy of independent living elderly, *J Am Diet Assoc* 91:300-304, 1991.
19. Weiss BD et al: Health status of illiterate adults: relation between literacy and health status among person with low literacy skills, *J Am Board Fam Pract* 5:257-264, 1992.
20. Davis TC et al: The gap between patient reading comprehension and the readability of patient education materials, *J Fam Pract* 31:533-538, 1990.
21. Davis TC et al: Rapid estimate of adult literacy in medicine: a shortened screening instrument, *Fam Med* 25:391-395, 1993.
22. Vellas BJ, Albarede JL, Garry PJ: Diseases and aging: patterns of morbidity with age: relationship between aging and age-associated diseases, *Am J Clin Nutr* 55:1225S-1230S, 1992.
23. Rosenberg IH, Miller JW: Nutritional factors in physical and cognitive functions of elderly people, *Am J Clin Nutr* 55:1237S-1243S, 1992.
24. Consultant Dietitians in Health Care Facilities: *Dining skills: practical skills for the caregivers of eating-disabled older adults,* Chicago, Ill, 1992, American Dietetic Association.
25. Lichtenstein MJ: Hearing and visual impairments, *Clin Geriatr Med* 8:173-182, 1992.
26. Cowart BJ: Relationships between taste and smell across the adult life span, *Ann NY Acad Sci* 561:39-55, 1989.
27. Schiffman SS, Warwick ZS: Effect of flavor enhancement for the elderly on nutritional status: food intake, biochemical indices, and anthropometric measures, *Physiol Behav* 53:395-402, 1993.
28. Niessen LC, Douglass CW: Preventive actions for enhancing oral health, *Clin Geriatr Med* 8:201-214, 1992.
29. Sullivan DH et al: Oral health problems and involuntary weight loss in a population of frail elderly, *J Am Geriatr Soc* 41:725-731, 1993.
30. Gift HC, Redford M: Oral health and the quality of life, *Clin Geriatr Med* 8:673-683, 1992.
31. Roy AT et al: Renal failure in older people: UCLA grand rounds, *J Am Geriatr Soc* 38:239-253, 1990.
32. Wilcox SM, Himmelstein DU, Woolhandler S: Inappropriate drug prescribing for the community-dwelling elderly, *JAMA* 272:292-296, 1994.
33. Montamat SC, Cusack B: Overcoming problems with polypharmacy and drug misuse in the elderly, *Clin Geriatr Med* 8:143-158, 1992.
34. Varma RN: Risk for drug-induced malnutrition is under checked in elderly patients in nursing homes, *J Am Diet Assoc* 94:192-194, 1994.
35. Trovato A, Nuhlieck DN, Midtling JE: Drug-nutrient interactions, *Am Fam Phys* 44:1651-1658, 1991.
36. Heymsfield SB, Williams PJ: Nutritional assessment by clinical and biochemical methods. In Shils ME, Young VR, eds: *Modern nutrition in health and disease,* ed 7, Philadelphia, 1988, Lea & Febiger.
37. Ham RJ: Indicators of poor nutritional status in older Americans, *Am Fam Phys* 45:219-228, 1992.
38. Kubena KS et al: Anthropometry and health in the elderly, *J Am Diet Assoc* 91:1402-1407, 1991.
39. Folsom AR et al: Body fat distribution and 5-year risk of death in older women, *JAMA* 269:483-487, 1993.
40. Launer LJ et al: Body mass index, weight change and risk of mobility disability in middle aged and older women, *JAMA* 271:1093-1098, 1994.
41. McEllistrum MC, Collins JC, Powers JS: Admission serum albumin level as a predictor of outcome among geriatric patients, *South Med J* 86:1360-1361, 1993.
42. Ferguson RP et al: Serum albumin and prealbumin as predictors of clinical outcomes of hospitalized elderly nursing home residents, *J Am Geriatr Soc* 41:545-549, 1993.
43. Kerstetter JE, Holthausen BA, Fitz PA: Malnutrition in the institutionalized older adult, *J Am Diet Assoc* 92:1109-1116, 1992.
44. Abbasi AA, Rudman D: Observation on the prevalence of protein-calorie undernutrition in VA nursing homes, *J Am Geriatr Soc* 41:117-121, 1993.
45. Albert SM: Do family caregivers recognize malnutrition in the frail elderly? *J Am Geriatr Soc* 41:617-622, 1993.
46. Breslow RA et al: The importance of dietary protein in healing pressure ulcers, *J Am Geriatr Soc* 41:357-362, 1993.
47. *Incorporating nutrition screening and interventions into medical*

practice: a monograph for physicians, Washington, DC, 1994, Nutrition Screening Initiative.

48. *Nutrition interventions manual for professionals caring for older Americans,* Washington, DC, 1992, Nutrition Screening Initiative.

49. Moyer WR: Social services to assist nutrition, *Prim Care Clin* 1:85-105, 1994.

50. Gatz M, Smyer MA: The mental health system and older adults in the 1990s, *Am Psych* 47:744-751, 1992.

51. Thompson MP, Morris K: Unexplained weight loss in the ambulatory elderly, *J Am Geriatr Soc* 39:497-500, 1991.

52. Rovner BW et al: Depression and mortality in nursing homes, *JAMA* 265:993-996, 1991.

PRETEST ANSWERS
1. c
2. b
3. d

POSTTEST ANSWERS
1. d
2. c
3. c
4. c
5. a

CHAPTER 10

Pharmacotherapeutics

TIMOTHY J. IVES

OBJECTIVES

Upon completion of this chapter, the reader will be able to:

1. Discuss some of the primary principles of altered pharmacodynamics in an older population and its effect on drug dosing regimens.

2. Discuss the effect of altered renal or hepatic function on drug dosing.

3. Perform a medication history on an older patient.

4. Write a prescription for a medication that contains all of the necessary features.

5. Describe the barriers to drug compliance that potentially confront an older patient when attempting to use a medication properly: dosing frequency, dosing formulations, adverse drug reaction profile, potential drug interactions, physical impairment (e.g., visual, auditory, mental status, or hand-grip functions), and caregiver services related to pharmacotherapy (e.g., drug administration).

6. Understand the impact of iatrogenesis and adverse drug interactions on the quality of life for an older patient.

7. Identify and discuss common medications that have been attributed as causes of the following conditions: depression, mental confusion, constipation, urinary retention, incontinence, dehydration, congestive heart failure, gout, cardiac dysrhythmias, and angina pectoris.

PRETEST

1. Which one of the following statements concerning medications in old age is false?
   a. Nineteen percent of hospitalizations in those over age 60 are due to medications.
   b. Congestive heart failure reduces gastric motility, leading to an increase in the ulcerogenic potential of NSAIDs.
   c. The dose of most cephalosporins does not need to be adjusted for renal function.
   d. Phenothiazine accumulation and half-life in elders is increased because of the relative increase in adipose tissue in the elderly.
2. Which one of the following statements concerning medications in old age is false?
   a. The reduction in total body water (TBW) increases the toxicity of digoxin.
   b. If the serum albumin is reduced, the anticoagulant activity of warfarin (Coumadin) is increased.

   c. Generic substitution is probably unwise for digoxin and the tricyclics.
   d. Medication compliance is reduced in elders compared with younger adults.
3. A 68-year-old woman with congestive heart failure is taking digoxin, 0.25 mg orally, every morning. At her yearly office visit, her physician notices that her serum creatinine level is 2.4 mg/dl, an increase from 1.5 mg/dl only 15 months ago. As a part of her presentation, she complains of fatigue and episodes of mental confusion. A recent serum digoxin level (trough) was 1.9 ng/ml. If no other factors are contributory, what actions(s) should be considered with respect to her digoxin dose?
   a. Make no changes.
   b. Increase the dose.
   c. Decrease the dosing interval.
   d. Reduce the dose.

The principles of medication use in an older population are presented in this chapter. Iatrogenesis attributable to drugs in an older population is also discussed. Basic pharmacotherapeutic monitoring parameters for older patients are provided.

▼ *PEARL LASSITER*

An 80-year-old African-American widow who lives with her daughter, Pearl Lassiter comes to your office with multiple chronic medical problems, including polypharmacy. Currently, her chief complaint is of being a nervous wreck, and she wishes she could just turn off her mind. These problems are reported by her daughter to be of at least 2 years in duration. The daughter is eager for another medical opinion. Because Mrs. Lassiter has had multiple gastrointestinal procedures, however, the daughter would like a review of her old records before further testing is undertaken. The family has agreed to obtain her medical records from other physicians for review before her clinic appointment. The daughter also believes that the patient would be better off if she took fewer medications.

Mrs. Lassiter's medical history includes a splenectomy, hysterectomy, appendectomy, hemorrhoidectomy, cardiac dysrhythmia, irritable bowel syndrome, depression, hypertension (controlled), recurrent urinary tract infections with frequency, urgency, and stress incontinence, anemia, occipital headaches, osteoarthritis (predominantly in the right knee), chronic left upper quadrant pain, and generalized weakness. Currently, she has been experiencing hearing difficulties, burning stomach, dry mouth, and decreased appetite (but she drinks En-

sure Plus in unknown quantities). She has also tried a gluten-free diet without success. Her current medications are sucralfate (Carafate) 1 g orally three times a day, cimetidine (Tagamet) 300 mg orally four times a day, enteric-coated aspirin 325 mg orally every day, atenolol (Tenormin) 100 mg orally every day, digoxin (Lanoxin) 0.125 mg orally every day, alprazolam (Xanax) 0.5 mg orally every day, naproxen (Naprosyn) 500 mg orally three times a day, flavoxate (Urispas) 200 mg orally three times a day (taken off and on), oxybutynin (Ditropan) 5 mg orally twice a day, dicyclomine HCl (Bentyl) 10 mg orally three times a day for diarrhea, furosemide (Lasix) 40 mg orally every morning, KCl 10 mEq orally every day, and Tylenol #2 1 to 2 tablets orally as needed for pain.

STUDY QUESTIONS

- *What potential drug-related problems do you see in this patient?*
- *In terms of adverse drug reactions or drug interactions, what concerns do you have for this patient?*
- *Do you have any further questions that you would like to ask the patient or her daughter?*

▼ *ANNA KOZLIEWSKI*

Anna Kozliewski is an 88-year-old, 96-pound, widowed Caucasian woman who was admitted to the local nursing facility approximately 1 year ago. Her admitting diagnoses were a previous right cerebrovascular accident with left residual pa-

ralysis, chronic atrial fibrillation, congestive heart failure, hypertension, renal insufficiency, and recurrent urinary tract infections.

Her current medications are digoxin (Lanoxin) 0.25 mg orally every day, chloral hydrate 500 mg orally every night (may repeat once nightly), phenazopyridine (Pyridium) 100 mg orally three times a day, aspirin 650 mg orally every 3 to 4 hours as needed for headache, clonidine (Catapres) 0.1 mg orally three times a day, hydrochlorothiazide 50 mg orally every day, methenamine mandelate 500 mg orally twice a day (she has been taking this medication for 4 months), and gentamicin 80 mg intramuscularly every 8 hours for 7 days (she is currently on the second day of treatment). A review of Mrs. Kozliewski's recent laboratory data reveals the following results of recent blood studies: a digoxin level of 1.8 ng/ml, serum potassium of 2.8 mEq/L, hemoglobin of 9 g/dl, hematocrit of 32, creatinine of 3.0 mg/dl, and glucose of 110 mg/ml. Her serum iron is low with an elevated total iron binding capacity. Her most recent urine pH was 9.0; microscopic examination revealed more than 100 WBCs per high-powered field. A sputum culture contained no growth, and a urine culture contained Escherichia coli and enterococci organisms with both pathogens being sensitive to methenamine and gentamicin.

Review of her most recent progress notes from the hospital reveals an average blood pressure of 140/88 mm Hg and a pulse over the past 3 weeks in the range of 45 to 60 beats per minute, with regular rhythm. She has had non–position-dependent edema 2+ of the ankles. Over the last 2 days, she has not eaten; she has merely nibbled at her meals. Her sensorium has been normal over the last few weeks except for recent worsening of hearing impairment. A generally withdrawn individual, Mrs. Kozliewski complains (mostly to her daughter, and mostly in Polish) of extreme tiredness in the morning, pain in her right foot in the joint of her great toe, and weakness in both legs.

STUDY QUESTIONS

- *Which of Mrs. Kozliewski's symptoms might be attributable to her drug regimen?*
- *What recommendations would you give the patient and her family?*
- *Would you alter the pharmacotherapy in any way?*

EPIDEMIOLOGY

Older patients, an estimated 6.7 million Americans, are at increased risk of drug-induced disease. This group comprises approximately 12% of the population but consumes over 35% of the medications used in this country today.[1] These medications are not limited to prescription drugs; over-the-counter (OTC) products account for two of every five drugs used by older patients and therefore comprise a potential source of adverse drug events (Table 10-1). Approximately 19% of hospital admissions for patients aged 60 years or older are due to drugs.[2] Older patients are particularly susceptible to drug reactions caused by altered pharmacokinetics, multiple diseases necessitating multiple drugs, problems with adherence to medication regimens, and inappropriately ordered drug dosages and schedules.

PHARMACODYNAMICS AND PHARMACOKINETICS

Pharmacodynamics is concerned with the effect of a drug at the targeted receptor site. Older persons react differently to medications because of factors such as multiple chronic disease states or altered receptor effects. While drug concentrations are measured in the plasma and not within the specific receptor sites (i.e., in specific organs), a given serum drug level often will yield a greater or longer pharmacological response in an older patient than in a younger one because of altered receptor sensitivity associated with aging.[3]

Pharmacokinetics (the quantitative processes of drug absorption, distribution, metabolism, or elimination) may produce higher serum concentrations at the site of action in older patients, even with unchanged receptor sensitivity. With a knowledge of basic pharmacokinetic changes associated with aging, more effective drug regimens can be designed. Estimating the time until equilibrium (i.e., when the rate of drug intake is equivalent to the rate of drug elimination) can help to determine the optimal dosing interval.

Table 10-2 shows a summary of some of the pharmacokinetic features peculiar to drugs commonly used in older patients. The following sections more fully describe the effect of drugs on the basic pharmacokinetic processes in older patients.

Absorption

Most drugs are absorbed by passive diffusion, a process that is unaffected by age. However, with reduced gastric acidity in older persons, the bioavailability of some oral solid formulations (tablets or capsules) and some specific drugs (e.g., aspirin) is reduced because their absorption depends on the gastric pH.

Conditions that lead to decreased gastric motility in older patients (e.g., congestive heart failure—CHF), can prolong the time a drug is available for absorption. Most drugs are absorbed in the duodenum, and CHF may often reduce absorption if reduced intestinal motility is caused by mucosal edema. With decreased gastric motility, drugs with ulcerogenic potential (e.g., nonsteroidal antiinflammatory drugs—NSAIDs) remain in contact with gastric mucosa longer. Decreases in intestinal blood flow may cause a decrease or delay in the absorption of many drugs. Also, with an increase in duodenal diverticula, greater bacterial colonization of the intestine may cause malabsorption of drugs.

Table 10-1   Drugs That Should Be Used With Caution Because of Particular Iatrogenic Risks

Drug	Adverse Effect	Recommendation
Barbiturates	Erratic and paradoxical effects	Use alternative drugs. A prolongation of the half-life occurs by an unknown mechanism. These are not drugs of choice in older patients.
Benzodiazepines (long-acting: diazepam, chlordiazepoxide)	CNS depression caused by prolonged $t_{1/2}$	Reduce the dose and reevaluate the need for the medication.
Digoxin	Increased toxicity	Base the initial dose on lean body weight; base the maintenance dose on creatinine clearance. The half-life is prolonged as kidney function decreases.
H_2 blockers	Mental confusion or disorientation	If possible, try to avoid use in older patients; alternative agents that do not possess this effect (e.g., antacids or sucralfate) are available.
Heparin	Increased incidence of bleeding	Monitor response; avoid other drugs that may impair platelet aggregation. The effect is more common in women and in patients over age 60.
Iron preparations	Poor response	Increase the dose. The effect is probably due to impaired gastrointestinal absorption or poor bioavailability of some generic products.
Levodopa	Hypotension, syncope, disorientation	Decrease the dose. The mechanism is unclear.
Lithium carbonate	Increased toxicity	Monitor serum levels; reduce the dose as needed. The mechanism is unclear.
Phenothiazines	Increased extrapyramidal symptoms	Start with a low dose and titrate slowly. The reaction is related to dopamine receptor supersensitivity.
Phenytoin	Greater neurological/hematological toxicities	Reduce the dose as effects seen are probably due to an increased percentage of *free* drug (unbound to serum proteins) and the total serum level (free plus bound) may be misleading.
Propranolol	Increased CNS/cardiac adverse effects	With a prolonged $t_{1/2}$, titrate the dose carefully. The mechanism is unclear.
Tricyclic antidepressants	Confusion, disorientation	Reduce the dose; effects usually occur within the first 2 weeks.
Warfarin	Enhanced activity	Reduce the dose; monitor the response. Home guaiac tests may be helpful.

Distribution

Distribution, the movement of a drug throughout the body to the appropriate receptor sites, can be affected by the aging process. A decrease in cardiac output reduces organ and tissue perfusion. In addition, with increasing age there is a 10% to 15% decrease in total body water and lean body mass.[4] As a result, water-soluble drugs with poor distribution into adipose tissue (e.g., digoxin, aminoglycosides, propranolol, and cimetidine) will have a reduced volume of distribution (V_d), increasing the serum drug concentration when normal adult doses are used. Conversely, body fat increases with age. Male fat increases from an average of 15% during young adulthood to 36% at age 75, and female fat from 33% to 45%. As a result, the V_d for some lipid-soluble drugs (e.g., barbiturates, benzodiazepines, or phenothiazines) may increase dramatically as they accumulate in adipose tissue. This increases the half-life and produces a prolonged duration of action or adverse effects (e.g., cognitive impairment) for these and other lipophilic drugs.[5]

Understanding changes in the protein binding of a drug is vital to correctly interpreting a serum drug level. A decrease in serum albumin and protein binding occurs in 15% to 25% of patients 60 years or older.[6] This means that drugs that normally are highly bound to plasma proteins (e.g., phenytoin, diazepam, tolbutamide, warfarin, digoxin, and aspirin) will have increased serum concentrations or free fractions with any decrease in serum albumin. When this occurs, a normal total serum drug concentration can be seen in the face of clinical toxicity, because a larger proportion of the drug is in an unbound (i.e., active) state.

Table 10-2   Pharmacokinetics of Individual Agents

Drug	Consideration
Aspirin	Both the duration of action and $t_{1/2}$ may be greatly increased at high doses.
Opiates	Blood levels are generally higher with prolonged analgesia.
Antibiotics	Those eliminated primarily by the kidney (penicillins, aminoglycosides, cephalosporins, and tetracyclines—except doxycycline) may have a longer $t_{1/2}$ and higher steady-state blood levels.
Antihypertensive agents	Propranolol has higher blood levels and a longer $t_{1/2}$. Methyldopa and clonidine are primarily renally eliminated and may have a prolonged $t_{1/2}$.
Digoxin	May have both increased $t_{1/2}$ and serum levels.
Tricyclic antidepressants	May have higher blood levels due to hepatic effects.
Phenothiazines	Blood levels may be higher.
Benzodiazepines	Oxazepam and lorazepam kinetics are unaltered and both have a shorter $t_{1/2}$ than other benzodiazepines (no active liver metabolites).
Theophylline	The $t_{1/2}$ may be prolonged.
H_2 blockers	The $t_{1/2}$ may be prolonged and steady-state blood levels higher. May cause confusion at higher doses.
Oral hypoglycemic agents	Predominately renal elimination (except chlorpropamide). Tolbutamide has the shortest $t_{1/2}$ with a more rapid clearing. Chlorpropamide may cause prolonged hypoglycemia and generally is not recommended in the elderly population.
Phenytoin	Steady-state blood levels may be higher.
Thyroxine	Metabolic clearance may be prolonged.

Metabolism

For drugs predominantly eliminated by hepatic metabolism, age-related changes are variable. As a result, the need to alter a drug dose with advancing age is difficult to predict in the absence of overt liver disease. Hepatic mass, hepatic blood flow, and mixed oxidase (cytochrome P_{450}) enzyme activity are known to decrease with age. This results in reduced drug metabolism and a decreased first-pass effect (high hepatic metabolism and extraction during passage from the portal circulation into the systemic circulation). This can lead to increases in the serum drug levels and clinical effects of certain drugs (e.g., propranolol, metoprolol, meperidine, lidocaine, verapamil, nitrates, acetaminophen, and tricyclic antidepressants) in older patients, often necessitating a decrease in the dosage.

With a decrease in the number and affinity of hepatic microsomal enzymes (phase 1 oxidation), there is a prolonged duration of action of certain drugs (e.g., benzodiazepines, warfarin, and phenytoin), and a decrease in dosage is usually indicated. Without a sensitive test of hepatic function, the full implications of these observations are not available, but it should be realized that changes in dosing may be required to obtain intended therapeutic outcomes. Serum drug levels can be helpful in monitoring several potentially toxic drugs (e.g., phenytoin) that are used frequently by older patients.

Excretion

Drugs that are largely dependent on renal blood flow and glomerular filtration rate for excretion (e.g., digoxin, lithium, aminoglycosides, penicillin, and chlorpropamide) must be reduced in dosage when the creatinine clearance is diminished. Glomerular filtration rate decreases with age for many renally excreted drugs (e.g., penicillins, cephalosporins, and aspirin), averaging a 40% decline between ages 20 and 80 years. For drugs or their active metabolites that are renally excreted, nomograms have been used to approximate the age-related decline in renal function, and dosages can be adjusted accordingly.

CASE DISCUSSIONS

In the case of Mrs. Lassiter, several of her prescribed medications were being used to treat drug-related adverse events caused by medications that were being used to treat her medical conditions. For example, the use of naproxen or aspirin may be a cause for the need of gastrointestinal medications such as cimetidine or sucralfate.

Although her medication regimen (e.g., digoxin) was designed for a patient with normal renal elimination, Mrs. Kozliewski's reduction in creatinine clearance (serum creatinine level of 3 mg/dl) may be a contributing factor to her symptoms, based on a decrease in renal elimination of some of these agents. Contributing to the need for this adjustment is the reduction in renal blood flow and perfusion that commonly occurs with increasing age.

PHARMACOTHERAPEUTIC CONSIDERATIONS

By providing an open atmosphere where patients can freely ask questions with respect to medication use, physicians make an improvement in the quality of life possible for many elderly patients.

Guidelines

The following guidelines may serve to optimize pharmacotherapy in older persons:

1. Older patients should be continuously evaluated for previously undiagnosed and treatable conditions that may affect or be affected by pharmacotherapy. An estimated 6.64 million Americans aged 65 years and older are using medications that place them at high risk for adverse drug events.[7] In many cases, iatrogenesis resulting from medications is also the cause of symptoms seen by primary care physicians (e.g., falls, mental confusion).

2. Be aware of the total cost to the patient for all of the medications (prescribed or OTC) that they are taking. This point is especially important for patients living on fixed incomes, and it may serve to improve adherence to pharmacotherapeutic regimens.

3. A careful medication history (Box 10-1) that includes the use of prescription, OTC, and social drugs may aid in clarifying the diagnosis.[8] With an estimated 19 million older persons using OTC products, this aspect of the medication history is important.[9] In an age of increasing self-medication, particularly with a growing trend toward shifting of medications from prescription to OTC status, be sure to ask about OTC drug use in older patients. Also, physicians should be aware of the patient's adverse drug reaction status.

4. As a part of the clinical decision-making process (Box 10-2), the clinician should consider whether any pharmacotherapy is necessary. If a medication is required, clear therapeutic endpoints should be determined for each patient. "Start low, go slow" is a good general rule to follow. If there is any question about dosage, the physician should start with 25% to 50% of a normal adult dose and increase gradually, titrating the dose to the desired clinical response. Small initial doses and frequent observations through office or home visits will provide a more accurate dosage titration than following some arbitrary dosing recommendation.

 "Start low, go slow" but be sure to increase the medication to an effective dose.

5. Dosage forms that can be easily self-administered (e.g., liquids or suspensions) should be used, as some patients may have problems swallowing tablets or capsules. If a product is unavailable commercially as a liquid or syrup, the pharmacist can often prepare such a formulation. Patients should be encouraged to take their medications standing up (if possible) and with plenty of liquids (if appropriate).

6. Older patients should be treated with as few drugs, including nonprescription medications, as possible. Drug regimens should be reviewed at least twice a year and when a new medication is prescribed or a dose is changed. Medications that have not been taken regularly, are duplicative, or for which an indication no longer exists (especially chronically administered medications) should be discontinued. Although many older patients do not want to waste anything, the physician should encourage patients to properly dispose of unused or outdated medications in which the date of filling of that prescription exceeds 1 year.

7. Encourage patients to bring all of their current medications with them to each office visit so you can review the medications currently being taken, how they are being taken, and whether their pattern of use matches the dosing regimen that was prescribed. A pill count can be used to verify the information given by the patient and to check the supply. Discourage the sharing of medications between older patients and their family and friends. Frank and open discussions with the patient should always accompany these monitoring methods.

 Encourage the patient or family member to bring all medications to all office visits.

Prescription Writing

The prescription is an important interaction between the patient and the physician. Unless properly written and communicated to both the patient and the pharmacist, a prescription can contribute to noncompliance and iatrogenesis. Prescriptions must be written legibly. A physician who has poor handwriting should print or type all prescriptions. Ink or indelible pencil should be used, particularly on prescriptions for controlled substances. Only one prescription should be written per order blank. The major components of a prescription are as follows (Figure 10-1):

Date. The date is required on all prescriptions for schedule II medications, which must be filled within 72 hours of writing. Also, prescriptions for schedule III and IV medications can be filled for only 6 months after they are written.

Patient's Name and Address. This information is required on prescriptions for schedule II drugs and should be a standard practice for all patients. More important, it will avoid potential confusion, especially in families with several people taking medications.

Inscription. The inscription is the body of the prescription containing the name and the strength of the drug.

Subscription. The subscription is the direction to the pharmacist, detailing the amount of medication to be

BOX 10-1
Components of a Medication History

As a part of the entire medical history, a review of the use of medications is warranted. The following points may serve as a format for use:

Current Prescription Medications:

To assess patient knowledge and compliance, be sure to include the dose and the specific dosage regimen as well as how long the patient has been taking the medication and for what reason.

Current Over-The-Counter (OTC) Medications:

Ask questions about OTC drug use based on specific organ systems or symptoms. One approach is to start at the head and work downward. Don't forget vitamin use and contraception methods for *both* men and women.

Previous Prescription or OTC Medications:

This may include medications the patient considers important enough to remember. This may also give you better insight into the patient's medical history.

Social Drug Use:
Alcohol

Assume that everyone drinks and ask the patient: "How much do you drink?" not "Do you drink?" Although the patient may not drink alcoholic beverages at present, be sure to ask about past drinking habits. Alcoholic products include beer, wine, hard liquor, and moonshine.

Tobacco

Ask about cigarette, pipe, cigar, snuff, and chewing tobacco use. If not currently using any tobacco products, be sure to ask about any previous use.

Caffeine

Coffee, tea, cola drinks, other soft drinks (e.g., Mountain Dew or Mello Yello), and even chocolate contain caffeine, which can alter sleep habits and may cause nervousness in some people, old or young.

Other social drugs

(e.g., marijuana, cocaine): Don't be judgmental; you are only obtaining information to benefit the patient. Also, don't assume that only young people use/abuse these agents.

Home Remedies:

One of the primary ingredients in most home remedies is alcohol. Always ascertain *why* these remedies are used.

Immunizations:

Make sure that the patient's immunization status is up-to-date, including influenza or pneumococcal vaccines. Ask if the patient has received a tetanus booster in the last 10 years.

Allergies/Adverse Drug Events:

Is there any history of an allergic reaction to drugs, foods, and the environment? Be sure that patients (and you) know the difference between an allergy and an adverse reaction. If the patient's medical chart indicates an allergy to a drug that is clearly an adverse reaction, be sure to make the appropriate changes. When in doubt, be cautious.

Drug Interactions:

After compiling all of the above drug data, try to determine if the potential for any drug interaction(s) exists.

Compliance Assessment:

If a patient is having a problem complying with the medication regimen, attempt to find out why this is happening: Is it forgetfulness, multiple (three or four times) daily doses, lack of knowledge about the disease state being treated, or inability to pay for the prescription? Ask patients how often they may forget to take their medications over the course of a week and why this occurs. Encourage patients to bring *all* of their current medications to each office visit ("Brown Bagging") to check the supply of medication (with a pill count), consider the risk of polyphysician use or polypharmacy, and review dosing instructions with them.

Ask patients if they have ever stopped taking a medication. If so, ask why they did so; they may have a good reason (e.g., an adverse drug reaction). Are any of the patient's medications causing problems (e.g., GI upset with NSAIDs) or worsening the patient's medical condition (e.g., β-blockers worsening CHF)? Always consider medications when a patient experiences an *acute* change in central nervous system or psychiatric status.

Medication Administration:

Are any special devices (measuring spoon, oral syringe, etc.) required to administer the medications? Mental status, eyesight, hearing, dexterity, socioeconomic status, and support systems should be assessed at every opportunity. Asking the patient to read the label on a prescription vial is important to assess literacy and visual problems. Does the patient have any problems with cognition?

Ask patients where they store their medications to prevent deterioration (e.g., storing insulin in a warm or hot area). Most people still store their medications in the two worst places in the home: the bathroom and the kitchen. Both rooms have high humidity (enhances the breakdown of the medications) and easy access to children, particularly in multigenerational families living under the same roof.

Summary:

Review the information obtained with the patient to make sure that it is correct. You may wish to ask the patient if there is anything with respect to medication use that you have forgotten to ask them. This allows the patient to add any other information to the history that he or she may have forgotten to mention initially. Also, it allows the opportunity to express concerns (e.g., cost) or fears (e.g., adverse drug effects) about the use of the medication(s). Ask if the patient has any questions about the medications (or drugs in general) that he or she would like to ask *you*.

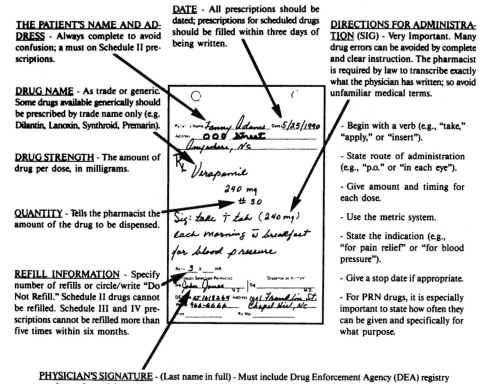

THE PATIENT'S NAME AND AD-DRESS - Always complete to avoid confusion; a must on Schedule II prescriptions.

DRUG NAME - As trade or generic. Some drugs available generically should be prescribed by trade name only (e.g. Dilantin, Lanoxin, Synthroid, Premarin).

DRUG STRENGTH - The amount of drug per dose, in milligrams.

QUANTITY - Tells the pharmacist the amount of the drug to be dispensed.

REFILL INFORMATION - Specify number of refills or circle/write "Do Not Refill." Schedule II drugs cannot be refilled. Schedule III and IV prescriptions cannot be refilled more than five times within six months.

DATE - All prescriptions should be dated; prescriptions for scheduled drugs should be filled within three days of being written.

DIRECTIONS FOR ADMINISTRA-TION (SIG) - Very Important. Many drug errors can be avoided by complete and clear instruction. The pharmacist is required by law to transcribe exactly what the physician has written; so avoid unfamiliar medical terms.

- Begin with a verb (e.g., "take," "apply," or "insert").

- State route of administration (e.g., "p.o." or "in each eye").

- Give amount and timing for each dose.

- Use the metric system.

- State the indication (e.g., "for pain relief" or "for blood pressure").

- Give a stop date if appropriate.

- For PRN drugs, it is especially important to state how often they can be given and specifically for what purpose.

PHYSICIAN'S SIGNATURE - (Last name in full) - Must include Drug Enforcement Agency (DEA) registry number and practicing address, the last two of which can be preprinted on the prescription blank. Signing on the "Product Selection Permitted" line allows generics to be dispensed. For Medicaid recipients to get a brand name drug, the words "brand name is medically necessary" should appear on the prescription, along with a signature on the "Dispense As Written" line.

FIG. 10-1 Sample prescription. (Modified from Sloane PD, Slatt LM, Curtis P, eds: *Essentials of family medicine,* ed 2, Baltimore, 1993, Williams & Wilkins.)

BOX 10-2
Questions to Ask in Deciding Whether or Not to Prescribe a Drug for an Older Patient

Is the treatment necessary?
Is this the safest drug available?
Is this the most appropriate dose, route of administration, and dosage form?
Is it being administered appropriately?
Is it effective?
Is it acceptable to the patient?
Do the benefits outweigh the risks?
Is it available generically?

---

dispensed and any auxiliary devices to be used in its administration, such as "Dispense 120 ml with an oral syringe." Weights and measures in a prescription should be specified with the metric system. Antiquated terms such as drams, scruples, grains, or even ounces are not recommended for use. A commonly used measurement is the teaspoon (5 ml); however, measurements can vary considerably (from 3.5 to 7.5 ml). Calibrated devices, such as measuring spoons and oral syringes, allow for a more accurate delivery of the medication and should be recommended in prescriptions for suspensions and liquids.

Transcription. Transcription refers to the directions to the patient. In Latin, it is abbreviated as *SIG,* however, as this is an antiquated term, the word *Label* is currently preferred. The directions to the patient should always be written in English, for the pharmacist always types the prescription label in English. Using Latin abbreviations such as BID, AC, or QHS is convenient but may confuse the patient.

The directions may contain instructions as to the amount of drug to be taken, the timing and frequency of dosing, the route of administration, and the duration of therapy. Other information, such as shaking well before use, refrigerating, or administering on an empty stomach, should be included here. Pharmacists have auxiliary labels containing this information; these can be attached to the prescription container. Notations such as take as directed or take as necessary (PRN) should be avoided because they are confusing to patients; directions should be specific about the frequency, indications, and dosage of both routine and PRN drugs. Directions for use should always begin with a verb such as take, apply, or insert. Also, directions to patients should remind them of the purpose of the prescription by using such phrases as "for pain relief" or "to relieve itching."

Refill Information. Refill information should be noted on every prescription. Prescriptions for schedule II drugs cannot be refilled, and prescriptions for schedule III and IV drugs cannot be refilled more than five times within 6 months. Unless a physician wishes to specify refills, he or she should circle or write "do not refill" to prevent forgeries for extra refills.

Signature. The physician's personal signature (last name in full) is required, as well as his or her DEA registry number and practicing address, the last two of which may be preprinted on the prescription blank.

Prescribing by Trade Name or Generic Name

Physicians can write for each medication by either its trade name or its generic name. Medications that are available generically can be produced and sold by any pharmaceutical company, thus potentially lowering the cost of a prescription to the patient. The bioavailability of different drug formulations is not always the same, however, as has been documented by case reports of altered clinical outcomes when a drug was changed from one brand to another. Cardiovascular agents, psychotropic agents, anticonvulsants, theophylline, furosemide, and oral anticoagulants are among the drugs in which these concerns have most commonly arisen (Box 10-3).

Although available generically, the agents listed in Box 10-3 should be prescribed by their trade name only, by signing the prescription on the "Dispense as Written" side. Reasons for this recommendation include variable bioavailability, poor quality control, formulation differences, and a narrow therapeutic index. There are significant product differences in bioavailability among different companies' formulations of the same agent. Because of this possibility, interchanging brands is never recommended. Drugs with a narrow therapeutic index are frequently those that can be monitored by serum drug levels (digoxin, phenytoin, etc.).

Compliance with Medication Prescriptions

Pharmacotherapy is often compromised by a lack of full compliance by the patient. While it is well known that the rates of adherence to medication regimens in an older population are similar to other age groups, compliance by older patients correlates primarily to the number of medications that are being taken.[10] Further, in some populations, up to 29% of older patients do not take any prescription or OTC medications, in spite of the fact that their health is noted to be fair to poor.[11] From 25% to 50% of geriatric outpatients make mistakes in taking their medications as prescribed.[11] Unintentional noncompliance is common and is often caused by complex regi-

---

BOX 10-3
Drugs with Bioequivalence Problems: generic substitution may be unwise for these drugs (Reference Brand Products in Parentheses)

Digoxin (Lanoxin, Glaxo-Wellcome)
Digitoxin (Crystodigin, Lilly)
Warfarin (Coumadin, DuPont Pharma)
Dicumarol (Dicumarol, Abbott)
Conjugated estrogen (Premarin, Wyeth-Ayerst)
Transdermal nitroglycerin systems (Nitro-Dur, Key, or Transderm-Nitro, Summit)
Quinidine gluconate (Quinaglute, Berlex, or Duraquin, Parke-Davis)
Phenytoin (Dilantin, Parke-Davis)
Carbamazepine (Tegretol, Geigy)
Primidone (Mysoline, Wyeth-Ayerst)
Valproic acid (Depakene, Abbott)
Chlorpromazine (Thorazine, SK-Beecham)
Thioridazine (Mellaril, Sandoz)
Any tricyclic antidepressant unless it is a branded generic product
Chloramphenicol (Chloromycetin, Parke-Davis)
Erythromycin base (oral tablets only)
Nitrofurantoin (Furadantin or Macrodantin, Procter & Gamble)
Theophylline (Sustained-release oral tablets)
Furosemide (Lasix, Hoechst-Roussel)
Levothyroxine sodium (Synthroid, Boots)

---

mens; a lack of understanding of the illness, drug, or regimen; or poor instructions.[13] Intentional noncompliance may also be common, particularly among patients with stoic personalities. Denial of their illness and dissatisfaction with the physician or pharmacist also contribute to intentional noncompliance.

> *To encourage compliance and simplify life, try to make most medications twice daily (or once daily if possible). Tell patients if all their medications can be taken together—they usually can.*

To help ensure compliance, the physician should simplify drug regimens as much as possible and coordinate drug administration with the patient's daily routines. If possible, once- or twice-daily dosing regimens should be used. A single daily dose at bedtime is sufficient for many medications and may be less expensive. With antihypertensive or antipsychotic agents, taking the dose at bedtime may help to cover the sedative and orthostatic hypotensive effects that are commonly experienced by many older patients.

Regardless of age, patients cannot comply if they do not understand or remember. Clear, comprehensive, and easily understood oral and written instructions about the proper use of a medication are therefore essential for good patient compliance. Providing patients (or someone responsible for them) with an understanding of the purpose of each medication may increase compliance with the physician's general instructions and with the specific comments on the proper use of the medication. Many older patients fear experiencing an adverse drug reaction, especially if they think it could have a negative impact on the quality of their lives or if it could be life threatening. Patients or their caregivers should be provided with information on some of the adverse consequences that may be experienced with the use of a medication and what to do if one occurs.

Physicians can help ensure compliance by asking if the patient has access to a pharmacy, can afford the prescription, and can open the containers provided by the pharmacist. Older patients with hand grip problems should be made aware that they can request easy-to-open closures on prescription vials and bottles from the pharmacist. Not having to open childproof safety caps on prescription vials will aid in reducing medication errors in the older population. Because many older patients with multiple medical conditions and multiple medications commonly spend from $125 to $150 on a monthly basis, prescription costs often can be lowered by prescribing generic products when available and appropriate. Several drug classes lend themselves well to generic substitution. These include antacids, antibiotics, antihistamines, topical anesthetics, thiazide diuretics, topical corticosteroids, and vitamins. Clinicians should always try to stay abreast of the costs of medications to the patient, since this may be one of the most important factors in maintaining adherence to pharmacotherapeutic regimens.

Patient Education

The importance of contracting with the patient for a therapeutic partnership cannot be overemphasized. Physicians should always be alert to the possibility of noncompliance and should tell patients what to do if doses are missed. To achieve therapeutic goals, the use of positive feedback and rewards have been shown to be beneficial. The physician may need to enlist family support to accomplish the desired outcome.

All patients should be given the following information about each medication: (1) the name of the drug, (2) its purpose (i.e., the condition it treats), (3) how and when it should be taken (and when to stop taking it), (4) what food, beverages, and other drugs to avoid while taking it, (5) how to store it properly, and (6) what adverse effects may result (are they serious, short-term, long-term, etc.?).

Explain the medication to the patient; if the patient cannot understand, be sure that a family member or other caregiver knows what the drug is designed to do, what it may do, and how to call you if something unexpected develops.

Patients should be provided with a list of explicit and clearly written dosage instructions. Helpful aids include diary charts, calendars for recording daily drug administration, and compact pill boxes that can contain the doses for an entire day or week. Such memory aids are important for patients of any age who are taking multiple medications. Other important issues to cover include encouraging refills on time, especially when medication discontinuation would cause a worsening in the patient's condition (e.g., drug withdrawal syndrome seen with β-blockers or other cardiovascular agents); instructing patients where to store their medications to prevent deterioration (e.g., not storing insulin in a warm or hot area); and encouragement of return or disposal of old unused medications.

Special attention should be given to patients with impaired intellect, illiteracy, poor vision, and diminished hearing when attempting patient education or writing instructions for use with their prescription or OTC medications. Relatives, friends, visiting health professionals, and local pharmacists can be used to help the patient with his or her pharmacotherapeutic regimen. Community pharmacists can provide useful information about prescription and OTC medications and can help to prevent drug interactions and irrational drug use.

When available, patient education materials on the medications being prescribed should be given. Pharmacists can also provide these materials when the prescription is dispensed. The use of a medication diary or calendar to record daily drug administration will often enhance compliance. Other health care personnel (i.e., pharmacists, nurse practitioners, physician assistants, and dietitians) can assist with patient education and help eliminate barriers to compliance. Finally, patients should be encouraged to bring *all* of their medications with them to every office visit.

POSTTEST

1. All of the following drugs are metabolized via the first-pass effect of the liver except:
   a. Potassium penicillin V
   b. Verapamil HCl
   c. Lidocaine HCl
   d. Propranolol HCl

2. How would you manage postural hypotension in a 74-year-old male patient who is currently taking atenolol (Tenormin) for hypertension?
   a. Increase the dosage.
   b. Decrease the dosage.
   c. Instruct the patient to stand up slowly.
   d. Instruct the patient to discontinue the medication immediately.

3. Mrs. Jones returns to your office for her annual visit. The only medication that she is currently taking is verapamil (generic) 80 mg orally three times daily for hypertension. This medication was prescribed for her at her last visit a year ago. Upon examination, she states that while she can easily afford the medication, she often forgets to take a dose when scheduled. What option(s) can you provide her to improve her compliance with her antihypertensive regimen?
   a. Switch to an extended-release dosage formulation.
   b. Change to a similar therapeutic agent that is dosed less frequently.
   c. Schedule the dosing with an activity related to her daily routine.
   d. Have a discussion with her about her feelings about her diagnosis of hypertension and her quality of life while taking the medication.
   e. All of the above.

4. When obtaining a medication history in an older patient, which of the following is least important?
   a. Nonprescription drug use
   b. Social drug use
   c. Diet
   d. Medication regimen compliance

REFERENCES

1. Department of Health, Education and Welfare: The drug users: task force on prescription drugs, Washington, DC, 1967, US Government Printing Office.
2. Beard K: Adverse reactions as a cause of hospital admission in the aged, *Drugs Aging* 2:356-367, 1992.
3. Feely J, Coakley D: Altered pharmacodynamics in the elderly, *Clin Geriatr Med* 6:269-283, 1990.
4. Greenblatt DJ, Sellers EM, Shader RI: Drug disposition in old age, *N Engl J Med* 306:1081-1088, 1982.
5. Greenblatt DJ et al: Physiologic changes in old age: relation to altered drug disposition, *J Am Geriatr Soc* 30:S6-S10, 1982.
6. Owens NJ, Silliman RA, Fretwell MD: The relationship between comprehensive functional assessment and optimal pharmacotherapy in the older patient, *Drug Intell Clin Pharm* 23:847-854, 1989.
7. Willcox SM, Himmelstein DU, Woolhandler S: Inappropriate drug prescribing for the community-dwelling elderly, *JAMA* 272:292-296, 1994.
8. Ives TJ, Anastasio GD: Ambulatory drug therapy. In Sloane PD, Slatt LM, Curtis P, eds: *Essentials of family medicine*, ed 2, Baltimore, 1993, Williams & Wilkins.
9. Helling DK et al: Medication use characteristics in the elderly: the Iowa 65+ rural health study, *J Am Geriatr Soc* 35:4-12, 1987.
10. Botelho RJ, Dudrak R: Home assessment of adherence to long-term medication in the elderly, *J Fam Pract* 35:61-65, 1992.
11. Chrischilles EA et al: Use of medications by persons 65 and older: data from the Established Populations for Epidemiologic Studies of the Elderly, *J Gerontol* 47:M137-M144, 1992.
12. German PS et al: Knowledge of and compliance with drug regimens in the elderly, *J Am Geriatr Soc* 30:568-571, 1982.

PRETEST ANSWERS

1. c
2. d
3. d

POSTTEST ANSWERS

1. a
2. b
3. e
4. c

CHAPTER 11

Rehabilitation

KENNETH BRUMMEL-SMITH

OBJECTIVES

Upon completion of this chapter, the reader will be able to:

1. Define rehabilitation and discuss its role in primary care.

2. Discuss the steps involved in rehabilitation and how they are affected by aging.

3. Discuss the role that various allied health care providers play in rehabilitation.

4. Discuss the choice of sites for provision of rehabilitation interventions and their Medicare/Medicaid/insurance reimbursement.

5. Discuss the methods for assessment of rehabilitation potential.

6. Given a patient with dominant hemisphere stroke, nondominant hemisphere stroke, hip replacement surgery, leg amputation, and arthritis:
   a. Review the functional impairments that have resulted in disability.
   b. Outline a realistic rehabilitation plan.
   c. Discuss the psychosocial aspects of care.
   d. Discuss the alterations in approach depending on the site of care.
   e. Discuss the types of assistive equipment applicable to each condition.

PRETEST

1. A 78-year-old woman is admitted for stroke rehabilitation. Which one of the factors below is most likely to influence her chances of returning home?
   a. The degree of neurological defect
   b. Her insurance status
   c. The degree of functional impairment
   d. Her social support system
2. What percentage of elderly persons are likely to be able to walk independently after a below-the-knee amputation?
   a. 10%
   b. 25%
   c. 50%
   d. 75%
   e. 90%
3. Which of the following is a potential benefit in the elderly of a hip prosthesis over pinning a fractured hip?
   a. Less blood loss
   b. Lower incidence of postoperative deep vein thrombosis
   c. Less anesthetic risk
   d. Earlier ambulation
   e. Reduced pain
4. Which of the following walking aids is preferred in patients with Parkinson's disease?
   a. A pick-up walker
   b. A straight cane
   c. A front-wheeled walker
   d. Standard crutches

Rehabilitation is as much a philosophy of care as it is a set of techniques or interventions designed to enhance the functional abilities of disabled persons. This philosophy holds that functional capabilities are modifiable, even in the oldest person.

Older people's fears are often expressed as relating to loss of function, such as becoming dependent on their families or being placed in a nursing home. One of the most important goals of geriatric health care is the promotion of function. Therefore rehabilitation is one of the foundational aspects of geriatric care.

One of the most common mistakes that primary care providers make is to assume that rehabilitation is something provided in special care units. In reality, rehabilitation is an approach that can be applied to the hospitalized patient, the older man seen in the office, the elderly woman visited in the nursing home, or the couple living at home.

Rehabilitation is comprehensive; it addresses a person's medical, psychological, and social problems so that the ability to live more independently is enhanced. It is less involved in treating disease than in promoting the person's ability to perform activities of daily living, get out into the community, enjoy leisure time, or return to work. Rehabilitation is a natural and necessary adjunct to comprehensive assessment.

> Rehabilitation is not only practiced in special units: it is an approach or philosophy that can be applied anywhere and anytime to help a person achieve his or her true potential.

Disability is common as one ages. Forty percent of disabled people are over age 65 years, and 63% of these are over age 75.[1] The majority of strokes, amputations, and hip fractures, conditions that often demand rehabilitation intervention, occur in elderly persons. One or more chronic conditions can be found in 86% of older persons, and over 50% of individuals over age 70 have limitations in daily activities.[2] Because families provide the bulk of care to frail elderly persons, higher levels of disability place a greater burden on the caregiving system. When families burn out, institutionalization often results, and health care costs rise. Therefore a lack of attention to disability in old age may adversely affect the patient, the family, and even society.

It is important to keep in mind certain definitions relating to disability. An impairment is any alteration in physical or physiological function at the organ level. Impairment of physiological function is extremely common in old age. However, when the impairment is of such a degree that it causes an alteration in the person's daily activities, it is called a disability. When a person with a disability is prevented from fully expressing his or her potential, usually because of societal barriers, the person has been handicapped (Box 11-1). Older persons with disabilities may be handicapped by a society that does not provide payment for a wheelchair, by a system that does not allow access to rehabilitation services, or even by their own ideas that being sick or physically impaired is normal at their age. Such an attitude has been termed the right to dependency.

▼ GEORGE PAUL (Part I)

Mr. Paul, an 80-year-old man with a recent left hemisphere stroke, has been admitted to an inpatient rehabilitation unit.

BOX 11-1
The Relationship of Impairment, Disability, and Handicap

Impairment: organ level
Disability: person level
Handicap: societal level

(His acute care is discussed in Chapter 45.) It has now been 18 days since his stroke. His speech is limited although he follows commands correctly. He had a nasogastric tube placed in the acute unit. His right arm and leg have begun to develop some mild muscle movements although they are as yet without voluntary control. A Foley catheter is in place. His wife visits daily, and it is clear that she is under a great deal of stress in coping with his new disability.

▼ MARIA HERNANDEZ (Part I)

Ms. Hernandez is a 65-year-old woman who had a right internal capsule hemorrhage leading to left hemiparesis. Initially her blood pressure had been difficult to control, but by the time she was discharged to the nursing home it was generally in the range of 110/60. (For a more complete discussion of her acute care, see Chapter 45.) She was sent to the nursing home because she was not thought to be a good candidate for inpatient rehabilitation because of her apparent cognitive deficits and severe left-sided neglect.

STUDY QUESTIONS
- What characteristics of Mr. Paul and of Ms. Hernandez are likely to be important in determining the type of rehabilitation needed?
- What factors most strongly affect a patient's prognosis for return to independent living?

PROCESS OF REHABILITATION

The process of rehabilitation is often different for older people when compared with younger people with the same diagnosis. Although the steps of rehabilitation are the same regardless of age, certain aspects of those steps are often quite different when caring for older persons.

Step 1. Stabilize the Primary Problem

Achieving stability is often elusive when the older person has multiple interacting medical conditions. For instance, ambulation is a function highly desired by most patients with stroke. Yet walking with a hemiplegic gait requires significantly more energy expenditure than walking with a normal gait. For the younger survivor of stroke, this may not be important, but for many 80-year-olds, underlying heart or lung disease may interfere with this goal.

Step 2. Prevent Secondary Complications

Secondary complications are much more frequently seen in older patients. The more common are discussed briefly below.
- Malnutrition often goes undetected in medical settings and worsens with longer hospitalization.
- Confusion is commonly seen. Multiple medications, environmental deprivation, and the effects of illness may worsen an already present, but subclinical, cognitive impairment.
- Contractures occur when a limb is not regularly stretched (range of motion exercises); within 3 weeks it may be impossible to recover the full range of motion.
- Deconditioning, characterized by loss of strength and endurance resulting from prolonged bed rest, begins after a few days in bed. Recovery of the lost function takes many weeks.
- Depression is almost a normal experience in reaction to the development of a new disability. Although it is common, it should not be accepted as untreatable.
- Incontinence can develop whenever mobility is restricted.
- Pneumonia often is related to prolonged bed rest or, in the case of stroke, swallowing dysfunction.
- Pressure sores develop rapidly in older persons, especially those with poor nutrition.
- Whenever a person lies in bed for a long time, and especially when certain diseases or conditions such as stroke or hip fracture affect leg function, the likelihood of deep venous thrombosis rises significantly.

Step 3. Restore Lost Function

The crux of rehabilitation is helping to restore lost functional abilities. Recovering the ability to dress, walk, or return to enjoyable activities is of major importance to disabled persons. Although the condition that caused the loss of function may never resolve, the person can still achieve an independent or less assisted lifestyle.

Step 4. Promote Adaptation of the Person to His or Her Environment

This area of adaptation is likewise different in older persons. They may not have the ability or resources to adapt to their environment, yet changes often make the difference between independent and institutional living. They may not believe they can learn to live with a disability.

Step 5. Adapt the Environment to the Person

A parallel adaptation process can involve changing the environment. For example, a person with a hip fracture may have adequately learned how to use a walker for mobility, but the bathroom door at home is too narrow to allow use of the walker. Widening the doorway will solve the problem.

Step 6. Promote Family Adaptation

Almost 85% of care is provided by the family.[3] These caregivers may be quite old themselves, have significant illnesses, and are often under a great deal of stress.

Hence, there are many reasons why rehabilitation with older clients may be different and more difficult than when working with others. These differences are summarized in Figs. 11-1 and 11-2.

> *Frequent interruptions to rehabilitation of elders include confusion, the multiplicity of medical problems, deconditioning, and depression (a normal experience when newly disabled).*

▼ GEORGE PAUL (Part II)

After 2 weeks on the rehabilitation unit, Mr. Paul's albumin level is 3.1 mg/dl, and his complete blood cell count shows a mild normochromic, normocytic anemia. His only source of nutrition is tube feeding. The speech therapist asks if the tube can be removed and a bulbar training program instituted.

STUDY QUESTION

- *What features of geriatric rehabilitation make a team approach essential? Who are the essential members of the rehabilitation team?*

REHABILITATION TEAMS

One feature that makes rehabilitation different from many other medical systems is its team orientation. Al-though most medical care is multidisciplinary in nature, rehabilitation requires a more formal process. Thus, in addition to seeing their patients individually and communicating through notes written in the patient's chart, interdisciplinary team members meet regularly to discuss patient problems and functional deficits, to decide on a comprehensive therapeutic plan, and to discuss goals by which patient progress will be measured. Regular team meetings are also important to allow staff members or the patient to bring up problems and seek solutions.

> *Rehabilitation is truly "interdisciplinary": consultants in rehabilitation are generally from disciplines other than medicine.*

Unlike traditional medical care, in which the consultants are other physicians, the team members in rehabilitation are experts in various therapeutic approaches. The primary members of the team are rehabilitation nurses, physical and occupational therapists, and speech pathologists. Others often include pharmacists, psychologists, and recreation therapists.

In inpatient rehabilitation, another crucial team member is the nurse. Besides providing important nursing care, the nurse ensures that the techniques learned in the physical or occupational therapy departments are reinforced and practiced. Having prolonged patient contact during the day, the nurse plays a crucial role in supporting psychological adjustment to disabilities. The nurse also plays an important role in training family members about caregiving skills.

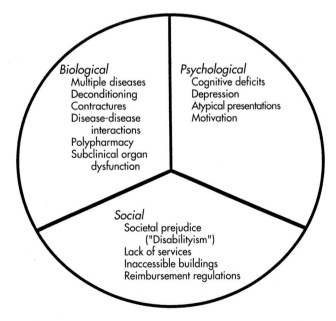

FIG. 11-1   Age-related factors that may affect rehabilitation.

FIG. 11-2   Disease-related factors that may affect rehabilitation.

Physical therapists assess strength, range of motion, endurance, and mobility skills. They are primarily concerned with promoting ambulation and transfers. They may use electrical stimulation to enhance function of weak muscles or to relieve pain. Physical therapists spend much of their time teaching patients to walk with canes or walkers or to use a wheelchair. Finally, they work closely with orthotists, who fashion braces for weak extremities, or prosthetists, who create artificial limbs.

When a patient has deficits in performing basic or instrumental activities of daily living, an occupational therapist can assist in retraining. Perceptual and sensory evaluations, as well as cognitive retraining programs, are also within their purview. An occupational therapist can help the primary care provider evaluate the patient's ability to drive a car, for example.

Speech pathologists not only assist the aphasic patient in achieving communication but can also help with cognitive assessment and evaluation of swallowing function (some occupational therapists and even physical therapists can also assess swallowing disorders).

Recreation therapists are especially helpful in geriatric rehabilitation. The ability to find leisure activities that are satisfying and enjoyable can significantly help many older persons adjust to disability.

The physician provides medical expertise and often serves as team facilitator. Because medical care tends to be arranged hierarchically, the physician must be careful not to inhibit the free flow of information and expertise in the team. The physician working in a team needs attention to group dynamics, respect for the other team members, and good communication skills. In most rehabilitation settings the physician with primary responsibility for the rehabilitation program is a specialist in physical medicine and rehabilitation. However, in many geriatric programs a geriatrician leads the team. Regardless, there is still a vital role for the primary care physician to play in managing the patient's medical care, relating to the family, and providing continuity of care once the rehabilitation program is complete.

 In rehabilitation the physician often serves as team leader, but not always.

SITES FOR REHABILITATION

Rehabilitation can be provided in any health care setting. Regardless of the setting, however, a standard requirement for third-party reimbursement is that the interventions will lead to improvement of a patient's functional status, not simply maintenance. Each setting has specific benefits and limitations, as well as special reimbursement requirements, so it is important for the primary care provider to be aware of the differences.

The patient's home is a logical site for much rehabilitative care for several reasons. The person's ability to negotiate and make use of his or her true living environment can be assessed and enhanced. There is no need to provide transportation to the provider's setting. Patients often feel more comfortable in their own surroundings. Finally, the patient's ability to carry over newly learned techniques to the next session can be assessed. However, there are limits as to how often the team members can visit the home, with Medicare allowing only a few weeks' home rehabilitation. Hence, the appropriate patient for home rehabilitation is someone who may benefit from outpatient care but because of transportation problems, limited endurance, or personal choice desires a home program.

The outpatient clinic is a wise choice for patients with less severe deficits than those seen in hospital settings but who still require access to more equipment or ancillary services than can be obtained in the home. Often, the stimulation of being around others with similar problems enhances patient motivation. Group programs, which have been shown to be positive for older patients, are also available. Again, Medicare has certain limits on the duration of therapy provided. For many elders, transportation to the clinic may be a significant barrier.

Since the advent of diagnosis-related groups (DRGs), many elderly patients are being discharged from hospitals at a more dependent level. This would seem to indicate a stronger role for rehabilitation interventions in the acute care hospital. Unfortunately, functional disability often goes undetected and is in fact promoted in the acute hospital.[4] Whenever possible, patients' function should be encouraged by having them sit in chairs, walk to the bathroom or diagnostic studies, and feed and dress themselves.

Specialized rehabilitation centers may be freestanding hospitals or departments within acute care hospitals. As of 1991, they are DRG exempt, which means that Medicare reimbursement is provided for each day of care rather than as a fixed payment based on diagnosis. To qualify for treatment in a rehabilitation center, patients must be able to tolerate 3 hours of therapy per day, 6 days a week, and have the potential for significant functional improvement. A physician who is knowledgeable about and skilled in rehabilitation must closely monitor all patients and treat any medical problems that arise. The rehabilitation team must meet weekly, establish goals, and document progress toward those goals. Depending on the disability, patients may be in the rehabilitation hospital for as little as 1 week for a hip replacement to as many as 6 months for a spinal cord injury.

One other important site for providing rehabilitation is the nursing home. Physical, occupational, and speech therapy are available through Medicare, provided that the patient has recently been in an acute hospital at least 3 days and the patient's functional disabilities are expected to improve with expert intervention. (Medicare will not fund therapy in any setting that is oriented only to maintaining the patient's level of function.) The majority of people admitted to rehabilitative nursing homes return home, usually within 2 months. An ideal patient is one who has medical limitations that prohibit him or her from tolerating 3 hours of therapy per day in an inpatient unit, but who temporarily needs both skilled nursing and physical or occupational therapy.

> *Medicare will not fund therapy designed to maintain the level of function; there has to be documented improvement.*

▼ MARIA HERNANDEZ (Part II)

The patient care team at the nursing home evaluates Ms. Hernandez. Physical, occupational, and speech therapists are asked by the director of nurses to see the patient. The primary physician is informed that Medicare will cover the cost of nursing home care as long as she can be shown to be improving.

ASSESSMENT OF REHABILITATION POTENTIAL

One of the most important roles for primary care providers is the identification of older persons who may benefit from rehabilitation. This process is called assessment of rehabilitation potential. In many ways this assessment is similar to the comprehensive assessment process described elsewhere in this book. The Barthel Index[5] has been used to evaluate patients with stroke for rehabilitation. Using a maximum score of 100, researchers have shown that patients scoring above 60 have good rehabilitation outcomes, whereas those scoring below 21 are likely to be unsuccessful in achieving independence.[6] Unfortunately, there is limited information about the use of this instrument with conditions other than stroke. The main areas assessed are cognitive, physical, psychological, social, and economic.

Cognitively, the patient must be able to retain new information learned in therapy. This usually precludes rehabilitation for patients with moderately severe dementia. The patient's physical status must be stable enough to allow participation in exercises without undue risk. Depression is not a contraindication to rehabilitation; a person's motivation and desire for rehabilitation may be limited at first but usually improve with support and counseling. Social supports are critical to rehabilitation outcomes. Those with no support systems are at the greatest risk. Finally, economic resources often determine whether a patient can be accepted into a rehabilitation program or which site for rehabilitation will be used.

STROKE REHABILITATION

Stroke is the most common problem leading to rehabilitation in the United States. Rehabilitation should begin within the first few days after the stroke to prevent secondary disabilities from occurring. Patients and families need information about the relatively good outlook for survivors of stroke. With rehabilitation, approximately 10% of survivors recover full physical function, 40% have some mild-to-moderate loss of function, and another 40% have significant functional losses. Only 10% are likely to need institutional care. Recovery of motor function is virtually complete within 6 months after a stroke, while sensory, speech, and swallowing function may take as long as 2 years to recover completely.

Stroke rehabilitation is divided into three phases: acute, rehabilitation, and long-term care. Management of the acute phase is discussed in Chapter 45. Major rehabilitation interventions take place in the rehabilitation and long-term care phases.

Rehabilitation Phase

The rehabilitation phase usually begins when the patient is medically stable, often 5 to 10 days after a stroke. The various members of the team assess the patient's deficits and needs. Together, team members develop a care plan based on goals that have been discussed with the patient and the family. It is important to know what the family's goals are at the beginning of the rehabilitation program. This discussion with the family unit is crucial to appropriate planning because the family's capacity to provide care often determines discharge outcomes.

Motor strengthening, endurance training, and skill building in managing transfers and mobility are usually in the purview of the physical therapist. Motor recovery usually follows a sequence of functional changes (Fig. 11-3). After an initial flaccid paralysis the affected limb develops a flexor pattern synergy; that is, the limb flexes at multiple joints when movement is attempted. Later an

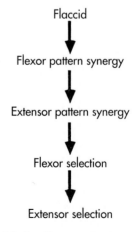

FIG. 11-3   Pattern of motor return.

extensor pattern synergy develops, followed by flexor selection. At this stage, the person may be able to flex isolated joints voluntarily but may still go into a synergy pattern when attempting extension. Finally, extensor selection occurs.

These patterns may either help or hinder the patient's functioning. For instance, a flexor pattern of the leg makes ambulation impossible, whereas an extensor pattern may facilitate the person's walking even with weak muscles. Not all patients follow the sequence described in the preceding paragraph; some progress only one or two steps, and others skip steps. Facilitation of useful patterns and alleviation of harmful patterns are key components of physical and occupational therapy and are crucial to recovery.

In hemiplegic stroke, balance training begins early: first with static sitting, later progressing to standing, then walking balance. Strengthening programs are carried out by all allied health therapists. Once the patient has good (4/5) strength (Table 11-1), can balance on the unaffected side, and can advance the affected leg somewhat, gait training begins. It is important for the patient to stand up when being tested for leg strength because that often facilitates otherwise weak muscles.

Various assistive aids are often used in stroke rehabilitation. Leg braces support weak muscles and may facilitate use of spastic muscle groups. The ankle-foot orthosis (AFO) is the most common type used in stroke. Two basic types exist: a polyethylene, molded brace and a metal, adjustable brace (Figs. 11-4 and 11-5). The first type is lighter, more cosmetically appealing, and easier for some older persons to don. However, it provides less stability, cannot be adjusted if the patient's status changes, and is less useful when spasm is present. Although the adjustable metal brace is less cosmetic, heavier, and harder to don, it provides much more stability, can be adjusted as neurological function changes, and can be used even when spasms are present. In most centers, a physiatrist prescribes the appropriate orthotic device, an orthotist fashions it, and a physical therapist trains the patient to use it.

Gait training usually starts with maximum assistance from two therapists. Gradually the patient is advanced to the parallel bars and then to hand-held equipment.

A variety of assistive devices can help patients with stroke as they learn to ambulate. Regular walkers are often difficult for the patient to use, since they require use of both hands. A special hemi-walker (Fig. 11-6) is used for those patients needing more stability. A four-prong cane (Fig. 11-7) is less cumbersome than the hemi-walker but provides less stability. Single point canes are infrequently prescribed for older survivors of stroke because they are unsafe for those who have balance and coordination problems.

Most older patients require training in the use of a wheelchair, if not as the primary mode of ambulation, then as a supplement for longer distances. There are hundreds of sizes and types of wheelchairs; a physical therapist should always be involved in prescribing one.

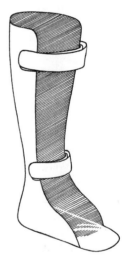

FIG. 11-4   Polyethylene, molded brace (AFO).

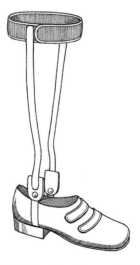

FIG. 11-5   Double-adjustable, upright brace (AFO).

Table 11-1   Quantitative Strength Measurement

Label	Score	Criterion
Normal	5/5	Examiner cannot break contraction
Good	4/5	Examiner can just break contraction
Fair	3/5	Patient can move joint against gravity, but not against resistance
Poor	2/5	Patient can move joint, but not against gravity
Trace	1/5	Muscle contraction is evident, but movement is not
Absent	0/5	No muscle contraction is evident

▼ GEORGE PAUL (Part III)

Mr. Paul has progressed in muscle movement to an extensor pattern synergy. The physiatrist and physical therapist determine that a metal AFO will help him walk more safely and with less energy consumption. A temporary brace is used while the orthotist fashions a permanent one. Mr. Paul currently can ambulate 20 m with a hemi-walker for balance.

Training in activities of daily living is primarily the function of the occupational therapist (OT). Sensory and perceptual deficits are major hindrances to achievement of independent functioning. Besides providing strengthening and building endurance, the OT offers reeducation in dressing, clothing modifications, and training in the use of special equipment such as weighted utensils, reachers, rocker knives (Fig. 11-8), clothes hooks (Fig. 11-9), and many others (Box 11-2). Many catalogs are available describing adaptive equipment.[7,8]

The use of resting splints on the wrists to prevent contractures or lap boards or arm troughs on wheelchairs to prevent subluxation of the shoulders is also decided on by occupational therapists. Cognitive retraining is an important component of the OT's role when working with the survivor of stroke.

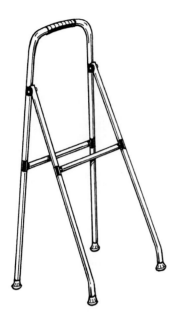

FIG. 11-6   Hemi-walker.

▼ MARIA HERNANDEZ (Part III)

Evaluation by the occupational therapist reveals that the patient's cognitive deficit is evidence of right brain dysfunction. The patient's neglect of objects on her left side interferes with her ability to participate in activities of daily living. An aggressive program to adapt to these limitations is begun.

BOX 11-2
Aids for Activities of Daily Living

Feeding: rocker knives, cutting boards, plate retainers
Dressing: Velcro closures, buttonhooks, sock donners, tilted mirrors, clothes reachers
Toileting: grab bars, raised toilet seats, Versa frames
Bathing: tub bench, grab bars, hand-held shower hose, long-handled brush
Grooming: tilted mirror, built-up handles

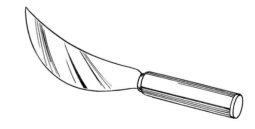

FIG. 11-8   Rocker knife.

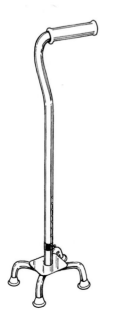

FIG. 11-7   Four-prong cane.

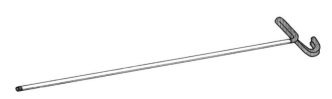

FIG. 11-9   Clothes hook.

Speech therapists are almost always involved in stroke rehabilitation. Even patients with nondominant lobe damage may benefit from their help. Through language retraining or use of alternative communication methods such as picture boards, they assist patients in regaining the ability to communicate. Speech therapists also participate in cognitive and bulbar retraining programs. Cognitive retraining involves special educational interventions to help compensate for the survivor's diminished mental abilities. Beginning with simple repetition and extending to expanded use of associative memory, cognitive retraining helps patients with stable neurological deficits develop better cognitive skills. Bulbar retraining involves techniques to reeducate swallowing musculature to help patients prevent choking and aspiration.

Aphasia is common after left hemisphere damage. Broca's aphasia, sometimes called motor aphasia, refers to a difficulty in producing speech. Comprehension of speech is often normal in Broca's aphasia, but the patient is unable to either think of or articulate words. Wernicke's aphasia is fluent but usually nonsensical. A type of sensory aphasia, it usually is associated with an inability to understand others. Many survivors of stroke have a mixture of these two types. Some patients also have dysarthria, difficulty articulating words caused by the effects of the stroke on vocal musculature. Because comprehension is normal, language training is quite helpful.

▼ GEORGE PAUL (Part IV)

Mr. Paul has a pure Broca's aphasia. Because Mr. Paul is unable to produce language, the speech therapist develops a picture book for him to use to communicate. His mood noticeably improves once he is able to make others aware of his needs, although he still becomes frustrated on occasion.

The rehabilitation nurse is perhaps the central therapist in the care of the survivor of stroke. Geriatric patients often have significant nursing needs, such as medication management, monitoring effects of treatment, and managing cognitive or behavioral problems. In addition to attending these needs, the rehabilitation nurse also encourages patients to practice techniques learned from other team members. The nurse works closely with family members to enable them to become better caregivers. Many nurses also provide training in the self-use of medications.

Strokes affecting the nondominant hemisphere have some special features. Surprisingly (since aphasia is absent), these patients often do more poorly in rehabilitation than those with dominant hemisphere injuries. Constructional apraxia and neglect of the affected side are two of the major factors contributing to this poor performance. Patients with nondominant hemisphere stroke generally have difficulty understanding visual-spatial arrangements. As a result, they are unable to orient themselves properly to perform motor tasks, a condition referred to as constructional apraxia. For example, the affected person may not understand the way a button goes through a buttonhole or how a shirt sleeve fits over the hand. Neglect of the affected side is frequently seen because the patient does not appreciate sensory input from that side. Patients with nondominant hemisphere strokes also tend to have emotional incontinence, crying easily for no apparent reason. In addition, they are often unable to recognize familiar faces. Finally, they are frequently unaware of their deficits. This lack of awareness can significantly impede their ability to rehabilitate.

In all patients with stroke, special attention must be paid to preventing secondary complications. Table 11-2 shows some of the measures that can prevent or minimize common complications. Depression is frequently seen during this stage; because of aphasia or emotional incontinence it may be difficult to recognize. Sometimes there is simply too much attention given to the physical problems to realize the person has become depressed. Support, counseling, and judicious use of antidepressant medication may all be necessary. For a more detailed discussion of stroke complications, see Chapter 45.

▼ MARIA HERNANDEZ (Part IV)

The charge nurse notices that Ms. Hernandez's blood pressure consistently is below 110/70 mm Hg. The patient seems to be lethargic. Her medications include captopril 25 mg twice a day and hydrochlorothiazide 25 mg every day. She notifies the primary physician. A decision is made to discontinue the captopril gradually. Two weeks later, the blood pressure averages 140/85 mm Hg and the patient is much more alert.

Table 11-2   Reducing the Risk of Secondary Complications of Stroke

Complication	Management Approach
Pressure sores	Turning, keeping area dry, nutrition
Malnutrition	Special foods, exercises, positioning, tube feeding
Venous thrombosis	Stockings, mini-dose heparin
Contractures	Range of motion exercises
Pneumonia	Food changes, positioning, intubation
Nerve palsies	Proper body positioning
Conjunctivitis	Eyedrops, taping
Depression	Counseling, medications
Confusion	Reduction of drug intake, reality orientation, family presence

A common problem that is encountered among patients with stroke during the rehabilitation phase is dysphagia (difficulty swallowing). Malnutrition sets in rapidly in patients who are unable to feed. Aspiration can also occur. The gag reflex is a poor predictor of those at risk for aspiration; even those with a strong reflex may aspirate. Hoarseness of voice is a more reliable sign. Videofluoroscopy during swallowing will demonstrate those likely to aspirate. Initially, attempts to promote safe swallowing can be made by speech or occupational therapists. However, often a decision must be made whether a nasogastric or gastric tube is going to be used. A tube facilitates better nutrition, but almost half of patients with either type of tube still aspirate. Fortunately, most patients recover their ability to swallow after some time.

One of the most important aspects of the rehabilitation phase is family training. Because the family provides the bulk of care, they need to be trained. All aspects of care need to be discussed, demonstrated, and tested. The family's emotional responses to the patient's disability should be elicited. Family members often have unrealistic expectations that can be clarified by information and by offering an opportunity to vent their own reactions and fears.

Long-Term Care Phase

The long-term care phase of stroke rehabilitation begins when the patient is discharged from the hospital or nursing home. A significant amount of rehabilitation continues after the patient goes home. Home modifications must be installed to allow access to all needed areas. Doors may have to be widened for wheelchairs to pass. Generally, doors 32 to 34 inches wide are sufficient. Ramp installation may be needed; ramps must be 12 inches long for every inch of rise. The bathroom usually requires the installation of grab bars near the toilet and the bathtub, a raised toilet seat (Fig. 11-10) with arms, a bath bench, and a hand-held shower hose. Kitchen modifications are often necessary. Stairs may need hand rails mounted.

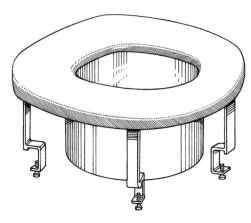

FIG. 11-10 Raised toilet seat attachment.

Safety in the home is of paramount importance. The ground floor is the safest level. If possible, provide a method of calling for help should a fall occur when the patient is alone. Many local hospitals have services in which an older person can rent a beeper to wear around the neck for such an emergency. Catalogs are available through which electronic aids, such as remote-control appliance switches, special phones, and emergency dialers, can be purchased.[9]

Adjustment to a major disabling condition may take as long as 2 years. Ongoing support from family, friends, and the primary care provider is important to fully successful adaptation. Stroke support groups, individual or family therapy, or a day health care center may be necessary at various times.

It is important for the primary provider to bring up the subject of sex. Fears that sexual intercourse will cause another stroke are unfounded. Simple reassurance suffices for most patients; a few need further counseling.

The resumption of social activities is the final test of stroke rehabilitation. Unfortunately, the survivor is all too often made to feel unwanted in social situations. Society remains largely discriminatory toward disabled people. Some communities have independent living centers that can be especially helpful in finding a new circle of understanding and supportive friends. Access to transportation services can also be arranged.

REHABILITATION AFTER AMPUTATION

▼ GARNER ROCHE (Part I)

Your patient, Mr. Roche, is a 74-year-old widower who has a long history of smoking, hypertension, and mild emphysema. For about 8 years, he has complained of pain in his left calf muscles after walking three or four blocks. In the last 2 years he has also developed angina pectoris when he walks more than two blocks. In spite of good control of his hypertension, in the last few weeks he has noticed a loss of sensation and darkened color of the great, second, and third toes on his left foot. Noninvasive testing of his lower extremities revealed an ankle/brachial index of 0.58 of the left popliteal artery and 0.27 of the dorsalis pedis and posterior tibial areas. Right dorsalis pedis was 0.60. An orthopedic surgery consultant has recommended a left below-the-knee amputation.

STUDY QUESTIONS

- *As Mr. Roche's primary care physician how can you help prepare him preoperatively for a successful course of rehabilitation afterward?*
- *What elements of Mr. Roche's medical history may impede successful ambulation after his amputation?*

Seventy-five percent of amputees are over age 65 years. In this age group, peripheral vascular disease is the most common cause. Care of the elderly amputee is complex because such patients usually have associated conditions like diabetes mellitus, hypertension, cardiac insufficiency, and contralateral vascular problems. The role of the primary care provider is to help decide on the type of amputation and to manage the medical and psychological sequelae.

Most amputations are below-the-knee (BK). This is the preferred surgical option because the success in achieving ambulation with a prosthesis is over 75% in the geriatric age group. Above-the-knee (AK) amputations are associated with a higher mortality and a dismal success rate in becoming ambulatory because of the extreme energy costs. In fact, the energy cost of walking with two BK amputations is less than that of one AK amputation (Table 11-3).

▼ GARNER ROCHE (Part II)

Mr. Roche agrees to the surgery in principle. However, he wants you to talk to his daughter first. After explaining the surgery, the risks, and alternatives, they decide to proceed with the recommended procedure. Before surgery, he meets the physical therapist to learn quadriceps exercises and is taught to lie prone. At first, he only can tolerate lying prone for 3 minutes. But after 2 days of practicing he can manage 12 to 15 minutes without discomfort. He also admits feeling quite depressed that he is losing a part of his body. A psychological consultation is arranged.

Following his surgery, Mr. Roche is able to learn proper transfer techniques, stump management, and use of a prosthesis. However, he finds that with ambulation both angina and claudication in his remaining leg develop sooner than before. Hence, he uses the prosthesis about the house and uses a wheelchair for longer distances, such as going shopping. Because he owns an automatic shift automobile, he is able to continue driving.

Before the amputation, all patients need optimization of their medical status, training in the exercises that will be used after the surgery, and psychological preparation. Range of motion exercises begin the day of surgery. Having the patient lie prone for 10 to 15 minutes two or three times a day helps to prevent contractures. Strengthening of the hip extensors and the upper body is also important. The second day after surgery, the patient can begin isometric quadriceps contractions. It is vitally important to prevent flexion contractures at the knee, because they increase energy costs and hamper use of a prosthesis. To help prevent contractures, the head of the bed should be kept flat and pillows should not be placed below the knees.

After the stump has healed, the patient must be trained in its care. Massage, stump wrapping to remove edema, inspection for evidence of infection or pressure, and routine hygiene must be learned.

Many elderly amputees use wheelchairs for traveling longer distances, so training in their use is needed. Therapists also can help these patients develop better balance and single-limb standing.

The permanent prosthesis is usually fitted around 6 to 8 weeks after surgery. This delay allows for stump shrinkage and healing. Often a temporary pylon prosthesis is used after 2 weeks to promote ambulation and prevent deconditioning. The most common type of permanent prosthesis uses a patella-tendon-supracondylar (PTS) socket with a solid-ankle, cushioned-heel foot (SACH). Most elderly amputees also use a strap connected to a waist belt for attachment. It is lightweight and easy to don. The cost of such a prosthesis may be as high as $2500.

Many patients adjust well to a prosthesis. These patients need training in prosthesis use, plus a brief rehabilitation to train them in the use of a wheelchair, transfers, and stump care. Some amputees are not able to learn to use a prosthesis for walking. At particular risk are those with significant cognitive impairment, prior immobility, contralateral vascular disease, weakness or sensory loss (e.g., stroke), or joint destruction.

Phantom sensations are often felt in the missing limb after an amputation. They occur in most amputees but are painful in only a minority. Significant discomfort usually resolves over time but can be disabling. The treatment of phantom limb pain is difficult; nonsteroidal antiinflammatory drugs are probably the most efficacious. Neuromas can also form at the amputation site. Local massage, injection with a steroid-anaesthetic mixture, or excision usually relieves the problem. Skin breakdown generally arises from a combination of inadequate attention to stump care and a poorly fitting socket. Socket fit may change with weight changes, especially weight loss.

HIP FRACTURE

▼ MABEL GREENE

Ms. Greene is an 80-year-old widow with a history of moderately severe osteoarthritis of her hands. Living alone in a one-story house, she has one daughter who lives about 300 miles away. One day she trips on a throw rug in her home and falls and injures her right hip. A subcapital fracture of the right femur is seen on x-ray. After her fluid status is stabilized, an orthopedic surgeon places a bipolar prosthetic device.

Table 11-3   Energy Costs of Amputation

Type of Amputation	Increase in Energy Required to Ambulate
Unilateral below-the-knee (BK)	25%-30%
Bilateral below-the-knee (BK)	40%-60%
Unilateral above-the-knee (AK)	65%-100%

While she tolerates the surgery well, Ms. Greene has poor endurance with therapeutic exercises. Therefore you send her to a local skilled nursing facility for a trial of rehabilitation. Upon admission she needs assistance with a front-wheeled walker.

Because of her arthritis of the hands, Ms. Greene is unable to use a regular walker effectively. Forearm troughs are added, and after much training, she becomes able to ambulate independently. She is discharged home with the services of a home health aide and a home chore worker. Her daughter is able to contract with a local handyman to install grab bars in the bathroom, a raised toilet seat, and a bath bench with a hand-held shower hose attachment. The throw rugs are discarded.

Many elderly patients benefit from rehabilitation after surgical repair of a hip fracture. This is especially true when patients have preexisting osteoarthritis or cardiopulmonary disease and whenever unsupervised exercise is contraindicated. Generally, the earlier the patient can begin ambulation training with weight bearing, the better the long-term prognosis. It is difficult for older persons to walk while they are only lightly stepping on their involved foot (toe-touch weight bearing). Hence, the surgical approach that allows early weight bearing is preferred (Table 11-4).

The patient with a hip fracture should be medically stabilized before surgical repair. As early as possible postoperatively, range of motion exercises of the uninvolved extremity can begin. The day after surgery the patient can sit up, quadriceps exercises can be initiated, and isometric contractions of other muscle groups can be started. Excessive motion may lead to joint disarticulation, however, because hip replacement surgery involves stretching and cutting of muscles that stabilize the joint. Therefore postoperative patients must be taught not to flex the hip more than 90 degrees and to avoid excessive abduction or adduction of the joint.

Supervised ambulation can begin on the second postoperative day, using a walker or a cane. Patients need to have their walkers fitted. Proper use of a walker involves advancing the walker 20 to 30 cm, then moving the weak leg first. Canes should not be used if either the ipsilateral upper extremity or the contralateral leg is weak, since

Table 11-4   Weight Bearing Recommendations After Hip Surgery

Type of Surgery	When to Begin Weight Bearing
Pinning	6-8 wk
Comprehension screw	2-3 days
Prosthetic replacement	1-2 days

no more than 25% of the patient's weight should be placed on a cane. When going up or down stairs, patients must keep the good leg higher (up with the good, down with the bad). It is difficult to carry objects safely when using a walker, so many people use a bag attachment.

ARTHRITIS

The key to arthritis management is prevention of secondary complications. Muscle weakness, contractures, uncontrolled inflammation, and anatomic derangement all contribute to pain and disability. Rehabilitation of the patient with arthritis begins with patient education. The person must learn daily joint protection techniques such as opening jars correctly, resting between household chores, and proper body alignment. Daily range of motion exercises and lying prone are recommended.

The cornerstone of treatment is pain management. With pain the patient cannot carry out a home rehabilitation program. A combination of oral and intraarticular medications, heat, massage, and rest is needed. Patients must be taught to recognize the fine line between rest and disuse. Intraarticular injections of steroids should probably be limited to two per year.

Equipment to be used in the home can promote independence. Many of the devices described in the earlier section on stroke can be used by patients with arthritis. Shoes with a large toe box and Velcro closures are often helpful. Early referral to orthopedists skilled in joint replacement is also advised; age alone is not a reason to refuse surgical repair.

PARKINSON'S DISEASE

▼ *VICTOR SARTORI*

Mr. Sartori is a 68-year-old man with Parkinson's disease for 10 years. He has been gradually declining in his activities of daily living (both basic [ADL] and instrumental [IADL]). He currently takes carbidopa/levodopa (Sinemet) and trihexyphenidyl (Artane). He also is depressed about his decline in function. A day rehabilitation program is available locally, and you refer him there, where he is seen by the physical and occupational therapists and a psychologist. A training program is begun with both individual and group therapy. The psychologist begins counseling oriented toward his adjustment to his disability. However, after 6 weeks the psychologist recommends a trial of antidepressant medication, and this seems to help somewhat. After 3 months of visits to the day health center, he is discharged, independent in ADLs and supervised in most IADLs.

Early in Parkinson's disease, rehabilitation may be of some benefit. The greatest benefits appear to come from group therapy. Patients can learn therapeutic exercises and methods for stretching and lying prone. In addition, they can participate in gait and balance training. For instance, patients can be taught to keep their heads up when walking and lift their feet when in the swing phase of ambulation. Regular range of motion exercises are helpful, but patients may become bored doing simple repetitive movements. Some believe dancing and singing to be of value.

Care should be taken when prescribing walking aids for patients with Parkinson's disease. Standard canes should be avoided because the tip of the cane tends to drift between the feet, threatening to provoke a fall. Pick-up walkers may exaggerate the retropulsion some Parkinson patients feel, causing backward falls. A front-wheeled walker is the preferred piece of equipment.

Home modifications that may be helpful include toilet equipment, rails on stairs, removal of shag and throw rugs, and bathtub benches. Speech therapists can also help these patients by using drills to increase their depth of breath between phrases, to modulate their tone, and to clarify speech articulation.

DECONDITIONING

All persons become deconditioned with bed rest and immobility. Older persons are particularly prone to this, since their time in bed in a hospital is typically longer than that of younger persons. Their families, and even they themselves, may believe they deserve time in bed after a long and stressful life. But losses in muscle strength and endurance begin shortly after a person takes to bed, and generally recovery from such losses takes twice as long in the elderly patient.

> *Bed rest is almost never indicated in elderly patients: it leads to deconditioning, which can be irremediable and fatal.*

Deconditioning is characterized by an elevated resting pulse, an exaggerated pulse or blood pressure response to minimal exercise, orthostatic hypotension, and easy fatigability. An increase in heart rate greater than 20 beats above resting during simple activities such as transfers is suggestive of deconditioning. Recognition of deconditioning is difficult in the presence of comorbid illnesses such as cardiac or pulmonary disease, malnutrition, dehydration, or infections.

To be considered a community ambulator, a person must be able to walk at 50% of normal velocity (normal = 70 m/min) and safely climb a curb. Many elderly patients cannot do this, even without specific conditions limiting their mobility, such as stroke or Parkinson's disease.

Treatment of deconditioning begins with stretching and strengthening exercises. Shoulder rotation, hip extension, knee extension, and ankle dorsiflexion are particularly important, because these are usually impaired by bed rest. Sitting tolerance is then addressed. Increasing periods spent in a chair will usually suffice, but occasionally the use of a tilt table will be required. Ambulation is then begun with or without an assistive device. Physiological monitoring by a physical therapist is needed to check blood pressure, pulse, and dyspnea level. A simple test of dyspnea can be made by asking the patient to count to 15 during physical activity. Dyspnea levels can be recorded on a scale of 0 to 4 (Table 11-5). All elderly patients who have been at bed rest for greater than 1 week should be considered deconditioned.

CONCLUSION

Rehabilitation techniques and approaches can be used in any geriatric health care setting. Given that many older persons fear losing their independence above all else, even death, the primary care provider should help disabled patients achieve the highest level of function they can.

Table 11-5   Measurement of Dyspnea by Having the Patient Count Aloud to 15 During Physical Activity

Response	Dyspnea Score
No breaths taken while counting	0
Patient hurries the count	1
One breath	2
Two breaths	3
Unable to finish (or three breaths)	4

POSTTEST

1. An older person would be considered handicapped when which one of the following factors is present?
   a. Renal function is significantly reduced.
   b. Manual muscle testing shows a strength level of 1/5 in the upper extremity.
   c. He or she uses a walker for community mobility.
   d. Services of a daytime attendant are required.
   e. He or she cannot attend a senior citizens' meeting because of a rule against the use of wheelchairs.

2. Typical duties of the occupational therapist in stroke rehabilitation include which of the following (more than one answer may be correct)?
   a. Training in ambulation
   b. Teaching dressing techniques for the lower body
   c. Driver's safety evaluation
   d. Bathroom transfer techniques
   e. Use of functional electrical stimulation for the upper arm

3. Which one of the following features is characteristic of nondominant stroke survivors?
   a. Prominent aphasia
   b. Lack of awareness of their deficits
   c. A high incidence of depression
   d. Swallowing problems and aspiration
   e. Visual field defects

4. A 78-year-old man was admitted to a rehabilitation program 3 weeks ago after having had a stroke with left hemiparesis. In the acute hospital his hypertension was difficult to control. For the first week of rehabilitation he did well, but over the past few days he has become increasingly somnolent and refuses therapy, saying that he is too tired. His medications include captopril, verapamil, and hydrochlorothiazide for hypertension and glipizide for diabetes. On examination his blood pressure is 105/60 mm Hg, his pulse is 80 and regular, his respirations are 18, and his temperature is 97.8° F. He has 2/4 strength on his affected side. Fine crackles are noted in both lung bases with no evidence of peripheral edema. Electrolytes, blood count, and renal function tests are normal. At this point your next step should be to do which one of the following?
   a. Begin tapering his antihypertensive medication to raise the blood pressure to 140/90 mm Hg.
   b. Order a ventilation-perfusion lung scan to rule out a silent pulmonary embolism.
   c. Start empirical antibiotic therapy for presumed pneumonia while awaiting the results of blood and sputum cultures.
   d. Start an antidepressant that has a low incidence of anticholinergic side effects.
   e. Order a repeat computed tomography scan of the brain to rule out a new stroke.

5. Which of the following features of amputation in the elderly is (are) true?
   a. Phantom limb pain occurs in a minority of patients.
   b. A prosthesis is useless in patients who will not walk.
   c. A pillow should be placed under the patient's knees to prevent skin breakdown.
   d. Energy costs of walking with an above-the-knee amputation are so high that many elderly are not able to ambulate safely with a prosthesis.

REFERENCES

1. Wedgewood J: The place of rehabilitation in geriatric medicine: an overview, *Int Rehabil Med* 7:107, 1985.
2. Brummel-Smith K: Introduction. In Kemp B, Brummel-Smith K, Ramsdell J, eds: *Geriatric Rehabilitation,* Boston, 1990, College-Hill Press.
3. Brody E: Informal support systems in the rehabilitation of the disabled elderly. In Brody SJ, Ruff GE, eds: *Aging and rehabilitation,* New York, 1986, Springer Publishing.
4. Warshaw G et al: Functional disability in the hospitalized elderly, *JAMA* 248:847-850, 1982.
5. Barthel DW: Functional evaluation: the Barthel index, *Md State Med J* 14:61-65, 1965.
6. Granger CV, Albrecht GL, Hamilton BB: Outcome of comprehensive medical rehabilitation: measurement by PULSES profile and the Barthel index, *Arch Phys Med Rehabil* 60:145-154, 1979.
7. *Enrichments: catalog for better living,* Bissel Healthcare Co, PO Box 579, Hinsdale, IL 60521.
8. *Comfortably yours: aids for easier living,* 52 West Hunter Ave, Maywood, NJ 07607.
9. *Selected products for people with special needs: catalog,* Radio Shack.

PRETEST ANSWERS
1. d
2. d
3. d
4. c

POSTTEST ANSWERS
1. e
2. b, c, e
3. b
4. a
5. a, d

CHAPTER 12

Ethics

MARY KANE GOLDSTEIN

OBJECTIVES

Upon completion of this chapter, the reader will be able to:

1. Discuss the role of the patient's age in ethical decision making about provision of medical care.

2. Discuss decisions concerning code status with patients.

3. Understand the approach to medical decision making with an incompetent patient.

4. Describe some common constraints on personal autonomy experienced by the frail patient.

5. Explain the concept of "conflict of interest" and describe some common conflict situations in medicine.

PRETEST

1. Which one of the following statements is false?
   a. The current legal standard in the United States is that a competent adult may refuse even life-saving treatment.
   b. If a power of attorney is not described as durable, it will generally lapse should the patient become incompetent.
   c. If a patient's wishes to refuse treatment become known after a treatment has been started, treatment cannot generally be withdrawn.
   d. Active termination of life is condoned, although not legalized, under strict guidelines in the Netherlands.
2. Informed consent involves all except which one of the following?
   a. The patient will have full disclosure of all aspects of the tests and treatment, their risks and benefits, and the alternatives.
   b. The patient must have the capacity to comprehend.
   c. The physician will be rendered free from liability.
   d. The patient must be free from any coercion.
3. Which one of the following statements is incorrect regarding cardiopulmonary resuscitation (CPR)?
   a. Septic patients who undergo a cardiac arrest are likely candidates for a successful resuscitation.
   b. Patients with cancer are no less likely than those without cancer to respond to initial resuscitation.
   c. Ventricular dysrhythmia carries a better prognosis for successful CPR than does asystole.

Ethical principles now widely recognized include: (1) the final choice of implementation of any medical recommendation remains with the patient; (2) when a patient's wishes are unknown in an emergency situation, the assumption is in the direction of preserving life; and (3) it is not ethically necessary to offer medically futile treatment.

Although these principles clarify some medical situations, physicians and other health professionals remain largely unprepared for many challenges. The implementation of a balanced approach, appropriately weighing the patient's autonomy and the physician's benevolence, is difficult to achieve in an era of rapidly evolving medical technology. The availability of procedures with potentially great benefits, but also the prospect of causing a protracted terminal phase with poor quality of life, is increasingly a cause of anxiety to many individuals. Professionals serving older persons need to maintain currency with the rapidly evolving ethical, societal, and legal directives on such issues.

The past decade has seen a growing emphasis on the formalization of ethical principles; there have been courses in ethics in a variety of professional schools, congressional attention to ethical principles for our lawmakers themselves, and open consideration of bioethics in fields such as genetic experimentation and termination of life-sustaining treatment. These cultural pressures to make ethical decision making more explicit have affected medical practice at a time when the physician's work is increasingly scrutinized by review boards, state quality assurance committees, and third-party payors. In addition, patients themselves have become more educated about health matters and often challenge medical decisions. As a result of these trends, primary care physicians must, both for reasons of personal professional integrity and as a response to societal scrutiny, become more conscious of the manner in which they make decisions about medical care.

 It is ultimately the patient's decision, and no one else's, whether or not to act on any medical recommendation.

This chapter focuses on the ethical issues most often raised in care of the elderly patient. Topics to be covered include age as a factor in decision making; limitation of treatment in the mentally competent patient; treatment of the terminally ill; medical decision making when the patient is mentally incompetent; challenges to patient autonomy; conflicts of interest; and the responsibilities of the practitioner in settings with limited resources. It is not possible to discuss all areas in depth; references are provided to guide further reading.

AGE AS A FACTOR IN MEDICAL DECISION MAKING

▼ WILLIAM HOPKINS (Part I)

Mr. Hopkins, an 89-year-old man who has been living at home with his wife and is in relatively good health, develops exertional chest pain. Based on history and physical examination findings, you believe he has a crescendo angina syndrome. The unofficial policy at the local hospital has been to *withhold angioplasty or coronary artery bypass grafting from patients older than 75 years.*

CASE DISCUSSION

You are confronted with the decision whether to limit workup and treatment because of age alone. You might attempt to avoid this dilemma by using a mathematical medical decision analysis model; however, at some point in the model it will be necessary to assign a weight to the value of continued life and the age question will surface again.

With the rapid expansion of the frailest elderly segment of our population and the escalating costs of medical care, consideration of age rationing is not a frivolous academic pursuit, but rather a vitally important area for public policy debate. Informal age rationing is surely a widespread practice. A famous comparison of the British and American medical care systems[1] describes the age rationing of dialysis and other procedures in the United Kingdom. General practitioners, aware of the limited resources and not wishing to refer to the hospital patients who will be unable to receive further treatment, tell patients that no further treatment is appropriate, rather than telling them that a treatment exists but is unavailable to them because of their age.[2] Limitation of treatment based on age is also common in the United States. Until recently, most drugs and treatments were not tested in the elderly, so practitioners could say with honesty that evidence supporting the efficacy of particular treatments in older persons was lacking. The high prevalence of multiple organ system illness in the elderly ensures that most physicians have personal experience of poor treatment outcomes. There is often an unconscious assumption that the elderly are frail and unlikely to do well with invasive treatment.

There are also philosophical arguments that openly support rationing based on age. Major arguments for age rationing have been reviewed, and rebuttals provided[3] to a number of them: (1) that there is decreased productivity by the elderly (yet, we value life in and of itself, not merely for the productivity of the person); (2) that respect for the elderly is consistent with limitations of medical care (but also requires forms of social support and justice that are lacking in the overall medical care delivery system); and (3) that differences in treatment based on age, unlike those based on sex or race, are consistent with a principle of equality, because over time all are treated equally if the young receive more medical care than the old (but this may not be the case if the older person being deprived of treatment was also deprived in youth under a different system). The most widely debated of the age rationing arguments[4] includes giving meaning to the late stages of life by assigning a role to the elderly of conservators of the future. In this role, the

elderly focus, not on preservation of their own lives, but on assisting the young to develop a good future for society. This position has been strenuously opposed by most senior advocacy groups, for fear that the argument will be simplistically translated by government finance agencies into strict age limitations on treatment.

What medical information can assist in making age-related decisions? Longitudinal studies of aging have found tremendous diversity among the aged. The following myths of aging should be abandoned: that different people age at the same rate and a single age cutoff for a given group could thus be determined; that a biological age can be assigned to an individual, implying that an individual's organ systems age at the same rate and that all organ systems in all individuals inevitably deteriorate over time. With such biological diversity among the elderly, we should be wary of generalizations based on age. In regard to surgical risk, there is probably a small degree of risk attributable to increased age itself, but the major component of the increased risk of the elderly is due to coexistent morbidity. Thus, in evaluating the probability of a good medical outcome, each case should be considered on the basis of the individual's overall health, with chronological age as only a small factor.

> *As medical technology extends what can be done, the challenge is to decide what should be done.*

CASE DISCUSSION

In approaching a case such as Mr. Hopkins, it is essential to separate the medical from the ethical considerations. The medical considerations should be evaluated in an age-blind fashion, with an objective review of pulmonary function, renal function, and other factors. If the medical risk is comparable to risks undertaken in younger patients, the remaining question is an ethical one: how much is prolongation of this aged person's life worth? The patient's assessment of the value of treatment should then take a prominent place in the decision.

▼ WILLIAM HOPKINS (Part II)

Mr. Hopkins is admitted to the hospital. The social worker on the team learns that Mr. Hopkins' greatest concern is that the angina will limit his ability to discharge his household obligations as usual. This is sufficiently distressing to him that he prefers to undertake the risk of further study and possible treatment, rather than continue to limit his life-style. He considers himself to be in generally good health except for the angina. You agree. He undergoes angiography and eventually a coronary artery bypass graft procedure. His postoperative course is complicated, and he spends several morose weeks in the hospital, wondering aloud if he has made the right choice. After discharge, he returns to his former level of activity and at a 6-month checkup declares that he is delighted with the result.

CASE DISCUSSION

Mr. Hopkins' case illustrates a sentiment frequently expressed by fit older patients: they wish continued treatment if it will maintain them at their present level of function, but they do not wish treatment that will keep them living in a disabled state. Practitioners should be careful to distinguish a request for treatment with a specific expected outcome from a request for any and all life-prolonging treatment.

LIMITATIONS OF TREATMENT IN THE MENTALLY COMPETENT PATIENT

▼ *LEO FALAKIS (Part I)*

Mr. Falakis is a 92-year-old widower whom you have admitted to the hospital for treatment of urosepsis. He is delirious on admission, but after several days of antibiotic treatment he is alert and coherent. When removal of his urinary catheter is attempted, he develops a large residual volume in the bladder, and a urological consultant recommends a prostatectomy. Mr. Falakis refuses the procedure and also states that if he becomes septic again he does not wish to have further antibiotic treatment.

The refusal of treatment by an apparently competent patient sometimes presents a dilemma to the practitioner. When the patient is hopelessly ill, limitations of treatment seem reasonable and are emotionally acceptable to most practitioners. When the patient is not terminal, however, the refusal of treatment for a remediable problem can be unsettling. Ethical medical practice is based on finding the balance of several ethical principles.[5] The principle of benevolence, of doing good for the patient, urges the provision of straightforward, clearly beneficial treatments. In balance with this, however, is the principle of autonomy, which calls for respect of the individual's right to control actions on his own person. When these two principles are in conflict, ethical consensus and legal precedent in this country give greater weight to honoring the individual's autonomy. The tradition of the right to protect one's person from invasion by others (the right to avoid unconsented touchings) has a long history in English common law and in U.S. legal precedent. The current legal standard in this country is that a competent adult may refuse even lifesaving treatment.[6] One consideration is that health care providers may overvalue health, relative to the value given it by the general public in comparison to other individual values. Ultimately, only the individual whose life is to be affected has the right to assign a value to medical treatment and to give or withhold consent for medical care.

> *Although the patient clearly has the right to refuse treatment, the physician is then obligated to be sure the patient is fully informed and capable of consenting freely.*

There is, however, an important caveat here. The physician has the obligation to be sure that the patient is fully informed and is freely consenting. Under the doctrine of informed consent, this is usually taken to involve three requirements (Box 12-1): (1) the physician must fully disclose the nature of all proposed tests and treatments, the alternatives to these tests and treatments, and the risks and benefits of both the proposed tests and treatments and of the alternatives; (2) the physician must ensure that the patient has the capacity to comprehend the information being presented; and (3) the patient must be free of coercion. The following sections describe some of the pitfalls to be avoided.

When a patient refuses a seemingly straightforward recommendation, a full reevaluation of the situation should be undertaken, with attention to each of the three components of informed consent: (1) has the patient received adequate information? For example, does the patient have misconceptions about the pain or danger of the proposed plan? Does the patient fully understand the negative consequences of withholding treatment? (2) Is the patient able to understand the information presented? Have hearing impairments, language difficulties, reading problems, or other barriers to communication with the competent patient been fully addressed? Has the patient's mental capacity been assessed? and (3) Is the patient free of coercion by family or hospital staff?

The following are examples of each of these problems and possible resolutions:

1. Vivid presentation of relevant information may lead a patient to change his or her mind. For example,

---

BOX 12-1
Elements of Informed Consent*

Full disclosure†:
    Nature of the disease or condition
    Proposed tests and treatments
    Alternative treatments
    Risks and benefits
Patient must have the capacity to comprehend
Patient must be free of coercion

*The doctrine of informed consent has evolved and varies somewhat from one jurisdiction to another.
Term *informed consent* first used in *Salgo v. Leland Stanford Jr. Univ. Bd. of Trustees,* 317 P.2d 170 (Cal. Ct.App. 1957).
†Elements of full disclosure described in *Natanson v. Kline,* 350 P.2d 1093 (Kan. 1960).

a patient may initially refuse amputation of a gangrenous foot because of a belief that loss of the foot will result in nonambulatory status. A meeting with a well-functioning amputee of the same general medical condition may dispel this fear. Information may also dispel patient misunderstandings about the nature of the procedure and its likely effects. Patients should be encouraged to express their concerns so that they can be directly addressed. Some patient concerns may include a combination of mistaken and realistic beliefs. For example, a patient concerned about becoming a burden to the family may on the one hand overestimate the likelihood of disability resulting from the planned treatments; on the other hand, this may represent a quite realistic expectation of an outcome that the patient has a legitimate right to avoid.

2. Patients are sometimes unaware of their own hearing deficits, or reluctant to reveal their poor comprehension of English, or their degree of illiteracy. Use of portable hearing amplifiers, interpreters, and oral rather than written presentation can improve comprehension. A patient from a non-Anglo culture may have hesitation about accepting unfamiliar treatments. Presentation of information in a culturally appropriate format, particularly with the assistance of a member of the patient's cultural group to provide interpretation, may reveal that the patient truly does wish the treatment. Depression may cloud competency, although there is great potential for abuse if physicians override patient wishes on the grounds that a nondepressed patient would have chosen the therapy.

3. There are many forms of subtle coercion. Unfortunately, the elderly are sometimes victims of fiscal abuse, even by members of their own family. Older persons may quite reasonably decide on their own to limit their treatment but should not be coerced into this by offspring eager to preserve their inheritance. Health care providers may use subtle coercion to convince patients to accept care against their will, for example, by withholding desired treatments such as pain medication until consent is given for aggressive treatment, by exaggerating the negative consequences of treatment refusal, or by overstating the likelihood of a positive outcome.

Physicians must remember that, although they are the authorities regarding medical treatment, it is the patient who is the source of authority for decisions to accept or refuse medical treatment.[7] Physicians should evaluate medical situations and make recommendations, but the final choice of implementation of the recommendation remains with the patient. Emergency situations in which the patient's preferences are unknown and unobtainable in a timely fashion are an exception to this rule. When patient wishes are unknown, the presumption is in the direction of preserving life. If it should happen that the patient's wishes later become known and the patient or his or her appropriate proxy requests it, treatment may be withdrawn.

▼ LEO FALAKIS (Part II)

After ensuring that the patient is rested and free of pain, you and a psychiatrist skilled in working with the elderly jointly interview Mr. Falakis. You review the plan for a prostatectomy, emphasizing the frequency with which the procedure is done in older individuals and the expected beneficial outcome. The patient states that he has had a long life and that he thinks that it has had its ups and downs but that overall he is satisfied with it. He has seen most of his friends and relatives age and die, and in many cases he has followed his friends' children to the grave. He has been a member of a small Greek Orthodox community, most of whose members have now passed away. He feels ready for his life to end, and he is adamant that he does not want to while away for years in a nursing home. He feels that if it is God's will that he develop another infection, he is ready to return to his Maker. You screen him both for cognitive impairment and for depression and find none. You also arrange for the patient's pastor to visit with him. The patient consistently maintains this position over several visits.

CASE DISCUSSION

Steps are taken to ensure that the patient is making an informed decision. First, the patient is made as comfortable as possible to minimize extraneous factors pushing him toward a limited life. The facts of the situation are reviewed in the presence of another professional capable of assessing the patient's comprehension (in this case a psychiatrist, although this function could be filled by another member of the health care team). The patient's reasoning is explored. Possible interfering factors such as depression are ruled out. Finally, the patient is assessed over several days and found to have a consistent response. In this situation the competent patient's wishes should be respected. The patient should be encouraged to put his wishes in writing and to communicate them to friends and family. The physician should also make clear that other forms of medical care the patient wishes (e.g., home nursing care for his catheter) will be available and that he has the right to change his mind without any prejudice against him. A plan should then be developed for handling the next episode of illness so that the patient receives symptom control and does not feel abandoned by the medical system.

ISSUES IN THE TREATMENT OF THE TERMINALLY ILL

Treatment of terminally ill patients requires some special considerations.[8] When caring for patients with terminal illness, physicians should routinely initiate discussions about life-sustaining treatments during nonemergency phases of illness. Patients should be encouraged to designate proxy decision makers (see Advance Directives) and to express their wishes in writing. The physician should follow a flexible care plan, adjusting treatments to the patient's changing condition and desires. Special attention should be given to adequate pain relief. Medication necessary to control pain at the end of life should not be withheld even if it risks depressing respiration. Symptom control should include attention to skin care, dyspnea, and nausea. Plans for the site of death—home, nursing home, hospital—should be discussed, and availability of medical support in the final hours should be arranged.

Assisted Suicide and Euthanasia

Ethical opinion on the propriety of assisted suicide is divided,[8] and a full discussion of the topic is beyond the scope of this chapter. Medical students and house staff rarely have sufficient experience to make such a grave decision and certainly should not provide medication to hasten death in a patient they barely know, as was described in the infamous "It's Over, Debbie" article.[9] Even more controversial than assisted suicide is euthanasia, in which the physician goes beyond providing the patient the means for suicide to actually performing a procedure that causes death. While condoned under strict guidelines in the Netherlands and widely discussed worldwide, euthanasia and assisted suicide are illegal in most countries.

RESUSCITATION AND CODE STATUS

▼ RHONDA BICKFORD (Part I)

Mrs. Bickford, a 72-year-old widow, is about to enter the hospital for an elective cholecystectomy. She requests that she be placed on no code status during her hospitalization. The surgical house staff question why they are undertaking surgery on someone who doesn't want to go on living.

Another set of special considerations arises regarding no code or do not resuscitate orders. There is a general presumption in our society that everyone is on full code status. A substantial amount of our public medical education effort is given to the attempt to educate every adult in cardiopulmonary resuscitation (CPR); it is assumed that no one who dies in public should go without a resuscitation attempt. The demonstrable efficacy of resuscitation of cardiac victims in the coronary care unit, or in a witnessed arrest out of hospital, has lead to the application of resuscitation measures to all hospital patients unless a specific no code order is written. When this treatment for cardiac patients is extended to other hospital patients (e.g., those with cancer, end-stage renal or cardiac disease, or pneumonia), the rate of success of the resuscitation procedure drops dramatically.

For older individuals with chronic disease the success rate of in-hospital CPR is poor. CPR may be painful and may prolong hospitalization only for death to result within a short time. In the few cases in which the older person survives to hospital discharge, the majority of patients experience major functional and neurological impairments that may be burdensome to them. Some believe that while CPR is a blessing for some elderly, it may be a curse for many others.[10] On the other hand, age alone is a poor predictor of resuscitation outcome, and age alone should not preclude the use of CPR.[11] Murphy et al. report that the only elderly patients in whom resuscitation is beneficial are those with a witnessed arrest, with ventricular tachycardia or ventricular fibrillation, and with restoration of sinus rhythm in 5 minutes.[12] These authors state that they think that insufficient research on healthy elderly exists to determine whether age independently predicts outcome. A summary of several studies of CPR is presented in Table 12-1.[13-17] It is important to remember that retrospective studies of patients who receive CPR may have serious selection bias: patients have been preselected to have CPR administered or withheld. The great variation in findings of different studies may be explained in part by this. For example, if CPR were performed on all patients who experienced a cardiac arrest in the catchment area of the Boston Five Hospital study, but were withheld from some chronically ill patients in the Seattle study because the emergency medical system was not called, the Boston study would be biased toward a poorer outcome than the Seattle study. To evaluate the outcome of CPR, studies with consistent criteria for provision of CPR are needed.

Many elderly people mistakenly believe that the effectiveness of CPR is over 50%.[18] Physicians should provide patients with information about the poor outcomes of resuscitation for in-hospital arrest for most patients over age 70 years. Recommendations to patients should take into account knowledge of which patients are most likely to benefit. Many elderly, when informed of their options, choose to be placed on no code status. Other persons may choose to remain on full code status, and their wishes should also be honored.

Survival after CPR is particularly poor for nursing home patients. Some geriatricians have called for policies that set "Do Not Attempt Resuscitation" as the default for nursing home settings.

▼ RHONDA BICKFORD (Part II)

In further discussion, Mrs. Bickford states that she understands that her general health status, apart from her gallbladder problem, is good. She wishes to have her surgery, to avoid future cholecystitis. If, however, during surgery or her postoperative period, she undergoes a cardiopulmonary arrest, she understands that there is a significant chance that she will not recover full function. She states that she feels that life

Table 12-1   Some Studies of Cardiopulmonary Resuscitation

Population	Results	Comments
294 university hospital patients with in-hospital CPR[13]	14% survived to discharge; pneumonia, hypotension, renal failure, cancer, and homebound life-style associated with in-hospital mortality; no survivors to discharge with pneumonia or CPR >30 minutes; 93% mentally intact at 6 mo.	Age alone did not influence prognosis.
140 teaching hospital patients with CPR; prearrest morbidity evaluated from chart[14]	55% successful CPR, 24% discharged alive overall; significant association of mortality with age >65; hypotension and azotemia, but none absolutely predictive of fatal outcome.	Age was associated with ultimate survival, not success of CPR.
1,405 age >70 and 1,624 age <70 out of hospital arrests in Seattle[15]	27% of old vs. 29% young resuscitated and admitted to hospital; 10% vs. 14% discharged alive; of 140 age >70 discharged, 112 went home.	Success for out-of-hospital arrests is similar for old and young.
503 age >70 with CPR at five Boston hospitals[16]: 2 acute care; 2 chronic care; 1 long-term care; 244 were out-of-hospital arrests	22% survived initially but only 3.8% to hospital discharge; only 1.8% with little or no impairment; only 0.8% of out-of-hospital arrests left hospital alive; survivors had ventricular arrhythmias and short CPR.	Authors state poor outcomes for elderly may have been due to concomitant illness; profile of patient with futile CPR: impaired organ system; dependency; unwitnessed arrest; asystole; or electromechanical dissociation.
399 CPR efforts in 329 Veterans hospital inpatients[17]; 77 CPR efforts were in patients age >70	In older patients, 31% had successful CPR, but none lived to discharge.	Presence of sepsis, cancer, increased age, increased medication doses, unwitnessed arrest; all were predictive of poor outcome.

must end at some point and that she would rather die suddenly from an arrest than live in a functionally disabled state. She is told that sometimes there is a brief pause in the heart's rhythm that can be restarted with no loss of perfusion to the brain. She says that if something of that sort happens during the operation, she would like to have her heart restarted, but that if there is difficulty reviving her, she does not want to go on breathing machines or other prolonged life support, which she saw happen to a friend of hers. It is then explained that during the surgery she will already be maintained by a ventilator. After further discussion, she clarifies her position to say that, if in the doctor's opinion there is a good chance of her returning to her usual function, she will accept emergency treatment, but that if the doctor believes that continued resuscitation attempts will result in brain damage, the resuscitation should be stopped. If she is mentally unresponsive, she does not wish to be maintained on a ventilator for more than a few days.

In considering a request for no code status, the physician should review the patient's general medical condition and discuss the possible outcomes of alternative actions with the patient. Undergoing elective surgery is clearly not inconsistent with a decision to refuse more extensive treatment. This should be discussed with the surgical team. Patients should be asked to put their requests in writing and to appoint individuals to make decisions for them should they be unable to do so themselves. The precise order to be written on the chart depends on the availability of the primary physician, the involvement of house staff, the code policy of the hospital, and other factors. The order may be changed several times during the hospitalization, as the patient moves from preoperative status, to recovery room, to open ward. It is impossible to either have a discussion or write an order that will anticipate all possible medical situations that may arise, but with clear communication of the patient's wishes, his or her general intent may be respected. Good communication between physicians is also important: the primary care physician must clearly convey the patient's wishes to cross-covering colleagues, surgeons, house staff, or other physicians involved in the patient's care.

> *Everyone on the team (including family members) must realize that "do not resuscitate" implies nothing about intensity of treatment while the patient is alive.*

▼ *RHONDA BICKFORD (Part III)*

The physician explains to Mrs. Bickford that unforeseen circumstances may arise and asks her to discuss her wishes with her husband and to make a formal proxy appointment for use if she should become mentally incapacitated. The physician also offers to meet with her husband or other family members if they wish. Mrs. Bickford executes a durable power of attorney for health care under state law, appointing her husband as her proxy decision-maker. She writes into the document her wishes regarding medical care. The physician writes a note in the medical record describing the situation and briefly discusses the plan with the surgical attending. The surgeon, having encountered this situation many times in the past, understands the patient's position and plans to discuss it with the house staff as a teaching point. Mrs. Bickford undergoes surgery and recovers uneventfully. Her durable power of attorney for health care remains on her office and hospital charts in case of future problems.

CASE DISCUSSION

This patient is a generally healthy woman who has a good chance of surviving CPR. Mrs. Bickford's physician was willing to respond flexibly to her wishes. He helped her to understand the actions for which she was giving or withholding consent. He then communicated this information to the key person—the surgeon—who would be giving orders in the operating room and recovery room.

In some cases, patients have extremely detailed requests, with specific consent or refusal of a series of treatments including intravenous therapy, antibiotics, ventilators, and defibrillation. Some hospitals encourage the listing of specific procedures that may or may not be used; other hospitals regard this as too confusing for the physician who must provide treatment of an arrest in the emergency setting. Physicians should seek information from the hospital administration about any local guidelines that are available.

"Do not resuscitate" or other limitation of treatment orders also will vary with the patient setting. A long-term care patient with probable Alzheimer's disease should have chart orders that cover use of intravenous therapy, transfer to hospital, and use of antibiotics, as well as resuscitation. Even a patient living at home may, in some communities, be able to use a do not resuscitate order. There is a growing movement, organized by county emergency medical services, to allow homebound patients to keep do not resuscitate documents so they can avoid an inadvertent resuscitation by emergency personnel.

MEDICAL DECISION MAKING FOR THE POTENTIALLY INCOMPETENT PATIENT

▼ *PAULINE McCOLLISTER (Part I)*

Ms. McCollister is a 73-year-old nursing home resident with hypertension, coronary artery disease, stroke, arthritis, renal insufficiency, foot deformity from childhood polio, and a hearing impairment. She is disoriented at times. She has lived in the nursing home for 10 years and rarely leaves the chair beside her bed. She has recently developed urinary incontinence, and you wish to perform a catheterization to determine her postvoid residual urine. She refuses the procedure.

Medical decision making with an incompetent patient should proceed as in Fig. 12-1. The first step is to determine whether the patient is in fact incompetent.

"Competency," as a legal term, has a precise meaning. The courts consider all adults competent unless judged otherwise by a court of law. Competency is also task specific—one is competent to handle finances or to make medical decisions and may be judged competent for one task but incompetent for the other. In the more customary medical sense, competency is roughly equivalent to having mental capacity for the task at hand.

 Competency is task specific; a patient can be competent to make one type of decision and not competent to make another.

To obtain informed consent, the physician must assess the patient's capacity to comprehend the information being presented and make a rational judgment about it. Most patients give evidence of their competency during the routine medical encounter in the questions they ask and the comments they make. When this evidence is lacking or when competency is questioned by a family member, another health care professional, or some other involved party, a more formal assessment should be undertaken. If the patient is already under medical care, one should first optimize the medical treatment, relieve the patient's discomforts, reduce distractions during the assessment, and minimize doses of sedatives to allow for greatest alertness.

The focus of a formal competency assessment is not only on mental status testing, but on the problem at hand. Accordingly, the patient should again be fully informed about the medical matter under discussion and should be encouraged to ask questions until he or she feels the situation is fully understood. The physician should then assess the patient's thought process in reaching a decision.[19] A patient should not be judged irratio-

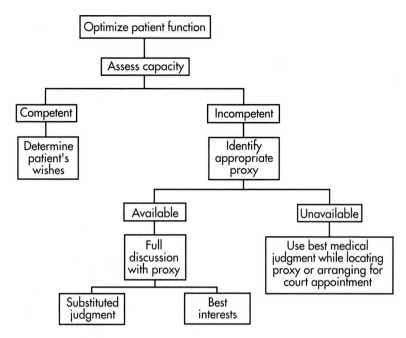

FIG. 12-1   Algorithm for medical decision making with an incompetent patient.

nal for disagreeing with the physician; rather, the process by which the patient's decision flows from the patient's values and stated premises should be examined. If the process is rational, the result should be accepted.

Even for a patient who has good cognitive function and understands the problem at hand, there may in rare cases be an impairment of competency caused by depression.

▼ PAULINE MCCOLLISTER (Part II)

During mental status testing, Ms. McCollister performs poorly on standard orientation questions. She can give neither the phone number nor the address of her residence, she misstates the year by 1 year, and she does not know who is the president. She can, however, give a full account of each patient who has been in the bed next to hers over the years, including the most recent. She can also identify all the staff, and she accurately states their shifts. She can describe other ward business in accurate detail. When asked to explain her present decision, she gives several reasons. She states that the urinary leakage is not bothering her now and that if it does in the future she will reconsider. She explains that she has always been a very private person and that she particularly dislikes and objects to any examination of her private parts. She has never had sexual intercourse and has never permitted a pelvic examination to be done, and she sees no reason to change her behavior now. She says she has seen a good many people come through the nursing home and die, and she has outlived them all, keeping her own counsel. She knows that the doctors mean well, but she thinks that a catheterization would be very invasive and she is unwilling to accept it. She

realizes that she has a number of medical problems and that any one of them could worsen at any time. She is willing to bide her time and see if the urinary problem becomes worse.

CASE DISCUSSION

This discussion illustrates that a patient may perform poorly on some mental status test items, but still retain the capacity to incorporate new information of importance, such as ward routines. The patient also demonstrates an ability to explain herself in a logically consistent manner. She should be considered competent to make this decision about the catheterization.

Advance Directives and Proxy Appointments

When the physician has determined as a result of careful assessment that the patient lacks decision-making capacity, an appropriate proxy decision maker for the patient must be identified. In most areas, state law governs the appointment of a proxy and specifics should be discussed with local legal counsel. Ordinarily, the next-of-kin is permitted to function as proxy for the patient who has become incapacitated. In some cases a conservator for the patient has been legally appointed for an incompetent patient. Where the patient has taken steps to appoint a legally recognized alternative proxy, that person should be consulted regarding the patient's medical care. This situation often arises when a close friend who is not linked to the patient by marriage, for example, a gay or lesbian companion or an old friend, is identified in advance by the patient as having priority over the family-of-origin. Many states have established special statutes that describe the components of a valid proxy appointment. Other states have allowed proxy appointments to be made under the general durable power of attorney laws that all states have. *The Power of Attorney Book*[20] provides information on state law and samples of documents to use without consulting an attorney. Choice in Dying (200 Varick Street, New York, NY, 10014, 212-366-5337) maintains information and forms for each state. State laws are frequently changed, and information should be rechecked regularly.

Substituted Judgment. After identification of the proxy, the physician must obtain informed consent from the proxy as if the proxy were the patient. The proxy must be instructed as to what basis to use for the decision. Proxies should be encouraged to do what the patient would have wished done (i.e., to make a substituted judgment). This should prompt a search for meaningful signs of what the patient would have wished. Where possible, a life trajectory of the patient's decisions should be sketched out and current decisions made in accordance with that trajectory.

> *Whether or not the family member is the official proxy, the family member must realize that he or she is helping assist the team to know what the patient would have wanted had he been able to communicate.*

The decision of the United States Supreme Court in the case of Nancy Cruzan allowed the State of Missouri to set a standard of evidence for the patient's prior wishes of clear and convincing.[21] This is a level of evidence somewhere between preponderance of the evidence and beyond a shadow of a doubt.[22] In other words, while not requiring the degree of legal certainty it would take to convict a murderer, it is considerably higher than the level of certainty required to find a physician liable for malpractice. While oral statements could under some circumstances meet the standard, the court decision encourages the use of written statements of wishes by competent persons. Such written statements, known as advance directives, are of several types. One form, known as the living will, is a general statement of the person's wishes for future medical care. It is considered informative and does not hold the force of law. An example of the Florida state living will in 1993 is shown in Fig. 12-2. An alternative is proxy appointment (see also discussion above) by designation of a health care surrogate or by Durable Power of Attorney for Health Care (DPAHC),[23,24] which allows a competent person to designate who should be the proxy decision maker for health matters should the person become mentally incapacitated. In most states, some form of health care surrogate or DPAHC is recognized either under specific legislation or via a general DPA statute. A sample of the Florida health care surrogate form is shown in Fig. 12-3. (State forms are frequently revised, and the current version for the correct state should be obtained.) One advantage of the DPAHC is that it has the force of law: the physician is expected to follow the instructions of the appointed proxy, if given in good faith. The physician is also in some states protected from civil and criminal liability when following such instructions. The DPAHC also allows for flexibility in response to unanticipated circumstances. When appointing the proxy under DPAHC, patients should express any specific wishes they have (e.g., limitations of feeding tubes, intravenous therapy, or antibiotics) as well as giving general instructions to the proxy.*

Copies of the document should be given to the proxy and to the patient's personal physician. Physician offices and hospitals should maintain a system of placing such documents on charts and of identifying charts which have them, so that they will be readily available at the time of a patient's illness.

Best Interests. Often, there is no evidence of the patient's prior wishes, so substituted judgment based on what the patient would have wished is not possible. In these cases the decision must be based on the best interests of the patient, as determined by the appropriate proxy. The assessment of best interests includes consideration both of prolongation of life and of the burden of treatment.[25]

Ordinary vs. Extraordinary Treatments

The terms "ordinary" and "extraordinary" have been used extensively in moral discussions, especially by Roman Catholic theologians, usually with the understanding that ordinary treatments must be offered (by the physician) and accepted (by the patient) to avoid wrongdoing. Extraordinary treatments were considered to be those that involved excessive expense, pain, or other inconvenience[26] or had little chance of success given the patient's condition. In the Quinlan case,[27] the New Jersey Supreme Court invoked the concept that judgments about treatment were to be based on the degree of in-

---

*However, great care should be taken about the specificity of such instructions. Several preprinted versions of living will and health care proxies suggest procedures that should be considered and discussed with the proxy. These often include certain treatments about which there is much societal prejudice despite their extreme usefulness in certain situations, such as electroconvulsive therapy (ECT) and antipsychotics; also, the technology is changing so fast that some extraordinary-sounding treatments are already routine. Certain treatments that may be precluded by such directives are often used for temporary maintenance during recoverable illness (e.g., tube feedings following stroke but before recovery of swallowing function). The important point is to have the patient clarify to the proxy the general nature of the patient's feeling about intensity of treatment in irrecoverable or highly dependent situations, avoiding specifics that may become outdated (*Editor's note*, RH).

FLORIDA LIVING WILL

INSTRUCTIONS	

PRINT THE DATE

Declaration made this _____ day of _____, 19_____.

PRINT YOUR NAME

I, _____, willfully and voluntarily make known my desire that my dying not be artificially prolonged under the circumstances set forth below, and I do hereby declare:

If at any time I have a terminal condition and if my attending or treating physician and another consulting physician have determined that there is no medical probability of my recovery from such condition, I direct that life-prolonging procedures be withheld or withdrawn when the application of such procedures would serve only to prolong artificially the process of dying, and that I be permitted to die naturally with only the administration of medication or the performance of any medical procedure deemed necessary to provide me with comfort care or to alleviate pain.

It is my intention that this declaration be honored by my family and physician as the final expression of my legal right to refuse medical or surgical treatment and to accept the consequences for such refusal.

In the event that I have been determined to be unable to provide express and informed consent regarding the withholding, withdrawal, or continuation of life-prolonging procedures, I wish to designate, as my surrogate to carry out the provisions of this declaration:

PRINT THE NAME, HOME ADDRESS AND TELEPHONE NUMBER OF YOUR SURROGATE

Name: _____

Address: _____

_____ Zip Code: _____

Phone: _____

© 1993 CHOICE IN DYING, INC.

PRINT NAME, HOME ADDRESS AND TELEPHONE NUMBER OF YOUR ALTERNATE SURROGATE

I wish to designate the following person as my alternate surrogate, to carry out the provisions of this declaration should my surrogate be unwilling or unable to act on my behalf:

Name: _____

Address: _____

_____ Zip Code: _____

Phone: _____

ADD PERSONAL INSTRUCTIONS (IF ANY)

Additional instructions (optional):

I understand the full import of this declaration, and I am emotionally and mentally competent to make this declaration.

SIGN THE DOCUMENT

Signed: _____

WITNESSING PROCEDURE

Witness 1:

Signed: _____

TWO WITNESSES MUST SIGN AND PRINT THEIR ADDRESSES

Address: _____

Witness 2:

Signed: _____

Address: _____

© 1993 CHOICE IN DYING, INC.

PAGE 2

FIG. 12-2 Example of the Florida state living will. Choice in Dying provides statutory advance directives for each state free of charge, as well as other materials and services relating to end-of-life medical care. Callers can contact Choice in Dying at 1-800-989-WILL. (From Choice in Dying, 200 Varick Street, NY 10014, [212-366-5540].)

vasiveness and likelihood of success. The definition of extraordinary, however, has remained elusive in practice. While at one time the use of ventilators was extraordinary, they are now quite ordinary. Because of this difficulty, most medical ethicists have moved from use of these terms to discussion of whether treatments are morally obligatory or optional. Basic care, including shelter, clothing, and food offered by mouth, is obligatory. Strictly, medical treatments are considered optional, in the sense that they may be offered depending on the medical indications.

When the Family Wants Everything Done

Over the past 20 years the majority of cases of conflict between family and physician over intensity of care have been cases in which the family sought the right to limit treatment. In the last few years, as the right to limit treatment has become well established, there has been a shift in focus to the rare cases in which a physician wishes to limit treatment against the wishes of the family. Physicians sometimes invoke the argument that there is no ethical obligation to provide futile treatment. This argument is problematic because there are differing interpre-

tations of "futility." Physicians are not obligated to provide treatment that is outside usual medical practice (e.g., Laetrile treatment for cancer) nor to provide treatment that is useless (e.g., repeat courses of chemotherapy for a cancer that has proven unresponsive). When a treatment will prolong life and the question is whether the quality of life is worth continuing, however, the decision moves beyond the purely medical arena. If a family wishes to maintain a comatose patient on ventilator therapy, they are making a determination about the quality of life in a coma, and not about the efficacy of ventilator therapy. Opinion in the bioethics community is divided about appropriate management. Physicians should consult with their hospital ethics committee or the hospital administration about such cases.

Enteral Feeding

▼ EDWIN MORLEY

At the age of 91, your patient Mr. Morley suffers a stroke, which causes left hemiparesis and difficulty speaking. The stroke progresses, and Mr. Morley becomes unresponsive and unable to swallow. His family feels certain, based on prior ex-

FIG. 12-3   Example of the Florida state health care surrogate designation. Choice in Dying provides statutory advance directives for each state free of charge, as well as other materials and services relating to end-of-life medical care. Callers can contact Choice in Dying at 1-800-989-WILL. (From Choice in Dying, 200 Varick Street, NY 10014, [212-366-5540].)

plicit discussions with the patient, that he would not want to have treatment that would be likely to leave him in a severely disabled state. The family declines treatment with intravenous fluids or enteral feeding tubes, and the patient dies several days later.

CASE DISCUSSION

This case presents one of the most difficult decisions in geriatric practice: whether or not to use an enteral feeding tube for a patient with an acute stroke.

An area of particular difficulty in decision making for the incompetent patient is use of enteral feeding tubes.[28] Patients who are mentally competent may of course make this decision for themselves, and long-term tube feeding is often used effectively in patients with swallowing problems after treatment for head and neck tumors, multiple sclerosis or amyotrophic lateral sclerosis, or other neurologic disorders. For incompetent patients, most physicians in this country also do not hesitate to place a feeding tube for short-term treatment in potentially reversible swallowing disorders. For example, in the first week after a stroke, the likelihood of recovery is often uncertain and a feeding tube may prevent malnourishment for the short time until swallowing function resumes. Many families and physicians are uncomfortable withholding an enteral feeding tube in this situation because the prognosis is unclear. If the patient has left explicit instructions, however, it is permissible to limit treatment in this way.[29]

Another difficult decision is that for the patient who has irreversible or progressive mental impairment and for whom a feeding tube will prolong nonsentient life. For example, when a patient with severe Alzheimer's disease reaches the point of being unable to accept hand feedings, a decision about use of a feeding tube must be made. The proxy must consider what the patient would have wished in this situation. Any available information, such as conversations with friends and family about similar cases in the past, should be used to reconstruct the patient's wishes. Many patients have indicated clearly that they would not want to receive continued treatment in this situation, and in these cases it is appropriate to withhold use of the feeding tube. Consensus is growing that tube feedings should be likened to other medical interventions and not considered part of routine care.[30] Hand feedings should continue to be offered and mouth care provided to alleviate any discomfort of a dry mouth.

> The clinician can help families with intensity of treatment decisions by clarifying what is generally regarded as reasonable in the circumstances.

Intravenous Fluids

When a decision to withhold life-prolonging treatment while providing symptom control has been made, special considerations arise concerning intravenous fluids and antibiotics. It is acceptable to withhold these treatments on request of the appropriate proxy decision maker when life prolongation is no longer the appropriate goal (e.g., in terminal illness or advanced dementia). In end-stage dementia, when cognitive functions are lost, it is unlikely that patients experience discomfort with dehydration. On the other hand, there are situations in which a dying, but alert, patient will be more comfortable with the provision of intravenous fluids, and these should not be withheld simply because the patient has refused more aggressive therapy.

CHALLENGES TO PATIENT AUTONOMY

▼ FRED DOOLEY (Part I)

Your patient, 82-year-old Mr. Dooley, has experienced a gradual decline in physical function over the past 5 years. He has had several small strokes with some residual weakness and is now unable to walk more than a few steps without assistance. He has been totally dependent on his wife for assistance in his instrumental activities of daily living for the past 2 years. He also asks his wife to help him with the basic activities of dressing, grooming, and feeding, although it is unclear whether he truly needs assistance in these areas. A fall precipitates an emergency room visit. He is found to have acute pneumonia and is admitted for treatment. After a week in the hospital, he is close to his baseline level of function, and discharge plans are being made. Mrs. Dooley says that she is unwilling to accept her husband back home. She maintains that he presents too heavy a care load for her, and that he must be placed in a nursing home. The patient, who is mentally competent, although physically disabled, insists that he wants to go home.

CASE DISCUSSION

Here is a sadly familiar scenario: a family caregiver at the end of her emotional and physical ability to provide care is at odds with the patient who wishes to exercise his autonomous right to return to his own home.

Patient Opposition to Placement

The placement of a competent patient in a nursing home against his or her will presents a painful dilemma to the health care professional. Social workers and discharge planning nurses struggle along with physicians to find adequate responses. As with other ethical dilemmas, a first step is to attempt to find a third alternative that is satisfactory to both parties. In some cases, alleviating caregiver stress can make home placement acceptable once again to the caregiver with provision of more in-home supportive services (e.g., housekeeping aides, home health aides, Meals-on-Wheels), self-help support groups or individual counseling for the caregiver, or further aid for the caregiver from the extended family or community. In other cases in which the caregiver simply cannot cope, even with increased support, the patient can be given an alternative to nursing home care that is more attractive (e.g., a residential care arrangement). In some cases, however, none of these alternatives resolve the problem, and a true dilemma remains. It is clearly unacceptable to physically place a competent patient in a nursing home against his or her will.

Some members of the health care team may begin to take sides either to blame the caregiver for his or her unwillingness to care for the patient or to blame the patient for being uncooperative with placement plans. Such decisions easily evoke strong personal emotions on the part of professionals, often pitting the final chance of the patient to live out his life in his own home against the last chance of the spouse to find some relief while still enjoying a modicum of good health. There may also be institutional pressure to free up the hospital bed. The conflict of a patient's right to return to his or her own home and the spouse's right to refuse overwhelming burdens of caregiving is difficult; it is made even more difficult if health professionals take rigid positions.

The staff should work at keeping an open mind, remembering the rights of both patient and caregiver. A practical approach might be a day pass at home for the patient in order to demonstrate to the patient his management difficulties (or convince the hospital staff that it will be possible to manage). Support for the caregiver may limit caregiver burden. Family counseling may be needed. Other family members, if available, may help.

When all these approaches fail to yield a resolution to the conflict, assistance from an outside source, such as a senior ombudsman program or a hospital ethics committee, should be sought.

▼ FRED DOOLEY (Part II)

The geriatric nurse and social worker meet with Mr. Dooley in several sessions. The geriatric nurse obtains precise information about Mr. Dooley's functional care needs and explains to the team exactly what assistance he will need from a caregiver for him to be maintained in his home. The social worker obtains the patient's permission to contact other family members, and he locates a son who has not been active recently in his father's care. Stimulated by the concern shown by the geriatric team, the son visits his father in the hospital and agrees to participate in family caregiving. Mr. Dooley also agrees to short respite-care nursing home admissions every 3 months. Arrangements are made for a medical evaluation for Mrs. Dooley. Her physician agrees that she is too frail to do heavy lifting and that she needs assistance with housework. She joins a caregiver self-help group, and with this support, she decides to accept a variety of in-home supportive services and her son's help. Arrangements are made for close follow-up. Mrs. Dooley is told that this arrangement is only temporary: Mr. Dooley is in a decline, and new arrangements will need to be made as the situation changes. Both Mr. and Mrs. Dooley are advised to consider the possibility that a nursing home placement will be unavoidable at some time in the future.

Autonomy and Disabilities

In both the home and institutional care there are many constraints on the autonomy of the elderly with disabilities.[31] While an older person who is mentally competent should be able to make his or her own decisions, one who has functional disabilities will often depend on others to carry out the plans. For example, a wheelchair-bound patient who is too weak to do independent transfers cannot get to the bank without assistance. The patient may think (in most cases accurately) that the person providing the assistance is doing a favor and that some obligation to that person has been incurred. The patient is also unable to function in privacy: a trip to the bank or the lawyer's office may lead to questions from inquisitive staff or residents. Caregivers, both formal and informal, must work at remaining sensitive to the patient's privacy and the patient's right to make independent decisions, even if they are not in accord with the caregiver's wishes.

▼ FRED DOOLEY (Part III)

In the caregiving support group, Mrs. Dooley learns how to set limits for herself in the tasks she performs to care for Mr. Dooley. She realizes that her past practice of tending to his every whim cannot continue and that she will be able to allow him to stay home longer if she maintains the limits. She also realizes that she would have felt a great burden of guilt had she placed her husband in a nursing home against his will.

Mr. and Mrs. Dooley bring their family together to discuss the situation. Mr. Dooley states emphatically that he dreads the prospect of a nursing home. He asks the family to support him in staying at home and to honor his wish that he not receive any life-prolonging treatment if his condition worsens. The family rallies to take turns in helping with caregiving. A few months later, Mr. Dooley has a large left cerebral stroke. While in the hospital, he dies from a pulmonary embolus. One year later, at a family gathering, Mrs. Dooley states that she is happy that they were able to allow Mr. Dooley to spend his last months at home as he wished.

Home care was a possibility for the Dooley family, and the relatively short period of care did not overburden this particular family's resources. Mr. Dooley was mentally competent and able to participate in decision making about his site of care. In this case the spouse and family were eager to provide the best care for the patient. In other cases the spouse, sometimes the victim of years of abuse by the patient, is truly unwilling to cooperate in a care plan. In such a situation the exact plan that avoids infringing on either spouse's rights must be worked out with the help of experienced social workers and sometimes an attorney.

This section has focused on the right of the competent but physically frail patient. Similar issues arise with the care of demented patients. When a patient is demented, the proxy takes into consideration the patient's wishes but ultimately may have to decide on the site of care. A spouse of a demented patient may feel considerable guilt about a nursing home placement; however, the ethical problem of denying a competent patient the right to live in his or her own home is not an issue. Physicians must often help families to reach the difficult decision of placing a demented patient in a nursing home because home care is excessively burdensome.

Restraints

The use of physical and chemical restraints is another area of management of elderly patients fraught with difficult ethical questions. Restraints are rarely considered in fully competent patients but are frequently used in acute hospitalized patients with delirium and a consequently fluctuating level of competence. Physical restraint of a patient should be used only when the patient is a danger to himself or to others and only when all other means of behavioral management have been exhausted. The use of a restraint by a health professional creates an obligation for the professional to attend carefully to the negative consequences that may follow restraint by monitoring them and working to prevent them: increased agitation, pressure sores, immobility, incontinence, constipation, and impaction. The presumed benefit of restraint should be carefully weighed against the risks of complications and the insult it presents to patient dignity. Restraints are sometimes used to permit other therapy (e.g., intravenous lines) to continue. The restraint may sometimes be avoided by reconsidering the necessity of the restrictive therapy. Chemical restraint by use of psychoactive pharmacological agents must also be prescribed with caution and only when for the clear benefit of the patient.[32] As a practical matter, physician refusal to write a sedative or major tranquilizer order without providing alternatives for the staff in management of a combative patient will lead to a breakdown of care. Close cooperation between the physician and the nursing staff is necessary to work out ward routines that minimize the need for patient sedation.

CONFLICTS OF INTEREST

Primary care practitioners should have a basic understanding of the concept of conflict of interest. This term is used to refer to a situation in which an individual has responsibilities that pull in different directions. Physicians have a responsibility to act in the best interests of their patients' medical care. Physicians also control the ordering of medical tests. Physicians who have a financial interest in the laboratory to which they refer all their patients for tests are said to have a conflict of interest in the sense that their judgment about what is best for the patient may be clouded by their desire to increase income from the laboratory by referring all patients there for excessive testing.

Financial institutions and legal firms operate under complicated rules governing conflict of interest. Attention has only recently focused on conflicts of interest in the medical profession. Some of the major areas will be discussed here.

Incentives for Limiting Medical Care

Physicians who receive financial incentive for limitation of medical care, the arrangement in many health maintenance organizations and preferred provider organizations, must be careful not to allow their medical judgment to be affected by the financial arrangements. Not surprisingly, it has been shown that some financial incentives do influence the behavior of physicians toward patients.[31] To avoid abuse, the financial reward should be kept several steps removed from the point at which a decision is made about a particular patient. For example, arrangements in which all physicians in a group benefit by a small percentage at the end of a year if the entire practice has kept costs down may be acceptable. On the other hand, if a physician knows that by keeping a particular patient who is in front of him now out of the hospital he can receive a financial reward, the conflict of interest is probably too great to allow for objective medical decision making.

Incentives for Overuse of Medical Care

It must be remembered that fee-for-service financial arrangements contain powerful financial incentives toward overuse of medical services rather than limitation of medical service. Abuse of this system may range from recommending overly frequent office visits to ordering expensive and potentially dangerous invasive tests without clear necessity. A physician may order a particular piece of office equipment (e.g., a treadmill test setup) and then use it on many patients unnecessarily to make a profit. Such practices are clearly unethical.

Legislators have scrutinized the practice of dispensing drugs directly from the doctor's office. When physicians dispense their own medications, it is feared that they will not be subject to the limits imposed by having another professional review decisions. For example, they may charge an excessive markup on the drugs. In response to this, many primary care practitioners have pointed out that there are advantages to the patient of physician-dispensed medication such as one-stop shopping (important for functionally disabled persons and almost a necessity in some rural areas).

The general rule that should be applied is that business activities should be intended for the reasonable support of the practice and for the provision of high-quality care to patients.[34]

Pharmaceutical Marketing

Pharmaceutical companies have a legitimate interest in marketing their products, but companies may be expected to be biased in favor of their own products. For many busy practitioners the most available source of information about medications is the drug detail person sent by the pharmaceutical company. Physicians should seek independently developed drug information from other sources (e.g., reviews in standard medical texts and journals).[30] Physicians should not accept valuable gifts from pharmaceutical companies.

ALLOCATION OF RESOURCES

Physicians are often involved in decisions of allocation of scarce resources. When a new drug is developed but available only in small amounts, requests for it must be prioritized. Organs for transplant are always in short supply. Another form of scarcity of resource is financial limitation. A fixed pool of money may be made available to cover services, and within that constraint the physician must decide how to allocate the money. The physician may be involved at several different levels: as a primary care doctor caring for individual patients, as a community physician participating in review committees, and as a policy maker developing guidelines for allocation of care.

Thoughtful discussions have been published regarding microallocation decisions in medicine.[35] It is not always possible to have what seems to be a just outcome; one must focus on just procedure.

The primary care physician may wear several hats and may need to apply different rules in different roles. As the primary medical care provider for an individual patient, the practitioner should function as patient advocate. As member of a committee formulating guidelines for equitable distribution of limited resources, the practitioner may function as a utilitarian, attempting to maximize overall benefit. As a politically active citizen, the practitioner may advocate for changes in the distribution of resources. Physicians should be careful to avoid having one set of responsibilities encroach on another.

SUMMARY

In the past, it has been alleged that statements of physician professional ethics were little more than self-serving rules reining in the members of the profession to protect their own interests.[36] With the assistance of ethicists the profession of medicine is now taking great care to adopt genuine ethical codes and practices. In resolving the wide range of ethical dilemmas presented by work with the older patient, the individual physician should uphold this standard. Physicians should separate medical from ethical questions and use ethical analysis to resolve dilemmas. Consultation with other members of the health care team can provide important insights.

POSTTEST

1. Which one of the following statements concerning CPR is false?
   a. In a study of out-of-hospital arrests, success rates were similar for the young and old.
   b. Sepsis reduces the chances that CPR will be successful.
   c. Over half of patients over 70 years surviving resuscitation do not survive to hospital discharge.
   d. Whether or not a patient has cancer does not influence the success of CPR.
2. Which one of the following statements is false?
   a. Competency is legally defined only in terms of the task to be undertaken.
   b. Legislation exists in most states to ensure that a properly executed health care proxy has the force of law.
   c. A treatment would be described as ethically extraordinary if it were expensive.
3. Which one of the following is not an advance directive for medical care?
   a. A living will
   b. A durable power of attorney for health care
   c. A statement to relatives that no aggressive treatment should be done
   d. A purchase of a "medigap" insurance policy
4. Which answer best describes the ways a proxy decision maker should be instructed to answer questions about medical care?
   a. Think of what it would be like for you in that situation, and answer as you would for yourself.
   b. Ask other family members to think what it would be like for them in that situation, and answer on the basis of their response.
   c. Recall things the patient said while still unimpaired that indicate his or her opinions on such a situation.
   d. Make your own judgment as to what would be best for those in the family who are still healthy and competent, and answer on that basis.

REFERENCES

1. Aaron HJ, Schwartz WB: *The painful prescription: rationing hospital care,* Washington, DC, 1984, The Brookings Institution.
2. Aaron HJ, Schwartz WB: Rationing health care: the choice before us, *Science* 247:418-422, 1990.
3. Jecker NS, Pearlman RA: Ethical constraints on rationing medical care by age, *J Am Geriatr Soc* 37:1067-1075, 1989.
4. Callahan D: *Setting limits,* New York, 1987, Simon & Schuster.
5. Goldstein MK: Ethical care of the elderly: pitfalls and principles, *Geriatrics* 44, 1989.
6. Gostin L: A right to choose death: the judicial trilogy of Brophy, Bouvia, and Conroy, *Law Med Health Care* 14:198-205, 1986.
7. Ruark JE, Raffin TA: Initiating and withdrawing life support—principles and practice in adult medicine, *N Engl J Med* 318:25-30, 1988.
8. Wanzer SH et al: The physicians responsibility toward hopelessly ill patients: a second look, *N Engl J Med* 320:844-849, 1989.
9. It's over, Debbie, *JAMA* 259:272, 1988.
10. Podrid PJ: Resuscitation in the elderly: a blessing or a curse? *Ann Intern Med* 111:193-195, 1989.
11. Scheidermayer DL: The decision to forgo CPR in the elderly patient, *JAMA* 260:2096-2097, 1988.
12. Murphy DJ et al: Outcomes of cardiopulmonary resuscitation in the elderly, *Ann Intern Med* 111:199-205, 1989.
13. Bedell SA et al: Survival after cardiopulmonary resuscitation in the hospital, *N Engl J Med* 309:569-575, 1983.
14. George AL et al: Pre-arrest morbidity and other correlates of survival after in-hospital cardiopulmonary arrest, *Am J Med* 87:28-34, 1989.

15. Longstreth WT et al: Does age affect outcomes of out-of-hospital cardiopulmonary resuscitation? *JAMA* 264:2109-2110, 1990.

16. Murphy DJ et al: Outcomes of cardiopulmonary resuscitation in the elderly, *Ann Intern Med* 111:199-205, 1989.

17. Taffet GE, Teasdale TA, Luchi RJ: In-hospital cardiopulmonary resuscitation, *JAMA* 260:2069-2072, 1988.

18. Clarke DE, Goldstein MK, Raffin TA: Ethical dilemmas in the critically ill elderly, *Clin Geriatr Med* 10:91-101, 1994.

19. Appelbaum P, Grisso T: Assessing patients' capacities to consent to treatment, *N Engl J Med* 319:1653-1658, 1988.

20. Clifford D: *The power of attorney book,* Berkeley, Calif, 1988, Nolo Press.

21. *Nancy Beth Cruzan v. Director, Missouri Department of Health,* Missouri, 110 S Ct 2841, 1990.

22. Annas GJ: Nancy Cruzan and the right to die, *N Engl J Med* 323:670-673, 1990.

23. Gilfix M, Raffin TA: Withholding or withdrawing extraordinary life support, *West J Med* 141:387-394, 1984.

24. Steinbrook R, Lo B: Decision making for incompetent patients by designated proxy: California's new law, *N Engl J Med* 310:1598-1601, 1984.

25. Cassel C, Goldstein MK: Ethical considerations. In Jarvik LF, Winograd CH, eds: *Treatments for the Alzheimer patient—the long haul,* New York, 1988, Springer Publishing.

26. Kelly G: The principle of nonmaleficence. In Beauchamp TL, Childress JF, eds: *Principles of biomedical ethics,* New York, 1983, Oxford University Press.

27. *Karen Quinlan,* Supreme Court of New Jersey, 355 A 2d 647, 1976.

28. Lo B, Dornbrand L: Guiding the hand that feeds: caring for the demented elderly, *N Engl J Med* 311:402-404, 1984.

29. Goldstein MK, Fuller JD: Intensity of treatment of malnutrition: the ethical considerations, *Prim Care* 21:191-206, 1994.

30. Steinbrook R, Lo B: Artificial feeding: solid ground, not a slippery slope, *N Engl J Med* 318:286-290, 1988.

31. Cohen ES: The elderly mystique: constraints on the autonomy of the elderly with disabilities, *Gerontologist* 28:24-31, 1988.

32. Goldstein MK: Ethical considerations in pharmacotherapy of the aged, *Drugs Aging* 1:1-7, 1991.

33. Hillman AL, Pauly MV, Kerstein JJ: How do financial incentives affect physicians' clinical decisions and the financial performance of health maintenance organizations? *N Engl J Med* 321:86-92, 1989.

34. American College of Physicians Ethics Manual: Part I: History; the patient; other physician, *Ann Intern Med* 111:245-252, 1989.

35. Beauchamp TL, Childress JF: *Principles of biomedical ethics,* ed 2, New York, 1983, Oxford University Press.

36. Starr P: *The social transformation of American medicine,* New York, 1982, Basic Books.

PRETEST ANSWERS
1. c
2. c
3. a

POSTTEST ANSWERS
1. d
2. c
3. d
4. c

CHAPTER 13

Hospital Care

DENNIS W. JAHNIGEN

OBJECTIVES

Upon completion of this chapter, the reader will:

1. Understand the role of the primary care physician in the hospital environment.

2. Know a five-step process for medical decision making in the care of elderly patients.

3. Know the common sources of adverse events for elderly hospital patients.

4. Understand the principles of planned prevention of the common problems of hospitalized elders.

5. Know the elements of discharge planning.

PRETEST

1. Which one of the following statements concerning hospitalization of elders is false?
   a. The hospitalization rate for those over 65 is twice that of the younger population.
   b. Elderly patients assessed in the emergency room are twice as likely to be hospitalized as younger persons.
   c. Delirium during hospitalization is predictive of a 40% 2-year mortality.
   d. Pressure ulcers develop in nearly 5% of hospitalized patients.
2. Which of the following medications causes the greatest number of adverse drug reactions in elderly patients?
   a. Digoxin
   b. Theophylline compounds
   c. Blood products
   d. Corticosteroids
   e. Antibiotics
3. The person elderly patients most commonly wish to make end-of-life decisions regarding their care is which one of the following?
   a. The physician
   b. A friend
   c. Their children
   d. An ethics committee
   e. Themselves

The ongoing care of elderly patients is characterized by periods of clinical stability or slow change that are interrupted by abrupt illness with sudden decline in function. These events often require the full range and intensity of available hospital services. For persons over age 65 the annual rate of hospitalization is 396/1000, twice that of younger populations. For those over 75 years the rate is over 50%.[1] High-quality, timely acute care is essential for optimal clinical outcomes in geriatric care. The hospital environment is fast paced, and the primary care physician must be both knowledgeable and selective in using the many diagnostic and therapeutic resources available.[2]

While hospitalized, the elderly patient is vulnerable to a number of unfavorable events.[1,3] These include side effects of medication, falls, adverse effects of the diagnostic process, infections, and the complications of surgery. Bed rest can lead to a rapid decline in functional status, with increased joint stiffness, decreased muscle mass, bone demineralization, and declines in aerobic capacity, postural integrity, cardiac output, and baroreceptor reflexes. These changes have collectively been termed the "hospital deconditioning syndrome." The primary care physician needs to be aware of these risks and try to minimize them.[4]

▼ LEO ALEXANDER (Part I)

You are the physician on call for unassigned patients at your hospital's emergency department. Mr. Alexander is an 83-year-old black man who lives alone. He is brought to the emergency room by the landlord of the apartment where he lives. The landlord relates that Mr. Alexander has been "going downhill for a long time" and "acting crazy" for the last 2 days, causing a disturbance in the building by shouting and pounding on the walls of neighboring apartments. The landlord thinks that Mr. Alexander hasn't been eating much, and his apartment was "a mess" when the landlord went in. The landlord says that he doesn't think Mr. Alexander has ever seen a doctor or has any relatives. The landlord doesn't want Mr. Alexander to come back to the apartment "unless he behaves better."

In the emergency room, Mr. Alexander is found to be febrile (39° C) and tachycardiac (110 beats/min), and he has a BP of 120/68. He is disheveled, smells of urine, and appears to have recently lost weight. He is mildly confused with a lack of attention, agitation, and lack of orientation to person, place, or time. Pulse oximetry shows 85% saturation on room air, which corrects with oxygen at 2 liters/min. A chest radiograph shows dense consolidation of the right middle and lower lung fields. You admit Mr. Alexander to a medical ward for treatment of pneumonia.

STUDY QUESTIONS

- *Who will make decisions regarding how aggressive Mr. Alexander's medical care will be?*
- *What other medical information do you need to determine his prognosis and decide on appropriate medical treatment?*
- *What is the source of his confusion and how should it be addressed?*

CASE DISCUSSION

This patient presents a fairly common scenario: minimal prior medical care, evidence of a gradual decline in functional status, a poor social support system, and a set of acute medical disorders. His care is further complicated by the presence of delirium, which limits his participation in his own treatment, and by uncertainty regarding both his baseline competence and the severity of any underlying disorders.

The emergency department is a common point of entry to the hospital for elderly persons. In a large national study, elderly persons were 4.4 times more likely to arrive by ambulance, 5.6 times more likely to be admitted, and 5.5 times more likely to require intensive care admission than younger persons.[5]

For the primary care physician, this will likely be the first encounter with the patient. Certain information must be rapidly obtained.

How sick is the patient? How rapidly do decisions need to be made? In the absence of information to the contrary, an elderly patient should receive all appropriate care regardless of age. Is the patient competent at baseline or previously demented? Is the patient competent to participate in medical decisions at this moment or not? A patient may appear to be demented merely because of acute illness, emotional stress, or simply not hearing or understanding the interviewer. Delirium can accompany most acute disorders in an older patient and should initiate a search for its cause. While a demented patient can sometimes participate in his or her own medical decisions, a delirious one rarely can. Delirium is common among older hospitalized patients, with 40% being confused at some time during their hospital stay. Delirium does not indicate that there is underlying dementia (although it is much more common in patients with prior dementia), but it is a predictor of mortality (8% during the hospital stay, with a 40% 2-year mortality) and of morbidity (40% of survivors are institutionalized after 2 years). Also ask if there is evidence of an advance directive of some type or a durable power of attorney that names another as the spokesperson. Is a family member or close friend available to help make the difficult decisions that may possibly occur, if not immediately, at some time during the hospital stay?

> *Hospitals are dangerous places for elderly people: keep the admission short and start discharge planning on or before the day of admission.*

The primary care physician must attempt to be the patient's advocate and not simply a skillful medical practitioner throughout the patient's hospital stay. While high-quality medical knowledge is absolutely essential to achieve the best outcomes, the primary care physician must try to represent the patient's best interests throughout the course of his or her illness, even when specialists may be managing much of the care. This is true even when the patient may become the primary responsibility of a surgeon or an intensivist. In such circumstances the primary care physician can help provide continuity of strategy ("What is the objective?"), reassurance to the patient and family that "someone they know" is involved in the patient's care, and assistance in deciding the appropriateness of potential interventions. By remaining active in the patient's care, the physician can resume primary care at the appropriate point.

Recommending a course of action that respects the patient's wishes and values and reflects sound medical judgement can be difficult. A five-step process can be used that can blend these and other factors and lead to a unique "patient-specific" plan (Box 13-1). This information can be obtained from a competent patient quickly if necessary and can help avoid both undertreatment and overtreatment. It can minimize conflicts with patient, family, and other health professionals by making the goals of treatment explicit, with measurable outcomes where possible. This process recognizes limited goals, such as palliation, as legitimate in certain clinical circumstances. Studies of the preferences of elderly patients reveal the following hierarchy of who should make the decision regarding end of life medical care:

1. The patient
2. The physician
3. Family members
4. A close friend
5. A court-appointed official

For an incompetent patient, special efforts must be made to identify a spokesperson who can report on the patient's values and any prior discussions about their wishes for medical care, its intensity, and persistence. This will usually be a spouse or other family member, although occasionally a friend may serve as a surrogate. States vary in their requirement for court involvement in such circumstances.

▼ LEO ALEXANDER (Part II)

Mr. Alexander's diagnosis is pneumococcal pneumonia, and you treat him with intravenous ceftriaxone. Respiratory failure develops. No family is located. A pulmonologist advises against therapy "because of his advanced age."

STUDY QUESTIONS

- *What do you do now?*
- *What criteria should be used to determine intensity of treatment?*
- *Is either age or the absence of family a factor in the decision making about intensity of treatment?*

In the frequent situation of making intensity of treatment decisions with no available information, management must be in the direction of preserving life and treating the illness within reasonable medical limits. To make the best possible clinical judgment in such circumstances, as much information about prior functionality as possible and the prognosis of the current situation itself must be

Step 1   Try to Ascertain the Patient's Values

How does the person feel about the current quality of life? What does he or she expect from the remainder of life? Does the patient follow any particular religious guidance? Has he or she established a formal or informal advance directive regarding medical care or resuscitation? Does the patient have a health care proxy?

Step 2   Determine the Patient's Objectives

Patients may seek a range of outcomes from a medical encounter. These can include explanation, reassurance, cure, relief of symptoms, advice, sympathy, palliation, or simply validation.

Step 3   Determine the Medical "Facts"

An accurate assessment of the conditions present is essential to make reasonable recommendations. An overall prognosis, natural history of the disease with and without treatment, and options for therapy, along with risk elements, are all needed. Patients and families often have misunderstandings about the efficacy of medical treatments and need the physician to provide forthright explanations.

Step 4   Make a Recommendation

Based on knowledge of the patient's values and wishes and the medical options available, make a recommendation. This need not include every possible option. Futile therapies need not even be suggested. This recommendation should be negotiated with the patient and, when appropriate, with the family. The competent patient takes primacy above family or other interested parties. Recommendations frequently change as a result of the course of illness and need to be frequently readdressed in the case of critical illness.

Step 5   Agree on a Plan and the Expected Outcomes

The expected outcome in any circumstance should be made explicit whenever possible. This helps avoid misunderstanding and disappointment and helps promote agreement among patient, family, and caregivers. If recovery or cure is anticipated, it should be stated; the same applies to symptom relief, rehabilitation, palliation, diagnosis, or health promotion. Fully document the plan in the patient chart so other consultants or members of the care team who may not have been part of the discussions can understand the reasoning behind a particular course of action.

taken into account. Age alone is clearly not a criterion. Concurrent, debilitating medical illnesses that might compromise treatment efforts would be factors to consider at any age.

Age alone is never a criterion in medical decision making.

▼ LEO ALEXANDER (Part III)

Because of Mr. Alexander's previous independence, the absence of a formal or informal statement of his wishes, and the presence of a potentially curable illness, you advocate strongly for intubation. You prevail. His blood oxygenation, serum electrolytes, and volume status all normalize. He is extubated after 2 days and transferred to a medical ward. The bladder catheter, which had been placed while he was in the ICU, is removed, but he is incontinent of urine and it is replaced. When he stands, he looks unsteady and the nursing staff are fearful that he will fall. He becomes agitated and uncooperative, and soft wrist and chest restraints are placed. He continues to call out, and haloperidol is given intramuscularly. This leads to adequate sedation.

STUDY QUESTIONS

- *What are some of the adverse events for which he is at risk?*
- *Whose responsibility is it to monitor and intervene to prevent such events?*
- *Who else should be involved in his care?*

Older hospital patients are much more likely than younger persons to have an adverse event not directly related to the cause of the hospital stay (Table 13-1). As many as 20% of these lead to increased length of stay.[4,7]

▼ LEO ALEXANDER (Part IV)

Mr. Alexander develops parkinsonian features. He stops eating for the next several days. At 1 week Mr. Alexander has profuse diarrhea that contains blood. A stage 2 pressure ulcer develops over his sacrum.

STUDY QUESTIONS

- What predisposed Mr. Alexander to diarrhea?
- What could have been done to prevent the pressure ulcer?
- What factors may have contributed to his loss of eating?
- Nursing staff are fearful of his falling risk: should he be mobilized nonetheless?

CASE DISCUSSION

The risk of falling is far outweighed by the fact that he is already showing signs of deconditioning. His lack of eating will quickly lead to a loss of energy and motivation. Deconditioning will prolong his stay in the hospital and may produce irreversible disability.

Confusion is observed in 20% to 50% of elderly patients during hospitalization stays. This can be stressful to the patient and family. Prompt recognition of the precipitating causes is important. Nonpharmacological measures such as leaving lights on and allowing a family member to remain in the room should be used first. Small doses of a short-acting benzodiazapine for patients with anxiety associated with their confusion can be effective. Neuroleptics such as haloperidol can be beneficial for some confused patients. Any of these medications can cause its own problems, and careful monitoring for the desired effects along with any side effects is important. Mechanical restraints should be avoided whenever possible. Their use may increase agitation and is associated with an increase in incontinence, pressure sores, and aspiration pneumonia.

Pressure ulcers develop in nearly 5% of hospital patients. Most occur in aged patients who are immobile, confused, malnourished, and incontinent of urine or feces. Recognition of those at risk is the most important preventive strategy. Turning the patient every 2 hours from a 30-degree left and right oblique position is the most effective prevention. Principles of pressure ulcer treatment are straightforward: relieve pressure, treat infection, remove eschar, cover with physiological dressing, optimize nutrition, and treat concurrent illnesses. Low air-loss and fluidized beds have a role in the treatment of deep ulcers, although they should not be routinely used as a preventive measure.

Many of the adverse in-hospital events are due to *medications*. Antibiotics are the most common source of adverse reactions in elderly patients; renal insufficiency, pseudomembranous colitis, skin eruptions, nausea, and vomiting are some of the more serious reactions caused by antibiotics. Parkinsonian features are a common side effect of psychotropics; these symptoms will usually resolve if the medication is promptly discontinued. Virtually any medication can cause an undesired reaction in an elderly patient; confusion is one of the most common side effects. (See Box 13-2).[6]

MULTIDISCIPLINARY CARE

The optimal care of an elderly person in the hospital is a team activity requiring the best discipline-specific skills, but they need to be coordinated so as not to be at cross purposes. The nurses caring for the patient and responsible for carrying out the physician's orders must understand the immediate and long-term goals of the care and participate in the care plan. Other physicians may be important in managing or advising about a specific aspect of the care. A dietitian may be critical in recognizing and proposing interventions needed to improve nutrition. A physical therapist may be essential to restore sufficient strength so that the patient is able to return home. A social worker is usually needed to identify both strengths and weaknesses in the proposed home environment that must be considered in the plan for care following hospitalization. Because of the numbers of individuals potentially involved, communication becomes critical. Efforts to visit patients together, hold regular team discussions, or write careful chart notes are essential. Early discharge planning is vital, since coordination of home care plans can take several days.

Table 13-1   Common Adverse Events in Hospitalized Patients

Incident	Percent of Patients With a Major Event
Infection	10.8
Surgery	9.2
Confusion	5.5
Drug reactions	5.1
Invasive procedures	2.5
Trauma	1.8
Pressure ulcers	1.5
Fluid balance	1.1
Any major event	22.0

From Jahnigen DW et al: *J Am Geriatr Soc* 30(6):387-390, 1982.

BOX 13-2
Drugs Causing the Most Adverse Reactions in Elderly Hospital Patients

Antibiotics
Theophylline preparations
Blood products
Sedative hypnotics
Antihypertensives
Analgesics
IV agents
Digoxin
Anticoagulants
Antiarrhythmics
Antiseizure medications
Insulin

From Jahnigen DW et al: *J Am Geriatr Soc* 30(6):387-390, 1982.

> *Everyone visiting the patient, especially the physicians, must consider and encourage mobilization, nutrition, and hydration on every visit.*

▼ LEO ALEXANDER (Part V)

You discontinue haloperidol, begin oral vancomycin, and order a low air-loss mattress. Saline dressings are applied. You order removal of the restraints, a dietary consultation, physical therapy assessment of the safety of his ambulation, and initiation of a strengthening program. The dietitian works with the nursing staff to implement a weight-gain diet with oral feeding. Mr. Alexander begins bedside physical therapy.

STUDY QUESTIONS

- *What are the next issues to be considered?*
- *What is Mr. Alexander's prognosis?*

▼ LEO ALEXANDER (Part VI)

Mr. Alexander has slow resolution of his confusion. His appetite improves, and he becomes able to feed himself. No evidence of a serious underlying condition is found. He does have chronic obstructive pulmonary disease (COPD) and improves on theophylline. He appears to be competent, although no formal assessment is performed. His diarrhea ceases, and he remains afebrile. Although his condition has improved, he remains weak and his balance is unsteady. He walks by holding onto the furniture. After 3 weeks in the hospital, he expresses a desire to return to his apartment. He is given the name of a community social work agency and advised to get Meals on Wheels. He is scheduled to have a physician office visit in 3 weeks. He is given prescriptions for an oral antibiotic for a urinary tract infection, oral theophylline, and an inhaler. One week later you hear that Mr. Alexander, having fallen in his apartment, has been brought to the emergency room once again by his landlord. The landlord says, "He's just as bad as before. Why didn't you help him? He isn't coming back to my place!"

STUDY QUESTIONS

- *What happened?*
- *Is this patient competent?*
- *Where were the several "continuity lapses" that could have prevented this from occurring?*
- *What do you do now?*

During the past decade the length of hospital stay has steadily declined, with many patients leaving before full recovery.[8] For persons without a strong family or other support network, the plan of care must be directed to the provision of assistance (e.g., safety, shopping, trans-portation, socialization, medical continuity, home services, meals, and similar issues).

For most elderly patients, discharge planning should begin at the time of admission. The living arrangements must be considered early on because many resources may need to be mobilized to make the plan viable. Some of the issues to consider in the discharge plan include:

- Patient wishes and values
- Social support system
- Financial resources
- Need for skilled home medical services
- Need for aides
- Prognosis
- Availability of community-based services
- Home modifications needed for safety
- Functional status on discharge
- Follow-up medical care
- Need for transitional living arrangement (nursing home, assisted living)

CASE DISCUSSION

Mr. Alexander's readmission represents a failure to prepare a thorough and realistic discharge plan. For example, this patient needed a thorough gait and balance evaluation before discharge. He had become severely debilitated while in the hospital. This decline in functional capacity is the aggregate result of decreased strength, balance, flexibility, energy, and alertness. Virtually all these problems are from disuse associated with prolonged bed rest. These decrements in functional capacity occur in people of all ages, but for frail persons this decline can exceed the threshold for safe ambulation.

Discharge planning needs to address the prognosis, expected outcomes, patient values and wishes, and the need for supportive services, therapies, nutritional treatments, and medications. It should clearly identify follow-up care plans and include information on emergency assistance. This should be fully written out and provided to the patient and caregiver, with oral explanations. If a home care agency is involved, the agency workers must be precisely instructed; they will be the main contact between you and the patient and the source of further services if necessary.

▼ LEO ALEXANDER (Part VII)

Mr. Alexander is readmitted with a broken hip. During this stay he undergoes surgical repair of the fracture. He receives aggressive oral nutritional supplementation. His medications are reduced. He is discharged to a skilled nursing facility under your care to continue his rehabilitation for 1 month. During this time he is evicted from his apartment. The social worker at the nursing home finds an assisted living apartment for Mr. Alexander that he likes and is able to afford. He does well in this setting.

▼ ABIGAIL HOOPER

Mrs. Hooper is 87 and has been a patient of yours for 10 years. She lives with her daughter and suffers from mild Alzheimer's disease, extensive osteoarthritis, osteoporosis involving her back, and non–insulin-dependent diabetes mellitus. She is frail and has recently lost 10 lb; her weight is now 98 lb. She has fallen twice in the past year. On one occasion she sustained a vertebral compression fracture that led to a 10-day hospitalization for pain control. She is seen in your office for evaluation of an upper respiratory infection that has been followed by the development of weakness, fever, and a purulent cough. She has not been taking fluids at home. On examination you conclude that she probably has pneumonia and requires hospitalization. Her family is concerned because during her last hospital stay she became severely confused and after discharge it took weeks before her strength returned.

STUDY QUESTIONS

▪ What factors are already present that might predispose to the same problem recurring with this admission?

▪ What can be done to anticipate and minimize these complications?

SUMMARY

The primary care physician has many vital roles in the hospital setting. If he or she is the primary attending physician, coordination of the many disciplines and many factors involved can be achieved more easily. In the tertiary care setting, or any setting where the personal physician is not primarily in charge of the case, the primary care physician has vital input concerning the patient's former status, baseline prior function, previously expressed wishes, and so forth that must be communicated to the frequently loosely associated "team" of many disciplines and backgrounds caring for the patient. The primary care physician must be aggressive in addressing issues of mobility, maintenance, and nutrition and in acting to prevent deconditioning. He or she must take the lead, along with the social services department, in coordinating a smooth transition at the time of discharge either into the community or into a temporary placement setting for a period of rehabilitation. On a case-by-case basis, these methods will reduce the startling morbidity and mortality of hospitalization for elders and the frequent readmissions and failure of community care for many of the most frail elders.

POSTTEST

1. Which one of the following factors concerning hospitalized elders is false?
   a. Confusion occurs in 20% to 50% of hospitalized elders.
   b. Fluidized beds should be used for routine prophylaxis of pressure sores.
   c. Studies of elders confirm that should they be unable to participate, they prefer the physician rather than a friend or family member to make end of life decisions on their behalf.
   d. Dementia is a factor predisposing to delirium.
2. An elderly patient is approaching discharge from the hospital. The family wants you to insist that she go to a nursing home because they are worried about her safety. The patient adamantly refuses to cooperate in these discussions. Which one of the following should you do?
   a. Follow the guidance of adult children.
   b. Hold a meeting among the hospital nurses, therapists, the social worker, and the patient and decide on the best placement.
   c. Determine if the patient is competent and if her wishes seem reasonable. If so, arrange a discussion with the patient and the family to attempt to reconcile the disagreement.
   d. Follow the guidance of the patient.
   e. Seek to have a court-appointed guardian named to act for the patient.
3. Which of the following is not an effect of bed rest in elderly persons?
   a. Bone demineralization
   b. Decreased aerobic capacity
   c. Decreased joint stiffness
   d. Decrease in resting blood pressure
   e. Impairment of baroreceptor reflexes

REFERENCES

1. Creditor M: Hazards of hospitalization of the elderly, *Ann Intern Med* 118:219-223, 1993.
2. Palmer R: Acute hospital care of the elderly: minimizing the risk of functional decline, *Cleve Clin J Med* 63:117-128, 1995.
3. Lefevre F et al: Iatrogenic complications in high-risk, elderly patients, *Arch Intern Med* 152:2074-2080, 1992.
4. Gorbien M et al: Iatrogenic illness in hospitalized elderly people, *J Am Geriatr Soc* 40:1031-1041, 1992.
5. Strange GR, Chen EH, Sanders AB: Use of emergency departments by elderly patients: projections from a multicenter data base, *Ann Emerg Med* 21:819-824, 1992.
6. Jahnigen DW et al: Iatrogenic disease in hospitalized elderly veterans, *J Am Geriatr Soc* 30(6):387-390, 1982.
7. Warshaw G et al: Functional disability in the hospitalized elderly, *JAMA* 248:847-950, 1982.
8. Inouye S et al: A predictive index for functional decline in hospitalized elderly medical patients, *J Gen Intern Med* 8:645-654, 1993.

PRETEST ANSWERS
1. b
2. e
3. e

POSTTEST ANSWERS
1. b
2. c
3. c

CHAPTER 14

Institutional Care

PHILIP D. SLOANE and FRANKLIN HARGETT

OBJECTIVES

Upon completion of this chapter, the reader will be able to:

1. Explain the differences between nursing home and residential long-term care in terms of population served, staffing, and financing.

2. Discuss the physician's role in long-term care, including the management of family issues commonly arising in the nursing home setting, common ethical problems, and the role of a medical director.

3. Discuss the following common medical problems in long-term care: management of dementia, acute infections, musculoskeletal disorders, falls, pressure ulcers, constipation, nutritional issues, dental care, and terminal care.

PRETEST

1. Your patient is an 85-year-old woman who was recently widowed and has no close relatives. Because of macular degeneration, rheumatoid arthritis, and a hip fracture that was pinned 9 months ago, she is unable to drive, cook, or do housework. She requires supervision with bathing but is able to dress, ambulate, and use the toilet independently. She scores 26/30 on the Mini–Mental State Examination.

    This patient is most likely appropriate for:
    a. Adult day care
    b. A residential care setting
    c. A nursing home
    d. A rehabilitation hospital

2. Which one of the following is most correct about physical restraints?
    a. They reduce agitation.
    b. They result in fewer falls, when used properly.
    c. Restraint reduction should begin with the hardest problem cases.
    d. Increased involvement in structured activity programs can reduce restraint use.

3. Which one of the following is most correct about nursing home patients?
    a. Injury is the most common reason for hospitalization.
    b. Empirical treatment of fever with antibiotics is rarely indicated.
    c. Vigorous prevention of falls can increase the pressure ulcer rate.
    d. Most pressure ulcers should be treated by encouraging them to dry.

The need for assistance with personal care or household activities is a hallmark of aging. The proportion of individuals requiring help with activities of daily living gradually rises from around 5% at age 65 to over 50% at age 90. With increasing disability comes the need for formal services. The expansion of home care has allowed a greater proportion of disabled elderly to remain at home; however, when needs are too great, residential long-term care is often required. In this chapter the two kinds of institutional long-term care are discussed, with a focus on issues of relevance to medical practitioners who care for patients living in these settings.

TYPES OF LONG-TERM CARE SETTINGS
Nursing Homes

Skilled nursing facilities, or nursing homes, are institutions that house persons requiring the care or supervision of a skilled nurse. They are licensed and regulated by state agencies, with considerable federal control through Medicare and Medicaid guidelines. Criteria for admission are imprecise to allow health providers and regulators to make decisions on a case-by-case basis; however, persons residing in nursing homes generally need assistance with at least one of the following activities: bathing, dressing, transfer, continence, ambulation, or eating.

The typical nursing home is organized into departments, which in smaller homes may consist of a single individual. The departments of social work, activities, administration, dietary services, housekeeping, and maintenance all tend to be small. Nursing is by far the largest

department. Within the nursing department a few licensed staff communicate with physicians, distribute medications, administer treatments, and supervise nursing assistants.

Non–Nursing Home Residential Care Settings (Domiciliary Care or Assisted Living)

A variety of long-term care options exist outside of nursing homes. These are called by different names and regulated differently from state to state (see Table 14-1). Those that offer significant supervision, assistance with personal care, and health services (such as assistance with medication) are generally termed board and care, domiciliary care, or assisted living facilities. Residents of these domiciliary care facilities tend to be somewhat less impaired than nursing home residents; however, all residents of domiciliary care facilities require some help or supervision with instrumental activities of daily living such as housework, cooking, managing finances, transportation, and shopping. Many also require help with activities of daily living. There is considerable overlap between the populations of nursing facilities and domiciliary care settings.

THE AIDE: PRIMARY CAREGIVER IN LONG-TERM CARE SETTINGS

The majority of care in nursing homes and residential care settings is provided by relatively unskilled caregivers, usually called nursing assistants or aides. The aide's work is primarily to assist residents with personal care. It is physically demanding, consisting of getting patients

Table 14-1   A Comparison of the Two Major Types of Long-Term Care

	Skilled Nursing Facilities (Nursing Homes)	Domiciliary Care, Board and Care, Assisted Living
Number of beds in United States	Approximately 1.5 million	Approximately 1.2 million
Major payment sources	Approximately 47% Medicaid, 46% private pay	Approximately 60% private, 35% Social Security disability
Services provided	Long-term stays for persons with chronic disabling conditions (the most common of which is dementia) who require care by licensed nurses	Long-term residence for persons who need some assistance and supervision but do not require the intensity of services provided in a nursing home
	Rehabilitation stays averaging 2-6 weeks for persons with acute problems (such as stroke or hip fracture) who require daily physical or occupational therapy	Long-term stays for persons who are on Social Security disability (SSI), many of whom are "deinstitutionalized" mentally ill persons
	Short-term respite stays for persons cared for at home, so that caregivers can get a break	Long-term care for persons who pay privately for services and have chosen a non–nursing home setting, but would qualify for nursing home care
Involvement of licensed nurses	24 hours/day	Variable, often supervisory
Medication administration	Medication administration by licensed nurses (usually practical nurses)	"Assistance with self-medication" provided by unlicensed staff (usually aides)
Percent of residents with moderate or severe dementia	60%	40%
Relationship with physicians	Legally required to have a medical director	Not legally required to have a medical director
	Most physician-patient visits take place in the home	Many physician-patient visits take place in physician's office
	Visits required every 1 or 2 months	Visits required annually

out of bed, washing them, brushing their teeth, grooming them, making their beds, changing their soiled linen, cleaning up after bladder and bowel accidents, monitoring them for falls, toileting them, and feeding them. The work is also psychologically stressful because during the course of the day aides often have to tolerate racial slurs, curses, hostility, and bitterness. The aides themselves often come from disadvantaged and unstable backgrounds. Thus it is not surprising that physical abuse by aides occurs occasionally, and psychological abuse, such as yelling at or insulting residents, is not uncommon.[1]

▼ *MINNIE CRAWFORD (Part I)*

Minnie Crawford, an 86-year-old with hypertension and mild dementia, is hospitalized for an impacted fracture of the right humeral neck. A widow, she has been your patient since moving in with her daughter and son-in-law 3 years ago. Two years ago, you hospitalized her briefly for a right anterior cerebral artery stroke, which left her with mild (4/5) weakness in the left lower extremity. She has been taking a diuretic for mild hypertension, and she complains of dizziness whenever she stands quickly. A typical blood pressure before hospitalization was 165/60.

In the emergency department you note some S-T abnormalities on the electrocardiogram, so you decide to admit her for observation. Since her shoulder fracture is stable, the arm is immobilized in a sling and swathe. Acetaminophen with codeine for pain is prescribed.

The following morning her cardiogram has stabilized, and myocardial infarction has been ruled out. You feel that the S-T abnormalities were due to mild hypokalemia, which you have corrected, and you plan to discharge her to home with frequent visits from a home health nurse. Her daughter objects, however, informing you that she and her husband had planned to go out of town for 3 days next week and that she does not feel Minnie can manage on her own with the fracture. She asks if you can place her mother in a skilled nursing facility for a week or two.

WHO RESIDES IN LONG-TERM CARE FACILITIES?

Residents of long-term care facilities tend to be old, sick, poor, and alone. Mean resident ages in nursing homes and domiciliary facilities range around 78 to 84 years. Virtually all residents have one or more sources of disability, such as Alzheimer's disease, multiinfarct dementia, stroke, severe chronic heart disease, osteoarthritis, amputation (usually secondary to diabetes), or chronic obstructive pulmonary disease (COPD). Lack of close relatives because of widowhood, divorce, never marrying, or not having children is a major risk factor for institutionalization. Low income is also a risk factor for in-

Table 14-2   Subgroups of Nursing Home Residents

Subgroup	Focus and Goals of Care
"Short stayers"	
Terminal, likely to die within 6 months	Comfort, pain relief, family support
For rehabilitation, likely to be discharged home within 3 months	Physical and occupational therapy, independence
"Long stayers"	
With medical problems (e.g., heart failure, osteoarthritis, COPD)	Medical management
With dementia	Behavioral management
With dementia and medical problems	Simplified medical regimen combined with behavioral management

stitutionalization. A higher proportion of white elders than black elders are institutionalized, apparently because of stronger extended family networks and the existence of more available at-home caregivers among black families. Risk factors for nursing home placement from a domiciliary care facility include dementia, hearing loss, and problems with basic activities of daily living.[2,3]

According to Ouslander, nursing home residents can be grouped into five types: short stayers for terminal care, short stayers receiving rehabilitation, long stayers with primarily medical problems, long stayers with dementia, and long stayers with both medical problems and dementia.[4] While patients do move from one group to another, this categorization is helpful to nursing home staff in setting goals and priorities for care (Table 14-2). For example, only some nursing home residents should be considered for health promotion activities such as mammography and cholesterol reduction; some (such as the terminally ill and those with advanced dementia) may be better off not receiving standard medical treatments such as antihypertensive care or antibiotics for infection.

PAYING FOR LONG-TERM CARE

Nursing home care is expensive, averaging between $30,000 and $50,000 per year and costing the nation a total of between $60 and $80 billion. Medicaid, an entitlement program for the impoverished, covers the costs of 47% of nursing home residents. Most of the remainder (46%) pay privately. Medicare pays only for short rehabilitation stays, which account for 4% of nursing home residents; private insurance pays for less than 2%.[5,6] Thus nursing home care is a significant burden both on private individuals and on state Medicaid budgets. Costs of physician care in nursing homes are reimbursed through Medicare Part B and, when applicable, through Medi-

caid; physician reimbursement for nursing home services by these public sources is quite modest.

Domiciliary care settings vary widely in cost but average somewhat less than nursing home care. Neither Medicare nor Medicaid pays for most domiciliary care, however. Traditionally, domiciliary care focused on younger persons with Social Security disability payments (SSI) or private funds; most older persons residing in domiciliary settings pay privately.

Nearly all nursing facilities charge considerably higher rates to private pay clients (often twice as much) than they are reimbursed by Medicaid. Thus facilities that have high proportions of private pay residents can provide better services and (often) a higher quality of care than those whose residents are primarily on Medicaid.

The threat of impoverishment by medical expenses in old age is quite real. The high cost of nursing home care, and its lack of inclusion under Medicare, can drain personal assets rapidly. Spending down of personal assets to $2000 is required for Medicaid eligibility; for married couples spouses are protected at an income at 150% of poverty levels and assets of at least $13,740 (as of 1992). Nursing home care is, however, often the last step in a series of costly encounters with the health care system. For this reason most nursing home residents who are on Medicaid entered the nursing home on Medicaid; however, one third of those entering as private pay patients spend down their assets and go on Medicaid while in the nursing home.[5]

> *Medicaid is the principal payor for nursing home care: of those who enter paying privately, one third spend down their assets to Medicaid-eligible levels while there.*

For persons concerned with paying for long-term care and preserving personal resources for a spouse or heirs, two strategies are available. Long-term care insurance, which is currently owned by only 4% of elderly, is slowly growing in popularity.[7] Owing to the escalating costs of nursing home care, however, purchasers (the mean age of whom is 68) cannot be sure that their policy will provide adequate daily payments to meet future nursing home charges. Some older persons attempt to preserve their personal resources through artificial impoverishment by transfer of assets to heirs. Medicaid eligibility boards look with disfavor at asset transfer, however; such transfers typically have to occur at least 2 years before application for Medicaid.

Medicaid programs and insurance companies are currently using two methods to reduce nursing home costs. The first is to base reimbursement on care needs, using a case mix reimbursement system analogous to hospital

Diagnosis Related Groups (DRGs). The most widespread nursing home case mix system is the Resource Utilization Groups (RUGs). Under the RUGs system, the more impaired the resident, the higher the reimbursement to the facility. The advantage of such a system is that it encourages facilities to take the heavy care patients who were difficult to place under flat rate reimbursement; the problem with such a system is that it provides a disincentive against homes helping patients improve, since improvement means lowered reimbursement.[8,9] The other method aimed at reducing nursing home costs attempts to maintain nursing home candidates at home by paying for whatever services are needed, up to a monthly cost ceiling. Unfortunately, neither case mix reimbursement systems nor community alternatives programs have been demonstrated to reduce nursing home costs.

> *Medicaid's policy of paying more for patients who require more care is unfortunately a disincentive to facilities to help patients improve.*

▼ MINNIE CRAWFORD (Part II)

After conferring with the hospital social worker, you inform Ms. Crawford's daughter that Medicare will not provide reimbursement for the nursing home stay, since a shoulder fracture does not require daily rehabilitation. A long discussion ensues, during which the daughter is adamant that Minnie needs to be institutionalized for the next 10 days or so, yet also expresses dismay at the idea of spending over $1000 for the stay. At last she agrees to pay for the nursing home admission, and Minnie enters as a respite patient into the nursing home where you are an attending physician.

Initially, Minnie is somewhat disgruntled, but she is befriended by the nursing home social worker who introduces her to the activities director. Two days later, when you visit to complete her admission paperwork, you find her smiling and actively participating in a reminiscence group. Your goals for care include keeping her mind active and engaged, watching for skin problems associated with the sling, having a physical therapist assess her and begin early rehabilitation (to avoid a frozen shoulder), and monitoring her for confusion or falls.

DEFINING AND ACHIEVING QUALITY CARE

Quality is an elusive concept in institutional care. As noted previously, goals of care depend on the problems and prognosis of the individual patient. Even death is not a bad outcome for many nursing home residents. There are, however, certain outcome goals that are reasonable for most residents. These include maximizing independence, autonomy, and physical function; provision of safety, security, and privacy; adequate nutrition; personal comfort; continuity with one's past; a sense of home; and maintenance of dignity, pride, and a sense of self-worth.[10] Table 14-3 provides examples of how these goals can be achieved and measured in long-term care facilities.

OBRA 87: The Nursing Home Reform Act

In 1987 Congress passed the Nursing Home Reform Act as part of the Omnibus Budget Reconciliation Act (OBRA). Implemented by a series of regulations in the early 1990s, OBRA has set standards designed to improve the quality of nursing home care. The following are among the regulations included under OBRA[11,12]:

- Mandatory training for nursing assistants (aides), 75 hours in length
- Comprehensive assessment of all residents using an instrument called the Minimum Data Set (MDS) and its associated Resident Assessment Protocols (RAPs)
- Preadmission Screening and Annual Resident Review (PASARR) to assure that persons needing active psychiatric treatment are not warehoused in nursing facilities
- Restriction on the use of and increased requirements for the documentation of psychotropic drug use
- Guidelines aimed at reducing the use of physical restraints

Whether or not OBRA has been successful in improving nursing home care remains the topic of considerable debate. Providers practicing in nursing facilities should be aware of OBRA requirements, which have become incorporated into nursing home regulations and survey processes.

> *OBRA 87 (the Nursing Home Care Reform Act) is entirely laudable in its motives, but the bureaucracy of its implementation is staggering. Whether it has improved nursing home care remains unclear.*

Minimizing Physical and Pharmacological Restraint

Research during the past decade has demonstrated that physical restraints increase rather than reduce agitation and rarely prevent falls or injuries. Thus it is now believed that physical restraints in long-term care often constitute an unjustified infringement on resident autonomy. At the same time there has been concern that psychotropic medications have been overused as methods of reducing agitation in long-term care. For this reason, organized

Table 14-3   Maximizing Quality of Life for Residents of Long-Term Care Facilities

Quality of Life Goals	Examples of Interventions	Measures to Assess Success of Interventions
Maximize independence, autonomy, and physical function	Avoid physical restraints Flexibility in mealtimes Provide glasses, hearing aids, and locomotion aids when needed Personal thermostats in rooms Exercise programs	Percent of residents restrained Percent of residents eating other than at prescribed mealtimes Rates of participation in interactions Get up and go test; timed ambulation
Provide safety, security, and privacy	Locks on drawers and closets Education and supervision of aides to prevent abuse and neglect Single rooms Small activity rooms for family visitation and entertaining guests Small unit size	Incidents of "lost" clothing Family satisfaction Rates of observed abuse Resident agitation rates
Nutritious and tasty food	Dentures available if needed Choice of food Tasteful food preparation	Resident's and family's satisfaction with meals Meal consumption Maintenance of weight at or above ideal
Personal comfort	Temperature comfortable for residents Treat pain adequately	Resident's satisfaction Resident's pain Minimal agitated behaviors related to pain (e.g., screaming)
Continuity with one's past activities and relationships	Involve family in activities Encourage bringing personal items into facility Provide activities that maintain normal social roles, such as cooking, housework, gardening	Family visitation rates Presence of mementos, own furniture, and knickknacks in rooms Participation in social role activities
Maintenance of dignity, pride, and a sense of self-worth	Beauty parlor on premises Staff assist residents in selecting clothes, putting on clothing, make-up, and jewelry Have residents participate in "work" activities such as greeting visitors, setting the table, and making beds Participation in social events that are fun, such as parties, dances, and games	Rating of personal appearance of residents Rates of participation in activities with meaning for the resident Rates of participation in social events Rate of smiling and laughing by residents

From Coons DH, Reichel W: *Am Fam Physician* 37:241-248, 1988.

efforts to minimize both physical and pharmacological restraints are considered important elements of quality care.

Physical restraints include vest, wrist, and ankle restraints, chairs with locking lap trays, waist restraints, and "safety belts" that cannot be opened by the patient. In addition, bedrails should be considered restraints when used to keep a patient from getting out of bed. Programs aimed at reducing physical restraints must offer alternatives:

- Increased involvement for residents in structured activities
- Psychosocial alternatives, such as active listening, therapeutic touch, and behavior modification
- Use of positioning devices such as wedge cushions and recliner chairs

- Environmental modifications such as carpeted floors and lowered beds
- Use of motion sensors and position monitors to alert staff when high-risk patients are attempting to get up
- Alterations in nursing care, such as additional observation, assisted daily ambulation, and regular toileting
- A search for and treatment of physiological causes of agitation, such as pain, constipation, and infection[13]

Successful restraint reduction programs are implemented in a manner that involves all staff, requires strong administrative support, and proceeds case-by-case beginning with "easier" cases first.

Pharmacological restraints can include antipsychotics,

hypnotics, sedatives, and antidepressants (when used for sedation). Drugs that should be avoided because the risks in frail elderly are unacceptable include long-acting benzodiazepines (chlordiazepoxide, diazepam, and flurazepam), diphenhydramine, meprobamate, short-acting barbiturates, muscle relaxants (cyclobenzaprine, orphenidrine, methocarbamol, carisoprodol), amitriptyline, and doxepin.[14,15] Some of the drugs that are considered more acceptable when used with discretion are listed in Box 14-1. Even when the least toxic agents are used, they should be prescribed for sedation or agitation reduction only if behavioral techniques have failed. (*Editor's note:* In practice, many patients require a combination of both behavioral techniques and careful, well followed up, pharmacological intervention; some patients, mainly those with truly psychotic features, *should* receive antipsychotics because behavioral management alone will not suffice.) In addition, antipsychotic agents must be prescribed in accordance with OBRA guidelines, as outlined in Box 14-2. As with physical restraints, the cornerstone of pharmacological restraint reduction is staff education and the provision of behavioral alternative treatments. In addition to those mentioned as alternatives to physical restraints, a wide variety of behavior management techniques are available.

> *Many potentially useful and humane drugs can be regarded (and condemned) as "restraints"; it is up to the prescribing physician to justify the usefulness of his or her prescription and to clarify that it is not being used merely as a restraint.*

THE PHYSICIAN'S ROLE IN LONG-TERM CARE

To some extent long-term care residents are a medically underserved population. This is not to say that they need more medical procedures, hospitalizations, and technological services; if anything, medicalization and dehumanization occur too often in long-term care settings. Rather, many long-term care residents lack the personal relationships and individualized attention that characterize the best primary medical care. There are many reasons for this: the logistics of traveling to a long-term care facility often reduces the number of physician visits, causing much decision making to be carried out over the telephone; Medicare and Medicaid reimbursements for physician services are low; and the facilities themselves often have such high rates of resident and staff turnover that meaningful, long-term relationships between staff, physicians, and patients are extremely difficult to develop.

Time management is an important element of nursing home work. Box 14-3 presents some suggestions for an efficient, effective nursing home practice.

BOX 14-1
Medications Considered Safest for Behavioral Symptoms in Older Persons

Antipsychotics

Haloperidol
Risperidone

Anxiolytics

Buspirone
Lorazepam
Oxazepam
Alprazolam
Triazolam

Antidepressants

Paroxetine
Sertraline
Nortriptyline
Trazodone

BOX 14-2
Guidelines for the Use of Antipsychotic Medications in Long-Term Care Facilities

Approved Indications

DSM-IV psychotic disorders, excepting delirium and dementia
Tourette's syndrome
Huntington's disease
Psychotic symptoms, such as delusions or hallucinations, in dementia
Psychomotor agitation interfering with provision of basic care and activities of daily living in dementia

Conditions for which Antipsychotics Are Not Indicated

Nonpsychotic behaviors that do not threaten others, such as pacing, wandering, uncooperativeness, crying out, screaming, repetitive mannerisms, or unsociability
Anxiety

From Smith DA: *Geriatrics* 45(2):44-56, 1990.

Working With Families

Most long-term care admissions involve two parties: the person who is institutionalized and his or her family. Often, it is the family that constitutes the greater challenge and occupies the majority of the physician's time. This is often quite reasonable; the majority of long-term care residents are poorly equipped to advocate for themselves, either because of dementia or because of weakness and

1. Limit your practice to one or two facilities in which you get to know the staff well and can influence policy (e.g., by serving as medical director).
2. Employ a midlevel practitioner. A physicians' assistant or nurse practitioner can manage routine patient care problems and serve as liaison between yourself and the nursing staff and families.
3. Be consistent. Have a regular day for rounds.
4. Prioritize your time on rounds. See the sickest patients first.
5. Develop protocols for common problems such as decubitus prevention, constipation, weight loss, falls, behavioral problems, and fever.
6. Train staff to limit after hours telephone calls to urgent medical problems. Provide mechanisms for staff to address nonurgent problems, such as a daily telephone call or regular rounds by yourself or a midlevel practitioner.
7. Speak with patients and families about advance directives soon after admission and whenever major status changes occur. Document these discussions in the medical record.
8. Communicate your expectations through discussions with staff, standing orders, and inservice programs.
9. Educate yourself about nursing home regulations, especially those that affect the provision of medical and nursing services.
10. Work as a partner with the nursing home staff. Learn their names. Be sensitive to the challenges they face. Seek to be a supporter rather than a critic, especially in public.

Modified from Anderson EG: *Geriatrics* 48(8):61-63, 1993.

immobility. Thus it is often the families who are the major decision makers and who attempt to look after the interests of their loved ones.

Physicians should encourage contact with families, even though it takes extra time. Institutionalized persons who have involved families are likely to receive more staff attention and to have medical problems detected earlier.[17] There are some general rules for working with families in the institutional setting:

■ The majority of physician contact is likely to be with one family member. This person usually will have been the primary caregiver before institutionalization. By signing the patient into the facility, this family member becomes the "responsible party."
■ Contact and then meet with families at admission and whenever there is a major status change. Try to clarify advance directives during these meetings.

■ Try to anticipate future events and discuss them in advance with families. For example, when a patient with dementia is beginning to deteriorate, meet with the family before the situation reaches a crisis. Discuss possible decision points (such as hospitalization or the use of antibiotics) before the issue arises.
■ Learn as much as possible about family dynamics. There are often complex interpersonal relationships within families, and these can lead to surprises. A common example of this is the son (or daughter) from out of town, who materializes during a crisis and insists on reversing decisions made by the physician and responsible party. The typical scenario occurs when an in-town daughter who visits her mother regularly is overruled by a sibling from far away who is unaware of the suffering the patient has already endured and insists on aggressive treatment of an end-stage case.

 In institutional care the family often constitutes the greatest challenge; it is up to health professionals to involve them in the care and to avoid an adversarial relationship.

Ethical Issues

Because of the population they serve, long-term care facilities must deal on a day-to-day basis with issues of informed consent and decisions to limit medical treatment. Issues unique to the nursing home include the low success rate of cardiopulmonary resuscitation, sexual expression among unrelated residents, and mistreatment of residents by staff. In general, medical staff should focus on the process by which ethical issues are decided, so that staff, residents, families, and medical practitioners are all involved. If all these parties are in accord about a decision, subsequent conflicts rarely occur.

Families should realize that it is humane for most nursing home residents to have do not resuscitate (DNR) status.

Institution of cardiopulmonary resuscitation (CPR) in the nursing home is generally futile; less than 2% of nursing home patients survive CPR and subsequent hospitalization.[18] The exception is the patient whose arrest is witnessed and who, at the time resuscitation is attempted, demonstrates ventricular fibrillation.[19] Consequently, it is probably most humane for the majority of nursing home residents to have do not resuscitate (DNR) status. For those who do not have DNR orders, it may be reasonable to initiate CPR only in those whose cardiac arrest is witnessed and to continue resuscitation only in those whose initial documented cardiac rhythm is ventricular fibrillation.[19]

Family members making surrogate decisions for their relative must realize that they are only trying to help decide what the patient would have wished in the circumstances.

Expressions of sexuality by residents often pose significant ethical challenges for staff and families. This is particularly true if the residents have dementia. Guidelines have been developed for such situations[20]; in general sexuality should be considered normal, but nursing home staff may intervene if participants are incompetent or threat of physical or psychological injury is present.

Medical Directorship

By law, all skilled nursing facilities must have a medical director. Generally, this is a physician who manages a significant proportion of the facility's patients and is paid on an hourly basis for the additional administrative responsibilities. The role of the medical director in a nursing home includes the following:

- Ensuring that physician care addresses legal and medical needs
- Organizing and supervising a quality improvement program for the facility
- Serving on required committees such as infection control, pharmacy, and utilization review
- Reviewing incident reports
- Assisting the facility in developing policies and procedures for health maintenance, routine laboratory testing, tuberculin screening, skin care, and research involving staff and residents
- Overseeing the health program for employees
- Conducting educational programs for employees, residents, and families
- Acting as a spokesperson for the facility in the community and with regulatory and other health care agencies[4]

A medical director who is committed and involved can have a tremendous impact on the health and well-being of residents in a nursing facility.

▼ MINNIE CRAWFORD (Part III)

Two weeks after she was admitted, you receive a call that Ms. Crawford has been refusing food and fluids for the past 24 hours and that she seems to be limping. On examination her rectal temperature is 101° F, her pulse is 110 beats/min, and her respiratory rate is 18 breaths/min. She has mild muscle weakness on the left side, including a minimal facial droop. Her chest is unremarkable, but bowel sounds are diminished

and a fecal impaction is noted on rectal examination. Urinalysis shows 30 to 50 WBCs per high power field.

You diagnose a urinary tract infection secondary to fecal impaction and a small subcortical stroke. You speak with the patient and her family; neither wants her to be hospitalized "unless it is absolutely necessary." You discontinue her PRN codeine, which she has continued receiving two or three times a day. You give her an injection of cefuroxime, then you prescribe oral cephalexin (she is allergic to sulfa drugs). She receives 1500 ml of intravenous fluid overnight. The next morning she is afebrile, eats all her breakfast, and seems less weak on the left side. You increase her daily aspirin dose from 1 to 2 tablets and ask the physical therapist to begin rehabilitation.

COMMON MEDICAL PROBLEMS IN LONG-TERM CARE SETTINGS

Long-term care facilities contain a population in which the medical problems of old age are concentrated. Thus they are settings in which expertise in geriatric medicine is particularly crucial. Professionals such as physicians, nurses, and physical therapists who work with long-term care residents should be vigilant for remediable health problems, of which there are many. The practice of medical care in the nursing home is challenging and highly complex. Many of the common problems in long-term care settings, such as incontinence, falls, immobility, and dementia, are dealt with in depth elsewhere in this text. This section focuses on problems or issues that are unique to long-term care, or that have not received adequate attention elsewhere in the book.

The major role of the attending physician at the nursing home is to be vigilant for remediable medical problems.

Management of the Patient with Dementia

More and more, long-term care facilities are becoming homes for persons with dementia. For this reason, management of dementia is a crucial aspect of effective long-term care. In the institutional setting, high-quality care requires an appropriate environment, care policies and practices, services, and personnel. Table 14-4 provides examples of some of the methods that can be used to manage persons with dementia so as to meet the goals of maximizing physical function while minimizing disruptive behaviors.

A recent innovation has been the development of special care units (SCUs) and nursing homes specializing in dementia care. The most common SCU is a moderate-sized, self-contained unit that seeks to serve persons with early and midstage dementia (who can walk and are able

Table 14-4   Examples of Techniques To Manage Dementia in Long-Term Care Facilities

Therapeutic Goal	Treatment Modalities

Manage disruptive behaviors without restraints	Disguised exits
	Limited exposure to triggering events
	  No intercoms and alarms
	  Staff instructed not to yell or talk loudly
	  Small living units with less commotion
	Wandering paths, natural barriers
	Use of diversion or distraction rather than confrontation
	Use of reassurance for anxiety
	Rechanneling of energy outlets through activities
	Environmental measures to reduce disorientation
	  Reduced ambiguity and choice (e.g., of food)
	  Visual access to toilet
	  Meaningful cues at doorway to indicate room
	Educated staff with consistent policies

Maximize independence in activities of daily living	Adequate staff time to support activities of daily living Regular toileting Diet control to minimize constipation Fluid restriction at night Finger foods, frequent snacks On-site kitchen Task breakdown or sequencing Starting the motion (e.g., brushing teeth) Walking program Activities that provide range of motion (e.g., dancing) Limiting choices (e.g., selecting clothing) Extra assistive devices (consult occupational therapist)

to communicate verbally to some extent); such units focus on keeping residents active and on maintaining mobility, continence, and feeding. A less common type of SCU is for persons with advanced dementia who are unable to walk and often fight or scream when personal care is attempted; this type of unit aims at providing gentle nursing care, conducting one-on-one or small group activities aimed at stimulating remaining senses, and providing humane terminal care. Family satisfaction tends to be greater with SCUs than integrated nursing home care; however, there is little evidence that patient outcomes are better in either setting.

Acute Infections

Infections cause the majority of deaths in the nursing home and are a major reason for hospitalization.[21] The lung and urinary tract are the most common site of serious infections; among discharged nursing home residents (including deaths), 49% have had pneumonia and 34% have had urinary tract infections.[22] Common non–life-threatening infections include conjunctivitis (which is often chronic because sagging lower eyelids provide a poor barrier to infection), herpes zoster, and candidiasis of the skin. The urinary tract is the most common source of bacteremia, followed by skin and subcutaneous tissue and the respiratory tract. The majority of bacteremic episodes are due to gram-negative organisms, and multiple drug resistance is common.[21] Management of these infections is discussed in relevant chapters of this text.

Management of fever in the nursing home is empirical.[23] In contrast to the community, where viral infections predominate, as many as one third of nursing home fevers, and the majority of fevers over 102° F, are caused by bacterial infection. In some cases a decision must be made concerning whether or not to treat with antibiotics; pneumonia and sepsis remain the "old man's friends"—relatively rapid and comfortable ways to die. If treatment is desired, rapid assessment and prompt treatment is essential.

Pneumonia (and other sepses) remain the "old man's friend"; families should be encouraged to discuss not treating should this benign exit from life present itself. Too often antibiotics are prescribed anyway, and life can thus be unnaturally prolonged.

Musculoskeletal Disease

Mobility is probably the single area in which medical care policies in the nursing home can have the most impact. An environment in which personnel frequently employ pharmacological and physical restraints, worry inordinately about falls, and "take care of" patients will end up with the majority of its residents in wheelchairs and unable to walk. In contrast, an environment in which personnel minimize restraints, encourage activity and exercise, and actively treat musculoskeletal problems will maintain independence in ambulation and transfer for years beyond that of mobility-poor settings.

Arthritis is extremely common in nursing facilities and is a common cause of immobility. Treatment should focus on physical measures, mobilization, and acetaminophen, since nonsteroidal antiinflammatory drugs are associated with peptic ulcer disease and renal complications.[24]

Falls and Pressure Sores

For many clinicians it is not customary to speak of falls and pressure sores in the same sentence. However, in the nursing home setting they are often two sides of the coin of dysmobility. People who have good mobility neither fall nor develop pressure sores. As soon as mobility becomes reduced, the risk of falls rises. People who have no independent bed mobility (i.e., cannot change position in bed) have the greatest pressure sore risk. The more emphasis is placed on fall safety, the more prone people are to pressure sores.

Pressure sores (decubitus ulcers) are areas of skin breakdown caused by ischemic infarction caused when the blood supply to an area of skin is occluded because of pressure between bone and an external surface. The external surface is usually the mattress or the seat of a chair. The harder the surface is, the less time until ischemia develops. Times to ischemic infarction range from less than 2 hours (on fairly hard surface) upward, depending on the surface. This is the rationale for turning patients at least every 2 hours when they are immobile. The majority of severe pressure ulcers encountered in the nursing home actually developed in the hospital.

Pressure sores are staged as follows: areas of skin reddening over bony prominences, which represent ischemia, are stage 1 pressure sores; ulcers that include only the skin are stage 2 pressure sores; ulcers that include the subcutaneous fat or muscle are stage 3 pressure sores; and ulcers that extend all the way down to the bone are stage 4 pressure sores. All areas of skin breakdown are colonized to some extent by bacteria; infection of the surrounding healthy tissue is less common.

Over the past two decades, pressure sore prevention has become routine in health care settings; pressure sores now tend to develop when a patient's condition changes and medical and nursing staff do not appreciate new needs quickly enough. Several scoring systems exist to rate a patient's pressure sore risk. Risk factors for pressure sores include immobility, lack of pressure sore prevention, acute illnesses such as stroke or pneumonia, any illness that reduces sensation in the skin (such as spinal cord injuries), sedative medication, urinary incontinence (which macerates the skin), and physical restraints. Effective prevention programs identify risk factors and initiate appropriate measures early.

Practically every clinician and every nursing facility has its own approach to treating pressure ulcers. Controlled trials indicate that attention to the pressure sore is the most important factor influencing healing. Beyond that, there are certain general principles:

- Most pressure sores heal best if kept moist
- Dead tissue should be debrided
- Pressure should be kept off the ulcer
- The wound should be cleaned regularly, but not with agents that kill granulation tissue (e.g., hydrogen peroxide).

Beyond these general principles, the effectiveness of specific treatments is often not clear.

Constipation

Long-term care residents are extremely susceptible to constipation. This is because they often have multiple risk factors. Risks for constipation include a prior history of constipation or laxative use, poor oral fluid intake, immobility, previous abdominal surgery, and many medications. Constipating medications include all anticholinergics, opiate pain medications, phenothiazines (and related medications), tricyclic antidepressants, antacids containing aluminum, calcium, diuretics, and iron.[25]

Table 14-5   A Bowel Management Program for Residents of Long-Term Care Facilities

Constipation Risk Status	Recommended Bowel Program
Low risk—can take fluids well, have little history of constipation, are taking few medications, or are reasonably mobile	Fluids: 1500 ml minimum Exercise: abdominal and pelvic exercises 1 ounce of fiber supplement recipe* Toileting: place on commode for 5-15 minutes after each meal Ambulate assisted or unassisted for a minimum of 50 feet twice a day
Moderate risk—some difficulty taking fluids or some history of constipation, on constipating medication, or have reduced mobility	Fluids: same 2 ounces of fiber supplement recipe* Exercise, toileting, and ambulation: same as above unless not tolerated by patient If no bowel movement occurs in 3 days, insert bisacodyl suppository. If no results, administer enema and reevaluate regimen
High risk—significant difficulty taking fluids by mouth or significant history of constipation, or chairbound or bedbound	Fluids: aggressive encouragement of ≥1500 ml 3 ounces of fiber supplement recipe* Exercise, toileting, and ambulation: same as above unless not tolerated by patient If no bowel movement occurs in 3 days, insert bisocodyl suppository. If no results, administer enema and reevaluate regimen

Modified from Karam SE, Niew DM: *J Gerontol Nurs* 20(3):32-40, 1994, and Stephany T: *Home Healthcare Nurs* 6(4):40-41, 1988.
*Fiber supplement recipe: 2 parts all bran cereal, 2 parts applesauce, 1 part prune juice. The resulting mixture tastes and spreads much like apple butter.

For this reason, all long-term care facilities should have an established protocol to prevent constipation. Table 14-5 provides one such protocol.

Nutrition, Hydration, and Maintenance of Weight

Weight loss, dehydration, and malnutrition are extremely common in the nursing home. Significant weight loss—a reduction of 5 pounds or more in a person who is not overweight—is frequent; the most common causes are depression, medications, cancer, and swallowing disorders.[26] Other causes of weight loss include poor-fitting or absent dentures and advanced dementia.

Long-term care facilities should monitor food and fluid intake daily and should weigh patients at least once a month. When intake is reduced or weight loss is documented, the patient should be assessed for reversible causes of poor intake, such as ill-fitting dentures, constipation, or medication. Often, reduced intake can be ameliorated by changing the diet to a simpler form, such as changing a regular diet to a soft diet or a soft diet to a pureed diet. Between-meal snacks and liquid nutritional supplements are also helpful. For persons who are unable to feed themselves, the most important factor in effective nutrition is adequate staff time to assist the patient. Except in the late stages of terminal illness, nearly all long-term care patients can take adequate food and liquid orally if the dietary formulation is optimal and staff take the necessary time to assist with feeding.

Dental Care

Oral health is an important and often neglected part of long-term care. Between 50% and 77% of nursing home elderly are edentulous; the remainder typically have many missing, broken, or decayed teeth. Between 27% and 75% of nursing home residents have gingivitis, and 50% to 62% have periodontal disease.[27] These dental infections can impair nutrition and cause chronic pain. In addition, many long-term care residents are unable to adequately brush and floss their teeth. In persons with dementia, mouth care is extremely difficult and can be even dangerous for the staff.

According to OBRA regulations, all nursing facilities are required to assess the dental status of each resident and to arrange for the provision of routine and emergency dental services. Ideally, this would be assured by a contractual arrangement with a dental director or consultant. Unfortunately, third party reimbursement for this difficult work is meager, and facilities often must seek out dental consultants who do nursing home work for the satisfaction of reaching an underserved population. Partial payment is sometimes available through private payment, Medicare (nursing facilities can charge Medicare residents an additional fee for dental services), Medicaid (approximately 20 states provide some dental coverage for adults under Medicaid), and posteligibility treatment of supplemental income.[27]

Health Maintenance

Screening and health maintenance in the nursing home must be individualized and based on the patient's medical status and prognosis. All new and prospective residents need to be screened for tuberculosis; because of the high prevalence of delayed immunological responses, the first tuberculin screen must involve booster testing and the use of controls.[4] Flu vaccination is also essential for all nonallergic residents, since group immunity is important to preventing epidemics. Beyond these measures the medical evaluation should include a history, physical examination, and laboratory testing based on these evaluations. Routine comprehensive laboratory assessment of nursing home residents is not recommended; it yields many positive results (17.2% of tests) but rarely results in patient benefit (0.2% of tests).[28]

▼ ROBERT JOHNSON

Mr. Johnson is a 71-year-old white man with advanced prostate cancer and chronic pain secondary to bone metastases. Several years ago he had a radical prostatectomy with radiation therapy, and he continues to receive hormonal therapy daily. He is admitted to the nursing home under your care from the hospital with a 30-lb weight loss over 12 months, new onset renal failure, and a pathological fracture of the proximal right femur. He has been confused, restless, and agitated. The family is anxious and somewhat angry with the care they received in the hospital. His wife states that he has pulled out his intravenous line several times and that he pulled out his urinary catheter, causing bleeding from his penis. His daughter and son are worried that he might attempt to get out of bed and sustain more injury. They are requesting that a restraint be used to prevent a fall. They also express concern about how the morphine pump will be managed and who will be responsible for medication management.

On examination he is disoriented and agitated. His temperature is 101.4° F rectally, pulse 110 beats/min, respiratory rate 38 breaths/min, and blood pressure 100/60 mm Hg. He does not respond to questions or follow commands. His mouth is dry; his pupils are small but react to light. Cardiac examination reveals a tachycardia and a 2/6 systolic murmur heard loudest at the apex. His abdomen is distended and somewhat tender without rebound. Rectal examination is significant for hard stool impaction, which is heme positive.

STUDY QUESTIONS

■ *What are the main issues to consider in caring for a dying patient like Mr. Johnson?*

■ *How would you evaluate Mr. Johnson for causes of confusion and agitation?*
■ *How do you respond to the family members' concerns regarding fall risk, self-injury, and pain management?*

TERMINAL CARE IN THE NURSING HOME

The definition of terminally ill is that death is inevitable and is likely to occur within some defined period of time, usually 6 months. Hopelessly ill is defined as having no reasonable expectation of recovery from illness, although not necessarily terminally ill. Elderly persons with advanced cancers, late-stage Alzheimer's disease, multiple strokes with dysphagia, and end-stage pulmonary, cardiac, and renal disease commonly receive terminal care in the nursing home.

The management of terminally ill and hopelessly ill patients requires the practitioner to have sensitivity to several features related to the care of the dying patient and to communication with family, friends, and members of the nursing home staff. The goal for the transition from the living state to death is comfort care. Communication is the paramount skill that must be practiced by the clinician; admission to the nursing home for terminal care requires clear communication with the patient and family regarding knowledge of diagnosis, prognosis, and medical care plans.

The primary diagnosis for the majority of patients admitted to the nursing home is obvious, especially if the issue is terminal care. The exceptions are long stayers in the nursing home for whom slow decline or a new event changes their status from hopelessly to terminally ill. These patients usually have advanced age, problems swallowing, or some other process limiting their ability to maintain life.

Prognosis is sometimes difficult; however, in many cases it will be obvious. Being honest with the patient may mean saying, "I am not sure how much longer this process will go on." Work with advanced dementia has indicated that one of the major determinants of length of life is the aggressiveness of the care; treatment of fever or use of artificial feeding will prolong life, but often in a state that many consider worse than death.[29]

> *Everyone in the nursing home should be good at terminal and palliative care; if they are not, major inservice education is required. Contracting with a hospice may help.*

Treatment plans should be discussed with the patient early in the terminal care process and before mental sta-

tus alterations, if possible. Often, however, it is the responsible party who must make the decisions during terminal care. Do not resuscitate status, a plan to forgo hospitalization, and decisions to avoid further diagnostic testing, artificial feeding (nasogastric or percutaneous gastrostomy), and antibiotics are all elements of the care plan that should be discussed, ideally before a critical event. For terminally ill patients these aggressive measures are usually not warranted; for the hopelessly ill patient with an unclear prognosis these decisions may require more discussion and thought.

Hospice services can often be provided as adjuncts to nursing home care. These can include more frequent monitoring of the patient and counseling for the family.

Symptoms associated with dying include restlessness caused by pain or fear, agitation, disorientation, and hallucinations. Respiratory symptoms include dyspnea and cough. Gastrointestinal symptoms may include anorexia, nausea, vomiting, diarrhea, constipation, and impaction. Other problems may include urinary incontinence, pressure sores, pruritus, dehydration, and inanition. When death is imminent, most patients with terminal illness develop labored breathing caused by metabolic acidosis, dehydration, or bronchopneumonia.

Since the goal of treatment is comfort, these symptoms should be managed actively to minimize stress on the patient, family, caregivers, and other nursing home staff. Acetaminophen for fever, enemas for impaction, oxygen or morphine for dyspnea, and condom or Foley catheters for urinary retention or incontinence are common therapeutic interventions in the dying patient. Complaints of thirst and dry mouth may be relieved with glycerine swabs, sips of liquids, and ice chips; parenteral fluids to relieve dehydration are not necessary for comfort. Food and administration of fluids beyond specific patient requests are usually not indicated as part of comfort care.

Pain control is an essential part of management of the end stage of life. If pain is present, pain control should be constant and not rely on PRN medication. Morphine sulfate is the narcotic of choice for treating severe pain; it can be given orally as an elixir (20 mg/ml), tablet (15 mg), or sustained-release tablet (30 mg). Patients who

Table 14-6 Commonly Used Drugs for Pain Relief in Terminal Illness

Drug	Typical Dose	
	Oral	Intramuscular/ Subcutaneous
Codeine	200 mg q4-6h	30 mg q3-4h
Morphine sulphate	40 mg q4-6h	4-10 mg q3-4h
Hydromorphone hydrochloride	7.5 mg q4-6h	1.5 mg q3-4h
Methadone hydrochloride	20 mg q4-10h	10 mg q3-6h

cannot drink or swallow can be medicated subcutaneously, intravenously, or by suppository. Hydromorphone is similar in effect and ease of administration and can be prepared in high concentrations (100 mg/ml) for high-dose parenteral use. Other opiates may be indicated in special circumstances, for example, methadone for the patient who needs a longer dosage interval. Frequent monitoring should be done to observe for breakthrough pain, oversedation, urinary retention, constipation, and nausea. Table 14-6 outlines the most commonly used narcotics and their typical doses.

Compassion requires an empathic response to concerns of family members during the death of a loved one. Reassurance that agitation and restlessness can be managed without physical restraint can be a very positive way of maintaining patient dignity.

POSTTEST

1. All but which one of the following is a major (>10%) payee of U.S. nursing home expenses?
   a. Medicare
   b. Medicaid
   c. Private funds
2. Which one of the following is most true about working with families of nursing home patients?
   a. Family members cannot sign a patient into a nursing home.
   b. Admission is not a good time to discuss advance directives, since it is often emotionally traumatic.
   c. Often, a relative from out of town forces physicians to change treatment plans.
3. Which one of the following statements is most correct about medical problems in long-term care facilities?
   a. Dental care is mandated by law and covered by Medicaid.
   b. Weight loss can often be corrected by changing the diet.
   c. Routine laboratory testing on admission often uncovers treatable medical problems.

REFERENCES

1. Foner N: Nursing home aides: saints or monsters? *Gerontologist* 34:245-250, 1994.
2. Salive ME et al: Predictors of nursing home admission in a biracial population, *Am J Public Health* 83:1765-1767, 1993.
3. Osterweil D, Martin M, Syndulko K: Predictors of skilled nursing placement in a multilevel long-term-care facility, *J Am Geriatr Soc* 43:108-112, 1995.
4. Ouslander JG: Medical care in the nursing home, *JAMA* 262:2582-2590, 1989.
5. Spillman BC, Kemper P: Lifetime patterns of payment for nursing home care, *Med Care* 33:280-296, 1995.
6. Cohen MA, Kumar N, Wallack SS: Long-term care insurance and Medicaid, *Health Aff* (Millwood) 13(4):127-139, 1994.
7. Butler RN et al: Health care for all: long-term care, the missing piece, *Geriatrics* 47:53-61, Nov 1992.
8. Fries BE et al: Refining a case-mix measure for nursing homes: Resource Utilization Groups (RUG-III), *Med Care* 32:668-685, 1994.
9. Coll PP: Nursing home care in 2001, *J Fam Pract* 36:431-435, 1993.
10. Coons DH, Reichel W: Improving the quality of life in nursing homes, *Am Fam Physician* 37:241-248, 1988.
11. Kelly M: The Omnibus Reconciliation Act of 1987: a policy analysis, *Nurs Clin North Am* 24:791-794, 1989.
12. Streim JE, Katz IR: Federal regulations and the care of patients with dementia in the nursing home, *Med Clin North Am* 78:895-909, 1994.
13. Werner P et al: The impact of a restraint-reduction program on nursing home residents, *Geriatr Nurs* 15:142-146, 1994.
14. Beers MH et al: Inappropriate medication prescribing in skilled-nursing facilities, *Ann Intern Med* 117:684-689, 1992.
15. Avorn J et al: A randomized trial of a program to reduce the use of psychotropic drugs in nursing homes, *N Engl J Med* 327:168-173, 1992.
16. Smith DA: New rules for prescribing psychotropics in nursing homes, *Geriatrics* 45(2):44-56, 1990.
17. Sloane PD, Ives T: Monitoring medications in the nursing home (editorial), *J Am Board Fam Pract* 8(3):249-250, 1995.
18. Murphy DJ et al: Outcomes of cardiopulmonary resuscitation in the elderly, *Ann Intern Med* 11:199-205, 1989.
19. Tresch DD et al: Outcomes of cardiopulmonary resuscitation in nursing homes: can we predict who will benefit? *Am J Med* 95:123-130, 1993.
20. Sloane PD: Managing the sexual behaviors of residents with dementia, *Contemp Long-Term Care* 66,69,108, October 1993.
21. Starer P, Libow LS: Medical care of the elderly in the nursing home, *J Gen Intern Med* 7:350-362, 1992.
22. Beck-Sague C, Bannerjee S, Jarvis WR: Infectious diseases and mortality among US nursing home residents, *Am J Public Health* 83:1739-1742, 1993.
23. Yoshikawa TT: Pneumonia, UTI, and decubiti in the nursing home: optimal management, *Geriatrics* 44(10):32-43, 1989.
24. Griffin MR, Ray WA, Schaffner W: Nonsteroidal anti-inflammatory drug use and death from peptic ulcer in elderly persons, *Ann Intern Med* 109:359-363, 1988.
25. Karam SE, Niew DM: Student/staff collaboration: a pilot bowel management program, *J Gerontol Nurs* 20(3):32-40, 1994.
26. Morley JE, Kraenzle D: Causes of weight loss in a community nursing home, *J Am Geriatr Soc* 42:583-585, 1994.
27. Henry RG, Ceridan B: Delivering dental care to nursing home and homebound patients, *Dent Clin North Am* 38:537-551, 1994.
28. Kim DE, Berlowitz DR: The limited value of routine laboratory assessments in severly impaired nursing home residents, *JAMA* 272:1447-1452, 1994.
29. Volicer BJ et al: Predicting short-term survival for patients with advanced Alzheimer's disease, *J Am Geriatr Soc* 41:535-540, 1993.

PRETEST ANSWERS
1. b
2. d
3. c

POSTTEST ANSWERS
1. a
2. c
3. b

CHAPTER 15

Home Care

JOSEPH M. KEENAN and KENNETH W. HEPBURN

OBJECTIVES

Upon completion of this chapter, the reader will be able to:

1. Describe the recent advances in home care technology.

2. Define the criteria that must be addressed in selecting patients for home care.

3. Describe the advantages of acute home care, postacute home care, and rehabilitation in the home setting.

4. Outline Medicare coverage of home care services.

5. Describe Medicaid coverage of home care.

6. Describe the role of the family caregiver in home care.

7. Describe the specific roles of the physician in home care.

8. Define the range of long-term care services available to home care patients.

PRETEST

1. Technological advances adapted to the home setting include:
   a. Dialysis
   b. Infusion therapies
   c. Ventilator care
   d. Sophisticated monitoring
   e. All of the above
2. All of the following are important in selecting a patient for home care except:
   a. Clinical stability
   b. Appropriate environment
   c. The age of the patient
   d. Caregiver support
   e. Financial support
3. Which one of the following statements is false?
   a. Medical malpractice actions involving physicians in home care are virtually nonexistent.
   b. Most older persons prefer long-term care in the home setting.
   c. Most home care, especially long-term care, is best provided by a multidisciplinary team.
   d. The most important health care system contact person for older persons is the public health nurse.

An overall goal of good geriatric medical practice is to maintain older persons in the familiarity, comfort, and dignity of their own home setting for as long as possible. If attempts to reduce the functional impact of illness in old age are to be successful, it is vital that all health professionals understand the significance of providing care in the patient's own home. Home care will play an increasingly central role in the delivery of health care to older persons. Recent growth of the home care field has expanded the professional roles of physicians, nurses, and other providers, with increased emphasis on care coordination and case management.

This chapter reviews the evolution of community-based care and practice in the past few years and highlights innovations in diagnosis, treatment, and monitoring.

RECENT GROWTH OF HOME CARE

Knowledge of the patient's own home situation is essential background information in comprehensive assessment and in effective ongoing health care management of most frail elders. This point is emphasized throughout this book. However, in recent decades factors including better access to transportation, widespread availability of the telephone, and increasing pressure on physicians to use their own time more economically have contributed to the decline of home care by physicians.

You cannot fully comprehend an older patient's situation unless you know where he or she lives.

There has been considerable growth in the home care field. The number of home care agencies has more than doubled in the past 7 years. The percentage of total home care visits that are to older persons is increasing: 67% in 1991, 69% in 1992, and 74% in 1993. Medicare home care benefits increased by 500% from 1988 ($2.1 billion) to 1993 ($10.5 billion), and Medicare expenditures are projected to reach $22.3 billion by 1999.[1,2]

The main stimulus to an increased emphasis on home care has been the pressure to contain health care costs. The implementation of the prospective payment system and of diagnosis-related groups (DRGs) by the Health Care Financing Administration (HCFA) in 1983 provided a major thrust in this direction. The average length of hospital stay for Medicare patients decreased by 24% between 1982 and 1986 for five diagnoses common in old age (congestive heart failure, acute myocardial infarction, pneumonia, cerebrovascular accident, and hip fracture).[3] Although some of this is owing to better prehospital workups and same-day admissions for surgery, this is mostly a result of shortening the period of convalescence. Thus the need has developed for home care services to increase, and to act as a safety net to provide care that is no longer being carried out in the hospital.

Managed care and health maintenance organizations (HMOs), emphasizing the reduction of costs, have also encouraged the use of home care as an alternative to hospitalization. There is clearly a financial incentive to cover services in the home that will obviate or shorten a hospital stay, such as infusion therapy. As managed care takes on the added risk of long-term care coverage as part of a capitated rate structure, home care services delivered in nursing home settings will help to contain hospital costs for this frail population.

Older persons and their family members do prefer home care,[4] independent of financial savings. Families are willing to participate in home care, even when professional services are provided.[5] Technological advances have made it possible to provide a wider range of clini-

Clinical stability: foreseeable deterioration or complications caused by illness or treatment must be able to be identified and managed in a timely fashion.

Caregiver support: there must be competent and reliable caregiver support available (family, friends, volunteers, etc.) to adequately and safely carry out the care plan and meet the basic needs of the patient.

Appropriate environment: the home setting must be adequate or adaptable to meet the needs of the patient and caregiver.

Availability of professional services: in-home professional support for education, assessment, and treatment must be available for scheduled and emergency care if complex or high-technology home care is planned.

Financial support: many home care services are poorly or not at all covered by Medicare and other insurers; eligibility for covered services should be evaluated and anticipated self-pay costs estimated before initiating home care.

cal services in the home: infusion pumps, dialysis units, ventilators, oxygen compressors, monitoring systems, and other technologies previously restricted to hospital settings are now available for the care of acute and chronic illness in the home setting. Two-way video systems allow remote monitoring of patients, including real-time observation of patients' activities, vital sign monitoring, and even auscultation of the chest and heart.[6]

SELECTING PATIENTS FOR HOME CARE

Modern home care includes a counterpart to all of the usual institutional settings of care. Acute care, postacute care and rehabilitation, long-term care, and hospice care are all available in the home if the circumstances surrounding the disposition of care meet appropriate guidelines. Proper targeting or selecting patients for home care is essential if quality and cost-effective outcomes are to be obtained. Five basic criteria or guidelines must be addressed in selecting patients for home care (Box 15-1).

The most important selection factor, and fortunately the one most familiar to physicians, is the determination of clinical stability. The physician is responsible medically and legally for patient care and therefore must anticipate, within reason, all eventualities that could threaten the desired outcomes of care. This determination frequently entails an assessment of the family caregivers with respect to competency, reliability, and motivation. In addition, the home environment must be evaluated and judged adequate to support the specifications of the care plan.

Physicians' awareness and sensitivity to cost of care issues have increased since the advent of the DRG payment system. However, this generally does not extend to knowledge of eligibility and coverage for professional services in the home. Physicians should be familiar with the local professional home care services that are available for their patients and the criteria that define or limit eligibility for financial support. The regulations and provisions of home care policy change frequently; a home care specialist or discharge planner can be invaluable in arranging services.

ACUTE HOME CARE

Because of the enormous potential for cost savings, acute home care, care planned in the home as an alternative to acute hospitalization, has been strongly supported by third party payers and HMOs. Hospitals have also gotten into the acute home care business. In part, it maintains a market share of the hospital business that is shifting out of their walls. Also, hospitals with acute home care services can often further reduce the length of stay of a Medicare patient, yet still receive the full DRG payment.

▼ *AUGUST SWENSON (Part I)*

Mr. Swenson is a 72-year-old retired salesman who lives with his wife in a well-kept, three-bedroom suburban home. He presents with a painful swelling in the calf of the right leg, with additional tenderness extending to the right popliteal and lower posterior thigh areas. Four days previously, Mr. Swenson was pulling weeds in his garden and, while backing up, stepped on the upturned blade of a hoe that had been lying on the ground behind him. The hoe handle sprang up, striking him in the calf. He experienced only moderate calf soreness until this morning, when he got out of bed and noticed that it was painful to walk on the right leg. He has no chest pain, shortness of breath, or recent cough. He and his wife have both enjoyed excellent health and are physically active. Your recent routine health examination showed him to be in good health. Physical examination now reveals findings consistent with acute deep vein thrombophlebitis (DVT) of the right leg. Pulmonary and cardiac examinations are normal and unchanged from recently. An outpatient venogram shows occlusion of the deep venous system of the right leg to the level of the midthigh. Baseline coagulation studies, complete blood cell count, and platelet count are within normal limits.

Acute home care, by definition, involves active medical management of a serious illness, and correspondingly, the physician's role is dominant and critical. The physician must exercise medical judgment and supervision of care just as if the patient were in the hospital. However, nurse clinicians and other home care professionals, in consultation with the attending physician, provide much of the in-home assessment and hands-on care of the patient. Ideally, the physician also personally performs assessment periodically in the home.

There are many situations in which a physician home visit is a useful and worthwhile practice, but none more so than the setting of acute home care. In-home personal assessment is always the most comprehensively informative way to obtain information about the patient, the environment, and the caregiver's capabilities.[7] The physical presence of the physician in the home is a powerful statement to the patient and family. The home visit instills confidence in the plan of care and enhances the family's respect and appreciation for the physician.

Home visiting by the physician is likely to improve the chances for the desired outcomes of care and, in the event of problems or complications, may well prove a useful risk management practice. Medical-legal actions against physicians involved in home care are virtually nonexistent. However, physicians should be aware, especially in the area of acute home care, that the potential exists for medical liability. Appropriate risk management should be practiced, including informed consent, good communication, and documentation of care in the medical record. The future potential of electronic medical records with access to information from all providers and sites of care holds great promise for better communication in home care.

▼ AUGUST SWENSON (Part II)

You tell the Swensons the diagnosis: deep vein thrombosis of the right leg secondary to the contusion of the calf. You discuss the risks and complications of DVT and its treatment, including the possibility of a pulmonary embolus, or hemorrhage from anticoagulation therapy. You outline the expected course including the caregiving tasks for a patient at bed rest for 5 to 7 days with a continuous heparin infusion and moist heat applied to the right leg. Since the clinical presentation is that of stable and uncomplicated DVT, you offer the option of having the full course of treatment in either the home or hospital, or initiating treatment in the hospital for a few days and completing it at home. Their preference is to receive the heparin therapy at home, but they are more comfortable initiating treatment in the hospital so that anticoagulation could be established in a safer setting. This also allows Mrs. Swenson a couple of days to arrange the home for care to be provided on the main level of the house and to schedule some caregiving help from their children. Mr. Swenson is discharged home on the second day of hospitalization on a continuous heparin infusion as well as oral warfarin sodium. The nurse clinician arranges to make daily home visits to supervise the plan of care, assess the resolution of the DVT, check the infusion, and draw daily coagulation blood tests. She also schedules home delivery of a hospital bed, commode, and infusion equipment while Mr. Swenson is in the hospital. You make a home visit on the second day after Mr. Swenson returns from hospital; there is improvement in the leg. All are reassured that it is going well. Mrs. Swenson kids you about how her husband is getting under her skin and she doesn't know how much longer she can keep him tied down in bed what with the weeds in the garden and all. Although impressed with her vitality and sense of humor, you still ask her privately if she is getting enough help. She appreciates the concern and reassures you that all is fine. Mr. Swenson has an uneventful recovery. Heparin is discontinued the sixth day after hospital discharge. Further follow-up is conducted at your office.

POSTACUTE/REHABILITATIVE HOME CARE

Postacute care differs from acute care in that the focus is on the restoration of function and the completion of convalescence rather than actively managing an acute illness. The patient has typically completed a course of hospital care and is a candidate for further therapy in the home setting. This is the type of home care that is most likely to qualify for Medicare coverage. Medicare eligibility criteria for home care are listed in Box 15-2.

Medical issues still dominate in postacute home care, and therefore the physician's role is important but more in balance with other professionals on the home care team. A nurse clinician or physical therapist may be much more intensively involved with patient care than the physician and may, in fact, be the main author of a care plan and assessor of clinical progress. When a Medicare case is opened and it meets eligibility criteria for home care, other services defined as nonskilled (e.g., home health aides, homemakers) may be integrated into the overall plan of care. This is an important area of service coverage for patients who live alone or have limited family support.

▼ WILLIAM WRIGHT (Part I)

Your patient, Mr. Wright, is a 74-year-old retired painter and widower who lives alone in his own home with his pet dog. He has lived in his present neighborhood for 52 years and has an extensive network of friends, fellow church members, and neighbors nearby, with his two children living out of town. He has peripheral vascular disease secondary to diabetes mellitus. A nonhealing foot ulcer has caused the vascular surgeon consultant to recommend a below-the-knee amputation of his left leg. His health is otherwise good, and he has previously been able to manage all activities independently, even driving a car. You discuss the upcoming surgery at length and specifically map out a plan with Mr. Wright for postacute care. The hospital home care nurse and physical therapist are contacted to anticipate and arrange the care setup and equipment needs: a hospital bed with trapeze, a wheelchair, a four-point walker, and a shower transfer bench. Mr. Wright's neighbors agree to take care of the dog during the hospital stay and provide for shopping needs and social support during convalescence. Mr. Wright's daughter is also contacted, and she is able to arrange to stay with him for the first week after hospitalization.

The postacute care and discharge planning for elective hospital care should begin early, preferably before hospitalization. Most elderly patients experience several transitions in settings of care following hospital discharge. Intermediate stages of convalescence may occur in a nursing home, transitional care unit, or rehabilitation hospital, sometimes punctuated with trials of home care in between.

Actual involvement of home care nursing or therapists before discharge is difficult because Medicare will not reimburse for that activity. Some home care agencies do the requisite advance planning but schedule a home visit on the day of discharge for the majority of patient contact. This day-of-discharge visit allows for a care plan that is developed from the direct assessment of the patient's current clinical needs, actual environment, and social supports, and the agency can be reimbursed for the visit.

Nursing and physical therapy are the most common skilled services used in the rehabilitation and postacute setting. Other skilled services may include speech therapy, stomal therapy, nutritional instruction, and occupational therapy. All of these services tend to be underused by physicians in planning for the aftercare of patients; perhaps the most underused is occupational therapy. It is precisely when other therapies have failed or plateaued in benefit that consultation from an occupational therapist can be most valuable. The concept of the prosthetic environment involves adapting the home to meet the limitations of the patient when that patient has reached the limit of physical recovery and adaptation.

▼ WILLIAM WRIGHT (Part II)

Mr. Wright is discharged after a 4-day hospitalization having had an uneventful surgical recovery. His wound is healing well, and a program to mature and form his stump for prosthesis is initiated. He had been up minimally during the hospital stay, but an active physical therapy program of ambulation with a walker, transferring, and use of the wheelchair is now started, with his daughter and the home care nurse involved at home. The nurse visits three times per week for dressing changes, assessment of wound healing, and review of exercise activities. A physical therapist and occupational therapist each make a one-time assessment early in the posthospital course to provide input into the rehabilitation plan. A rotation of friends and neighbors provide caregiving support to Mr. Wright's daughter. A neighborhood handyman volunteers to install some railings and handholds in the bathroom and stairways at the occupational therapist's suggestion. A home

---

BOX 15-2
Home Care Medicare Guidelines

All of these conditions must be met for home care services to be covered by Medicare.

Medicare Part A

Patient must be under the care of a physician and the plan of treatment must be established and supervised by the physician.

Patient must be homebound, which is defined as possessing one of the following characteristics:

Needs assistance to leave home

Requires considerable and taxing effort to leave home

Medical condition may contraindicate leaving the home

Most occasions of leaving home would be brief and usually for health reasons

Skilled service must be required on a part-time or intermittent basis.

Covered services are defined as noncustodial, and nonmaintenance; thus services are covered only if they are demonstrated to facilitate progress to a higher level of functioning.

Skilled service is defined as the inherent complexity of services or condition of the patient requires a professionally trained person such as a nurse or physical, speech, or occupational therapist.

Nonskilled personal care services may be covered if they are part of a care plan that involves skilled intermittent care.

Intermittent is defined as services being required less than 7 days a week.

Up to 8 hours per day, up to 28 consecutive days may be covered if the care is authorized as reasonable and necessary by the attending physician.

Longer periods of consecutive day care may be covered under special circumstances.

Provider must be a participating Medicare certified home care agency.

Medicare Part B

Durable medical supplies may be covered if the device is required to allow an impaired individual to remain comfortably at home.

Medical supplies must be prescribed by the physician.

Physician must state specific diagnosis necessitating the device, the prognosis, and the projected use of the device.

Medicare covers 80% of the cost of purchase or rental (whichever is cheaper) after the Part B deductible has been met.

Modified from Health Insurance for the Aged Act, PL 89-97, 101-102, 79 Stat. 286, 290-91 (1985), codified as amended at 42 USC 1395-1395xx (1982); and Medicare Catastrophic Coverage Act of 1988, PL 100-26.

health aide is scheduled to assist with personal care and a bath twice a week. By the end of the second week, Mr. Wright is functioning independently within the home, including bathing. By the end of the third week, he is ready for a prosthesis and attends the hospital for outpatient instruction by the physical therapist.

COMMUNITY- AND HOME-BASED LONG-TERM CARE

Community- and home-based care include the informal services of family and friends and are the most expanding areas of health care in the home. Traditionally, most long-term care has been provided in the home; this is not a renaissance area of home care. It has, however, received stimulus for new growth from recent developments in other areas of home care.

It has been estimated that for every person over 65 years old in a nursing home, there are up to four comparably frail elderly people being cared for in the community. Family caregivers provide approximately 80% of the care for these older people living in the community.[8] Demographic projections of our aging population and the expected numbers of frail and dependent older people predict a crisis in long-term care in the early 21st century. The Pepper Commission, the Bipartisan Commission on Comprehensive Health Care, urged the expansion of the coverage of home care services for long-term care as a key step in addressing this problem.[9] The evolving long-term care legislative proposals that are currently under consideration all advance home care as the central and fundamental component of future long-term care policy.

> *Relocation fosters confusion because of unfamiliarity; therefore try to keep the patient in the most familiar place available: his or her home.*

The dominant health problems in long-term care are in the areas of function, self-care, quality of life, and social supports. As such, the dominant provider roles are in the areas of personal care, nursing, and social work. Most of the medical problems of older persons are chronic and either stable or in slow decline. Nevertheless, good medical management is needed to maintain medical stability and prevent iatrogenic problems, such as inappropriate medications that could interfere with function or quality of life. The physician is an important member of the long-term home care team, but more as a consultant or advisor and less as a provider of services.

Physicians legitimately cite the lack of reimbursement for their consultative services as a major disincentive for increased involvement in home care. Recently, the American Medical Association added case conference and telephone management codes to the *Physicians Current Procedural Terminology (CPT) Manual*[10] to help develop standards for charging for that part of professional practice. It is important for physicians to put in the requisite supervisory and consultation time to maintain high-quality home care, and they must begin submitting appropriate charges for that service. Although many private insurance companies have been reimbursing physicians for care management activities, HCFA has steadfastly refused to pay for these services, claiming that they are included in the physician office and hospital visit charges. However, beginning in January 1995, HCFA will reimburse physicians for "care plan oversight" if the physician spends more than 30 minutes in that activity with the patient's caregivers in a 30-day period. Details and limitations related to charging for care plan oversight are being developed.

An important role of the physician in this setting is that of active advocate for the patient and family caregiver. The physician is the only health professional that virtually all older persons visit regularly, often many times in a year. Physicians are uniquely positioned in the long-term health system to provide patients and families with information about, or referral to, community-based services. The list of services is extensive and ever growing (Box 15-3). Unfortunately, most physicians are not very knowledgeable about available community services or about patient eligibility requirements.

The complex needs of older persons in the community, and the complex and ever-changing array of available services, have given rise to a new provider role, that of case manager. Any knowledgeable health professional

---

BOX 15-3
Long-Term Care Services Available to Home-Care Patients

Hospice
Respite care
Geriatric day rehabilitation hospital
Day care
Sheltered workshop
Congregate meals
Community mental health
Senior citizen center
Geriatric medical services, dental services, podiatry services
Legal services
Protective services
Visiting nurse
Homemaker
Home health aide
Chore services
Meals on Wheels

or even family caregiver can function as case manager, but the skills needed for ongoing assessment, coordination of services, and periodic reassessment often require a home care nurse or social worker in the role. Physicians usually do not have the available time or knowledge of community services to best provide case management. However, longitudinal experience with the patient and family makes the physician's input as consultant or advisor essential to the case management process.

▼ JUANITA GOMEZ (Part I)

Mrs. Gomez is an 82-year-old widow who lives alone in a one-bedroom apartment in a senior's high-rise facility. Her daughter, who lives in the same city but about 30 minutes away, calls you to express her concern about her mother's apparent decline. Neighbors in the high-rise provide a close social network for Mrs. Gomez. They have recently informed the daughter that Mrs. Gomez has been less involved in high-rise activities. The daughter states that she telephoned her mother this morning and when no one answered, she rushed over to check on her and found her on the floor apparently unable to get up by herself. You agree to stop by the apartment on the way to the hospital at noon to assess the situation.

Review of your chart reveals that Mrs. Gomez has Parkinson's disease with fair control of tremor and rigidity on a combination of benztropine mesylate (Cogentin) and levodopa-carbidopa (Sinemet). She also has chronic osteoarthritis of the knees and hips managed with as-needed ibuprofen. Her mental status has been good. In previous discussions, in addition to her preferences regarding advance directives and limitations for resuscitation, Mrs. Gomez has expressed a very strong wish to continue living in her apartment as long as possible. At the apartment, she is alert, oriented, and sitting comfortably in a living room chair. By her description, the falling problem has gotten progressively worse over recent months, causing her to limit her activities in the high rise. She never loses consciousness and so far has not hurt herself falling. She states that the falls almost always occur when she is trying to get out of her easy chair or bed. She feels her body freeze in midtransfer and she usually just drops back into the chair or bed. If she falls to the floor, the combination of the Parkinson's disease and osteoarthritis makes it difficult for her to get up. Otherwise, her health has been unchanged, and she generally feels well.

The assessment reveals normal vital signs, including sitting and standing blood pressure. Cardiovascular examination with portable electrocardiography and rhythm strip is normal. Neurological examination findings are compatible with Parkinson's disease, with significant muscle stiffness but no lateralizing findings. Joint examination shows stiffness and limited range of motion in hip and knees. The Mini–Mental Status examination results are normal at 27/30. As part of your functional assessment, you ask her to get up from the chair and walk

across the room. As she stands and is about to take her first step, she becomes akinetic, loses her balance, and pitches heavily back into the chair. She confirms that this is the pattern of her falling but says that once she manages to begin walking, she does not have any problems.

In the ensuing discussion with her and her daughter, the daughter expresses her growing concern about her mother's safety and ability to continue living alone; she would like your support in urging her mother to consider going into a nursing home. Mrs. Gomez repeats her strong preference to continue living in her apartment and lists all of the friends she has in the high rise who help look after her. The apartment is very pleasant with many well-kept flowering plants, a tidy kitchen area, and good access by elevator to the congregate dining and social areas of the high rise.

Many advances in long-term home care have been in the areas of environmental improvements to reduce functional barriers, new technology to facilitate care, and improved monitoring systems to enhance safety. The technological applications developed in this area have included mobile personal care robots, electronic and telecommunicated monitoring, and freestanding total care systems for the bed-bound. These systems provide bathing, whirlpool, flush toilet with bidet, automatic range-of-motion settings, and a decubitus-preventing mattress, all in a unit that is the size of a hospital bed. Automated medication reminder systems can help forgetful patients remember complex medication schedules. Personal radio transmitter call-for-help units linked by telephone to a hospital hotline or 911 can be worn by the patient and are as easy to use as a push-button garage door opener. Most long-term home care does not require high technology; these advances expand the option of home care to more patients.

Many useful environmental modifications are low technology, such as more manageable door handles and water tap handles, more accessible counter and cabinet space, and doors and rooms that are wheelchair-accessible, including a ramp into the home. The home care nurse, physical therapist, and occupational therapist all have an experienced eye for the environmental changes that can enhance safety and improve function.

Physicians play an important role in the process that patients and their families undertake when considering home-based long-term care. Technology increasingly provides impaired patients with acceptable levels of functional independence in their environment of choice. However, particularly for those who live alone, there is a higher degree of risk than living in a supervised environment. Nevertheless, quality of life and sense of personal control may be worth the risks and outweigh their own fears and the concerns of their families (and, in many cases, their physicians). In acute home care the responsible physician acts more authoritatively in management and supervision; in home-based long-term care the physician acts on behalf of the patient's autonomy by helping to clarify the issues of risk and independence presented by this form of care.

▼ *JUANITA GOMEZ (Part II)*

You explain to Mrs. Gomez and her daughter that, although it is not possible to promise a risk-free living situation, measures could be taken to improve her safety and function in the apartment. The cost of these changes would be less than the cost of a month in the nursing home. So, even if it did not work out on a long-term basis, it would not be an expensive trial. A referral is made to a home care agency for assessment and development of a care plan to support her desire to stay in her apartment. The visiting nurse arranges a buddy-system of checking in with other neighbors on the same floor of the high rise, and a regular phone contact each day with the daughter. The easy chair is exchanged for an electronic lifting model, which mechanically assists her to a standing position allowing her to take hold of a four-point walker for added balance. Similarly, a toilet seat lift, handholds, and a tub transfer bench are installed in the bathroom and partial railings on the bed for added balance and support. Regular weekly visits by a home health aide are initiated for bathing and special personal care. The nurse also requests an evaluation screening for eligibility under the 2176 waiver for expanded community-based long-term care assistance. Delivery of groceries and medications to the apartment is arranged, and free use of a wheelchair for outings is available through a high-rise social program. Her daughter visits regularly on weekends and, with the wheelchair, they can go on shopping and other outings together. The nurse learns that Mrs. Gomez is Roman Catholic and quite religious but that she has not been able to get out to church for several years. The nurse contacts the priest at her local church, and he is willing to include Mrs. Gomez in his weekly home rounds and bring her communion. He also arranges weekly visits from a member of the church prayer group who visits and says the rosary with her.

Most states have applied for and received the federal waiver authorized in section 2176 of the 1980 Omnibus Budget Reconciliation Act (OBRA), allowing Medicaid funds to be used for the maintenance of a Medicaid-eligible person in the community who is deemed to be at immediate high risk of nursing home placement.[11] This benefit is limited to the poor who have serious physical or mental disability. It is capped at the estimated per capita cost of nursing home care or a percentage of it. It can be a great benefit in maintaining a frail older person at home, since it is more flexible than Medicare funding for home care. Skilled services, personal care services, or even day care can be covered if they fit into an approved plan to maintain the patient at home.

Adult day care is an important adjunct to long-term home care, since many primary caregivers have other daytime responsibilities. Fifty-five percent of the caregivers of the frail elderly are also employed, and many have dependent children.[8] Day care can also provide social, nutritional, and recreational enhancement to the community-based care of an older person. Successful long-term care in the community must meet the needs of the caregiver as well as the patient. In fact, studies indicate that the determinants of nursing home admission have more to do with caregiver factors than patient factors.[12]

SUMMARY

Home care is expanding. Technological development that at one time shifted the emphasis of modern medicine to the institutional setting has come full circle; it now leads as a growth area in home care. As a result, increasingly complex care is being provided in the home, and more than ever physician involvement and leadership are needed. Physicians are the key health professionals for linking frail elders in the community and their family caregivers with the growing array of home care services.

Managing the care of the elderly, especially community-based long-term care, has become so complex that it often requires the contributions of several professionals working as a team. A new role has evolved for a coordinator of care, a case manager, that also includes functioning as an advocate for the patient and caregiver. The family caregiver is essential to the success of home care.

Physicians have a responsibility to become knowledgeable regarding home care so that their patients can enjoy full access to these services. Long-term care health policy is being rewritten to address the growing needs of our nation's aging population. Home care promises to be central in that policy.

POSTTEST

1. The dramatic growth in home care over the past decade has been stimulated by all of the following except:
   a. New health technology adapted to the home
   b. Patient and family preference for care in the home
   c. Cost containment efforts
   d. Broad-based support and involvement of physicians
   e. The effect of DRGs on the length of hospital stays

2. Which one of the following is not a requirement for eligibility for home care under Medicare?
   a. The care plan must be established and supervised by a physician.
   b. There must be a home care nurse or social worker as case manager.
   c. The patient must be homebound or at least have considerable difficulty leaving the home.
   d. A skilled service must be required on an intermittent basis.
   e. The home care agency must be Medicare certified.

3. Which one of the following statements is true?
   a. Families will significantly decrease their involvement in care if professional services are provided.
   b. A Medicare patient who requires posthospitalization personal care assistance (e.g., bathing, dressing, feeding) will be covered for services as long as a physician orders the care.
   c. Physician-ordered durable medical devices are covered by Medicare if required to allow an impaired older person to remain comfortably at home.
   d. The physician's role is more dominant in long-term care in the home than in acute or postacute home care.
   e. Discharge planning should be initiated as near to the expected end of hospitalization as possible.

4. Which statement is false?
   a. Occupational therapists help adapt the home environment to the physical limitations of the patient.
   b. Family caregivers provide approximately 80% of the care for frail community-dwelling elders.
   c. Proposed long-term care legislation advances home care as central to future health policy.
   d. Physicians make the best case managers for patients needing long-term care.
   e. Dominant health problems in long-term care include physical function, self-care, and quality of life.

REFERENCES

1. *Managed Care Digest,* Long term care edition, Kansas City, Mo, 1994, Marion Merrell Dow Inc.
2. Vladeck BC, Miller NA, Clauser SB: The changing face of long-term care, *Health Care Fin Rev* 14(4):5-23, 1993.
3. Rogers WH et al: Quality of care before and after implementation of the DRG-based prospective payment system, *JAMA* 264:1989, 1990.
4. American Association of Retired Persons, the Villers Foundation: *The American public views long term care,* Princeton, NJ, October 1987, Survey conducted by RL Associates.
5. Christianson JB: The evaluation of a national long term care demonstration, *Health Serv Res* 23:99, 1988.
6. American Telecare Systems, Edina, Minnesota.
7. Ramsdell J: The role of a home visit in comprehensive geriatric assessment, *Am Acad Home Care Physicians Newsletter* 1:1, 1989.
8. Brody SJ, Poulshock SW, Masciocchi CF: The family caring unit: a major consideration in the long-term support system, *Gerontologist* 18:556, 1978.
9. The Pepper Commission: The United States Bipartisan Commission on Comprehensive Health Care. Fact sheet distributed by the Office of the Pepper Commission, 140 Cannon House Office Building, Washington, DC 20515.
10. American Medical Association: *CPT Codes and Nomenclature,* Chicago, 1989, The Association.
11. 42 USC 1396-1396p (1982) and Health Care Financing Administration, US Department of Health and Human Services, Pub No 03156, *The Medicare and Medicaid data book,* 1983, at 27, Table 2.6; at 38, Table 2.14 (1983).
12. Collerick EJ, George LK: Predictors of institutionalization among caregivers of patients with Alzheimer's disease, *J Am Geriatr Soc* 34:493, 1986.

PRETEST ANSWERS
1. e
2. c
3. d

POSTTEST ANSWERS
1. d
2. b
3. c
4. d

CHAPTER 16

Terminal Care

JOEL POTASH

OBJECTIVES

On completion of this chapter, the reader will be able to:

1. Define terminal illness.

2. Understand the nature of palliative care as opposed to aggressive care in terminal illness.

3. Know the qualifications for, benefits of, and limitations of hospice care.

4. Develop a step-wise plan for pain control in the terminally ill.

5. Understand the importance of regular home visits by the physician to the terminally ill patient.

PRETEST

1. All of the following except which one are usually temporary side effects of the use of morphine?
   a. Nausea
   b. Constipation
   c. Hallucinations
   d. Sedation
   e. Respiratory depression
2. Hospice care for the terminally ill:
   a. Is only covered by Medicare
   b. Is not available to residents of nursing homes
   c. Requires a life expectancy of less than 12 months
   d. Only covers patients with cancer
   e. Allows patients to retain their own primary physician

3. Which one of the following statements is false?
   a. A "do not resuscitate" (DNR) order is not required to qualify for hospice care.
   b. Patients with continuing terminal pain should be wakened from sleep to administer oral doses of analgesic.
   c. To avoid overdose with analgesics, they should generally be given on an "as needed" basis in terminal patients.
   d. With cancer pain, acetaminophen should be continued, even if it has failed to control the pain, when mild narcotics such as oxycodone are initiated.

▼ ANNA ALDRIDGE (Part I)

Anna is an 81-year-old patient of yours who has survived successful operations for colon cancer, endometrial cancer, a parathyroid adenoma, and an aortic valve replacement. Two years ago she had a stroke and has a mild residual hemiparesis. Three months ago a biopsy during upper GI endoscopy revealed a gastric lymphoma. She had no evidence of metastases. Nine days after her second course of chemotherapy she is admitted to the hospital by her oncologist; she has fatigue, nausea, vomiting, anorexia, and difficulty breathing. Her hematocrit is 29, and she is in heart failure. An echocardiogram reveals moderate to severe mitral regurgitation, an intact prosthetic aortic valve, and an ejection fraction of 25%. The oncologist determines that she cannot tolerate further chemotherapy, and therefore her life expectancy is less than 6 months. He refers her to the hospice. She will be returning home from the hospital tomorrow.

▼ BARRY BLOKER (Part I)

Mr. Bloker, 66, calls your office on referral from the AIDS Care Center. His rectal cancer, previously treated with laser surgery, has recurred, and he refuses further surgery. A letter from an infectious disease specialist states that Barry has been human immunodeficiency virus (HIV) positive for 4 years and now has acquired immune deficiency syndrome (AIDS) with a T4 lymphocyte count of 200. He had non-Hodgkin's lymphoma 30 years ago treated with chemotherapy and radiation therapy. He had multiple resections of lymph nodes in his neck, groin, and supraclavicular areas. Ten years ago, he had Hodgkin's lymphoma, which was treated with chemotherapy and radiation therapy. A parotid gland cancer was irradiated 2 years ago. Last year possible pelvic metastases

were irradiated. He has a history of depression. His major complaints are pain in the right leg and lower back, depression, loneliness, and rectal pain that prevents him from sitting and walking. His referring physician feels that he is terminally ill and too weak to make visits to the AIDS clinic. Barry requests a home visit.

▼ CATHERINE CAMPINELLI (Part I)

Ms. Campinelli is a 75-year-old patient with progressive dementia, hypertension, and angina pectoris, who has lived in a nursing home for the past 2 years. She is a widow without children or close relatives. Admission to the nursing home occurs after hospitalization for severe angina and congestive heart failure. Because she is unkempt and has lost weight, the hospital social worker visits her apartment and finds bottles of medications, all nearly empty, in the cupboards and refrigerator. Ms. Campinelli thrives at the nursing home, where she receives her medicine regularly and eats her meals with other residents. She regains her lost weight, but soon after that, over a period of 6 to 8 weeks, she loses 15 lb and complains of nausea and upper abdominal pain boring through to her back. An abdominal CT scan reveals a mass. She has a bilirubin level of 7 mg/dl, an elevated alkaline phosphatase level, and a minimally elevated aspartate aminotransferase level (AST). Exploratory laparotomy reveals an inoperable pancreatic cancer. Now, 1 week later, she remains in the hospital on IVs. Her nausea has increased, she is unable to eat, and her bilirubin level is 12 mg/dl. Her pain is not controlled. The surgeon has ordered acetaminophen with codeine, 30 mg, 1 tablet every 4 hours PRN, and the nurses are reluctant to give her the medication unless she asks for it. The nursing home will not readmit her without a feeding or percutaneous endoscopic gastrostomy (PEG) tube. The patient is not believed to *have capacity either to consent to or to refuse medical treatment. She has had a do not resuscitate (DNR) order since admission to the nursing home. There is no health care proxy or living will. Her prognosis, with nutrition, is 3 to 6 months. Hospital policy is to provide artificial nutrition to patients unless there is clear and convincing evidence that they would not want it or death is imminent.*

STUDY QUESTIONS

- *What can you suggest to relieve the symptoms?*
- *What should you discuss with the patients at this stage?*
- *What services might help and how can they be financed?*

TERMINAL ILLNESS

The most common definition of a terminal illness is that of the hospice benefit under Medicare: a life expectancy of 6 months or less. While it may be relatively easy to predict an imminent death, deciding when a patient's life expectancy resulting from illness is less than 6 months is difficult. Oncologists have the most data and experience with the course of incurable illnesses, and their prognostication is often correct. The Karnofsky Performance Status (KPS) may be helpful. Cancer patients with KPS scores of 50 or less died within 6 months in one study.[1] Other predictors of terminal illness include weight loss, diminished food and fluid intake because of appetite loss or difficulty swallowing, and progressive dyspnea. Determining early terminal status of illness is more difficult in the end stage diseases of the heart, lung, and liver and in dementias and motor neuron diseases. Some predictors of terminal illness in AIDS include *Mycobacterium avium-intracellulare* infections, dementia, and cachexia.[1] Consultation with specialists can be helpful in determining the prognosis of an illness. However, the criteria for establishing a 6-month prognosis for life in most diseases other than cancer are yet to be developed.

CASE DISCUSSION

Anna Aldridge and Barry Bloker have been found to be terminally ill by an oncologist and by an infectious disease specialist, respectively. Anna is well known to you, since you are her primary physician. Barry is a new referral. In each case, you must evaluate the patient yourself to determine whether in your judgment he or she has 6 months or less to live. This determination of a 6-month life expectancy is a requirement for admission to a hospice, and it sets the stage for discussion of important medical, psychosocial, and spiritual issues surrounding dying. If you are uncertain about a terminal diagnosis, consult a specialist in the patient's disease who has experience in palliative care.

THE HOSPICE

Hospice care is an option available to all terminally ill patients under Medicare and most Medicaid third-party insurers and managed care organizations, although the benefits may differ in each case. Qualifications for hospice admission are listed in Box 16-1. The patient must elect the hospice program with the understanding that treatment is palliative, that is, to relieve pain and symptoms rather than to seek cure or to prolong life.[2] The primary caregiver (PCG), who assumes responsibility for the patient's care when the patient can no longer live independently, may be a family member, a friend, or a hired professional caregiver. Alternatively the patient may be enrolled in a nursing home with a hospice contract or a supervised living arrangement, such as an apartment or group home sponsored by a church or community organization to provide a residence for terminally ill patients who have no PCG or whose PCG is unable to provide or purchase the care the patient requires.

A DNR order is not required to qualify for hospice care. Some patients, especially those recently diagnosed as terminally ill, need additional time to decide on DNR status; others will not want resuscitation but are unwilling or emotionally unable to sign a DNR request. Many states offer an out-of-hospital DNR order that will be honored by emergency medical technicians (EMTs). In any event, it is unlikely that cardiopulmonary resuscitation (CPR) will be successful in restoring a terminally ill patient to a preexisting state of functioning, and it is likely that such a patient will not survive resuscitation, will die shortly thereafter, or will never leave the hospital.[3] It is imperative that you discuss DNR status with a patient with capacity or with the health care proxy or someone qualified to sign DNR requests in your particular state for patients without capacity.

The hospice patient is assigned a primary nurse who makes at least weekly visits to the home or nursing home. Hospice nurses provide 24-hour availability for home visits. Usually hospice care provides home aides to give personal care to the patient and to assist the PCG, according to the patient's needs: an average routine is 2 hours, 5 days per week. Hospice services may provide up to 24 hours of continuous home care in unusual circumstances such as a crisis or when the patient's death is impending. The patient or family may hire additional help privately or through insurance. The services of a hospice so-

---

BOX 16-1
Requirements for Hospice Admission

Life expectancy of less than 6 months
Availability of primary caregiver or nursing home or
    other supervised living arrangement
Palliative care plan
Concurrence of attending physician
Election of hospice by patient

cial worker or counselor and spiritual caregiver or minister may be elected by the patient. Nutritional services, physical and occupational therapy, and alternative therapies such as music or massage therapies may be provided if indicated. All hospices must provide trained volunteer family caregivers (FCGs) who give additional support for the patient or family, if desired.

Hospice care is reimbursed by Medicare on a per diem basis. All hospices have contracts with area hospitals to provide hospitalization as needed (e.g., for pain control). Hospices can provide respite care, often in a nursing home for a limited time to relieve the caregiver. The hospice is responsible for payment for all medicine for the terminal illness and for durable medical equipment such as hospital beds, commodes, walkers, and oxygen. Laboratory and other testing for the terminal illness, with prior hospice authorization, is also paid by the hospice. Ambulance services for transportation to the office or hospital are usually not covered. In an emergency the hospice nurse visits the patient and contacts the attending physician to establish a treatment plan.

Each hospice has a medical director with expertise in pain and symptom management who is available to consult with attending physicians. The hospice medical director or other hospice physicians supervise the hospice interdisciplinary team, which comprises a nurse, social worker, spiritual caregiver, and often a nutritionist.

The primary attending physician continues to bill Medicare for service and may bill under CPT code 99375 for phone management of the home hospice patient if it exceeds 30 minutes per month. Consultations (e.g., with an oncologist or cardiologist) related to the terminal disease must be paid for by the hospice and require prior authorization by the hospice. Unauthorized testing or treatments for the terminal illness are not covered by Medicare and become the patient's responsibility. The treatment of any coexisting disease is covered independently by Medicare, including the reimbursement of attending and consulting physicians.

CASE DISCUSSION

Anna is already enrolled in hospice services; you must be aware of the benefits and limitations of hospice care. You should discuss the hospice with Barry.

▼ ANNA ALDRIDGE (Part II)

You visit Anna at her daughter's home. She and her daughter have decided that it is unsafe for Anna to live alone. You have a report from the consulting oncologist. Anna has a DNR order to which she has consented. She does not have a health care proxy. As requested, her daughter is present. You do a focused history and examination.

- What should you and Anna discuss?
- What specifically do you need to ask her?

DISCUSSING TERMINAL ILLNESS

When discussing a terminal illness, the physician should first determine what the patient's understanding of his or her illness is and, in a cancer case, ask what the oncologist has told him or her. The patient's feelings about the information he or she has been given should be determined. The physician should also clarify that the patient understands his or her limited life expectancy even if the patient has signed a consent form for hospice care. Some people sign forms without reading or understanding them, or the patient may be in denial. The physician should ask how much medical information the patient would like to have. The ethical principles of autonomy and beneficence demand that patients receive truthful information about their illness and make informed decisions to accept or to refuse care as long as they have the capacity. Decision-making capacity should be assumed unless proven otherwise.

After determining the patient's understanding of his or her illness, the physician should determine what the patient's goals are. A common goal is relief from pain, but there are many individual preferences. If the patient does not bring this up, the physician should ask about hospitalization or the desire to stay at home. Activity needs should be determined: many people want to stay mobile; others are ready to rest and be immobilized in their final weeks or months. Obviously a discussion about the bald facts of the terminal illness itself can lead at some point (this is the beginning of an ongoing process) to discussion about religious beliefs, spiritual needs, the afterlife, and how family and friends are to relate to this situation. There may be family problems that the patient wishes to address, matters to resolve, and farewells. There may well be personal affairs to sort out: financial and legal or testamentary issues, for example, may still not be resolved. Religious preference leads to important differences in the view of what suffering, pain, and dying "mean" to the patient and family. The following case discussions review these aspects as they evolve in the three selected cases.

▼ ANNA ALDRIDGE (Part III)

Anna does not want to return to the hospital. While she is concerned about being a burden to her daughter, she looks forward to being with her two grandsons aged 3 and 5. She is fearful of pain, although her only current pain is from the arthritis. She wants assurance that you will relieve pain if and when it comes. She would like to feel stronger and wants to remain ambulatory. Her bedroom is upstairs. In the morning she can come downstairs slowly holding onto the rail, but she has to go up the stairs after supper on her hands and knees. She feels unsteady. She is very anxious and would like to sleep better. You talk about her appetite and how she is eating and about her bowel and bladder function. She is not suffering side effects from chemotherapy, nor is she suffering symptoms of congestive heart failure (CHF). She does not want a transfusion, yet the oncologist has suggested a complete blood count (CBC) every 10 to 14 days.

STUDY QUESTIONS

- List the goals of terminal care that she has already helped to define.
- What resources can be mobilized to address each goal?

▼ ANNA ALDRIDGE (Part IV)

Your discussion leads Anna to establish the following goals:

1. She wishes to remain at her daughter's home and not be hospitalized. A home aide is in place 2 hours daily on Monday through Friday. Her daughter is planning a trip to Cape Cod for a week in August. The hospice will put in a shift of home aides from 11 PM to 7 AM during that time or arrange for a week of respite care in a nursing home. The daughter decides to hire additional help privately so that Anna will not be alone. The private help is told that 911 or a rescue squad is not to be called in an emergency. The hospice phone number will be prominently displayed near all phones and on the refrigerator. A copy of the home DNR order will be readily available.

2. She wants to have pain controlled. You reassure her vigorously that pain, if it occurs, can be controlled at home using medication by mouth. You assure her that if this does not relieve the symptoms (although it does in the majority of cases), subcutaneous and other routes for pain relief will be used. You assure her that hospitalization is not necessary to ensure cancer pain relief and that the hospice nurse will check each week for symptoms and can be contacted any time.

3. She wants to feel stronger and to remain ambulatory. You suggest moving her bedroom downstairs, but she refuses. A nutritionist will visit and review her diet: a liquid dietary supplement may help. A physical therapist can visit at home and assess her strength and mobility and make suggestions. A walker will be helpful for her stability and to build her confidence. A stair elevator chair is not financially possible. You mention that transfusions may help maintain strength and activity if her anemia becomes symptomatic; she is not interested in transfusions.

4. She wants to sleep better. She agrees to try diphenhydramine (Benadryl) 25 mg or 50 mg after side effects are discussed; you assure her that alternatives are available.

5. She wishes to receive ongoing medical care. Since it would exhaust Anna to come to the office, regular home visits are indicated every month. You assure her that the hospice nurse will notify you of any changes in her condition, but the patient may call the hospice or your office directly at any time.

▼ BARRY BLOKER (Part II)

Since Mr. Bloker finds sitting and walking painful, you visit him at home. He looks cachectic, having lost considerable weight, and his memory is failing. He tells you that he was divorced 15 years ago and has two adult daughters, one of whom lives in the area. They are unaware that he is ill, and he insists that you not tell them. He refuses to tell anyone about his HIV disease except his housemate Tom. Tom and Barry jointly own their home. Tom works several jobs, but he is able to do the house cleaning and cooking. In the last 4 months Barry has lost interest in life and been tearful; he has a poor appetite and has trouble sleeping. He is Roman Catholic, but he is too "embarrassed" to call his priest.

STUDY QUESTIONS

- What else should be discussed, given his diagnosis?
- How will you help Barry to establish his priorities and plans, since he is clearly having a hard time with his diagnosis and situation?

CASE DISCUSSION

In Barry's case it is necessary to clarify his knowledge about the disease itself. His site of care (home, hospital, or elsewhere), his confidentiality, and his self-enforced remoteness from his family will all be management issues and should be discussed.

▼ BARRY BLOKER (Part III)

The rest of the interview does not go well. Barry is not forthcoming in discussion about how his disease came about, but it was apparently not related to blood transfusion. You review his treatment: he had been taking zidovudine (AZT), but he has stopped recently because of his concern about side effects.

He takes trimethoprim-sulfamethoxazole (Bactrim) for prophylaxis for Pneumocystis carinii, since his T4 lymphocyte count has dropped below 200. He has decided not to have further T4 counts. He has no history of opportunistic infections.

He does not have a DNR or a health care proxy, but he would not like to be placed on life support machines. He prefers not to go to a hospital in the case of an emergency or if he becomes too weak to care for himself. He will not consider nursing home placement. He has avoided analgesics for fear of side effects, but he does want pain control if it is needed. He continues to voice concern about his confidentiality.

As a result of your discussions, the following plans are agreed upon between you and Barry:

1. He wishes to remain at home. You clarify that the hospice will be able to provide him with home aides for 2 hours daily. A nurse will visit weekly and will respond 24 hours, 7 days a week, if needed. With that assistance he will be able to remain at home. He agrees to a hospice referral. Whereas the hospice will cover AZT and Bactrim if he is likely to have discomfort without them (e.g., because of secondary infections), you are unsure about the need for AZT.

2. He wants to be free of pain and to have symptoms controlled. You explain to him the rationale for pain relief in terminal illness (see below). You assure him about side effects. You mention that bone metastases could be irradiated to relieve pain. You inform him that x-ray and laser treatment of his protruding rectal cancer might make sitting more comfortable: the hospice would cover both with prior authorization. Barry is relieved to know that the hospice will pay for his pain medications, since his application for Medicaid has not yet been processed. You mention that he might not qualify for Medicaid because of his joint ownership of the house.

3. He wishes to be less lonely. You mention that a volunteer family caregiver from the hospice could visit. He would like someone to go to the bank for him each week. You mention an oral history project at the local university; two students could visit and record his oral history to leave for his daughters or friends. He would like that, but he asks that the students not be told of his HIV infection. Again you mention that at some point in the future he might want to contact his daughters, and you suggest a letter or phone call. He says he will think about it. You mention the priest, but he will not allow contact.

4. He wishes to protect his confidentiality. You assure him that physician and hospice records are confidential and cannot be released without his consent. The hospice needs to know the terminal diagnosis, as does the primary nurse, but confidentiality is protected at hospice team meetings. You inform him that aides do not need to be told the diagnosis, since they use universal precautions.

You refer Barry to the hospice. The admissions team (a social worker and nurse) visit him at home to make an assessment by appointment.

PAIN AND SYMPTOM CONTROL

The first rule of pain control is to believe the patient's complaint about pain; the second rule is to inquire about pain at every opportunity. It is helpful to ask the patient to use a scale to measure pain, such as 0 to 10 where 0 is no pain and 10 is unbearable pain. Terminally ill patients with chronic pain may not resemble patients with acute pain: vital signs may be normal and pupils may not be dilated. Terminally ill patients may barely move in order to avoid pain rather than appear restless as do patients with acute pain; their facial expressions may be placid instead of grimacing.

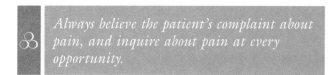

Always believe the patient's complaint about pain, and inquire about pain at every opportunity.

Control of pain and other symptoms in the terminally ill is often intensive but nontechnological.[4,5,6] In general, the analgesic regimen starts with acetaminophen, adding ibuprofen and progressing to narcotics if necessary. Whereas PRN medications may be helpful at first, the medication regimen should be established as a regular schedule to ensure good pain control and the prevention of pain rather than its mere relief. The objective is to avoid pain breaking through.

In terminal care, the objective is the prevention of pain rather than merely relieving it when it occurs. Pain and the fear of pain are to be removed.

There is almost no reason for failure to control pain in a terminally ill patient. The World Health Organization suggests a stepladder approach to pain control (Box 16-2). *Step one* is the use of nonnarcotics such as aspirin, acetaminophen, or nonsteroidal antiinflammatory drugs (NSAIDs). The first drug to use is acetaminophen, 325 mg, 2 or 3 tablets every 4 hours, up to 4 g per day, or ibuprofen 600 to 800 mg every 6 hours (acetaminophen *and* NSAIDs should be tried together; they have an additive effect). *Step two* is the use of mild narcotics such as codeine, oxycodone (Percocet is oxycodone with acetaminophen), or hydrocodone (e.g., Lortab and Vicodin), usually with acetaminophen. For example, the patient may be given acetaminophen with codeine 30 mg (Tylenol No. 3), 1 to 2 tablets every 4 hours; or oxycodone 5 mg with acetaminophen (Percocet), 1 to 2 tablets every 4 hours. Remember that all pain medications are given around the clock. Nurses and family must wake the sleeping patient to administer doses. *Step three* is taken if these medications are ineffective. Oral narcotics, usually morphine, which is generally effective, are given, and there is no upper limit to the amount that can be given. Oral narcotics can be as successful in controlling pain as subcutaneous, intramuscular, or intravenous narcotics. Once the effective dose of morphine has been reached, it can be converted to a sustained release preparation (see below). When initiating narcotics, the patient and family should be encouraged to discuss their concerns, which often include fears of addiction, sedation, and respiratory depression, as well as the imminence of death. Physicians have similar fears and may be hindered by inadequate education in pain control or restrictive state laws, such as triplicate prescriptions requirements for narcotics and antianxiety drugs. Most of the fears of the physician, patient, and family are unwarranted. Temporary side effects of narcotics include nausea or vomiting, sedation, and hallucinations; these usually resolve in a few days (Table 16-1). Constipation may be a serious and ongoing problem. Each patient in whom

Table 16-1   Frequency of Narcotic Side Effects

Side Effect	Frequency (%)
Dry mouth	39
Drowsiness	38
Constipation	35
Sweating	23
Nausea and vomiting	22
Agitation	16
Itching	10
None	24

From Enck RE: *The medical care of terminally ill patients*, Baltimore, 1994, Johns Hopkins University Press.

BOX 16-2
Pain Control: World Health Organization Stepladder Approach

Pain
↓
(Step One)
Nonopioid, ± adjuvant
(e.g., acetaminophen, then add ibuprofen, then consider tricyclic, etc.)
↓

Pain Persisting or Increasing
↓
(Step Two)
Mild narcotics, plus nonopioid, ± adjuvant
(codeine, oxycodone, hydrocodone, plus acetaminophen, plus adjuvants)
↓

Pain Persisting or Increasing
↓
(Step Three)
Strong narcotic, ± nonopioid, ± adjuvant
(short-acting morphine, converting to sustained release morphine [SRM], sustained release oxycodone [SRO], fentanyl patch, or morphine pump/infusion, etc.)
↓

Freedom From Cancer Pain

From *Cancer pain relief and palliative care*, Technical Report Series No 804, Report of the WHO Expert Committee, World Health Organization, 1990.

---

regular doses with narcotics are initiated needs prescriptions for nausea (e.g., prochlorperazine [Compazine] 25 mg suppository, q8h per rectum PRN) and constipation (e.g., senna 1 to 2 tabs hs, increasing as needed).

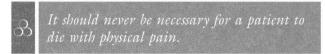

It should never be necessary for a patient to die with physical pain.

Physicians should always order a breakthrough dose of analgesic. For a patient taking morphine, the breakthrough dose can be calculated by dividing the total daily dose of morphine by 6. How often the breakthrough dose is used should be regularly checked: if three or more doses are needed in a 24-hour period, the basic analgesic dose should be increased.

Always be ready for "breakthrough pain" and order an appropriate analgesic dose.

Once the regimen of oxycodone or morphine is established, the dose may be converted to sustained release morphine (SRM: MS Contin, Oramorph SR) or sustained release oxycodone (SRO: OxyContin), which only need to be given every 12 hours. To convert to SRM/SRO, calculate the total daily dose of morphine or oxycodone in milligrams and give the same total milligrams per day divided into two doses at 12-hour intervals (Table 16-2). When SRM/SRO is initiated, it takes approximately 12 hours to become effective, so the shorter acting analgesic (oxycodone or morphine) is continued for 2 or 3 more doses at 4-hour intervals after the SRM is initiated. Note that SRM/SRO tablets cannot be crushed; otherwise the entire dose of morphine will be immediately released. SRM/SRO pills can be placed

Table 16-2   Conversion to Oral Morphine (mg)

Prior Oral Medication	Prior IM/SC Medication	Multiplication ×
Morphine		1
	Morphine	3
Codeine		0.15
Hydrocodone		1
Hydromorphone		4
	Hydromorphone	20
Methadone		1.5
	Methadone	3
Levorphanol		7.5
	Levorphanol	15
Meperidine		0.1
	Meperidine	0.4
Oxycodone		1
	Oxymorphone	30

IM, Intramuscular; *SC,* subcutaneous.

high in the rectal vault against the wall of the rectum (not in the stool), and it is effective by this route (although rectal administration is not included in the *Physicians' Desk Reference*).

In patients surviving longer or patients who cannot tolerate oral medication, the fentanyl patch (Duragesic) 25 to 50 μg every 72 hours can be used (see Table 16-3). A new patch takes up to 18 to 24 hours to become effective, so application of the patch should be overlapped with at least one or two additional doses of SRM (or more of oral morphine or oxycodone, if that is what is being converted from).

Table 16-4 summarizes the management of several other terminal symptoms. *Nausea* can be controlled by a number of drugs. Trimethobenzamide (Tigan) suppositories 200 mg every 6 hours or prochlorperazine (Compazine) suppositories 25 mg every 8 hours rectally can be instituted and changed to an oral route if successful; alternatives include promethazine (Phenergan) 25 to 50 mg qid by mouth and metoclopramide (Reglan) 10 mg orally half an hour before meals and at bedtime. Lorazepam (Ativan) 0.5 to 1.0 mg every 6 hours or haloperidol (Haldol) in a similar dose may be helpful. Scopolamine orally or sublingually (Donnatal) or hyoscyamine (Levsin) may be used.

Dying patients do not usually experience discomfort from undernutrition; a minority may experience discomfort from dehydration.

Placement of a gastrostomy (PEG) tube can extend life by allowing adequate nutrition. There is no need to place

Table 16-3   Morphine/Fentanyl Equivalency

Oral Morphine/day (mg)	Fentanyl Patch (μg/hr)
60	25
120	50
180	75
240	100

Table 16-4   Frequency of Symptoms and Management in the Last 48 Hours of Life

Symptom (Frequency)	Management
Noisy and moist breathing (56%)	Atropine or scopolamine (0.4 mg repeated q4-8h as needed) along with morphine (10-15 mg)
	Suctioning, change of position, and reassurance
Pain (51%)	Adjustment in opioid dosage
Restlessness and agitation (42%)	Methotrimeprazine (25-50 mg IM q4h as required)
	Diazepam (5-10 mg)
	Chlorpromazine (50 mg q4-8h)
	Midazolam (10 mg stat dose and then starting dose of 30 mg/day using continuous infusion)
	Lorazepam (sublingually in doses of 1-2 mg every hour as needed)
Urinary incontinence (32%) and retention (21%)	Padding
	Male external catheter
	Indwelling catheter
Difficulty swallowing (29%)	Rectal administration of drugs
	Continuous infusion of medications, preferably subcutaneous, via pump device
Dyspnea (22%)	Reassurance
	Bedside fan
	Diazepam (5-10 mg stat dose and then 5-20 mg at night)
	Morphine (5-10 mg q4h or doses of morphine titrated to achieve a respiratory rate of 15-20 respirations/min)
Nausea and vomiting (14%)	Antiemetics, such as haloperidol, administered by continuous infusion
Sweating and feeling of heat (14%)	Steroids
	Indomethacin (100 mg rectally)
Muscle twitching, jerking, and plucking (12%)	Diazepam
	Midazolam (5 mg stat dose and starting dose of 10 mg/day by continuous infusion as muscle relaxant; 5 mg stat dose and starting dose of 20 mg/day by continuous infusion for multifocal myoclonus)
Confusion (9%)	Reassurance
	Haloperidol (5-10 mg IM stat dose, then oral or IM 5-15 mg daily)
	Chlorpromazine (50 mg)

From Enck PE: *The medical care of terminally ill patients,* Baltimore, 1994, Johns Hopkins University Press.

a PEG tube in a terminally ill patient if he or she can eat at all, unless the patient requests it and has a reasonable life expectancy (e.g., a month). Dying patients usually do not experience discomfort from decreased intake of food, but patients and family need to discuss any concerns about starvation. If a patient has no food intake and only minimal fluid intake, death will usually occur within 1 or 2 weeks. Dehydration caused by poor fluid intake may cause a decrease in level of consciousness because of azotemia. Dry mouth is best treated by moistening of the lips and mucous membranes of the mouth, rather than by IV hydration. It is possible to give IV fluids at home by subcutaneous hypodermoclysis,[7,8] but this is rarely required. Whereas one recently published study[7] supports the common observation that it is not necessary to be well nourished, nor even well hydrated, to die with peace, comfort, and dignity, the possibility remains that some individual's restlessness, opioid intolerance, and discomfort (if present in the terminal stages) may be relieved by intravenous fluids.[8,9] However, the majority of terminal patients do not seem to require being well hydrated in order to be comfortable. In addition, an IV infusion can limit mobility, and ordering one can potentially subject a dying patient to repetitive, painful attempts to maintain it. Thus intravenous infusion in the terminal phase of life is not the standard of care, whereas oral hygiene, pain relief, and symptomatic relief of nausea and restlessness most certainly are. Unfortunately, many otherwise competent health professionals sometimes still fail to achieve even this.

> *Death accompanied by marked undernutrition and definite dehydration can be natural and dignified, but death accompanied by pain, nausea, or fright can never be.*

CASE DISCUSSION

Catherine Campinelli is obviously dying. Her cancer is inoperable and probably obstructing her common bile duct. A stent could be placed in her common bile duct by endoscopic retrograde cholangiopancreatography (ERCP) to relieve her jaundice, itching, and nausea.

▼ CATHERINE CAMPINELLI (Part II)

Ms. Campinelli's pain relief regimen begins with acetaminophen with codeine, 30 mg, 2 tabs by mouth every 4 hours around the clock in addition to Compazine suppositories, 25 mg rectally every 8 hours PRN nausea. Her pain decreases from 7/10 to 4/10, and her nausea is minimal. Oral feedings are initiated as tolerated. Her narcotic is changed to oxycodone with acetaminophen (Percocet) 2 tabs every 4 hours PO round the clock. The order for breakthrough pain is 2 tablets of Percocet every 2 hours PRN. Her pain is controlled for the most part (1-2/10); she needs two extra doses of Percocet per day. You decide to convert her to sustained release morphine (SRM) for more consistent, prophylactic pain relief. Catherine's current daily equivalent dose of morphine is 80 mg (5 mg of oxycodone × 2 tabs per dose × 6 doses per day + 10 mg × 2 for breakthrough). You order sustained release morphine, 45 mg by mouth every 12 hours. When sustained release morphine is initiated, it takes approximately 12 hours to become effective, so you continue her Percocet, 2 tabs, for two or three more 4-hourly doses. You order a breakthrough pain dose of Percocet, 2 or 3 tabs, or morphine 15 mg PO every 2 to 4 hours PRN. Catherine remains comfortable (pain is 0-1/10), is eating minimally, and takes two cans of liquid dietary supplement per day. The nursing home readmits her. Catherine eats less and less and then cannot swallow her pills. There is discussion with the nursing staff about why an IV or PEG tube is inappropriate when death is imminent. Catherine dies peacefully 6 days later.

ADVANCE DIRECTIVES

It is important to obtain advance knowledge of patients' wishes about DNR orders, their health care proxy or durable power of attorney for health care matters, and the use of artificial nutrition and hydration when they are no longer able to eat or drink sufficiently. Additionally, a values history[10] should be a part of the patient's chart. Knowing a patient's values about life, dying, and health care adds credibility to advance directives when the patient no longer has the capacity to participate in medical decisions. Patients may want to create a general living will and mention specific conditions, such as persistent vegetative state, or specific technologies, such as maintenance on respirators, in their advance directive. The Federal Patient Self-Determination Act (1992) requires hospitals and nursing homes to ask about the existence of advance directives and to offer assistance in their creation, if desired. Physicians should display forms for advance directives in the office waiting room and offer to discuss advance directives with all older or very ill patients. A copy of any existing advance directive should be placed in the patient's chart, and its existence noted on the problem list. Some states allow an out-of-hospital DNR order, signed by the patient or surrogate and the attending physician, which exempts EMTs from responsibility to resuscitate the patient. Any DNR order should be prominently posted in the home of terminally ill patients in case 911 or a rescue squad is called.

Families must remember that even if they have the authority of a directive or proxy, they are not making the decisions; they should express what the patient's wishes would have been, had he or she been able to express them.

USE OF ETHICS COMMITTEES AND ETHICS CONSULTATIONS

An ethics consultation or a meeting with the ethics committee can be sought in any case of dispute or doubt about the intensity of treatment, such as whether or not to recommend a PEG tube in a patient who is unable to eat sufficiently. With inoperable, terminal cancer, artificial nutrition and hydration (ANH) may merely prolong dying, pain, and suffering. Inability to drink or eat in the terminally ill is usually not associated with discomfort other than dry mouth; this is easily fixed with good mouth care. Many people in similar circumstances die comfortably at home without ANH in the hospice, the model of terminal care. Some nursing homes refuse to admit patients who are unable to eat without ANH. If necessary, ask to meet the ethics committee (however, smaller nursing homes may not have one). Nursing homes with hospice contracts are likely to accept terminally ill patients even when they are unable to eat or drink. If necessary, you can seek a court order to prevent institution of ANH if it appears to be incompatible with the good of the patient or to seek clear and consistent evidence of a patient's wishes; however, a favorable outcome through any court is not guaranteed.

FOLLOW-UP OF THE TERMINAL PATIENT

Terminally ill patients benefit from regular physician visits. Many are too weak or in too much pain to travel to the office. House calls are then indicated. It is appropriate to assess acute illnesses of terminally ill patients at home rather than in the emergency room if the patient or family wants to avoid hospitalization. Laboratory and other tests should be ordered only if they will effect a change in treatment plan. If the patient is enrolled in hospice services, testing should be authorized by the hospice; authorization will depend on whether testing will result in treatment leading to greater comfort. Many laboratories and imaging offices provide services at home. Under the Medicare option, any testing has to be authorized by the hospice and the determining factor will be whether the test would cause a change in treatment plan leading to greater comfort. Reassessment should include questions about pain and other discomfort, appetite, food and fluid intake, level of activity, sleep patterns, and bladder and bowel function.

▼ ANNA ALDRIDGE (Part V)

Anna's nausea remits with meclopropamide (Reglan), and her appetite improves. Her weight increases, and with the help of home physical therapy she walks down and up the stairs twice a day with little difficulty. She has difficulty sleeping, cries a lot, and hates to think about leaving her grandchildren. Sometimes she doesn't feel like eating but her daughter and her home aide coax her. She requires almost no pain medicine. She takes acetaminophen, 2 tablets, twice a day for her arthritis. Since her strength is improved, you do not order a CBC, although Anna is curious about her anemia. She is taking a multivitamin with iron.

Anna wants to continue her DNR order. She has not completed the health care proxy form, but she agrees to do so and asks her daughter to be her proxy.

DEPRESSION IN THE TERMINALLY ILL

In a situation of terminal illness, patients and physicians alike often feel that depression is "justified." However, it frequently responds to treatment. If there are sleeping problems, a low dose of a sedating tricyclic antidepressant such as amitriptyline can be helpful. Antidepressants often have a coanalgesic effect. Hospice services cover this medication. In addition, counseling or psychiatric consultations can be arranged for depression.

▼ BARRY BLOKER (Part IV)

After talking with Barry's doctor at the AIDS Care Center, you recommend that Barry resume his AZT. His rectal pain is finally controlled with oral morphine 30 mg every 4 hours around the clock. You change this to SRM, 100 mg every 12 hours PO. He uses 30 mg of morphine PO if he needs to sit for any duration of time (e.g., on the shower stool). He is much weaker. He is dictating his oral history and gains a realization of his many accomplishments. He asks the hospice minister to contact his priest; he hopes to receive communion. A family caregiver from the hospice comes weekly to do Barry's banking. Barry is embarrassed by the odor of his rectal seepage. He would like laser resection of his rectal cancer in hopes of improving his hygiene and his ability to sit. Both daughters have called; he has told them he is ill but not that he has HIV/AIDS. His housemate seems overwhelmed. You suggest increasing the home aides' presence to 6 hours daily during weekdays and 4 hours on Saturday and Sunday. The hospice agrees to your plan. You schedule rectal surgery.

A month after rectal surgery, Barry has less rectal discomfort but his weakness has progressed. He is confined to bed except for the use of a bedside commode. His memory is significantly worse. Tom asks about a T4 lymphocyte count. Although the T4 count would not affect Barry's treatment, Barry says that if the T4 count is much lower he is ready to stop fighting to live. You agree to the test. His T4 lymphocyte count is 50. His eating and drinking become minimal, and he asks you to visit to say goodbye. Two weeks later Barry dies at home. You attend calling hours at the funeral home and comfort Tom.

BEREAVEMENT CARE

It is not unusual for bereavement to last a year. Hospice services offer 13 months of bereavement care to the family and caregivers of deceased patients. After the patient's death, family members may benefit from a telephone call or card from the physician expressing sympathy and inquiring into their well being. It is important to allow families and caregivers to express their anger, guilt, and grief. Hospice services offer bereavement groups and individual counseling if desired, both without cost. It is important to remember that for many, pathological reactions to bereavement arise from dissatisfaction about the arrangements around the time of death and after death. The American Psychiatric Association (APA) has described the characteristics of normal bereavement to help clinicians distinguish this normal phenomenon in life from pathological processes such as major depression (with the implication that specific antidepressant therapy would then be helpful) (Box 16-3).

▼ *BARRY BLOKER (Part V)*

Three weeks after Barry's death, you receive a call from Karen, his youngest daughter; she is upset. Unknown to you, Karen cared for her father during the last 3 days of his life. She requested and received a copy of her father's death certificate, on which you had listed AIDS as the cause of death. She was unaware of her father's HIV/AIDS and is concerned about her exposure. Although she is a nurse, she did not use universal precautions. You invite Karen to your office for a meeting, at which you discuss your ethical responsibility to honor Barry's request for confidentiality. You discuss how HIV is transmitted. It is unlikely that caregivers of AIDS patients will get infected, but you recommend HIV testing and counseling from her own physician, now and again in 3 to 6 months. Karen agrees to have the hospice bereavement counselor contact her.

▼ *ANNA ALDRIDGE (Part VI)*

Anna continues to improve. On your fifth monthly home visit she does not appear to be dying. You suggest that she visit her gastroenterologist to see whether her lymphoma has disappeared. She agrees. Upper GI endoscopy with guided sonography reveals a normal stomach; her spleen and liver are also normal by sonography. You schedule a meeting in your office with Anna, her daughter, and the hospice nurse to dis-

---

BOX 16-3
Differentiating "Normal" Bereavement from Major Depression

In a reaction to the death of a loved one, consider a major depressive episode if the following occur:
Marked grieving symptoms, persisting 2 months after the loss
Guilt about things other than actions taken or not taken by the survivor around the time of death
Thoughts of death other than the survivor feeling that he or she would be better off dead or should have died along with the deceased person
Morbid preoccupation with worthlessness
Marked psychomotor retardation
Prolonged and marked functional impairment
Hallucinatory experiences other than hearing the voice or transiently seeing the image of the deceased person

Modified from *Diagnostic and statistical manual,* ed 4 (DSM-IV), Washington, DC, 1994, American Psychiatric Association.

---

cuss discharge from hospice care since Anna is no longer terminally ill. Hospice services will also meet with the family to make a discharge plan, and Anna will be referred to a home care agency for any remaining needs. The hospice clarifies to Anna and her family that she can be readmitted when she again becomes terminally ill.

SUMMARY

A carefully integrated approach to a patient known to be terminally ill, using the services of a hospice, can result in greatly enhanced care of the dying patient and of the bereaved family. Hospice care provides an enrichment of services, reimbursed by Medicare and Medicaid, to ease the dying process. The hospice medical director and staff are experts in the preventive approach to pain relief and the often dramatically escalating doses of analgesics necessary for preventing pain and distress. Symptomatic relief of associated symptoms, such as nausea, and more dramatic interventions if necessary to relieve intractable symptoms (although the prime objective is improving the quality and not the length of life) will be used in patients with such needs. Hospice care is associated with bereavement counseling both before and up to 13 months after the death. Anyone can refer a patient to a hospice, and should a patient cease to be terminally ill, he or she can withdraw from the hospice to have the care reinstituted later if necessary. Hospice care is increasingly important in the care of the elderly not only in the community but also in the many nursing homes that have arranged hospice services.

POSTTEST

1. Pain control can be achieved by oral medications in what percent of terminally ill patients?
   a. 25%
   b. 50% to 60%
   c. 75% to 85%
   d. 95% to 100%
2. Which one of the following is considered unethical in dying patients?
   a. Withholding artificial fluid and nutrition
   b. Withdrawing artificial fluid and nutrition
   c. Regular doses of narcotics for more than 4 weeks
   d. All of the above
   e. None of the above

3. Which one of the following is true about sustained release morphine tablets?
   a. They are ineffective when given rectally.
   b. They require a breakthrough dose of a short-acting narcotic PRN.
   c. They may be crushed if the patient has difficulty swallowing.
   d. They should be ordered every 12 hours PRN.
   e. They have an upper limit beyond which they are ineffective.

REFERENCES

1. Enck RE: *The medical care of terminally ill patients,* Baltimore, 1994, Johns Hopkins University Press.
2. Doyle D, Hanks GWC, MacDonald N: *Oxford textbook of palliative medicine,* New York, 1993, Oxford University Press.
3. Taffet GE, Teasdale TA, Luchi RJ: In-hospital cardiopulmonary resuscitation, *JAMA* 260(14):2069-2072, 1988.
4. *Physicians handbook of symptom relief in terminal care,* Santa Rosa, Calif, 1993, Sonoma County Foundation for Excellence in Medicine.
5. Twycross RG, Lack SA: *Therapeutics in terminal cancer,* New York, 1990, Churchill Livingstone.
6. *Management of cancer pain,* Clinical Guideline No 9, Rockville, Md, 1994, US Department of Health and Human Services.
7. McCann RM, Hall WJ, Groth-Juncker A: Comfort care for terminally ill patients: The appropriate use of nutrition and hydration, *JAMA* 272(16):1263-1266, 1994.
8. Fainsinger R, Bruera E: The management of dehydration in terminally ill patients, *Palliative Care* 10:55-59, 1994.
9. Craig GM: On withholding nutrition and hydration in the terminally ill: has palliative medicine gone too far? *J Med Ethics* 20:139-143, 1994.
10. Doukas DJ, McCullough LB: The values history: the evaluation of the patient's values and advance directives, *J Fam Pract* 32(2):145-153, 1991.

PRETEST ANSWERS
1. b
2. e
3. c

POSTTEST ANSWERS
1. c
2. e
3. b

UNIT II
THE MAJOR SYNDROMES

I am a very foolish fond man,
Fourscore and upward, not a hour more or less;
And to deal plainly,
I fear I am not in my perfect mind.
—Shakespeare, *King Lear*

What does it matter if he can't remember his grandchildren, as long as they can remember him?
—Wife of patient with Alzheimer's disease, Syracuse, 1995

He that conceals his grief finds no remedy for it.
—Turkish Proverb

Do not go gentle into that good night,
Old age should burn and rave at close of day;
Rage, rage against the dying of the light.
—Dylan Thomas, "Do Not Go Gentle into That Good Night"

It is better to wear out than to rust out.
—Richard Cumberland, quoting an 18th century sermon of Bishop George Horne

The quality of a life is determined by its activities.
—Aristotle, *Nichomachean Ethics*

And then he falls, as I do. . . .
. . . .
And when he falls, he falls like Lucifer,
Never to hope again.
—Shakespeare, *Henry VIII*

CHAPTER 17

Confusion, Dementia, and Delirium

RICHARD J. HAM

OBJECTIVES

Upon completion of this chapter, the reader will be able to:

1. Discuss delirium's clinical features and differentiation from dementia.

2. Describe the appropriate diagnostic workup and implied interventions for diagnoses found in a patient presenting with delirium or any change in mental status.

3. Define the syndrome dementia and its differential diagnosis.

4. Understand the role of family members and other caregivers in the presentation, nonpresentation, experience of early symptoms, and ongoing treatment of patients with dementia.

5. Describe the clinical criteria for dementia of Alzheimer's type (DAT) and vascular dementia (multiple infarct dementia, or MID), evidence to be sought that would be supportive of these diagnoses, and the clinical features that would be consistent and inconsistent with each.

6. Construct an appropriate diagnostic and management plan for patients presenting either an abrupt or an insidious onset of mental status change, including brain imaging, laboratory investigation, neuropsychological testing, and short screening tests suitable for the office setting.

7. Describe ways that the physician, other health professionals and nonhealth professionals, the family members, and other caregivers can interact to prevent or ameliorate the characteristic symptoms and problems of a progressive dementia including memory loss, indecisiveness, judgment problems, concurrent depression (including use of antidepressants), diminished driving skills, disorientation, unadaptability, personality change, hallucinations, disinhibition, diminished daily living skills, dysmobility, wandering, aggressiveness and agitation (including use of antipsychotic medication), catastrophic reactions, concurrent medical problems, sleep disorders, sundowning syndrome, repetitive behaviors and shadowing, delusions and illusions, paranoia and suspiciousness, living arrangements and placement, incontinence, lost lower extremity skills, undernutrition, legal issues, ethical concerns, and terminal care.

8. Defend the need for a philosophical approach that places appropriate decision making and autonomy with the patient and allows him or her to stay in the security of the home environment for as long as practical, weighing this against family and societal stress and the costs of care.

217

PRETEST

1. Which one of the following statements concerning dementia is true?
   a. A community study in 1990 showed the prevalence of findings suggestive of dementia to be 30% in people 80 years or older.
   b. The second most frequent cause of progressive dementia is multiple cerebral infarctions.
   c. The clouding of consciousness in dementia helps distinguish it from delirium.
   d. Preservation of abstract thought late in dementia is frequent.
   e. Undetected diabetes mellitus is one of the principal causes of apparent dementia.

2. Which one of the following statements is true concerning the differential diagnosis of dementia?
   a. Patients with depression tend to give vague, inaccurate answers to mental status questions.
   b. Seizures early in dementia suggest normal-pressure hydrocephalus.
   c. Medication side effects constitute one of the most important causes of reversible apparent dementia.
   d. An abnormal vitamin B_{12} test in dementia should be followed by a Schilling test before treatment.

3. Which one of the following is true regarding issues important to caregivers in dementia?
   a. Reminiscence therapy has been shown to improve behavior and well-being in patients with dementia.
   b. Power of attorney gives the designated person the right to make medical decisions for the patient.
   c. The living will is legally accepted as an indication of patients' wishes in most states.
   d. Having multiple family members with probable Alzheimer's disease does not increase the risk of the individual developing the disease.

4. Which one of the following is false concerning medical aspects of the dementias?
   a. It is generally more important to carry out brain imaging in the patient with early dementia than during the later phases of the illness.
   b. The most common reversible cause of changed mental status lasting several weeks is depression.
   c. Pick's disease can be clinically distinguished from Alzheimer's disease.
   d. Creutzfeldt-Jakob dementia is caused by a transmissible agent.

The aging brain is a vulnerable organ, exquisitely sensitive to changes in its environment: drugs, disease processes in other organ systems, environmental change, and many other factors greatly affect its function and thus the function of the whole person. Alteration in mental status is an important early sign of disease and of medication problems in elders, and it must be both noticed and efficiently acted upon. The syndrome delirium represents the most dramatic acute clinical manifestation of such influences on the brain.

The aging brain is also the site of one of the most common illnesses of the old, Alzheimer's disease. With a mean age of onset of about 81 years, it is the main cause of progressive decline of brain function in old age, characteristically causing a prolonged period of decline (about a decade or more) during which time there is progressive dependence on family members and the health care system. Alzheimer's is but one of many causes of the syndrome dementia. Accurate diagnosis is the first step of a long process, and it should be followed by years of skilled management involving dedicated health professionals and trained caregivers, who are frequently family members. The caregivers' ability to help minimize the effects of dementing illness on the individual is key to maintaining as much quality of life as possible and to postponing dependence, the most costly phase in both emotional and fiscal terms, for as long as possible.

The terminology for the dementias has recently been changing.[1] The APA nomenclature,[2] dementia of Alzheimer's type (DAT), is used here. Appropriate use of the word "Alzheimer's" helps professionals and society as a whole to appropriately address the many individuals whose lives will be affected by this particular type of dementia.

However, to the practicing physician, it has been clear for years that a change in brain function, the nature of which is often difficult to characterize, is in fact one of the most common manifestations of virtually any illness, medication effect, or other major change in an older person. The full clinical picture of a classic, agitated delirium can be the presentation of many illnesses in old age and is thus diagnostically challenging. Often the patient is unable to contribute to answering two vital and simple questions that are frequently overlooked by health professionals faced with a demonstrably confused older patient:

■ How long has this been going on?
■ How abruptly did it start?

A health care system responsive to the needs of Alzheimer's patients would have the characteristics most old and frail patients need: open, uninhibited access to services that address emotional, social, and physical needs, as well as overt acute illness; continuity, to allow familiarity and trust to develop not only between the patient and the physician but also within a widening circle of family members, professionals, and nonprofessionals; comprehensiveness, with services that emphasize health maintenance and prevention; respite services for the stressed caregivers; accountability (these patients more than other elders needs someone to take charge of their situation); home-based care (individuals with dementia generally function much better in familiar, secure surroundings); and appropriate dementia-specific skilled care environments during acute illness, for temporary respite, or for the final months or years, after home care has become impossible.

> *A health care system responsive to the needs of Alzheimer's patients would be responsive to the needs of most of the old and frail: accessibility, continuity, comprehensiveness, accountability, and availability of respite.*

▼ MAY HOMER (Part I)

Mrs. Homer is a 75-year-old woman not previously known to you, the emergency room physician. She presents around 11:00 PM one evening, having been brought in by the police after being found confused and attempting to make her front door key fit a similar apartment door to her own, but on a different floor in the apartment complex in which she lives. She had become abusive, confused, and frightened and looked pale, ill, and agitated; since they could not establish her correct address at that time, she has been brought to the emergency room. On examination, it takes several attempts to gain her attention to answer any questions at all, but once focused on a question she rambles on in a disorganized way, her speech sometimes incoherent. She is at times drowsy and falls asleep during the interview. When awake, she seems to be talking about things that are in the room with her and is unable to describe where she is, who she is, or where she lives. Her pulse is 96 and regular and her BP 145/90. She is at times agitated and diaphoretic and at other times quiet, withdrawn, and near sleep.

STUDY QUESTIONS

- Which specific laboratory studies or other investigations should be ordered now and why?
- If a family member or friend can be contacted, what particular questions should be asked?
- The officer accompanying her has mentioned Alzheimer's; a young trauma victim in pain from a reducible wrist fracture is waiting and other patients are backing up. Is Mrs. Homer's care urgent?

DELIRIUM: A MEDICAL EMERGENCY

Delirium is the acute effect of physical illness on brain function (Box 17-1).[3] It can be caused by intracerebral disease, but it is much more often due to acute illness or physiological change elsewhere in the body. It is the presentation of many serious underlying diseases and is often the result of several interacting diseases and their treatments. Delirium is largely or completely reversible, provided the causative illness can be identified and treated promptly. The causative illness may itself be life threatening.

Delirium is unfortunately often neglected as a medical emergency. It is common and is estimated to affect as many as 30% to 40% of all older persons admitted to the hospital.[4]

A danger for the clinician is to assume that there has been little change from the prior status and that the person is suffering "only" from (chronic) dementia. If there is no information about the prior history, it is best to assume that the confusion is of new onset and proceed accordingly.

> *A relatively acute onset with disorganized thinking and inability to maintain and shift attention is specific to delirium.*

Although some of the diagnostic criteria for delirium might be fulfilled in a dementia patient, the relatively acute onset (especially if there are hallucinations andother psychomotor changes), the disorganized thinking with rambling, irrelevant, or incoherent speech, and the

---

BOX 17-1
Diagnostic Criteria for Delirium

Disturbance of consciousness with change in cognition that is not better accounted for by a dementia
Develops over hours to days
Fluctuates during the course of the day
Impaired ability to focus, sustain, or shift attention
Cognition impaired (memory, orientation, language) or perceptual disturbance (misinterpretations, illusions, hallucinations)
Associated with sleep-wake cycle disturbance, disturbed psychomotor behavior (restlessness, hyperactivity, or decreased psychomotor activity; may be stuporous), emotional disturbance including fear, electroencephalograph (EEG) abnormalities (generalized slowing or fast activity)
Evidence that disturbance is caused by a general medical condition, substance intoxication or withdrawal, or multiple etiologies

From *Diagnostic and statistical manual of mental disorders* (DSM-IV), ed 4, Washington, DC, 1994 American Psychiatric Association.

inability to both maintain and shift attention are specific to delirium.

The most agitated states of delirium bring themselves to medical attention, but the psychomotor agitation, and perhaps the hallucinations or delusions, can lead to a "psychiatric" rather than a "medical" approach. Although such a patient may require the skills of mental health nursing, a calming one-on-one approach, or even sedative or antipsychotic medications, nothing should distract from the emergency nature of the medical investigation for the underlying cause or causes.[5]

The differentiation from psychosis can be difficult. In delirium, however, there is generally no prior history of psychiatric illness, the sensorium is clouded, and the onset is acute. In a true psychosis the patient is much more likely to have a clear sensorium, intact memory and orientation, and a history of prior psychiatric illness, generally from before the age of 65. The hallucinosis of delirium tends to be based around more familiar aspects of the patient's life, with delusions whose origins can be explained, whereas the hallucinations and delusions of a primary psychosis tend to be more bizarre and more out of touch with reality.[6]

An atypical presentation, the "quiet" delirium, with passive dysfunction (but still a marked change from the previous level of function) can easily be missed. All caregivers must be sensitive to functional change as an indicator of major illness in older persons. A change from persistent objectionable feistiness to unusual quietness could well represent the onset of such a "passive" delirium.

> *Be aware of "quiet" delirium: a change from objectionable feistiness to unusual quietness could represent serious illness.*

▼ MAY HOMER (Part II)

You order a chest x-ray examination and laboratory tests for Mrs. Homer: CBC, electrolytes, renal and hepatic function, blood alcohol, and urinalysis. Initial microscopy suggests a urinary tract infection, laboratory findings suggests dehydration, and the other results are normal. Your examination reveals no localizing or lateralizing signs in the CNS, but the patient is only intermittently cooperative, and her mental status fluctuates. She appears clean, well nourished, and not self-neglected, and there is no sign of injury or falling. You decide to observe her, initiate treatment of the urinary tract infection, and schedule a CT scan of the brain, largely to rule out the possibility of a subdural hematoma. Overnight Mrs. Homer improves slightly, but she is still confused the next day when her daughter is contacted. Mrs. Homer's daughter states that her mother was fully functional and not in the least confused or impaired in her memory, living independently at

home before this episode. The daughter had a normal conversation earlier the same evening with her on the telephone, although her mother did say that she was having trouble with urination. Hearing of Mrs. Homer's hospitalization, her neighbor in the apartment building visits and says that after dark some youths had been making a noise outside the apartments at about the time the outside lights at the complex were shut off each night. She had heard Mrs. Homer open her door and shout at the youths; she thinks Mrs. Homer probably went out and became lost from her apartment in the dark and panicked, as she had done once before.

STUDY QUESTIONS

- *Does Mrs. Homer fulfil the criteria for delirium?*
- *What specific precipitants can be identified already?*
- *On the evening of admission, should she be "left alone to get some rest," as one of the nursing aides suggests, or intensively observed for signs of deterioration?*

CASE DISCUSSION

Whereas the initial management was reasonably appropriate, several other etiologies have not been considered, including an acute myocardial event and the possibility of sepsis. The urinary findings may be coincidental, since she may have chronic problems with bacteriuria; if septic, she is in danger of acute collapse. If a head injury has contributed, acute deterioration is again the danger. The absence of much history makes it important to regard this as an acute, emergency case; meningitis, as well as subdural hematoma, would be clinically suspected if her situation should deteriorate or fail to improve promptly.

DELIRIUM VS. DEMENTIA

Delirium has been defined in the preceding section. There are some important differences between delirium and dementia. Dementia (Box 17-2) is not a diagnosis: it is the name of a syndrome, and it is mandatory to define the diagnosis. The essential clinical feature of dementia is that there are multiple cognitive deficits, sufficiently severe and persistent that they cause impairment in function, with a definite decline from a previously higher level of functioning. "Functioning" includes occupational as well as social functioning. The cognitive impairments always include memory plus at least one of the following: aphasia, apraxia (impaired ability to carry out motor activities despite intact motor function), agnosia (failure to recognize or identify objects despite intact sensory function), or disturbance in executive function (planning, organizing, sequencing, and abstracting). If all these things occur only during the clinical occurrence of an apparent delirium, then it is not "dementia." However, dementia, whatever the cause, is a predisposing factor toward delirium, so the two can coincide. And although dementia is usually irreversible or at least incompletely reversible and is generally chronic (by defini-

BOX 17-2
Clinical Features of the Syndrome Dementia

1. Multiple cognitive deficits, including memory impairment and at least one of the following: aphasia, apraxia,* agnosia,† or disturbed executive functioning (planning, organizing, sequencing, abstracting)
2. Cognitive deficits severe enough to impair occupational or social functioning
3. Cognitive deficits representing a decline from previously higher function
4. These deficits not occurring exclusively during the course of delirium

NOTE: Dementia is not a diagnosis.

Modified from *Diagnostic and statistical manual of mental disorders* (DSM-IV), ed 4, Washington, DC, 1994 American Psychiatric Association.

Apraxia is the inability to carry out purposeful movements even though there is no motor or sensory impairment; this includes the inability to use objects: for example, constructional apraxia (cannot copy simple drawings), motor apraxia (cannot use an object even though its nature is recognized), sensory apraxia (cannot use an object because its nature and purpose are not recognized).

†*Agnosia* is a failure to recognize sensory stimuli: for example, visual agnosia (cannot recognize objects by sight), tactile agnosia (cannot recognize objects by touch or feel), ideational agnosia (cannot make up the idea of an object from its components).

Table 17-1   Distinguishing Delirium from Dementia

Delirium	Dementia
Abrupt precise onset with identifiable date	Gradual onset that cannot be dated
Acute illness, generally days to weeks, rarely more than 1 month	Chronic illness, characteristically progressing over years
Usually reversible, often completely	Generally irreversible, often chronically progressive
Disorientation early	Disorientation later in the illness, often after months or years
Variability from moment to moment, hour to hour, throughout the day	Much more stable day to day (unless delirium develops)
Prominent physiological changes	Less prominent physiological changes
Clouded, altered, and changing level of consciousness	Consciousness not clouded until terminal
Strikingly short attention span	Attention span not characteristically reduced
Disturbed sleep-wake cycle with hour-to-hour variation	Disturbed sleep-wake cycle with day-night reversal, not hour-to-hour variation
Marked psychomotor changes (hyperactive or hypoactive)	Psychomotor changes characteristically late (unless depression develops)

tion it has to persist long enough and be severe enough to interfere with daily function), dementia is neither necessarily irreversible nor necessarily progressive. Persistent dementia from hypoxic brain injury, for example, may cause a true dementia, but ultimate resolution (even complete resolution) may occur. However, most of the causes of dementia are progressive, and the most common cause of progressive dementia remains Alzheimer's disease. The term dementia is not used for cognitive impairment associated with diagnosable psychiatric conditions, which must be considered. Dementia is not a medical emergency, whereas delirium is (Table 17-1).

Delirium is a medical emergency.

Thus the crucial questions to ask when suspicious of dementia, answers to which must generally be established from witnesses other than the patient, are the following:

- How long has this been going on?
- How abruptly did it start?
- Is this situation progressing, and if so, how fast?

▼ **MAY HOMER (Part III)**

Mrs. Homer's mental status slowly improves following rehydration and the initiation of treatment for the urinary tract infection. She is much less confused by the tenth day, and a geriatrician consultant confirms no evidence except for some mild short-term memory impairment to suggest dementia. Mrs. Homer is well oriented to time and place and wants to return to her own apartment. However, her immobility during hospitalization has led to her being unsteady on her feet; she needs the assistance of one person to get out of bed. Physical therapy is instituted, and she can safely walk 3 weeks after admission, when she is ready for discharge. Plans are made for follow-up to check for signs of dementia. A visit by the public health nurse is arranged, and Mrs. Homer's daughter also agrees to visit or call more regularly.

CASE DISCUSSION

Mrs. Homer's was a rather clear-cut case of delirium. Often there is not such convincing evidence of good prior function. The urinary tract infection, dehydration, and the fear of being locked out in the dark precipitated her abnormal mental state (delirium). As is often the case, slight cognitive deficits were present after the delirium resolved. It is therefore wise to follow up not only to check on coping skills, since this patient's frailty and unadaptability have been demonstrated, but to pick up any subtle signs of dementia, perhaps with mental status testing. Such testing in the hospital, away from the familiar home environment, is misleading, so a later assessment of mental status will be more realistic. Earlier ambulation dur-

ing the hospitalization could probably have led to the avoidance of her transiently diminished walking skills, but this precaution was overlooked in view of the acuity of the situation.

▼ GEORGE MACDONALD (Part I)

Mr. MacDonald is a 72-year-old man who is brought to you by his daughter. He has lived alone in the old family home, a five-bedroom house out of town, since his wife died 3 years ago. About 2 years ago an episode led to an emergency room diagnosis of a "small stroke." His daughter now describes that episode as consisting of transient facial weakness, weakness of his left arm, and slurring of his speech that lasted approximately 1 hour and had come to her attention by his calling on the telephone. She had thought that he might be drunk because his speech was slurred. She had gone to the house and found him in the described state. Apparently his blood pressure was normal at that time, and he recovered and was sent home. Nothing like that incident has occurred since, but Mr. MacDonald has always resisted seeing physicians and has had no medical attention since then. Mr. MacDonald's daughter describes the state of the house, the uneaten food she and her brother had supplied (and then had to clear out), and the piles of dirty laundry and old newspapers. Mr. MacDonald smokes, and there are burn holes in his favorite chair. Mr. MacDonald defends himself from these apparent criticisms and insists that his daughter is fussing. He describes his daily life in lively fashion and says he enjoys his home and eats well. He is friendly and relaxed. While he is getting ready to be examined, you take the opportunity to speak privately with his daughter. Seen alone, she feels able to describe in more detail the chaos of her father's life and home, which had always been neat and organized until a year or so ago. He had been rather withdrawn for a couple of months following his wife's death, but he had eventually started eating more, socializing a little with some old friends, and generally doing things for himself. (His wife had died slowly of cancer, at home, and he had already been doing many domestic chores for a year or two before her death.) Now Mr. MacDonald's health is failing, and his two children have to alternate calling by phone and visiting; they have spent several months preparing him to visit you today. Mr. MacDonald's daughter describes her father as difficult to help; some days he will hang up on her on the telephone. On at least two occasions he has made it difficult for them to visit him for several days at a time. His voice sometimes sounds slurred on the phone. As you leave the interview to examine Mr. MacDonald, your nurse informs you that his blood pressure is 180/115.

STUDY QUESTIONS

- *You have only 10 more minutes of appointment time: on what should the interview and examination of Mr. MacDonald be concentrated?*
- *What specific questions should be asked of the daughter?*
- *Are there already hints of a potential etiology?*

DEMENTIA: PRESENTATION

In general, patients subsequently demonstrated to have a dementia syndrome do not initially present themselves to the physician. The earliest symptoms can be subtle.[7] It is often said that a complaint of memory loss is more likely to come from a patient suffering depression than dementia, but this is misleading: patients with dementia are often quite aware of their problems. Insight is often preserved until quite late in these illnesses. However, it is generally another family member, a friend, or a neighbor who calls or visits the physician and often accompanies the patient to the office. Quite often the patient refuses to come; a home visit (without the patient's consent—the physician should be concerned here with beneficence, not civil liberty) is essential and extremely revealing in such circumstances.

> *Unless a physician is prepared to visit the home, many dementia patients will receive no medical attention.*

The patient may not realize his or her problems, or he or she may realize and react with denial. Family members will also try to explain away and ignore the subtle but ultimately progressive symptoms that they see in their family member, often out of respect, sometimes out of fear. Symptoms that others frequently notice include short-term memory loss, poor judgment, inability to handle complex tasks (such as balancing the checkbook), and increasing unwillingness or inability to initiate or take part in activities in a previously well-functioning individual. Often an apparent "personality change" with irritability, a loss of humor, or even hurtful remarks will draw attention to the problem. There is frequently a long period during which some family members have a sense that something is wrong and others do not; family disputes can occur at this stage. Occasionally the presentation is more dramatic: few or no symptoms will have been noticed, but suddenly the unadaptability characteristic of dementia is exposed by some event (e.g., a family holiday or hospitalization). In these more dramatic presentations, care must be taken to ask direct and searching questions in order to establish the insidious onset. The physician must be prepared to seek and question other witnesses or explore prior medical records.

> *In dementia, the preserved social skills can be misleading: the patient can "rise to the occasion" and appear "well."*

During the early phase of dementia a characteristic is the often astonishing preservation of social skills with the patient able to "rise to the occasion" at the office visit (or when an old friend visits or a family member comes from out of town). This ability to participate in simple conversation, preserved in long-term memory, can be very misleading. Family members feel that they are not going to be believed. Sometimes they are not believed by friends or other family members who say, "I really can't see anything wrong; we had a good talk just like before"; health professionals can make the same mistake and disbelieve the family's story. Formal mental status testing is usually revealing in these circumstances; however, office screening tests (as will be described in this chapter) may not be sensitive enough in the early phases. Observation over time becomes the diagnostic technique.

Patients who live alone or who only have the companionship of a frail spouse are liable to present to the physician later. Sometimes it is only the death or illness of a fragile spouse that reveals the cognitive difficulties of the patient.

Should physicians screen for dementia at routine health maintenance visits in patients over 80? "Testing" questions can be insulting to intellectually preserved older individuals and may reduce their enthusiasm for visiting the physician. Perhaps the most important thing is to be clinically alert so that the range of subtle hints (reduced activities, self-neglect, inadequate fluid or nutritional intake, increased accidents, etc.) lead to a consideration of this possibility.

In practice, the problem with detecting dementia is that vague, functionally impairing, general symptoms can be caused by many different illnesses in old age.[8] An acute major illness like pneumonia or myocardial infarction will often present as modified mental status; a chronically bleeding ulcer can give a convincingly progressive history of mental decline, as might the insidious effects of centrally acting antihypertensives or a persistent, unrecognized depression.

However, once the three questions are answered and it is established that the cognitive changes, while dysfunctional and progressive, are on a time line of weeks or months rather than days, the investigation can proceed in an orderly manner through the office and from the patient's home.

> Alzheimer's disease is not diagnosed "by exclusion"; there may be a period of diagnostic uncertainty, but the diagnosis confirms itself over time, provided that an accurate history and an objective, scored mental status test, sometimes repeated at intervals, are obtained.

▼ GEORGE MACDONALD (Part II)

During the remaining interview time, brief testing of mental status confirms that Mr. MacDonald does not know the year, his address, or age, although he remembers his date of birth. On examination he has some weakness of his left arm and his left hand grip, but no other localizing or lateralizing neurological signs. He has hypertensive changes in his fundi. His daughter says that she is unaware of his ever having had an alcoholic drink in his life, but you ask her to check the home.

STUDY QUESTIONS

- *Should antihypertensive medications be started today?*
- *How can this be followed up in view of the patient's unwillingness to be seen again?*
- *What investigations should be ordered today?*
- *What is the likely diagnosis?*

CASE DISCUSSION

In view of the history of likely transient ischemic attacks (TIAs), this blood pressure reading must be followed up. It may be elevated by the circumstances, and there is evidence of a normal blood pressure 2 years ago. Hypertension should not be diagnosed on one reading, but if Mr. MacDonald's BP should remain elevated, it should be treated. Noncompliance with medication is likely. The visiting nurse can check a series of BP readings at home, which gives the nurse access to the home for more general observations and follow-up. Full investigation of the likely causes of the apparent dementia and a more complete assessment of mental status, perhaps conducted in the familiar environment of Mr. MacDonald's own home, should be planned.

IS IT DEMENTIA?

Formal, objective testing of mental status using one of the standard validated instruments is extremely important, although many physicians untrained in the use of formal questionnaires for this purpose are naturally uncomfortable at first with the technique. Informal interviews can be quite misleading, and patients will soon become uncomfortable if they perceive that they are being "tested" during the course of what started off as a routine interview. Screening tests that can be used in the office setting do not test everything, of course; they test only those aspects of dementia that lend themselves to that format. The tests are culturally biased; adjustments must be made for physical disability, visual impairment, and literacy. But despite these provisos, a formal test will provide objective documentation, and it is particularly useful for demonstrating progression over time (or resolution on occasion). Since dementia of Alzheimer's type is the most common cause of progressive dementia, and since evidence of progression is important for the establishment of that clinical diagnosis, repetition of the test at intervals over time (generally of at least 3 to 6 months) can be diagnostically helpful. Whereas it is usually best to do the examination one-on-one with the patient (so that family members do not "help out"), it is important to review the results with family members; often the family have not realized how severe the problems were, or they have already fallen into the trap of feeling that the person is being awkward and uncooperative or feeling that the patient "won't," whereas in fact the patient "can't."

> *Family members first have to realize that the patient "can't" rather than "won't."*

Memory is naturally a central part of such tests. Patients with dementia may register information, understand, and respond, but then fail to enter it into memory, or they may enter it and are then unable to access it.

The most widely used screening tests for the presence of dementia are the Mini–Mental State (MMS) Examination,[9] (See Fig. 5-1) and the Short Portable Mental Status Questionnaire (SPMSQ) (Box 17-3).[10] The MMS has been widely adopted for screening patients for long-term care placement. A physician is not required to ad-

---

BOX 17-3
Short Portable Mental Status Questionnaire

1. What is the date today (month/day/year)? (All three correct needed to score)
2. What day of the week is it?
3. What is the name of this place? (Any correct description needed to score)
4. What is your telephone number? If you do not have a telephone, what is your street address?
5. How old are you?
6. When were you born (month/day/year)? (All three correct needed to score)
7. Who is President of the United States now?
8. Who was the President just before him?
9. What was your mother's maiden name?
10. Subtract 3 from 20 and keep subtracting 3 from each new number all the way down. (Whole series correct needed to score)

Error score (out of 10): Add one if patient is educated beyond high school; subtract one if patient is not educated beyond grade school.

Scoring: 0 to 2 errors—intact intellectual function
3 to 4 errors—mild intellectual impairment
5 to 7 errors—moderate intellectual impairment
8 to 10 errors—severe intellectual impairment

From Pfeiffer E: *J Am Geriatr Soc* 23:433-441, 1975.

---

minister such tests, but proper training is required for the test to be valid.

Many physicians feel uncomfortable using such instruments. Their use inhibits the normal free flow between patient and physician by which the history is generally obtained. Some of the questions seem naive. Insightful patients may be nervous of being tested or even be insulted, and a physician inexperienced in the use of these tests will contribute to these feelings. Prior interaction with the patient should have given some impression of the impairment and the patient's insight. Given a convincing history of problems and decline, it is much more likely that using a formal instrument will produce objective and useful information than that either physician or patient will be embarrassed by its use.

To avoid an awkward change from open interview to formal questions, it is best to regard the mental status test as part of the physical examination and to schedule it as such. Introducing the questionnaire (perhaps by discussing memory problems the patient is aware of) as "an examination of your memory" rightly implies that the mental examination is comparable to the physical examination with which physicians and patients are familiar and generally produces a calm and compliant atmosphere.

As well as being culturally and educationally biased, the tests may not be sensitive enough in the early stages, especially in an individual of high intellectual function. A valid score relies on effective communication and understanding between interviewer and patient: eye contact, concentration, and good hearing of instructions must be ensured, and the interviewer must be sure that the patient is making an adequate effort.

THE DEMENTIAS

Two discrete illnesses (which can occur concurrently in the same patient) account for the majority of individuals with progressive dementia: Alzheimer's disease, or, more correctly in current nomenclature, dementia of the Alzheimer's type (DAT), and vascular dementia, formerly known as multiple infarct dementia (MID). Vascular dementia has been estimated to be the cause of possibly 20% of all cases of dementia. However, at least one study implies that there are as many patients with multiple infarcts *and* Alzheimer's as an explanation of dementia as there are patients with multiple infarcts alone.

The nomenclature for dementias keeps subtly changing, although the word "Alzheimer's" is well established in the public eye and correctly reflects the pathological changes[11] that Alzheimer himself described in a young patient in 1907. The NINCDS/ADRDA* nomenclature,[1] which uses the term "probable Alzheimer's disease" as the highest level of certainty in terms of diag-

---

*National Institute of Neurological and Communicative Disorders and Stroke/Alzheimer's Disease and Related Disorders Association

nostic labeling in a living patient and the term "possible Alzheimer's disease" for situations of even less certainty, is still widely used; but the DSM-IV terminology—DAT and vascular dementia—are used in this book.[2]

The diagnostic criteria that suggest that a patient with a dementia syndrome has dementia of the Alzheimer's type are summarized in Box 17-4. The criteria for vascular dementia are summarized in Box 17-5. The diagnosis of Alzheimer's disease is not entirely "by exclusion," as is often implied. The diagnosis is generally highly suspected on the basis of history alone, and while the physician looks for potentially causative or (more likely) contributory factors, additional evidence of the presence of the characteristic inexorably progressive loss of brain function is obtained and documented.

Differentiating between DAT and vascular dementia

(while acknowledging that the two may coincide and that patients with multiple cerebral infarcts are not necessarily demented) has implications for the clinical management.[12-15] The significance of multiple infarcts or vascular changes is that they imply underlying cardiovascular disease: the prognosis of the patient depends on the cardiovascular status.[16] Patients with vascular dementia should (1) undergo careful evaluation of the cardiovascular system for signs of dysrhythmia or other factors that may precipitate emboli, (2) be considered candidates for daily aspirin to reduce platelet aggregation, (3) have their blood pressure controlled, if elevated, (4) cease smoking, and (5) not be allowed hypotensive episodes (e.g., during elective surgery or from potentially orthostatic medications).

Other illnesses in which dementia is the characteristic manifestation of the disease process include Pick's disease, Creutzfeldt-Jakob dementia, and Huntington's disease. These diseases are rare, but they must be considered. *Huntington's disease* is associated with characteristic manifestations of a positive family history of choreoathetoid movements associated with progressive dementia, with its characteristic autosomal dominant inheritance (half the offspring affected).[17] *Pick's disease* is probably clinically indistinguishable from Alzheimer's disease, although some clinicians feel that abnormally bizarre behavior relatively early in the illness is characteristic. This is predictable, since Pick's disease affects the frontal lobes first, and is in contrast to the temporoparietal distribution of Alzheimer's disease changes early in that illness. Although the diagnosis is generally confirmed only at autopsy, brain imaging (e.g., by single photon emission computed tomography [SPECT]) enables this diagnosis to be more strongly suspected premortem.[18] *Creutzfeldt-Jakob dementia*, rarer still, is

---

BOX 17-4
Diagnostic Criteria for Dementia of the Alzheimer's Type (DAT)

A. Multiple cognitive deficits with both of the following:
   1. Memory impairment (impaired ability to learn new information or to recall previously learned information)
   2. One (or more) of the following cognitive disturbances:
      a. Aphasia
      b. Apraxia
      c. Agnosia
      d. Disturbance in executive functioning (planning, organizing, sequencing, abstracting)
B. Cognitive deficits that cause significant impairment in social or occupational functioning and that represent a significant decline from previous functioning
C. A gradual onset and continuing cognitive decline
D. Cognitive deficits that are not due to the following:
   1. Other CNS conditions that cause progressive deficits in memory and cognition (e.g., cerebrovascular disease, Parkinson's, Huntington's, subdural hematoma, normal-pressure hydrocephalus, brain tumor)
   2. Systemic conditions that are known to cause dementia (e.g., hypothyroidism, vitamin B_{12} or folic acid deficiency, niacin deficiency, hypercalcemia, neurosyphilis, HIV infection)
   3. Substance-induced conditions
E. Symptoms not occurring exclusively during the course of a delirium
F. Disturbance that is not better accounted for by another Axis I disorder (e.g., major depressive disorder, schizophrenia)

Modified from *Diagnostic and statistical manual of mental disorders* (DSM-IV), ed 4, Washington, DC, 1994 American Psychiatric Association.

BOX 17-5
Diagnostic Criteria for Vascular Dementia

A. Same criteria as in DAT
B. Same criteria as in DAT
C. Focal neurological signs and symptoms (e.g., exaggerated tendon reflexes, extensor plantar response, pseudobulbar palsy, gait abnormalities, weakness of an extremity) or laboratory evidence indicative of cerebrovascular disease (e.g., multiple infarctions involving cortex and underlying white matter) judged etiologically related to the disturbance
D. Symptoms not occurring exclusively during the course of a delirium

Modified from *Diagnostic and statistical manual of mental disorders* (DSM-IV), ed 4, Washington, DC, 1994 American Psychiatric Association.

caused by a transmissible agent called a prion or "slow virus." The characteristic triad is dementia, myoclonus or other involuntary movements, and periodic activity on EEG, although as many as 25% of individuals with the disorder have atypical presentations. The onset is characteristically between 40 to 60 years of age, and up to 15% of cases may have a familial component. There may be a prodrome of varied mental symptoms followed by visual and motor problems along with a rapidly progressive dementia generally occurring over only months but sometimes over years. Typically there are characteristic changes on EEG.[19]

▼ **GEORGE MACDONALD (Part III)**

Follow-up visits to Mr. MacDonald's home require persistence because of his unwillingness but result in two further blood pressure readings, both elevated. On the second visit the nurse is able to obtain an MMS score of 20/30. Mr. MacDonald is isolated and lonely but is willing to receive services, once it is explained that he will not have to pay. His daughter, some old family friends, and the visiting nurse are organized so that, in rotation, they can assist him with compliance with the medication regimen (simplified to one aspirin and one long-acting verapamil per day). His daughter accompanies him for magnetic resonance imaging (MRI), which confirms several cerebral infarcts as well as small vessel changes. Working diagnoses of vascular dementia and hypertension are made.

STUDY QUESTIONS

- *What further steps must be taken to maintain Mr. MacDonald's state of health and safety?*
- *What further investigations should be carried out for contributory factors or even potentially causative factors, despite the presence of the multiple cerebral infarcts?*

CASE DISCUSSION

Although the diagnosis is reasonable based on the brain imaging and observations, it is essential that a patient with dementia be fully investigated for contributory factors. Especially in the case of an individual living alone, assistance for both daily activities and intercurrent illness should it occur (Mr. MacDonald is at risk in several ways) must be provided.

DEMENTIA: POTENTIALLY CAUSATIVE AND CONTRIBUTORY FACTORS

Physicians enjoy the hunt for a single diagnosis, for a cause that can be cured. Dementia, as with much of geriatric medicine, is not like that. There are frequently many factors and often several formal diagnoses contributing to the syndrome in any one patient.

The family (and often the patient) must understand the nature of the workup. Despite wide publicity to the contrary, some individuals still assume that brain imaging will positively diagnose Alzheimer's disease. It must be clarified that the workup is not intended so much to look for a "cause" as it is intended to rule out some rare serious possibilities and to anticipate finding some contributory factors that will make the dementia even worse if unaddressed. If families understand this, the situation of families going from physician to physician seeking more intense investigation could be more often avoided.[20,21] In a series of patients with newly diagnosed dementia, 14% were found to have potentially reversible causes. When followed up in 2 years, only one third of these, despite control of the potentially causative condition, had actually experienced a reduction in the progression of the dementia; in total, less than 5% of those with apparent dementia did not progress.[22] Of course, treatable or reversible conditions must be sought. Patients with cognitive difficulties, being less aware of symptoms, may have relatively more nonpresented, and thus untreated, illnesses. The causative or contributory factors in dementia must be considered not only at the initial presentation but at intervals throughout the course of the dementia. These factors should be reviewed in follow-up, perhaps every 3 years or so. They should also be considered in any patient with existing dementia who suddenly becomes worse.

The possible contributory factors can be summarized in a mnemonic based on the word *dementia* (Box 17-6). (The original author of this mnemonic is unknown, and I have added "environment" and "alcoholism," two important factors.) The first three letters cover the three areas that account, in published series,[22,23] for the majority of the potentially reversible causes of dementia: drugs, depression (emotional), and thyroid disorders (metabolic or endocrine).

Drugs

Virtually any prescribed or over-the-counter medication, and some substances in foods and beverages, are potentially (although unintentionally) psychotropic. Classic offenders include sedatives, anticholinergics, centrally acting antihypertensives, digoxin, and some β-blockers. De-

---

BOX 17-6
Causes and Aggravators of Apparent Dementia

D—Drugs
E—Emotional illness (including depression)
M—Metabolic/endocrine disorders
E—Eye/ear/environment
N—Nutritional/neurological
T—Tumors/trauma
I—Infection
A—Alcoholism/anemia/atherosclerosis

mentia increases the risk of noncompliance, of overdose, or of failing to take necessary supplements (such as potassium). However, appropriate medication must not be denied, even to patients with dementia. Mental status testing can sometimes be helpful in assessing the cognitive effect of a medication or in determining if there is relief of the cognitive deficit after the medication is stopped.

Depression

The "dementia syndrome of depression" describes the well-recognized phenomenon of depression presenting with cognitive impairment. Mental status screening tests can generally not distinguish this cognitive impairment of depression from that of dementia. The old term *pseudodementia* is less favored today, since the diagnosis in such a patient is depression and not dementia.[24] The family and patient need to be prepared for recovery, not progression, if depression is the diagnosis. This should be suspected in the clinical examination as a cause in any individual with a relatively recent onset (less than 1 year) or a rather abrupt onset of apparent "dementia." Remember that depression can develop over weeks, although developing over days or even overnight is more common. Also, some depressive states are more persistent than is typical.

Patients with dementia probably develop depression more often than nondemented people do.[25,26] This is predictable. Dementia is, after all, a generally progressive condition, often with preserved insight in the early phases and sometimes into the later phases, but there may be more physical or neurochemical reasons for the association. Depression should always be considered along with other medical causes in an individual whose dementia abruptly worsens, especially if there are positive answers to direct questions about sleep disturbance, diurnal variation in mood, appetite change, and constipation (i.e., the signs and symptoms, especially the "vegetative" ones, of a major depressive episode). Such direct questions are usually necessary, since such symptoms are often misattributed by the patient and family alike. Improvements in antidepressants, perhaps especially the introduction of the selective serotonin reuptake inhibitors (SSRIs) (especially sertraline [Zoloft] and paroxetine [Paxil]) make it wise to mount an enthusiastic and, if necessary, persistent trial of antidepressants in patients with dementia exhibiting a new onset of such symptoms. On the other hand, older medications, especially those with marked anticholinergic effects (virtually all of the tricyclics), are to be avoided. Deeply depressed patients with dementia and concurrent depression have been successfully treated with electroconvulsive therapy (ECT). Patients with later dementia who are deeply depressed sometimes respond to the phenothiazine antidepressant amoxa-

pine. Trazodone (Desyrel), with its tranquilizing properties, has also been successful, especially in situations where screaming agitated behaviors in a patient with dementia might be a symptom of depression.

Some older individuals whose depression has prominent symptoms of cognitive dysfunction, even though they had no recognized prior cognitive deficit, never fully recover, remaining somewhat cognitively impaired. Some of these individuals ultimately develop dementia when followed up over time.[26] Some such patients may have had previously unrecognized Alzheimer's disease that became more manifest when the depression first occurred. Perhaps the cognitive impairment caused by the initial depression is a manifestation of the vulnerability of a brain that is ultimately going to succumb to Alzheimer's disease. However, increasing knowledge about the physical, neurochemical changes in the brains of older individuals with depression is consistent with the idea that a cognitively impairing depressive illness leaves its physical mark permanently on an individual's brain function. It is not known whether treatment of such patients with antidepressants reduces the likelihood of persistent cognitive problems or their later occurrence.

The differentiation of depression from dementia (i.e., the features that help the physician distinguish a new-onset dementia from a new-onset depression[24]) are reproduced in Table 17-2. The nature of the patient's response to formal mental status questions is significant; the speed of onset and the prior functioning are vital evidence. The single most useful test to make this differentiation in cases of diagnostic uncertainty is formal testing by a neuropsychologist. Neuropsychological evaluation can be extremely helpful not only in accuracy of diagnosis but in helping the family and the patient with prognosis.

A number of questionnaires exist to help the primary care physician identify depressed patients.[27,28] The Geriatric Depression Scale[27] is a very simple "yes or no" questionnaire that demented individuals can complete and that does assist in establishing the degree of actual dysphoria in such patients, helping to identify depressed individuals who could be considered for antidepressant therapy.

Schizophrenia

Schizophrenia can have its onset in late life. An important aspect of the differentiation is that cognitive function is characteristically unimpaired in the psychotic patient. Chronic schizophrenics, especially older individuals who have been institutionalized for a large proportion of their lives, can superficially look as if they are suffering from dementia. However, there is generally a long history of psychiatric illness and the cognition will generally be unimpaired when tested (e.g., on the MMS). Such patients may develop dementia concur-

Table 17-2 Distinguishing Depression from Dementia

Dementia	Depression
Insidious onset	Abrupt onset
Long duration	Short duration
No psychiatric history	Often previous psychiatric history (including undiagnosed depressive episodes)
Conceals disability (often unaware of memory loss)	Highlights disabilities (in particular complains of the memory loss)
Near-miss answers	"Don't know" answers
Day-to-day fluctuation in mood	Diurnal variation in mood, but mood generally more consistent
Stable cognitive loss	Fluctuating cognitive loss
Tries hard to perform but is unconcerned	Often does not try so hard but is more distressed by losses
Memory loss greatest for recent events	Equal memory loss for recent and remote events
Memory loss occurs first	Depressed mood (if present) occurs first
Associated with unsociability, uncooperativeness, hostility, emotional instability, confusion, disorientation, and reduced alertness	Associated with depressed or anxious mood, sleep disturbance, appetite disturbance, and suicidal thoughts

Modified from Wells CE: *Am J Psychiatry* 36:895-900, 1979.

rently, of course. The difference in thought content between schizophrenia and dementia has been well described: "in schizophrenia . . . , sudden . . . inexplicable twists in the . . . thought content, . . . tolerance for conflicts, . . . conclusions reached on a logically unacceptable basis; in dementia, . . . expressed thoughts [with a more] meandering course—one can follow the progression of thoughts, but they appear to lead nowhere."[29]

The frequency with which chronically psychotic individuals are undiagnosed, living their lives in reclusive isolation, sometimes leads to the presentation of a patient with a long-term history suggestive of psychosis as a potential patient with dementia. This often occurs because old age, frailty, or illness finally unravels the patient's fragile living arrangements. Neighbors of such patients can usually describe how long the problem has been going on; often such individuals are accepted as eccentric recluses for decades before they come to medical attention. Physicians should suspect previously unrecognized long-term psychosis in the individual who has lived for years alone as a recluse and whose appearance suggests dementia but who, on testing, is intellectually better than anticipated.

Frequently, psychosis earlier in life is undiagnosed; the "eccentric" patient who has lived for years alone as a recluse or who tests intellectually better than anticipated is probably a previously undiagnosed schizophrenic.

Thyroid Disease

Hypothyroidism is often missed in old age; classical symptoms occur in many older persons who are in fact euthyroid. Hyperthyroidism often presents its classical picture in the old, but a proportion develop so-called apathetic hyperthyroidism. Both hypothyroidism and apathetic hyperthyroidism can look like dementia. In about half of patients with dementia *and* thyroid disease at presentation, the dementia progresses anyway, even when the thyroid disorder is treated. Laboratory screening is clearly essential.[22,23]

Metabolic Disorders

A large range of metabolic, and sometimes endocrine, changes can produce or worsen dementia, although few could alone produce a dementia syndrome. These changes include dehydration, protein-energy malnutrition (PEM), hypoglycemia (secondary to overtreated or underfed diabetes mellitus or to starvation), hyperglycemia (usually in a previously unrecognized diabetic), hypocalcemia (from hyperparathyroidism, multiple myeloma, or sarcoidosis), hypercalcemia (especially during the treatment of disseminated cancer, when it can cause a dementia-like picture or can mimic a major depressive episode), hypoxia (from chronic obstructive pulmonary disease [COPD], congestive heart failure, etc.), hypercapnia (generally associated with COPD), alkalosis or acidosis (both unlikely to present subacutely), hypernatremia (usually from dehydration or IV therapy), and hyponatremia (usually secondary to IV therapy, but also from inappropriate antidiuretic hormone secretion [IADH syndrome], which characteristically produces mental confusion in this age group), total body fluid depletion (from dehydration, diuretics, or bleeding), previously undetected renal or hepatic failure, some other endocrine disorders (Cushing's syndrome, hypopituitarism), and accidental hypothermia.

Eyes and Ears

Visual Problems. Visual problems are contributory rather than causative, although sometimes an individual with marked visual impairment, especially if there is hearing loss as well, is so sensorially deprived that the appearance of dementia may pertain.

Hearing Loss. Hearing loss is socially isolating and is associated with suspiciousness or frank paranoia in patients with or without dementia. It is a very significant contributory factor to the impairment of patients with dementia; it will make the dementia appear worse than it is. If the problem is not addressed, the patient will become functionally worse. Unfortunately, fitting and having the patient tolerate a hearing aid when dementia is already present is generally unrewarding and frustrating; hearing dysfunction must be picked up earlier in life and therefore should be screened for in the "young old."

> *Remember that there is a linear relationship between hearing loss and paranoia.*

Environmental Factors

Environmental Change. Environmental change upsets orientation and other aspects of cognitive function, even in some elders without prior demonstrable impairment. Mental status testing carried out in a new situation, such as the emergency room or on arrival in a nursing facility, will thus not give reliable results. Conclusions should not be made about a person's cognitive status, nor their behavior, until the period of relocation stress has passed; this frequently takes several weeks. Prescribing a psychotropic to cover such situations is acceptable, but it should be discontinued promptly (weeks at most).

Certain special situations, such as admission to an intensive care unit (ICU), emergency room visits, and even planned brain imaging or other x-ray examinations, necessitate special precautions. The "ICU syndrome" is disorientation that occurs as a result of sensory deprivation (and overload) in that situation; normal old people can look demented, and patients with dementia can be functionally worse in intensive care units or emergency rooms.

> *In an unfamiliar situation, normal old people can look demented, and patients with dementia can be worse: don't make a final judgment on cognition in a place that is unfamiliar or frightening to the patient.*

Environmental Toxins. Heavy metal poisoning, such as arsenic, lead, mercury, and magnesium, as well as chronic carbon monoxide poisoning, as can occur from exhaust fumes or from gas leaks, are rare factors that can contribute to dementia and should occasionally be considered.

Nutrition

Patients with dementia are at risk for malnutrition. Folate testing is still recommended in the dementia workup, mostly as a screen for malnutrition. Malnutrition itself, especially if there is marked wasting (cachexia) from protein-energy malnutrition, can cause a dementia. This should be discovered on physical examination rather than from laboratory tests.

Of the classic vitamin deficiencies, although vitamin C (ascorbic acid) deficiency can produce chronic mental changes, it is vitamin B_{12} deficiency (generally associated with pernicious anemia) that has attracted most attention as a potential cause of dementia. There is virtually no evidence that replacing vitamin B_{12} in a patient with dementia and a demonstrably low vitamin B_{12} level actually helps the dementia. However, most geriatricians believe it should be screened for in all patients with apparent dementia, and all would treat the deficiency as a potential contributory factor or at least to protect from long-term peripheral neurological damage.

Neurological Disorders

Normal-Pressure Hydrocephalus. Normal-pressure hydrocephalus (NPH) is a rare but potentially correctable cause of dementia, which therefore must always be considered. This syndrome can occur in the absence of head trauma and can be suggested by the appearance on brain imaging. Confirmation of the diagnosis, however, requires cisternography, which is not without risk and therefore must be carefully considered. NPH causes a classical triad of apraxic gait, urinary incontinence, and dementia. The neurosurgery involved is a shunt operation to drain the accumulating ventricular fluid; it must be done early in the course of the dementia.

Parkinson's Disease. Parkinson's disease is an important consideration.[30,31] Some patients with dementia have parkinsonian findings, generally occurring rather late in the dementia; this may represent further cerebral deterioration or, in the case of vascular dementia, the progression of the atherosclerotic process to the basal ganglia. Treatment of such patients with antiparkinsonian drugs is in general not rewarding, but if the symptoms are causing disability, such medications should be tried. However, a proportion of patients with Parkinson's disease undoubtedly develop dementia, and most believe that this is not just coincidental Alzheimer's disease but a specific dementing process associated with the Parkinson's disease.[31] It has been implied that some of the cognitive changes may be secondary to the long-term use of antiparkinsonian medications, especially levodopa, despite their obvious utility in relieving the parkinsonian symptoms. The occurrence of Parkinson's disease, dementia, and depression all in the same patient presents unique challenges in balancing risks versus benefits.

Tumors

Except for meningiomas, primary brain tumors are less common in the later years than earlier in life. A frontal lobe tumor or tumors, whether primary or metastatic, benign or malignant, including cerebral abscess (rare), may present as a dementia. Brain imaging can miss a small tumor, and there is occasionally justification for following up a negative brain image should unexpected deterioration occur. But some small tumors have no clinical significance. To rule out treatable tumors, it is generally recommended to complete brain imaging in any patient with dementia of less than 3 years' duration.[22,32]

Trauma

Brain injury can produce dementia.[33] Patients with dementia are prone to falling and thus head injury; they may not remember the incident because of the dementia. Cerebral atrophy, present in many older individuals, including some without dementia, allows movement of the brain within the skull, causing shearing forces on the blood vessels and predisposing to the development of subdural hematoma. Brain imaging can detect this. Many authorities believe that serious head injury is a predisposing factor to Alzheimer's disease, with the trauma somehow stimulating the development or initiation of the process. Brain injury from hypoxia (e.g., in individuals following cardiac arrest with delayed resuscitation) can cause a dementia with an unpredictable course, sometimes involving surprisingly late but slow recovery over months or years.

Unreported (or unrecognized) trauma elsewhere in the body and unrecognized tissue damage or infarction elsewhere (e.g., myocardial infarct, gangrene) characteristically worsens dementia.

Infections

Acute Systemic Infections. In elders, pneumonia, urinary sepsis, and intraabdominal problems such as cholecystitis and diverticulitis frequently lack the traditional signs of infection (tachycardia, leukocytosis, fever), producing instead cerebral symptoms. Such infections are a significant cause of delirium or "worsening" of a dementia.

Chronic Systemic Infections. Chronic systemic infections, such as tuberculosis and subacute bacterial endocarditis, should be considered as contributory or causative factors in dementia; they can be difficult to diagnose.

Infections of the Central Nervous System. Infections of the central nervous system are rare but must be considered. Tertiary syphilis should always be screened for. Although there is often debate as to what should be done about positive results, most physicians treat presumptively, possibly even bypassing the lumbar puncture if the serologic findings are positive. Whereas encephalitis and meningitis would obviously be considerations in a recent-onset confusion, chronic meningitides from tuberculosis and fungi do rarely occur and should be suspected if dementia coincides with unlocalizable, low-grade sepsis; they can potentially be confirmed on lumbar puncture.

Atherosclerosis

Vascular dementias are generally produced by atherosclerosis. One completed stroke would be an unlikely cause for the global cognitive impairment of dementia, unless associated hypoxic damage at the time of the incident had contributed to the clinical picture. In all patients with dementia, a history of *TIAs* should be sought. The significance of *Binswanger's disease* (small vessel atherosclerotic disease) and its associated white matter changes seen on brain imaging in relation to dementia is uncertain. Most physicians now believe that the periventricular white matter changes frequently seen on MRI have little significance, but some cortical white matter changes of small vessel disease may be significant; the MRI may be the only evidence of multiple cerebral infarcts as a possible cause of the dementia. Low-dose daily aspirin (81 mg/day) should be prescribed for its prophylactic properties if there is any evidence of cerebrovascular disease.

Congestive heart failure (not all atherosclerotic) can contribute to cognitive impairment; poor cerebral perfusion results. Some older people have little or no dyspnea, despite the presence of pulmonary edema. *Pulmonary embolism* can produce acute, or sometimes chronic, hypoxia and thus cognitive changes. *Myocardial infarction*, even if it does not produce CHF, can do the same. *Cardiac dysrhythmia* may contribute to embolization and could ultimately cause cerebral changes. These potential contributory factors make a thorough cardiovascular examination necessary, with electrocardiography and echocardiography at times, in all dementia patients.

Alcoholism

Alcoholism alone is a well-recognized cause of dementia. In all patients with dementia it must be clearly established whether there is or is not a history of alcoholism in the patient or in a son or daughter and whether there is continued drinking. Patients may resort to alcohol in reaction to the early symptoms of dementia. Some clinicians believe that the dementia induced by alcohol sometimes ultimately progresses even if drinking ceases. There is no doubt that cerebral dysfunction is worsened in any dementia patient if alcohol is used. If possible, no patient with dementia should consume alcohol at all.

Detecting the alcoholic is difficult: family observations are useful. A home visit may reveal signs of alcoholism. Malnutrition (or its laboratory signs, such as folate deficiency, low cholesterol, or reduced serum albumin) should increase clinical suspicion.

Anemia

Anemia obviously will worsen cerebral impairment. Anemia is a significant sign of underlying illness and must be investigated. With regard to vitamin B_{12} deficiency, it appears that it is the vitamin B_{12} deficiency that is neurotoxic, not the anemia.

▼ GEORGE MACDONALD (Part IV)

You order thyroid studies, a CBC, electrolytes, and liver and renal function tests; all are within normal range. But there are low serum albumin, folate, and vitamin B_{12} values, the latter being repeated and confirmed. You decide to treat the vitamin B_{12} deficiency and to improve nutrition through Meals on Wheels. Vitamin B_{12} injections ensure a nursing visit, enabling extra surveillance for compliance with antihypertensive medications and other recommendations. Mr. MacDonald's daughter contacts the rest of the family and communicates your thoughts regarding the relative risks and benefits of his staying in his own home. Since Mr. MacDonald wishes to stay there, they decide that at least for the time being the benefits of staying outweigh the potential advantages, including nutritional, of living anywhere else where more supervision could be provided.

CASE DISCUSSION

Mr. MacDonald appears to represent a classic case of multiple infarct dementia. He has probably had several (unreported) TIAs. The focus in his management will now be his cardiovascular system and his general health. He will need to be persuaded if possible to stop smoking and to comply with the antihypertensive regimen and the aspirin, and he will need assistance to look after himself and to maintain his compliance, nutrition, and other aspects of his care. His relatively young age is a factor: provided further infarction can be prevented, his cerebral function may stay stable. At present, he has some insight and is competent to continue most activities. Thus efforts to maintain him at home are very reasonable.

▼ GEORGE MACDONALD (Part V)

Over the next 6 months the serum albumin measurement does not improve, and it is feared that Mr. MacDonald is not taking all the food offered to him. No further TIA-like activity occurs. With increasing family support, Mr. MacDonald is able to remain in his own home for a period of just over 2 years, at which time, following a family conference concerning his decreasing ability to care for himself and at least two episodes of falling without injury or apparent TIA, he moves into an adult home, having deteriorated slightly to an MMS examination score of 15/30. Six months later, despite control of his blood pressure, regular aspirin, and good nutrition, he sustains a major brain stem infarction, is hospitalized, and subsequently dies.

▼ DORIS ARNOLD (Part I)

Doris Arnold is an 85-year-old woman, brought to see you by her son, a 52-year-old self-employed businessman. He has called you previously, expressing his concerns about his mother's failing mental powers. She is unaware of any problem, but she raises no objection to visiting the physician. She lives alone in the old family home, her husband having died 7 years previously. On further questioning, her son agrees that for several months, although less than a year, Mrs. Arnold has been having increasing difficulties in caring for herself, eating erratically, and often failing to bathe—changes that he attributed to old age. He says that on a recent family trip to Florida, she became very confused and agitated in the motel, and a local physician saw her and prescribed haloperidol 5 mg 3 times daily to calm her down. While taking this, she was quieter but even more confused, and she fell on two occasions without injuring herself and became incontinent of urine. She became progressively stiffer in her movements, and her son reduced the dose to one tablet at night. However, she has not improved much and has become incontinent of feces as well. He asks, "Is this Alzheimer's?" Although she is still living in the old family home, he says that he has already decided that his mother must move permanently into his own home because of her condition. His wife is 37 years old and head of the English department at a local high school. They have three children who are 4, 8, and 16 years old. The 8-year-old is in therapy for severe behavioral problems.

STUDY QUESTIONS

- What steps should be taken to establish the diagnosis?
- Are the son's plans premature or realistic?
- Critique the medical management so far.
- If this is Alzheimer's disease, what should the management plan be once the diagnosis is established?

▼ HAROLD FRANKLIN (Part I)

You have been Thelma Franklin's personal physician for many years. During a routine pelvic examination, she breaks down and weeps uncontrollably when asked about sexual activity. She describes a traumatic period of nearly a year during which her husband Harold, 68, who runs his own small business, has been much more sexually demanding; this was acceptable to her at first, but now it is getting embarrassing, with him making loud remarks, for example, when they are out to eat, about her poor sexual responsiveness. At a social occasion a few weeks ago, he became loud and abusive after no more drinks than "either of us might usually have." Several times he has gone out in the evenings, which is quite unlike him, driving alone in the car, sometimes returning with evidence of drinking. She thinks he may be having an affair and blames herself for her great involvement in voluntary activities and neglecting her husband and herself (she is somewhat over-

weight and takes an antihypertensive). She asks you if you know a good marriage counselor, but she doubts that Harold would come, since he has not seen a physician in years.

STUDY QUESTIONS

- What should you do next?
- You have known the family and their children for years: can they help?
- How can you even get to see Mr. Franklin?

CASE DISCUSSION

Doris Arnold's son is already asking, "Is it Alzheimer's?", and it is indeed a possibility. However, the history is short and permanent modifications in life-style must not be made until the diagnosis is clearer. Harold Franklin has not officially declared himself a patient yet, although you do care for the rest of the family. Something is clearly wrong, and Alzheimer's disease, at his age, does not head the list of family issues that need to be explored. His drinking and driving and the misery he is producing for his spouse make some intervention urgent.

HISTORY

The history alone may be specific enough and long enough, with sufficient characteristic manifestations, to make the diagnosis of Alzheimer's disease likely. The history taking must be focused and planned so that all relevant sources of information are used. The patient must be questioned, but other witnesses are needed: ideally, it should be someone living with the patient, or at least visiting on a regular basis, and personally unimpaired. Frequently, the history must be obtained piecemeal from a frail spouse (who may be embarrassed or even feel a need to defend the spouse from the implication of losing brain function), sons and daughters, or neighbors and friends, all of whom may bring their own interpretation of the severity and impact of the symptoms. (This is especially true of those who feel guilty about their distant location, unavailability, or poor relationship with the patient.)

> *Always arrange to see family members separately from the patient with dementia; never talk about such patients in their presence.*

Since most patients with dementia are more able to comprehend information (and mood, affection, and hostility) than to express it, physicians must not speak about them in their presence without involving them; doing so will induce suspiciousness or even paranoia, especially if there is hearing loss. Doing so would also be role modeling inappropriate behaviors to the caregivers. The family members may appropriately be constrained from ex-

pressing their observations frankly in front of their relative, so separate, private interview time must be arranged. Sometimes it will be necessary for a physician to briefly inform the family member (while the patient is changing for the physical examination, for example), or even tell them by telephone in advance, that he or she will have to speak with them separately. A separate, specific appointment may be ideal. It is absolutely vital that the family member have this private time both at the initial assessment and later on as the illness progresses; it is quite impossible to involve them therapeutically in the relationship if every comment is constrained by the presence of the patient. This may mean more actual appointments, but the time will be well spent. Medicare allows a billing code for discussion with family members about a patient in the patient's absence.

> *Patients with dementia are generally more able to comprehend than express. They understand affection, hostility, and impatience long after speech has been lost.*

Obtaining previous records and investigations is vital. Many patients with apparent dementia have already had some kind of workup and often seek the help of a new doctor because of their continuing deterioration or because they have not been taken seriously enough or been provided with the practical linkages with help that are so necessary to optimal management.

A medication history must be obtained; all medications, including over-the-counter, that are in the house should be brought in (the "plastic bag test"), even if this is an established patient of the physician's own.

> *Always check on all the medications; use "the plastic bag test."*

If not already known, a clear picture of the home situation must be obtained. The suitability and safety of the house for the patient's degree of functioning, the presence or absence of others in the home and their willingness or ability to help, the proximity and helpfulness of relatives and neighbors, the help available in an emergency, and the access to transportation and supplies must be known. Information can be concurrently obtained about financial status, the patient's average day, what he or she does or used to do, nutrition, alcohol consumption, and other daily habits (especially if a member of the team can actually visit the house). Patients with dementia should be helped to stay in the familiarity and security of their own home environment for as long as possible; judgments about that environment cannot be made unless its qualities and potential are known.

PHYSICAL EXAMINATION

Examination of any elderly patient should begin with observations of gait, balance, and mobility while the patient is still fully dressed. With the patient remaining fully dressed, but as part of the physical examination (and ideally performed in the examination room so that it is clearly separate from the interview), formal testing of mental status should be performed. Using an established instrument such as the MMS examination (see Fig. 5-1) is required for the reasons previously stated. It should also be recorded as part of the physical examination.

Dementia-specific aspects of the physical examination include the following:

1. Look for localizing and lateralizing signs in the central nervous system; at a minimum, the cranial nerves, the tone, power, and coordination of all extremities, and balance and gait must be carefully tested. Whereas the presence of primitive reflexes (sucking, grasping, and glabella tap) are suggestive of diffuse cerebral disease, they can be present in healthy old people. When dementia is diagnosed late in the course, this neurological examination may show the increased tone and uninhibited, brisk reflexes of cerebral disinhibition. However, these findings in an early case are more consistent with vascular dementia.

2. Signs suggestive of Parkinson's disease must be sought: cogwheel rigidity, bradykinesia, the nature of the facies, and the presence or absence of tremor should be noted.

3. Contributory factors must be sought: vision and hearing must be screened, a cancer-related examination should be done, and the cardiovascular system in particular must be carefully evaluated.

4. Other screening tests, such as pelvic and rectal examinations if due, should probably be postponed to a subsequent visit to assist in patient compliance with subsequent visits, since so many patients with dementia are unwilling to see the physician. However, some assessment of urinary incontinence and bowel difficulties (as well as personal hygiene) should be made, noninvasively, during the initial checkup. A brief musculoskeletal evaluation for range of movement and signs of painfulness or dysmobility should be made.

▼ DORIS ARNOLD (Part II)

On examination, Mrs. Arnold is pale, with tired, sunken eyes and a dry mouth with very neglected teeth. She smells of urine, and her clothes are soiled with urine and feces. Cardiovascular and chest findings are normal, as is the abdominal findings, except that she is extremely thin and has multiple firm masses palpable in the descending colon. On rectal examination she is leaking feculent fluid and has hard, rocklike feces in the rectum. She is cooperative during the examination, and you complete a thorough neurological examination. There are no localizing or lateralizing signs, and the cranial nerves are normal. Her tongue will not stay still, and she has cogwheel rigidity most notable in her upper extremities. She has an expressionless face and walks with a stiff and shuffling gait. Her feet are neglected, especially her toenails. She does not know where she presently is, and although she can relate her name and date of birth, she cannot figure her age and believes it is 1970.

STUDY QUESTIONS

- *Are these physical signs consistent with dementia, or could they be medication induced?*
- *What investigations should be carried out at this stage?*

CASE DISCUSSION

Mrs. Arnold appears to be suffering an extrapyramidal syndrome secondary to the haloperidol. Although the son is anxious to maintain the medication because his mother was so agitated before, it is clearly necessary to reverse the syndrome and to try her without medication. Since her increased confusion did appear secondary to the relocation and stress of the trip to Florida, it is reasonable to discontinue the haloperidol. Were no such evident precipitating factor present, temporary use of an anticholinergic agent such as benztropine (Cogentin) might have been justified, although the ultimate plan would still have been to discontinue the medication, which is probably worsening the situation in several ways. Formal mental status testing might be revealing, but the haloperidol may be impeding Mrs. Arnold, and a more reliable baseline will be obtained when it is out of her system.

▼ HAROLD FRANKLIN (Part II)

Although you have known the Franklins for some years, neither you nor Thelma can persuade Mr. Franklin either to seek counseling or to attend your office. The behavior continues for several months until one afternoon Harold drives his car off the road and hits a tree. He is not injured, but police investigation of his blood alcohol level leads to a court case, and he is banned from driving for 1 year. Humbled into coming for a checkup, he finally sees you, and you are frank regarding Thelma's concerns. He declares that he feels he has been "going crazy," and he finds it increasingly difficult to remember what he has done and who he should call; his business is failing as a result. Now he has trouble remembering things and has had to delegate much of the day-to-day running of his business to others.

Mr. Franklin is on no medication, and a physical examination reveals him to be in good shape. His Mini–Mental State examination score is 20/30, with poor short-term memory, in-

ability with serial sevens, and uncertainty regarding which year it is. (He jokes about this but is clearly embarrassed.) He denies that sexuality is a problem, saying that their sexual life has been poor for years. He says his drinking is not a problem; he feels he was unlucky to have been booked. He does agree to submit to brain imaging and blood tests.

STUDY QUESTIONS

- *What tests should be done at this stage?*
- *What diagnostic possibilities exist?*
- *What, if anything, should you tell the family?*

CASE DISCUSSION

It should not have been necessary for the misfortune of an auto accident to draw Mr. Franklin into medical attention. It was highly appropriate to use the opportunity to investigate and to make Mr. Franklin look squarely at his problems, which he seemed relieved to discuss. He and others would have been less exposed to danger had you approached him directly, before his accident. A phone call, a letter, or a "request to come for a checkup" neutrally delivered by your nurse could potentially have accessed him.

INVESTIGATIONS

Laboratory investigations to screen for contributory and causative factors and to look for associated problems such as poor nutrition should be completed in all patients. These investigations are summarized in Box 17-7. Any suspicion regarding the rarer contributory or causative factors (such as heavy metal exposure) would direct the screening appropriately.

Brain imaging is a rapidly changing technology; clinicians must remain alert to the specific indications for the various types.[32,34-36] Brain imaging is recommended in all patients with the dementia syndrome except for a discrete group of patients in whom the syndrome is diagnosed late in its course, in whom it is reasonably certain there has been no head trauma, who have had symptoms for at least 3 years, and who have a typical Alzheimer-like history: gradual onset, no early neurological signs or symptoms, and a smooth progression of symptoms (see Box 17-4). Families (and physicians) should realize that brain imaging rules out other possible contributory factors, but it does not "rule in" Alzheimer's disease. In particular, cerebral atrophy has little significance as an isolated finding: many older individuals with normal mental status have this. Progressive cerebral atrophy on serial scans is supportive of Alzheimer's disease; it is rare that such serial scans are obtained, and following the patient clinically would generally provide equally strong evidence. A familiar companion should always accompany a patient with dementia for brain imaging; even with the use of "open" MRI machines, short-term sedation with lorazepam, for example, is occasionally appropriate.

BOX 17-7
Suggested Investigations in Dementia

All patients:
  CBC
  TSH $\pm$ T$_4$ $\pm$ free T$_4$
  Vitamin B$_{12}$ and folate
  Serological test for syphilis
  BUN and creatinine
  Calcium
  Glucose
Most patients:
  CT scan or MRI of brain (except in those severely demented with history over 3 years, nonabrupt onset, no history of head injury, and no early localized neurological symptoms or signs)
  Electrolytes
  Liver function
  ECG, chest x-ray examination, urinalysis: often recommended baseline in all elders, not specific to dementia
Some patients:
  EEG
  SPECT
  Neuropsychological testing

Multiple infarcts may well be shown by these techniques, especially if MRI is used. Although the MRI appearance does not make the diagnosis, this would provide supportive evidence of vascular dementia being the likely diagnosis if there were other evidence of vascular disease.

There are four main types of brain imaging[32,34-36]:

1. Computed (axial) tomography (CT or CAT scan) is widely available. The injection of contrast improves definition but present (fifth-generation) machines, in experienced hands, give much better definition, even without contrast, than the original machines did. Contrast can be used only if renal function is known to be adequate; contrast increases the trauma and risk. Most clinicians regard a CT scan of the brain as an adequate "rule out" for space-occupying lesions of clinical significance (i.e., causative) in dementia. A CT scan is probably the equal of MRI in experienced hands. CT can identify moderate to large areas of infarction and can detect significant subdural hematomata.

2. MRI is sophisticated, more expensive than CT, and widely available.[35] No injection is necessary. The patient must lie still for at least 5 or 10 minutes. The traditional machines were much more claustrophobic and threatening than most CT scanners. Recently, "open" MRI scanners have been introduced and are clinically useful in dementia patients.

Most clinicians find MRI superior to CT for picking up microvascular changes, such as Binswanger's disease, or small infarctions, which may be especially sought in cases fulfilling the clinical criteria for vascular dementia or in cases where there is significant cardiovascular disease.

3. Single photon emission computed tomography (SPECT) is a technique becoming more widely available, in which radioactive material highlights brain activity (not just structure). Whereas neither CT nor MRI provides other than exclusionary evidence of Alzheimer's disease, there is increasing evidence that the SPECT scan can support the diagnosis itself[36] by demonstrating symmetrical metabolic changes in both the temporoparietal areas; such changes are characteristic of Alzheimer's disease. SPECT may help diagnose Pick's disease, since such patients have bilateral frontal impairment with relative sparing of the temporoparietal areas in the early stages. This is a secondary investigation that should be performed subsequent to a CT or MRI; it is developing a place as supportive evidence in situations of diagnostic uncertainty. Of course, a normal or noncharacteristic SPECT does not rule out Alzheimer's disease.

4. Positron emission tomography (PET), like SPECT, provides information about cerebral function. Although it has been available longer and the literature on diagnosis of Alzheimer's disease with this technique is compelling, its high cost and special equipment needs make it available only as a research tool.[37,38]

Neuropsychological testing is the single most useful diagnostic test for establishing a diagnosis with some certainty. Relatively expensive and time consuming (and not universally available), it is to be used in selected cases. Neuropsychological testing is especially helpful in a person of high intellect who tests "normal" on screening mental status tests in the office yet appears to have something cognitively wrong from the history. It is also useful for helping distinguish between depression and dementia as etiologies of cognitive impairment and for helping to distinguish vascular and traumatic causes at times. The neuropsychologist can more precisely define the nature of memory deficit in patients in whom memory disorder is the main problem; this leads to a more precise definition of coping skills and reminder and mnemonic techniques.

▼ DORIS ARNOLD (Part III)

Following your explanation that the haloperidol may be making things worse, it is discontinued, and Mrs. Arnold moves promptly into her son's home. You urge him to discuss the implications of this more fully with his wife and children, since the relationship between his wife and his mother was never good and the family is already stressed by three children in school, one of whom has had severe behavioral problems for more than 2 years. Both parents describe themselves as workaholics, and there is no one in the house during the daytime. The son's decision stands, and you are able to arrange a visiting nurse for fecal disimpaction and surveillance for an improved diet and sufficient fluid intake. Your nurse assists the son in contacting a local day care program for his mother to attend several days a week. While making these arrangements, laboratory tests including thyroid studies, vitamin B$_{12}$, folate, VDRL, CBC, urinalysis, BUN, creatinine, and serum proteins are conducted. Mrs. Arnold's hemoglobin is 11.2 with normal indices and BUN is elevated at 42, but creatinine is normal and her albumin is 3.5. At an office visit 2 weeks later, when Mrs. Arnold has been off haloperidol for over 2 weeks, she has a Mini–Mental State examination score of 10/30, with impairment in most parameters tested. The son tells you that although his mother can physically bathe, dress, eat, and walk around independently, she needs constant reminding to do all of these things. They get into fights about her choices of clothing and her assertion that she need not bathe, and on at least two occasions she has been incontinent of urine "just because she will not go to the bathroom when we tell her." A CT scan is obtained, showing marked bilateral cortical atrophy but no other abnormalities. Unfortunately, Mrs. Arnold responds to the visits to the day program with hostility and confusion, overwhelmed by seeing "so many people" and becoming disoriented and confused in the new setting. After several attempts, the director of the day program advises the son that it is not helping his mother and that she is too confused to gain from their program. During the fifth week of Mrs. Arnold's living in the son's home, he declares to you that he believes his wife and family can no longer tolerate his mother's presence. He has already made inquiries for her to go and live in an adult home; unfortunately, they will not accept her because of her behavioral disturbance in the day program, current level of care need, and occasional incontinence.

STUDY QUESTIONS

- Have all appropriate attempts been made to educate this family about the management of Mrs. Arnold's problems?
- If a nursing home bed were available tomorrow, what problems would be anticipated in placing Mrs. Arnold promptly into the new environment?
- If, as is more likely, such an alternative is not available for several months, how can the management of this stressful situation be improved?

CASE DISCUSSION

By stopping the medication, managing the bowel problem, and working on Mrs. Arnold's nutrition, dehydration, and functional incontinence, some improvement can be anticipated. However, she is still very confused and dependent on paid help or the family for her self-care skills. She has barely had time *to get over the stress of relocation, and the family must learn and understand this. They have not given Mrs. Arnold enough time, nor have they taken the time to acquire the necessary skills to help her behaviorally. The period of several months before alternative placement becomes available (and it is questionable whether she even needs to be placed in a nursing home) must be used to educate the family in the optimal handling of the manifestations of her illness.*

▼ HAROLD FRANKLIN (Part III)

All tests for contributory factors are negative, including a CT scan of the brain. Mr. Franklin's daughter, aware of her mother's concerns about her father's drinking, driving, and sexuality, is appalled when you say that you are considering the possibility of Alzheimer's disease. She had thought he was suffering "the male menopause" and feels strongly that a second opinion should be sought. Because of the complexity of these family stresses and the continuing denial of certain of the problems by Mr. Franklin, you refer Mr. and Mrs. Franklin to an Alzheimer's diagnostic center in the next town.

STUDY QUESTIONS

- What are the other diagnostic possibilities?
- Can anything further be done to confirm the diagnosis at this stage?
- If this is Alzheimer's disease, how would you explain the implications of this diagnosis to the family members?

EXPLAINING ALZHEIMER'S DISEASE TO THE FAMILY
Naming the Diagnosis

Once the diagnosis of dementia of Alzheimer's type is made, the name "Alzheimer's" should be given to the illness and related to the family as such. The feeling that "bad news never comes too late" may be a part of many physicians' reluctance to give this illness its name, and premature labeling would indeed be inappropriate. However, the naming of the illness opens up information and help for caregivers and gives the legitimacy of a definite illness, dispelling the misconception that the patient "won't" when in fact he or she "can't." There are often family concerns about telling the patient the diagnosis. Although many patients with Alzheimer's disease are spared painful intellectual curiosity about what is wrong with them because of the cognitive impairment itself, early patients generally have insight, and many have sufficient intellectual capacity that they read about the illness and realize that they are developing its symptoms. Self-presentation of patients with actual Alzheimer's disease does occur. Some such patients may be so concerned that they are "losing their minds" or developing "mental illness," with its associated stigma, that they are re-

lieved to be given the diagnosis of Alzheimer's disease; this at least gives them something concrete to focus on. Early patients of high intellect, aware of the diagnostic possibilities, can sometimes be therapeutically (or at least psychologically) helped by support groups of similar individuals or by cognitive rehabilitation techniques to exercise the preserved mind. Sadly, the old anecdote that people developing Alzheimer's disease do not know what is happening is simply not true. In rare cases it is reasonable to withhold the naming of the illness when the patient has a particularly morbid fear about Alzheimer's disease itself. But, as with truth-telling about cancer and other illnesses, the availability of specific treatments and approaches makes it less and less appropriate to disguise the diagnosis from patients who are cognitively intact enough to want to know.

> *Many patients with Alzheimer's disease are spared painful intellectual curiosity about what is wrong with them because of the cognitive impairment itself. Specific treatment approaches make it wrong to disguise the diagnosis from patients who are cognitively intact enough to want to know.*

Describing the Cause

Many family members have read a good deal regarding Alzheimer's disease, and the primary care physician must be an up-to-date resource regarding its causes and the considerable amount of research work currently in progress. Much publicity attaches to every step forward in research because of the reasonable hope that defining the cause will ultimately lead to treatment and a cure. Families who are naive about the interpretation of research must be guarded against quackery and against having false hopes elevated. All must realize that specific treatment does not follow automatically or quickly, even as the causative factors are becoming defined. Whereas the possibility of patients with early Alzheimer's disease participating in experimental or new drug treatments is quite strong if they live close enough to a major center, those with more advanced disease are unlikely to be helped by anything developed in their lifetime.

The *genetic* research on Alzheimer's disease is among the most exciting and most recent work. A genetic predisposition in certain patients has long been recognized, but only recently was a genetic predisposition to late-life onset (the most typical form) been shown. Studies in the late 1980s linked changes at chromosome 21 with familial Alzheimer's disease; this was at least consistent with the knowledge that trisomy 21 (Down's syndrome) appears to predispose to the inevitable development of Alzheimer's disease in the late life of Down's syndrome patients (i.e., in their late 40s or early 50s). By the early 1990s, some familial cases associated with changes at chromosome 14 had been identified,[39] but it was in during 1991 to 1993 that changes at chromosome 19, associated with both the familial and sporadic forms, were described.[40] Then, in 1994, studies were published that led to the discovery that apolipoprotein-E (apo E) is involved in both protection from and the risk of developing the disease[41,42]: the presence of the genetic form called apo E4 increases the risk, and a rare form, apo E2, appears to be protective.[42] More recently, the discovery was made that individuals homozygous for apo E4 (inheriting one gene from each parent) not only had a greater chance of developing the disease but appeared to have a slightly earlier onset.[43] Obviously, new work is emerging constantly, and primary care physicians must be advised to keep abreast of the latest developments in this area. These developments are exciting, but sadly, they will not affect the immediate treatment prospects of current patients. Recent implications that education as such might actually increase synaptic activity and therefore "protect" against Alzheimer's disease are beginning to be investigated.[44,45]

Much other work on defining the cause of Alzheimer's disease continues. The role of β-*amyloid,* present in the center of the Alzheimer's plaques,[46-48] has been considerably researched, with much work about the precursor proteins (which are also markedly elevated in Down's syndrome). There is work with *nerve growth factor* to preserve the neurons from their progressive death, which is the essential feature of the disease.[49,50] Research continues to increase our knowledge of the *neurochemical* effects of Alzheimer's disease.[51] The latter is most likely, in the short term, to produce specific therapy, although such therapy could be said to address the effect rather than the cause of the disease. A long series of work on the significance of cholinergic mechanisms[52,53] led to the logical introduction of the only specific medication yet approved in this country for the treatment of Alzheimer's: *tacrine* (Cognex). The use of this medication is described in detail below.

Medication for Alzheimer's Disease

Tacrine (Cognex) is the only medication specifically approved in this country for the treatment of Alzheimer's disease.[54-56] (Hydergine is now discredited.)[57] The concept that increasing one of the neurotransmitters (acetylcholine) known to be reduced in Alzheimer's disease would help cognition is based on an extensive literature about the relationship between loss of cholinergic activity in the brain and the actual intellectual dysfunction of Alzheimer's disease. There is interesting research into smoking, with its positive effects on learning ability,[58] and there are many studies showing intellectual improvement when choline is enhanced.

Tacrine is basically an anticholinesterase, with the special quality of crossing into the brain and thus actually working to preserve available brain choline.[59] (Choline is available in health food stores, so family members need to understand the blood-brain barrier.) Undoubtedly, tacrine can reduce or at least postpone the progression of memory loss and other cognitive dysfunction in some patients with Alzheimer's disease, occasionally with actual improvement in memory function but more often with the production of at least a plateau or a slowing of the speed of decline. It is indicated in only the early and middle phases of the disease, and the cost of treatment is significant.

The approved prescribing protocol for tacrine is rigid[60]; a starting dose of 10 mg qid for 6 weeks is increased to 20, then 30, then 40 mg qid at 6-week intervals. The maximal allowed dose is 40 mg qid and it is the dose at which cognitive improvement was demonstrated in a proportion of patients in the trials that led to the accelerated release of this medication and its approval by the FDA. A safe, short-acting medication, it has to be given 4 times daily, and it is best absorbed if given between meals. Inevitably, compliance is a problem, and the administration of this medication is challenging if the person still lives alone, as many suitable subjects do. Since improvement is not anticipated until the second 6 months of taking the medication, a clinical decision as to whether or not tacrine is helping should generally not be made until it has been in use for at least a year. A blood test is required every 2 weeks until the patient has been on the maximal dose for 6 weeks, and after that it is required quarterly. Blood tests are necessary because of elevations in liver enzymes, which if recognized (and the dose is appropriately reduced) result in no permanent liver damage.[61] Families should be reassured on this point: this medication appears to be safe. The blood test requirement is an extra stretch for already stretched families. There is no way of telling who will respond and who will not, and families must realize that more than half of the individuals who get to the maximum allowed dose of tacrine will not be helped, which is frustrating after generally a year or so of effort with compliance and blood tests. However, in the controlled studies over 40% had some benefit relative to the predicted course of the disease. In one trial the mean response to 3 months of tacrine treatment was, on average, comparable to reversing 6 months of disease progression; there also is the occasional "dramatic responder." Many families given this information are desirous of trying the medication. Taking tacrine does use up some of the (limited) energy of the family; it generally involves a commitment by the family because of the issue of maintaining compliance. Family members must be counseled that other treatments must continue while tacrine is being tried: behavioral management, continuing education of the family, attention to the environment, stimulation of long-term memories, and attention to the organization of social and other experiences that the patient will enjoy are some of the ways in which a family can practice treatment that will definitely benefit the patient.

Some families decide that the efforts of compliance and the disruption caused by blood tests and other procedures are not worth the effort, especially if the individual's progress is slow or has reached a plateau and the situation is satisfactory or if efforts to maintain compliance will effectively undermine the person's capacity for living alone. Where the family's energy is already being stretched in attempts to maintain the patient in his or her own home (which, although associated with some risk, is often very much what the patient desires and is undoubtedly beneficial in increasing orientation because of the familiarity and security of "home"), it is often hopeless to attempt compliance with a medication that needs to be given so frequently. A twice-daily form is currently being researched, but it is not available yet. However, a trial of tacrine is not mandatory in all patients with Alzheimer's disease, and families should not feel that they have failed to achieve optimal treatment if it is not organized. But it must always be considered, and consideration should occur relatively early in the disease.

Clinical questions about potential interaction with medications that are anticholinergic (including many antidepressants and antipsychotics) are not fully answered, but such medications can be safely given with tacrine if necessary. One method is to initiate and stabilize associated depression (generally using a nonanticholinergic drug) before initiating tacrine. It is of interest that tacrine has some qualities of the antidepressants, but these qualities are not thought to be tacrine's prime mode of action.

Several other medications are in the process of clinical trials at this time: *selegiline,* a monoamine oxidase inhibitor (MAOI), which has already been approved for its potential neurological protective effects in Parkinson's disease; *indomethacin* and another NSAID, *ibuprofen,* may, by reducing the inflammation surrounding the amyloid core of Alzheimer's lesions, protect against neuronal damage[62]; *estrogen,* which seems likely to have a preventive or even therapeutic role, and *antioxidants,* including the readily available vitamins A, C, and E, which may be a safe and inexpensive way to protect neurons against damage from metabolic processes over time, but whose efficacy has not yet been proved. The Alzheimer's Association's Information and Referral Service provides critical updates regarding current studies in which willing patients may participate. For some patients this is therapeutic even if they are given a placebo; both patient and family feel that they are contributing to necessary research. The current studies include propentofylline, which may

help the survival of brain cells; a study of prednisone; and ongoing studies of physostigmine. The calcium channel blocker nimodipine is being studied to see if it relieves cell damage, and metrifonate and other anticholinesterases are also under clinical investigation.

Primary care physicians must guard against premature prescriptions of these medications, several of which are available already for other indications. For example, many clinicians are aware that indomethacin crosses the blood-brain barrier: the depression and confusion it can produce in older patients using it for the treatment of their arthritic pain is well recognized. But since the benefits of these medications are not known in Alzheimer's disease, the risk-benefit ratio is obviously not known either. Pretending that an individual has another indication for selegiline or indomethacin, for example, is unprofessional and dangerous. These drugs should be used only for approved indications until there is proper data to guide physicians in the use of these medications for Alzheimer's disease.

Educating the Caregiving Family

People cope better with something that they understand. Caregivers immediately need access to information, through both books[63-65] (which are not best for everyone) and support organizations such as the Alzheimer's Association. (Another justification for identifying this illness to the family is that they can look for help in the phone directory under that name.) However, family members have the potential to go beyond merely "coping" to become well-informed, capable managers.[66] In the account later in this chapter of the behaviors and manifestations seen in Alzheimer's disease and the other progressive dementias, the role is described of a family member becoming skilled and, in effect, a part of the therapeutic team, treating, preventing, and reducing the functional impact of the manifestations of this disease as the illness progresses. The need for the family members to gradually take over aspects of the patient's life must be emphasized while recognizing that patient autonomy should be respected and that the patient may retain competence for certain decisions until late in the illness.

 Family members often suffer unnecessarily because they project their own, cognitively intact feelings onto the patient; fortunately, dementia generally prevents patients from fully perceiving their situation.

In giving information and directing caregivers to where they can find help, the physician must emphasize his or her own availability. It is wise to schedule follow-up appointments rather than to wait for each crisis. This makes it possible to institute an anticipatory approach, for example, recognition of sleep disturbance and other behaviors early, when intervention is more likely to be beneficial; early consideration of legal issues, financial concerns, and testamentary capacity; and preparation of the family for the need for, and cost of, increased services and ultimately, in many cases, placement into a long-term care facility. Continuing availability of the physician and his or her staff and the Alzheimer's Association and other community services enables this anticipatory approach to be used, and it spares the family from becoming overwhelmed by the prospect of the many things that will need to be done over time.

When giving the diagnosis of Alzheimer's disease, the physician should emphasize the preservation of skills, such as long-term memory, and of many other aspects of the individual's life and personality, even late in the illness, such as the appreciation of joy, love, the company of children, music, memories, food, warmth, comfort, sex, affection, activities, outings, and many other life-enhancing factors.[66] That patients with dementia can often understand what is being said even if they do not understand the words and can comprehend feelings better than they express them must be clarified and reinforced. If properly appreciated, these facts make an enormous difference to the caregiver's enthusiasm and commitment. Many do not know the natural history, having the impression of a condition more rapidly progressive to total dependency than is usually the case. The physician should also mention the naturally occurring (though rare) plateaus, usually of a year or less but occasionally longer, in which cognitive status does not deteriorate.

> *Although Alzheimer's disease is a progressive illness, each symptom does not simply intensify with time: many troublesome symptoms resolve as the illness progresses.*

Another important point to emphasize to caregivers is that although the illness is progressive, each symptom does not simply intensify with time. For example, wandering may be a major problem for a time, but it generally becomes less a problem later in the disease. Psychological upset in response to the patient's realization of failing cognitive powers decreases as awareness decreases. Periods of agitation, disturbance, or depression, indeed any of the problematic behaviors and other upsets that may occur during a progressive dementia, are phases that often resolve over time, sometimes because of the progression of the illness. The man who will not give up his car or gun will later forget and be passive and "easy" about such things. Many individuals feel that they will inevitably be overwhelmed, anticipating that each difficulty will add to the prior difficulties as the disease progresses. The physician and his staff need to continually reinforce that, as with the "difficult" child, the disturbed phases and the difficulties often pass.

CAREGIVER STRESSORS

Alzheimer's disease is stressful in itself: it is a long illness with progressive dependence.[67,68] In addition to this, watching a near relative deteriorate, sometimes behaving in ways that mimic or exaggerate his or her prior characteristics, including the undesirable ones, is more stressful for caregivers who are family members than those who are not.[69]

Caregiver characteristics that increase stress include the caregiver's own frailty, since many caregivers are spouses. In view of the frequent onset of this illness in the 80s and beyond, even a caregiving daughter or son may be retired and either be or feel old themselves.[70]

Many caregivers are men, but the majority are women: wives, daughters, and daughters-in-law. The majority of caregiving younger relatives also have careers and frequently have obligations to their own children. Thus much burden and responsibility falls on these individuals of the "sandwich" generation (or, as someone has commented with black wit, the "club sandwich" generation, with two generations on one side and one on the other—all with their own demands).[71]

> *There are two special groups of problem caregivers: overinvolved daughters and denying sons (as well as some overinvolved sons and denying daughters, of course!).*

The known familial predisposition to Alzheimer's disease adds to the stresses. Physicians can appropriately confirm that familial predisposition is less a factor than "living long enough to be at risk." Many people are indeed genetically predisposed, and that fact has been widely publicized. But even for those with a history of Alzheimer's disease in the family, genetic testing cannot give a certain enough prognosis for risk to warrant any change in life-style or plans by a family member.

Other factors that stress caregivers include disturbed sleep, aggressive or abusive behavior by the patient, physical dependence on the caregiver for activities of daily living (ADLs), incontinence, and ingratitude; a major factor for many is the combination of guilt and sadness at watching progressive decline in one who, in most cases, the caregiver was close to and who is becoming "not the person I knew." It is because of this last issue, the pain of watching deterioration in someone near and dear to the caregiver, that the physician must encourage the caregiver to find help (even if it is necessary to pay for it). Someone less emotionally involved may find the day-to-day tasks easier. Day programs, services in the home, and, ultimately, placement in an adult home or skilled facility can in part be encouraged based on this correct premise. At an early stage in the illness it is important to discourage family members from rash promises based on misperceptions (e.g., "I promise to never put you in a nursing home"); placement is often both necessary and positive later in this illness. Temporary respite placement is of great value in maintaining the caregiver by allowing vacations and the opportunity to preserve a life of his or her own. Later, if there is marked physical dependence, having others take care of the physical needs in a skilled facility can free the family member to focus on emotional and social support. Once the patient is unaware that he or she is no longer at home or is failing to recognize his or her spouse or caregiver, it is probably time for somebody else to take over much of the care, so the family member can start constructing (or reconstructing) a life of his or her own for the time, which is drawing inexorably nearer, when the patient will be gone.

> *Never make rash promises to an older relative, such as "I promise never to put you in a nursing home" or "I promise never to give you tranquillizers, ECT, or a feeding tube." In time, "extraordinary" treatment becomes "ordinary."*

▼ HAROLD FRANKLIN (Part IV)

Two months after the initial ban on his driving, Mr. Franklin is seen at the Alzheimer's diagnostic center. More detailed neuropsychological assessment, in particular assessment for depression, reveals many dysphoric features. The center describes him as positive on the Geriatric Depression Scale, and a detailed and careful history reveals that some problems with memory and calculation were present for several months before the more recent onset of depressed feelings, sleep disturbance, loss of appetite, and diminished sexual performance. The diagnostic picture is clouded by his continued drinking; the center links Mrs. Franklin with Al-Anon and, through her, attempts to reduce his alcohol consumption. Mr. Franklin refuses sexual counseling. Management with an antidepressant is initiated, since it is thought that he has developed a major depressive episode in response to the realization of his declining cognitive powers. Thus the diagnoses are major depression, possible dementia of Alzheimer's type, and alcoholism. In view of the likelihood of the second of these diagnoses, the family is given literature and urged to contact the Alzheimer's Association for support and help.

STUDY QUESTIONS

- *What problems can be anticipated in the short and long term, and how will you help the family to be prepared for them?*
- *What else could be done at this stage to ease the situation and reduce Mr. Franklin's impairment?*

CASE DISCUSSION

Mr. Franklin's continuing use of alcohol will impair his cognition, depress his mood, and in general disrupt his life more. Positive efforts should be made to reduce or eliminate the alcohol consumption. Tacrine and SPECT were not available at the time this case occurred; they would now be considered. Given the mixed etiology of Mr. Franklin's difficulties, a SPECT at this point, if it had been available, could have been useful, since, if it showed the characteristic symmetrical bilateral temporoparietal changes, it would support Alzheimer's disease as the likely etiology. Provided Mr. Franklin's liver passed the alanine aminotransferase (ALT) screen, a trial of tacrine would then have been reasonable.

▼ DORIS ARNOLD (Part IV)

Mrs. Arnold has now been living with her son and his family for 2 months. Although she is on a waiting list for skilled nursing home placement in the area, it is not anticipated that she will be able to be placed for several months. You organize a family conference that includes all three of the children, and you briefly and simply explain the illness and the need for all of them to understand better how to reduce confusion and disruption for her. "But she doesn't even remember our names," says the middle child.

You direct them toward the local chapter of the Alzheimer's Association, which provides straightforward literature to explain the illness, and the son and his wife attend a support group. They read about the illness, and the 16-year-old, at her high school teacher's suggestion, completes a school project on the illness and presents it to her class. This involvement reduces the otherwise completely negative disruption of having grandma at home, which has greatly modified the children's social life. In some ways the family is functioning better, especially the middle child, who spends time with his grandmother. Specific directions to avoid confrontation, to ease clothing choices and the associated arguments by leaving only one suitable outfit in her closet for the weather expected that day, and continued firm reminding to urinate regularly, which decreases the incidence of her incontinence, reduce much of the stress.

Six months later, Mrs. Arnold has deteriorated still further and now does not even recognize her son. She has progressed to needing physical assistance with dressing and bathing. A bed becomes available at the skilled care facility, and she moves in. The move is carefully planned, and she takes some of her furniture and personal treasures with her to ease the transi-

tion. The first few weeks are difficult, but she settles in. She stays there with regular visitation, especially from the oldest grandchild, for less than 2 years; during this time she deteriorates considerably, requiring feeding and assistance with transfers. At the time of Mrs. Arnold's admission, her son had discussed both resuscitation status and the approach to illness. At that time he had greatly desired her to be treated intensively whatever happened and to be resuscitated. One year later, Mrs. Arnold's condition is deteriorating following two episodes of aspiration pneumonia caused by choking episodes. Both episodes settled with antibiotic treatment, but the first of them involved a hospitalization during which she became more confused. You again discuss her resuscitation status with her son. He revises his opinion, remembering that his mother had always said that she did not wish to be dependent on anyone and that she particularly had feared medical machines. Thus when she develops a third episode of pneumonia after nearly 2 years in the facility, it is agreed that she will not be hospitalized. Although initial treatment with an oral antibiotic is commenced, she succumbs to the pneumonia without hospital transfer. Despite her initial hostility, the daughter-in-law becomes a volunteer for the Alzheimer's Association and is instrumental in organizing a respite program for caregivers in the community.

CASE DISCUSSION

Although Mrs. Arnold's dementia progressed quite quickly, her institutional placement was postponed by skilled handling, and both she and the family were given a period of stressful but also meaningful time together. Her grandchildren gained from her presence. If placement had been achieved earlier, the hostility and resentment over Mrs. Arnold's care might never have been resolved. The changing attitude of the son, from guiltily wishing to do everything to more sensibly realizing that, without a specific directive from his mother, decisions regarding intensity of treatment and resuscitation should be based on what was known of her wishes, demonstrates appropriate change in attitude as the illness evolves and the family becomes more experienced. In this case the course of the illness was short and the family's resources limited relative to her rapid dependency.

▼ SARAH GOODCHILD (Part I)

You receive a phone call from Lynn, the 58-year-old daughter of Mrs. Sarah Goodchild, a patient of yours whom you have known for some time. Three years ago she experienced a somewhat abrupt onset of functional and memory impairment with self-neglect, and you successfully identified depression and treated her for 1 year with an selective serotonin reuptake inhibitor (SSRI). The apathy and lack of motivation that particularly characterized her depression resolved satisfactorily, and at follow-up visits she seemed to be coping well. She lives alone; her husband died 9 years ago. The daughter's concern now is that she has noticed, especially during the past 2 years, that her mother's memory for appointments and events, and even her mother's household skills, has been diminishing. Although you had reassured her that her mother did not appear to have Alzheimer's disease about 2½ years ago when the depression was successfully responding to your management, she is concerned that this may indeed be the problem now. Her mother denies any problem. Lynn feels sure that her mother will not mention memory problems at her next visit, when you are to follow up on her mild hypertension.

At Mrs. Goodchild's next visit you ask about memory, and she denies any problem. You gently point out that her daughter is concerned about her memory, and she agrees to a short memory test; you administer a Mini–Mental State examination. To her embarrassment, she scores only 17/30 on this, with poor short-term memory and orientation to time, plus visuospatial impairment. However, she does not appear to be experiencing any of her prior symptoms of depression, since specific inquiries for diurnal variation in mood, sleep problems, and change in appetite or bowel habits are all negative. By telephone, her daughter confirms that the changes she has noted have been very slowly progressive, but she is able to give numerous instances of progressive worsening; Lynn has to handle her mother's checkbook, Mrs. Goodchild is much more unkempt, she is not feeding herself well, her standards of home care are slipping, and she has had a couple of small fires in her kitchen. Lynn has read about tacrine (Cognex) and wonders if her mother would be a candidate for it.

STUDY QUESTIONS

- What investigations will help to confirm the diagnosis?
- If this does appear to clinically be Alzheimer's disease, is she a suitable candidate for specific treatment?

CASE DISCUSSION

Clearly a workup for contributory factors is essential. In view of the already moderate degree of dementia, a SPECT may well provide confirmatory evidence of Alzheimer's disease and help in decision making about the role of tacrine. However, compliance is an issue, since this patient denies the problem and lives alone.

▼ SARAH GOODCHILD (Part II)

Your investigation for contributory factors is negative. Mrs. Goodchild is borderline hypertensive, but the MRI shows only nonspecific white matter changes. Lynn has a conference with her several siblings, who agree that Mrs. Goodchild's previously involved grandmothering of her many grandchildren has sadly diminished; they feel strongly that tacrine should be tried. Although between them they could visit frequently, compliance with the medication will be problematic. However, Mrs. Goodchild has hinted that she is lonely and would consider living with her daughter Lynn, who has plenty of space; they have an excellent relationship.

To improve diagnostic certainty rather than simply await further deterioration, a SPECT is ordered; it shows symmetrical, bilateral temporoparietal perfusion deficits, characteristic of Alzheimer's disease. Based on this information and her history, a plan to relocate is implemented, a screening ALT test is obtained and is within normal limits, and tacrine is initiated.

Whereas Mrs. Goodchild experiences transient nausea on initiation of the medication and at each dose change, this is minimized by giving the medication with meals for the first 1 or 2 weeks after each dose change. Otherwise her clinical course is smooth, and at the end of a year, she is happily settled into her daughter's home. She subjectively does not appear to have lost memory function, and she enjoys the company of her grandchildren, all of whom she can still name. Formal testing with the Mini–Mental State examination shows a plateau, with a score of 18/30. One year later the plateau is maintained and the medication continues at 160 mg per day, with quarterly blood tests. Her prior depression has not recurred.

CASE DISCUSSION

Mrs. Goodchild's case is of interest in demonstrating the modest predictive importance of an episode of cognitively impairing major depression. Such patients should be followed in case they have persistent, or even progressive, cognitive deficits. Some authorities would have recommended more prolonged therapy with the antidepressant. However, this appeared to be not a recurrence of the mood disorder but a more an insidious, and subsequent, onset of progressive cognitive dysfunction. Whereas the clinical diagnosis of dementia of Alzheimer's type could have been established by simply watching and waiting (and was highly likely even at her re-presentation), the SPECT provided supportive evidence. Without attentive family members (in this case leading to the possibility of relocation to a more supervised setting), compliance with the medication would have been problematic, even if her cognitive deficits had been less severe. Given the speed of onset a "wait and see" approach would have been unwise. The likelihood that the tacrine induced this plateau is high. A coincidental, naturally occurring plateau could have been the explanation, but these are unfortunately rare. This patient should probably continue on the medication until definite signs of cognitive slippage confirm that she is beginning to stop responding to the medication. When that occurs, withdrawal over several weeks is advisable. Even so, there may be a temporary downswing in cognition but with a return to baseline within weeks. The utility of serial numeric measurements of mental status (using the same instrument each time) is well demonstrated by this case.

MANAGING ALZHEIMER'S DISEASE

Each separate manifestation of Alzheimer's disease as it progresses can be positively approached with a treatment plan. The plan should incorporate activities for the physician, the family members, and often for the patient.[72]

The plan should include a preventive approach to the symptom or the behavior, either preventing the symptom from worsening or preventing or reducing its impact on the patient or caregiver. Most of this treatment is not a prescription of medication, although some medications are indicated and will be described. Most of the treatment involves educating the caregiving family members, and sometimes other health-related professionals, in the appropriate management. The family members actually participate in the therapy. Ideally, the caregiving family members manage the patient under the direction and consultation of the physician and other health professionals.

Early on, family members must become familiar with the services available, including the different health professionals (social workers, nurses, dietitians, etc.) and non–health professionals (such as lawyers) that they will need to access. The complexity of the provision of care and the payment system has led to the evolution of the case manager or care manager. Increasingly, both in organized systems of care such as Medicaid and health maintenance organizations and also privately for individual families with the means, these individuals can assist families to access and pay for services and help them to understand their eligibility for services and to make good judgments about the use of their own and the patient's resources as a means of reducing the impact of the illness and ensuring appropriate care. The objectives of the treatment plan are to have a skilled, rested caregiver (which means organizing appropriate respite and support), to reduce the disruption to both the patient's and caregiver's lives, and to postpone the morbidity and dependency that often characterize the last years of many of these patients' lives. Keeping the person at home until death can be wonderfully satisfying and may involve hospice care in the terminal stages. However, this may be an impossible aim; there may be tremendous family stress, and guilt should not be laid on the caregiver whose family member needs institutional care.

A few families do not respond to their moral obligation and will even abandon their relative. Abuse, passive or active, fiscal and otherwise, may occur. In the majority of cases, astonishing devotion and personal and financial resources are brought to bear by family members.[73]

Sometimes one or several family members are pathologically overinvolved. Sometimes a son or daughter will seek to make amends for a lifetime of unsatisfactory parental relationship in the final years; in such situations, "burnout" of the caregiver or inappropriate decisions (generally doing more than is appropriate or inducing dependency) are the dangers. Sometimes a spouse of a patient will sacrifice more of his or her life and personhood than is reasonable; in such instances the near fanaticism of the family member can be difficult to incorporate into a teamlike approach, since no professional effort will approach the unrealistic standard of care to which the caregiver aspires. The health professional team in such difficult family circumstances must focus on the priorities of caring for the patient, who must not be exposed to excess danger through denial of disability (e.g., allowing driving or walking outside independently when cognitively incompetent to do so), on the safety of others (e.g., giving up driving), and on the reasonable use of medical resources (e.g., the use of gastrostomy tube feeding when the prognosis for life is short and prolongation of life is not in the patient's best interest, even if the family is not ready to "let go").

MANAGING THE SYMPTOMS AND BEHAVIORS OF ALZHEIMER'S DISEASE AND THE OTHER DEMENTIAS

Most of the rest of this chapter details the management of the symptoms and behaviors commonly seen in patients with dementia (Box 17-8). These symptoms and behaviors are presented in approximately the order in which they characteristically become problems and demonstrate the use of an integrated approach involving professionals and family members.

Memory Loss

Short-term memory loss is often the first symptom noticed. Many people attribute this to "old age," and indeed impaired short-term memory may be a feature of "normal aging."[74] However, by the time that it becomes clear that the memory losses are progressing (generally after more than a year has gone by), the family and patient realize that something more than normal aging is occurring. Short-term memory loss is extremely disabling. Yet many simple techniques can be used to reduce the impact of the

---

BOX 17-8
Objectives of the Management of Progressive Dementias

Preserving function, including physical, social, and self-care skills, for as long as possible

Accessing preserved long-term memory for enjoyment and validation

Maintaining patients in the security and familiarity of their own homes for as long as possible

Appropriately and actively using psychotropic medications and behavioral management techniques

Discussing the patient's preferences for resuscitation and high-technology maintenance while still cognitively able

Appointing a health care proxy or writing advanced directives while still able (and completing the will and doing estate planning)

Carefully planning all relocations, whether temporary or long-term

---

memory loss on the individual's daily life: "Post it" notes, reminder lists, reminders by family members, and most especially a personal notebook (one notebook in which everything that needs to be remembered can be noted) should be used. Techniques that nondemented individuals use to improve memory, such as word association or making a focused effort to learn, may have application; but in general, once the memory loss is clearly being caused by a dementia, it is more likely that "forcing," which induces anxiety, will not help memory and may even cause distress. The best technique is to replace the short-term memory loss with reminders. Computer programs have been used as mnemonics and will undoubtedly have increasing application in the future.

> *The best technique is to replace short-term memory loss with reminders, for example, a single notebook in which everything that needs to be remembered and could possibly be forgotten can be written down.*

The caregiver must be sensitive to the degree of memory loss to judge how much notice to give of upcoming plans or activities; too much forewarning may result in an anxiety state rather than pleasant anticipation, yet giving no warning may not be best either and may result in surprise and disruption. Short-term memory loss can occasionally be used to advantage. For example, when driving must be given up, confrontation with the unwelcome fact can often be postponed indefinitely. Memory loss is also the basis of repetitive behaviors, such as asking the same question over and over; such behavior can be extremely trying. When this becomes the behavior, distraction techniques (introducing another subject or activity), withdrawal techniques (the person who is continually being requestioned withdraws for a few minutes, then comes back with a fresh activity or subject), or actual confrontation ("You have asked me that many times before; let us talk . . .") may be used.

Especially in old age, there is a huge quantity of long-term memory to access. Even when access to long-term memory is becoming impaired, techniques to help the person access this enjoyable fund of memories, use them, and give the patient a sense of his or her reality and validity as a person can be helpful. Reminiscence therapy has been specifically shown to improve the quality of life and calm behavioral upsets including sleep disturbances. Family members should take the time to collect old photographs, records, television shows, video tapes, and other things from the past that can be enjoyed and give structure and a sense of relevance to the patient. Often these memorabilia can be viewed again and again. (I have had two patients who were helped late in their illnesses by "The Honeymooners" reruns.) Companies specializing in nostalgia and memorabilia have produced material specifically to assist with this type of therapy.

> *Even though access to long-term memory is impaired, there is so much long-term memory in an older person that accessing it, using it, and enjoying it can all improve the quality of life for the patient and family, but the family will have to set things up in order to make it happen.*

It is important to realize that poor memory is not necessarily associated with failure to understand. Patients may clearly understand what is said to them but fail to remember the information long enough for it to be useful. Much frustration for professionals and caregivers could be avoided if this were realized.

> *Patients with dementia may clearly understand but still fail to remember.*

Documenting the degree of memory loss and frequency of memory lapses is important not only in showing progression but also in documenting a major crisis: the point at which the patient fails to recognize or remember the primary caregiver (often the spouse).

Poor Judgment and Indecisiveness

The inability to make decisions, even simple ones such as what to wear can be disabling from the earliest stages of progressive dementia. The caregiver must become skilled in cueing and in reinforcing what to do in subtle ways so that confrontation and conflict are avoided. Poor judgment, manifested by disastrous financial decisions, inappropriate shopping or food choices, or wearing the wrong clothes for the weather, can obviously have serious consequences. But the caregiver must allow the patient a sense of autonomy and encourage involvement in decision making whenever possible. Giving too many alternative choices or too much input is one of the mechanisms leading to "catastrophic reactions" (see below). Thus the caregiver must be alert to the need to take over functions slowly and subtly and to avoid the unnecessary presentation of choices.

> *Given a choice between something familiar (staying in the chair) and an "unknown" activity (a trip to the shops), the patient will tend to do the familiar activity ("he refuses to go out, even when we offer").*

Lack of Motivation

Family members often feel that the patient lacks motivation and often interpret this as a conscious "giving up" or a sign of depression. This may be true, but a patient with preserved insight (which can occur until quite late in dementias) will realize that certain things are disturbing or overwhelming and therefore to be avoided. A patient with early dementia will know the discomfort of being at a gathering where he or she could not remember the names of familiar family members. The patient will remember how overwhelmed and confused he or she was in a restaurant, facing too many choices and with so much distraction. Closely accompanying dementia patients through such situations can improve these experiences, encouraging continuing socialization that may otherwise be given up prematurely. Abstract capability is generally lost early, so it is difficult to conceptualize something in the abstract. Given a choice between the secure and familiar (sitting in a chair in a comfortable room) and the unfamiliar or threatening (even if it has the potential for pleasure—a trip to the shops, a drive in the car, a vacation), the safe, boring, and familiar may well seem more attractive. An early principle for family members to establish is that instead of asking *if* the patient wants to do something, it may be necessary to simply tell *when* it is time to do it (sometimes reducing forewarning, even of major events, can reduce the ruminating and anxiety at the prospect of something unknown and potentially disrupting). When it is time to do something, the patient must be cued in every possible way: a hand on the elbow, body language suggesting that it is time to get moving, the presence of others heading toward the same activity—these are the kinds of cues that will help a patient with dementia go along with activities that ultimately will give the patient pleasure. The patient would likely refuse to go along if challenged with a choice. Some caregivers find this hard because it sounds patronizing. If properly understood, it improves quality of life and relationships.

> *Don't ask patients with dementia if they want do something, tell them when it is time to do it. (Then cue them, doing everything to make it appear the inevitable thing to do.)*

> *Patients with dementia lack abstract capability, so how can they conceptualize a new place to live? Naturally they will tend to refuse the prospect of relocation; it is a reasonable fear of the unknown and literally inconceivable.*

Disorientation and Unadaptability to New Environments

Disorientation starts early and gets worse. Time and place orientation by the caregiver and a familiar environment can help. Familiarity becomes even more important later in the illness. Hospitalization, institutionalization (even if it is for temporary respite), and even the temporary relocation of going to the hospital or the doctor for tests may all require careful planning, with a calming constant and familiar companion to explain and guide the patient. Going to relatives for the weekend or going on a vacation can be more disruptive than it is worth. On the other hand, some patients do tolerate moves and are even stimulated by change, perhaps more in the earlier phases. Adjustment reactions can be severe and may mimic psychosis; major tranquilizers may be appropriate for their symptomatic management (but only temporarily, for example, for 3 to 6 weeks).

Prevention is better than trying to control emotional outbursts. Familiar objects from home that can be transported into emergency rooms, intensive care units, and places that are going to become home can ease the transitions. A "buddy system" at the time of a relocation is important. One accompanying individual can steer even a quite demented person through the complexity of a potentially disrupting social or family occasion. A patient with early disease can thus still enjoy a quality of life that might otherwise be denied.

 Familiar objects from home can ease transitions; photographs of the patients as they "were" will help staff and visitors to see patients as people.

Personality Change and Disinhibition

It is stressful for families to watch the deterioration of someone close to them. Sometimes the changes are exaggerations of previously suppressed traits; sometimes they are quite unlike "the person we knew." Behaviors may range from embarrassing social remarks and behavior to sexual acting out and, occasionally, exhibitionism or shoplifting. These may be the presenting symptoms. Many have difficulty managing all this with the necessary degree of tolerance and humor. Sometimes the caregiver has taken on the role in a subconscious attempt to resolve a previously poor relationship; exaggeration of prior personality traits in the patient will make this especially difficult. The use of reminiscence to allow the past relationship to be recalled and enjoyed has been mentioned previously.

Nutritional Problems

Even in the early stages of dementia, nutrition is problematic. The lack of judgment to make good choices and the observation that faced with a bewildering variety of foods a dementia patient will choose nothing (as frequently happens when trays are presented in hospital settings) lead to the principles of early management of eating in dementia. These principles are summarized in Box 17-9. As the disease progresses, undernutrition generally becomes a major problem. Clearly it is a principle to maintain oral feeding for as long as possible; caregivers must become "experts" at spoon feeding. Increasingly, hospitals and institutions are instituting volunteer training programs to spoon feed elders, many of whom are suffering dementia as the main cause of their feeding difficulty. A summary of practical hints to help in feeding patients with dementia is given in Table 17-3.[90]

 Maintaining oral feeding (frequently by spoon feeding) for as long as possible is the most important nutritional intervention in Alzheimer's disease.

Sexuality

Many older individuals hesitate to talk about sexuality to the physician; many physicians are unprepared to discuss sexuality, especially in their older patients. Yet it is clear that sexual activity may be a rewarding part of relationships; even quite late in dementia it can be calming for both partners. Disinhibition or even aggressiveness may be a problem, however, and a frail spouse may need special advice (or the patient may need sedation) if sexual demands are inappropriate or too aggressive. Physical contact or an embrace may be vital for the comfort and reassurance of the patient. At the other end of the sexuality spectrum, it may be necessary to counsel a spouse not to be repulsed at masturbatory activity (especially in men). (I still treasure the case of a straitlaced farmer's wife who kept her demented husband quiet for hours with the same sexy video!)

BOX 17-9
Nutritional Advice to Families Caring for Early Dementia Patients

1. Provide fewer choices at meals; give small servings; provide individual nutritional snacks throughout the day.
2. Reduce stimulation at mealtime; turn off the television or radio and focus on enjoyment of the food.
3. Go to restaurants that are familiar, and go early for lunch or dinner when fewer people are around; talk to the owner or waiters* and ask them "to go with the flow" if something embarrassing should occur.

*Or use the ADRDA "business card," which says, "Excuse my companion who has Alzheimer's disease."

Table 17-3   Feeding the Patient with Late Dementia: Practical Hints

Problem	Interventions
Poor attention/concentration	Talk through the steps, place utensils in hand, make food visible
Combative/food throwing	One food at a time, sit on nondominant side, offer rewards, use unbreakable dishes held in place with suction cups
Constant chewing	Soft foods, small bites, tell patient to stop chewing
Distractable/indecisive	Constant environment, no distractions, limit choices, one food at a time
Forgets to swallow	Upward stroke on larynx, tell to swallow, feel the swallow before next bite offered
Too restless/pacing	Sit beside patient, exercise before, offer finger foods, use covered and spouted cups
Apraxia (cannot use objects correctly)	Make eating a series of simple steps, use verbal cues, finger foods, limit utensils and cups
Bites utensils	Vinyl-coated spoons, do not fully insert, massage arm and leg muscles to promote relaxation of bite, tell not to bite
Can't/won't chew	Check if dentures fit, alternate placement of food on different sides, between gum and cheek, etc., tell to chew
Doesn't remove food from utensil	Place small amount of food on front of spoon, tell to close lips, withdraw spoon as lips begin to close, use "pusher" spoon
Keeps food in mouth	Cool spoon with ice between bites, press on top of head with open palm to trigger swallowing, vary texture of food
Open mouth/food falls out	Spouted cup, blot lips, lip closure exercises (popsicle, etc.)

Communication Disorders

A good general rule is to assume better comprehension than expression in the patient with dementia. No one should speak about any older patients in their presence without specifically involving them. Aphasia is a common early feature of dementia, and there is some evidence that marked early difficulty is associated with a more rapid decline in Alzheimer's disease. Word-finding difficulties can be frustrating to the patient, so the caregiver must become skilled in understanding the patient's wishes. The role of memory loss in impairing communication (the patient understands but fails to store the information and thus may as well have not heard it) has been mentioned previously. The aphasia of Alzheimer's disease is generally of the receptive type (Wernicke's aphasia), which is associated with the temporoparietal areas (the areas initially affected in Alzheimer's disease). In receptive aphasia the patient cannot recognize sensory symbols and speaks fluent nonsense with a natural cadence. As the frontal lobes become involved in Alzheimer's disease (or if vascular problems or Pick's disease affects the frontal lobes), an expressive aphasia (Broca's aphasia), in which the understanding of speech is worse than the understanding of writing, will occur.

Repetitiveness and Shadowing

Constant repetition of the same questions can be an early symptom. Sometimes there is shadowing, with the insecure, demented patient following the caregiver around and depriving the caregiver of any privacy or rest. Aborting such behaviors consists of the caregiver withdrawing for minutes only and returning with a fresh subject or activity. A direct approach to repetitiveness sometimes helps: "You've asked me that twenty times before; the answer is . . . Let's talk about (something else). . . ."

Emotional Lability

Emotional lability of the pseudobulbar type is more associated with vascular dementia or poststroke states. In this condition the emotional response to any kind of stimulus is tears and apparent emotional upset or sometimes inappropriate euphoria. It is characteristic of this state for the patient to be easily distracted from the inappropriate emotional response; moving the patient's attention to something else sometimes "turns off" the response. However, more persistently dysphoric states can look like, or even be clinically indistinguishable from, an unusually dysphoric episode of major depression; in this case a trial of antidepressants may be justified.[24,26]

▼ *HAROLD FRANKLIN (Part V)*

Within 2 months of starting the antidepressant, Mr. Franklin's mood improves and his sexual disinhibition in public becomes much less of a problem, but it is clear that Mr. Franklin cannot maintain his business. He hands it over to his partner in exchange for a financial settlement. After taking the antidepressant for 6 months, he is less depressed but his cognitive status has diminished further still, and he continues to obtain alcohol and get drunk from time to time. He needs to be reminded to change his clothes and bathe, although he can physically carry out all such functions.

STUDY QUESTIONS

- *What can be done to improve his ADL function?*
- *How can his persistent alcoholism be addressed?*
- *What can be done now to help with his management later on?*

CASE DISCUSSION

As Mr. Franklin deteriorates, he will be more dependent on others for his alcohol supplies. It should therefore be increasingly possible, provided the family addresses the problem with determination, to reduce and eliminate his alcohol consumption. This may help his cognition and depression and may improve his self-care skills. Before he becomes cognitively worse, the family should set up a health care proxy and discuss intensity of treatment issues with Harold. It will be important later to know his opinion of being "maintained on machines," for there is no doubt that he will be incapable of making health care decisions on his own behalf soon. While he is still competent, wills and other financial arrangements should be completed. Extended family should be informed of his deterioration to allow resolution of any unfinished business, emotional or fiscal.

Diminished Self-Care Skills

Loss of ADLs and IADLs will occur as dementia progresses. Since the relationship between ADLs and cognitive impairment is not completely predictable, it is helpful to record dependence or independence in the common ADLs and IADLs at regular intervals. The precise functional dependency will need to be known when in-home services or placement become issues.

Indecisiveness may underlie some functional difficulties; with dressing, for example, problems can sometimes be resolved by having only one complete outfit in the closet at a time. IADLs such as telephoning can be simplified using telephones that encode commonly used phone numbers; similar techniques can help the patient use the microwave and television for as long as possible.

Although it may be quicker to do things for an individual rather than to let him or her struggle on, the danger of taking over too early is that each skill, once taken over, is unlikely to be regained. The individual must be encouraged to at least finish each task, even if each has to be set up and started for him or her. Later, when feeding is the only self-care skill remaining, positive efforts will be needed to preserve this in the event of hospitalization; hospitalized patients with advanced dementia quickly decondition and become more dependent, never achieving their prior baseline.

Maintaining function in dementia means recognizing that if the caregiver or others get things started, the patient may be able to finish an activity with considerable satisfaction.

Driving

Driving is a special problem in dementia.[75,76] Patients with mild dementia, provided that they have good visuo-spatial skills, seem to be safer drivers than males in their early 20s,[77-79] but once it is clear that there is a progressive dementia, it seems reasonable to plan on discontinuing driving. Even with mild dementia, visuospatial impairment mandates discontinuing driving. Impaired judgement, memory difficulties, and the natural worsening of cognition make giving up driving, although an undoubtedly unfortunate loss of independence and self-image, in the public interest and eventually necessary in all progressive dementias. The family should be advised to use any excuse to get the car off the road and the keys away from the patient. The physician has at least a moral obligation to report an individual who continues to drive when unfit. Usually such problems can be overcome by gaining the support of the family; hiding the car keys, postponing driving until "tomorrow" (which never comes), and (in particularly difficult cases) removing the distributor cap or even selling the car are all possible approaches.

When it is necessary for the patient to give up driving, take advantage of the memory loss. Tell the patient, "You cannot drive until tomorrow," but tomorrow never comes.

Delusions and Illusions

Delusional thinking in dementia is often based on attempts to rationalize phenomena around the patient, such as a light on the wall or moving shadows. Hearing loss often contributes to delusional thinking, allowing the disordered mind to misinterpret what is said and leading to suspiciousness and paranoia. The caregiver must be counseled to not argue about delusions and to avoid behaviors that will induce suspiciousness, such as talking about the person with dementia in front of him or her or just outside the door. Sometimes the delusions are complex, with a psychotic flavor. Family members must realize that such delusions must never be inappropriately reinforced; the individual should be gently corrected, but if conflict is obviously going to result, the subject should be changed. The same approach should be used with hallucinations (see discussion below).

Don't argue with a patient about delusions or hallucinations: they are "real" to the patient, but don't nurture or reinforce these thoughts either.

Hallucinations

It is now recognized that hallucinations, generally visual but occasionally auditory and generally benign and non-threatening, occur in all phases of dementia. Commonly, as with true psychosis, the patient seems to realize that the objects seen or heard are not really there; often merely reassurance that "the mind is playing tricks" is enough, for the hallucinations of dementia do not have the directive or frightening quality associated with the hallucinations of psychotic illnesses. However, hallucinations may be disruptive or unpleasant, and if so, they can sometimes be effectively resolved by the use of antipsychotics; such hallucinationary activity is usually sensitive to low doses of antipsychotics. The family may need reassurance, since these symptoms appear to be more like "mental illness" (which has a stigma) than other dementia symptoms.

Diminished Mobility

As judgement and perception diminish, maintaining mobility can become dangerous. Some of the loss of mobility associated with dementia may be secondary to efforts to keep the patient "safe." Often the patient's own insight is what leads him or her to become more cautious. Other patients with dementia present problems of excess mobility and wandering. Maintaining a range of mobility and a daily exercise program is important in preserving well-being, physical health, orientation, and probably, good sleep patterns.

Late in the illness, the neurological problem of increased tone in the lower extremities becomes a physical handicap to mobility.

▼ HAROLD FRANKLIN (Part VI)

More than 2 years after Mr. Franklin's initial presentation, the depression is behind him and his drinking has finally moderated after a family conference at Al-Anon made the entire family firmly resolved never to supply the alcohol. A health care proxy has been signed, and wills and life insurances are in order. Harold is still living at home, on his own for much of the day, and Mrs. Franklin has taken a full-time job to maintain the family's finances. She calls you because, for several weeks, although Harold seems to do all right in the day, by the evening he is increasingly agitated. By around 11 PM he becomes unreasonable, won't get ready for bed, and rambles on loudly about many topics. Mrs. Franklin believes he spends most of his afternoon asleep in the chair. The interrupted nights are exhausting her. Reexamining Mr. Franklin with the Mini–Mental State examination, you note that his score has dropped to 12/30. He does not appear overtly depressed, and in fact he is socially well preserved during the interview.

STUDY QUESTION

■ *What steps (including medication) can be taken to correct this trying situation?*

Insomnia and Sundowning

Disturbed nights are one of the most common "last straws" for caregiving relatives, precipitating requests for placement. Demented patients who are up at night are in danger of falling and fracture. The caregiver who is deprived of sleep will not be equal to the challenges of the next day.

Patients with dementia characteristically start to suffer a disrupted sleep pattern similar to that of an alcoholic. Periods of awakening are prolonged, and periods of deep sleep are less.

In addition, many patients suffer day-night reversal, a sleep phase syndrome, which, if recognized early enough, may be correctable; the technique is to postpone the patient's time of initiation of sleep (it can never be brought forward, since you cannot force sleep) in an effort to maintain day-night rhythm. Correcting day-night reversal is difficult, so a preventive approach is recommended: daytime naps should always be kept short. Exercise or activity in the morning or early afternoon is associated with better sleep patterns.

Sometimes a disrupted night is preceded by a virtually psychotic state called the *sundowning syndrome,* which is characteristic of the middle and late phases of dementia.[80] Occasionally this responds to minor tranquilizers and behavioral management alone, but minor tranquilizers can make the situation worse. Sundowning is one of the few indications for the use of antipsychotics in selected patients. Before trying medications in a patient with dementia who is clearly more agitated as night falls, caregivers should be advised to try simple measures such as a night light, a calm and fulfilling evening, perhaps some familiar television or music, minimal disruption and noise, exercise in the morning or early afternoon, and the sense of the presence of others rather than isolation or darkness to reduce the primitive fearfulness that appears to predispose to this syndrome. Experienced hospital nurses know of these techniques and place sundowning patients with dementia outside of their rooms and near the nursing station, where there is the security of activity, light, and companionship.[81]

Occasionally, minor tranquilizers have a role in simply initiating sleep, particularly for a short period of time, in newly changed circumstances, as an adjunct, or in efforts to correct day-night reversal. Chloral hydrate, very short-acting benzodiazepines, and zolpidem (Ambien) are generally recommended. Naturally, they should not be used for long.

▼ HAROLD FRANKLIN (Part VII)

Management of the insomnia includes increasing companionship and activity in the day and environmental changes (night light, radio), but it also requires thiothixene (Navane) in low doses. After 2 months of taking the medication, Mr. Franklin lets himself out of the house one day and is brought back by the police after having been intercepted by a supermarket manager for attempting to walk out of the store with bread and eggs for which he had not paid. On being challenged, he became hostile and agitated. On questioning, it appears Harold has been going out for walks during the daytime and has so far not become lost. On reassessing him, you find his mental status remains at 12/30. The Franklins' daughter calls, saying that this is an unsafe situation and that her father must be institutionalized soon in view of the danger he is in.

STUDY QUESTIONS

- *Does this incident mean that Mr. Franklin should be in a nursing home?*
- *Can anything be done to control wandering behaviors?*

CASE DISCUSSION

Increasing behavioral manifestations in a patient with dementia still living at home should lead to consideration of a day program to provide useful and therapeutic activity. The possibility of the thiothixene causing motor restlessness (akathisia) should be considered. At the very least, Mr. Franklin should wear identification at all times; it would be wise to enroll him in the Safe Return program of the Alzheimer's Association (see below).

Wandering and Falling

Daytime and nighttime wandering is a middle-phase phenomenon. It must be recognized that as the disease progresses, patients often become so disorganized that they cannot persist in this activity. Wandering should be distinguished from self-directed, reasonable walking behaviors, which are therapeutic. However, the danger of getting lost or of being unable to cope with changed circumstances means a careful balancing of the patient's ability with the risks involved.

> *Control wandering if possible, but at least make sure the patient has identification (or a Safe Return bracelet) at all times.*

How much can be done about wandering depends on the environment available for the person to walk in. All patients with dementia should wear identification at all times, either stitched into their clothing or as a bracelet: the Alzheimer's Association runs a national identification program called Safe Return. The patient wears an identification bracelet with a toll-free number and code so that wherever the patient is found, there is telephone access to the caregiver or other responsible individuals. Perimeter control can be instituted in the home situation by disguising exit doors with screens or markings on the

floor (as has been the practice in institutional settings) or by simply using complex locks. This negative approach can be balanced by the positive one of simply providing somewhere to do the walking (as many institutions fail to do). Tranquilizers help little and may add postural hypotension or other balance disorders to the difficulties already present, and phenothiazines and haloperidol can cause a dyskinetic action called akathisia, which is an irresistible urge to move about. Simple solutions such as placing the mattress on the floor can reduce some falling tendencies. Sometimes wandering can be inhibited simply by distracting activities. One of this author's caregivers found that her husband would stay still, fascinated by the television—but only if there were young women on. So she bought videotapes, considering this a better alternative than restraining him or placing him in an institution.

Patients with dementia are at increased risk of accidents and falling because of misperception of their environment. From an early stage it is important to make the environment safe, with adequate lighting, an uncomplicated, uncluttered environment, and safe flooring and other arrangements in the bathroom and kitchen.

▼ HAROLD FRANKLIN (Part VIII)

Nearly 4 years into Harold's illness, the family has become organized around his disabilities, and he remains at home most of the time, attending the day program 3 days a week. He is still able to be left alone safely in the house from time to time. His wandering phase has stopped, assisted greatly by attention to perimeter control in the house, which was accomplished with complex locks and some disguising of the doors. The family has also been careful to ensure a place where he can walk, fenced and gated, in his own yard. The family members are distressed and surprised when, at the family Thanksgiving dinner, Harold becomes agitated and angry and strikes one of the grandchildren with the walking cane he has adopted recently. Assisted to his room, he is calmed by one of the thiothixene capsules he still takes at night for his sundowning.

STUDY QUESTIONS

- *Should the family now avoid involving Mr. Franklin in family activities?*
- *What advice can be given to prevent this from happening again?*

Aggressive Outbursts and Catastrophic Reactions

Aggressive outbursts can occur early, secondary to the frustration of the patient. Alcohol and minor tranquilizers can aggravate this by increasing disinhibition. Occasionally the caregiver is physically abused. Such aggressiveness may be hidden from health professionals because of embarrassment and shame. Sometimes the aggressive outbursts are part of a generally agitated state, which occurs usually rather late in the illness, with the patient in a state of continuous, meaningless mental activity that can sometimes be perceived even when he or she is at rest or near sleep. Such individuals probably need a low dose of an antipsychotic for control of their thoughts; this will help bring the outbursts under control, too.

> *Don't give too much warning about upcoming events: the patient may not be able to handle the anxiety of anticipation.*

Frequently the aggressive outbursts are intermittent and situational, and continuous treatment is not justified. The term *catastrophic reaction* has been coined to describe outbursts that are the result of the individual being overwhelmed by too much sensory input or by decision-making needs, especially when such a situation is complicated by concurrent illness or medication. Such verbal, emotional, or physical outbursts often occur on family occasions (when it is stressful to see so many people who are familiar, who should be remembered, and who "might expect me to remember their names . . ."). They also commonly occur during hospitalization or with other relocations. Occasionally the patient is goaded by a frustrated caregiver. Careful counseling about the avoidance of such situations, early recognition that such a reaction is coming, and use of techniques to distract and calm the patient can be taught to the caregiving family members.

> *Avoid overwhelming the patient by having too many things happening at once: arrange one-on-one meetings whenever possible.*

A special problem is the handling of dementia-related emergencies of *uncontrollable aggression*. What should the family do when the patient becomes uncontrollable; where should they go for help? Unfortunately the advocacy that has led to the recognition that Alzheimer's disease and the other dementias are not to be regarded as "mental illnesses" (i.e., they do not carry the same stigma) has effectively closed off the availability of mental health services to such patients. Because mental health services are being cut back anyway, it has become useless to look to them for the assistance they have historically provided for people who are agitated and require a caring environment with experienced mental health nurses. Regional emergency psychiatric services will not handle such patients unless they have a second, definable "psychiatric" diagnosis as the cause of their symptoms, and many of course do not. Ambulance services will frequently decline transportation of unwilling patients to the hospital, so families must often turn to the police force. It may seem absurd to have to ask for uniformed police to take a patient to the hospital, and it is tempting to mimic the great APA slogan "Depression: it's an illness not a weakness" with the phrase "Alzheimer's: it's a disease not a crime!" Nonetheless, family members must be advised that should the patient become so uncontrollable that he or she is dangerously agitated, the police must be called and asked to take the patient to the emergency room in hopes of persuading the medical system, the emergency room physician, and the primary care physician, if available, to attempt admission to an environment where behavioral medication can be titrated and there can be environmental and medical interventions.

Incontinence

Urinary and fecal incontinence can occur as a result of dementia; the patient's awareness and motivation to respond to the need to urinate or evacuate are lost. However, full consideration of all the potential causes of incontinence must be made. Diapers are recommended as a first aid procedure (and often as a long-term solution) but must not substitute for adequate investigation. Failure to treat a simple precipitating cause, such as a urinary infection, a diuretic drug, or (in the case of bowel incontinence) a fecal impaction, devastatingly increases the level of care needed for an already dependent patient and may greatly reduce the alternatives available for placement. When the incontinence is due to a lack of awareness or to simply failing to toilet on a regular basis, then a simple toileting regimen (going every 2 hours or more often if necessary to maintain dryness) should be combined with encouraging the individual to empty the bladder fully each time (double voiding in females and males; this is facilitated by having male patients sit to urinate, if they will). In an attempt to "catch" bowel movements, it is useful to take advantage of the gastrocolic reflex (i.e., sit the patient on the toilet within a half hour of breakfast, lunch, or dinner, when evacuation is most likely) and perhaps add a few exercises (abdominal crunches if the patient can do them) just before the attempt. Patients with dementia have an increased number of uninhibited bladder contractions because of the lack of cerebral inhibition, the dementia itself being one factor inducing the "unstable bladder."

Dysphagia and Other Late Nutritional Problems

Dysphagia is classically associated with stroke activity, and many health professionals are familiar with the necessity to provide supplementary feeding through a nasogastric or gastrostomy tube or intravenously, until swallowing function recovers. The dysphagia that occurs in dementias is generally not self-limiting, although in the vascular dementias it may be. Usually in dementias, difficulties with swallowing function are liable to be persistent. If it is clear that a dementia patient is having trouble swallowing, evidenced by unwillingness to attempt eating, choking or coughing during feeding, or actual episodes of aspiration with pneumonia, it is vital that the patient be evaluated fully by a speech therapist for swallowing function. Depending on the stage of the illness, it is appropriate for a modified barium swallow to be carried out so that specific recommendations can be made about the consistency of food, positioning of the patient, and appropriate techniques for feeding (this is generally a phase when the individual has to be fed). There are many ethical issues surrounding what to do if an individual can no longer swallow, but before such decision making every effort must be made to maintain spoon feeding as long as possible. Maintenance of oral feeding has recently received increased emphasis (Table 17-3). More widespread use of these techniques in hospitals, homes, and nursing homes could improve the nutritional status of many patients with dysphagia or late dementia and postpone or render unnecessary the consideration of more invasive methods such as gastrostomy tubes.[82,83]

There is no absolute ruling on the matter, but it is becoming increasingly clear and is generally the ethical consensus now that nasogastric and gastrostomy tube feeding is not necessarily in the best interest of a patient with late dementia, close to the time of death. However, the decision has to be individualized, and not only must the patient's wishes be respected (this is when an advanced directive, completed when the individual is competent, is invaluable), but also the feelings of family members and staff must be considered. They will need support if a decision is made, as it occasionally must be, to allow the individual to waste undernourished as he or she progresses into the remaining few weeks to months of his or her dementia. Although it is clear that a dignified death can be achieved even if a person is undernourished or even underhydrated, recently concern has been expressed that some dehydrated patients are restless as a result of the dehydration; intravenous fluids are a possible comfort measure in such individuals, although they are not necessary in the vast majority of terminal care patients with dementia. Some consider it an "extraordinary" treatment to sustain the nutrition of an individual close to death from dementia when awareness of thirst and hunger has long receded.

Late Dysmobility and Other Problems

Late in dementia, disinhibition of lower extremity tone leads to increased flexor tone, with the potential for contractures. Before this, spasticity of the lower limbs may make walking physically difficult or impossible. Seizures do occur in late dementia; they rarely warrant specific anticonvulsant management.[84] The downward spiral of uninhibited incontinence, spasticity, progressive immobility, a tendency to fecal impaction, skin breakdown, respiratory stasis, infection, swallowing problems, and the danger of aspiration combine with other problems to render the patient in need of expert terminal care. Hospices are increasingly involved at this stage in the care of patients with dementia, both in the home and increasingly in nursing home settings. A special problem is the "6 months or less" prognosis rule for hospice care, since it is so difficult to predict how close to death a dementia patient is.[85] Some guidelines do exist, based on current clinical experience (Box 17-10).

▼ HAROLD FRANKLIN (Part IX)

Ten years after his initial diagnosis, Mr. Franklin remains at home. He has slowly lost his functional independence, and a year previously his wife Thelma retired from her job to stay home and care for him. The phases of wandering and sundowning are now behind him, but he has become incontinent of urine, seeming unaware of when he needs to urinate. Thelma is full of praise for disposable diapers, which enable her to cope with this distressing symptom. Over the next year, Harold becomes increasingly immobilized, with stiffening in his lower extremities; he eventually becomes bedbound. He begins to lose weight. Efforts are made to modify his diet, but he requires spoon feeding. Although his mouth can be kept comfortable, he is unable to take sufficient calories by mouth to maintain his weight.

As his health care proxy, and confident from their prior discussions that Harold would not wish to be artificially maintained, Mrs. Franklin decides that gastrostomy feeding is not

---

BOX 17-10
Terminal Stages of Alzheimer's or Other Dementias

Limited vocabulary (six words or less)
Absence of smiling
Inability to walk without substantial assistance
Inability to sit up independently
Difficulty eating or swallowing
Recent weight loss
Decreased consciousness or coma
Bowel or urinary incontinence
Recurrent respiratory or urinary infections
Inability to hold up the head or track objects with the eyes

Data from *The Jacob Perlow Hospice Newsletter*, New York City, 1992; *Hospice care for people with Alzheimer's disease*, Alzheimer's Association; and Hanrahan P, Luchins DJ: *J Am Geriatr Soc* 43:56-59, 1995.

a consideration. You realize that without sufficient caloric input his prognosis is probably less than 6 months, so you initiate hospice services to supplement the existing visiting nursing services; a hospital bed, a bedside commode, and other resources are made available by hospice care to assist in his terminal nursing care. A "nonhospital DNR" is written, so that there will be no confusion or 911 calls, and you counsel Thelma about what to do when he finally dies.

Twelve years from the initial diagnosis, Mr. Franklin dies quietly at home following a short febrile illness that, as a result of previous discussion, is not treated, since you and Thelma both feel confident about Harold's previously expressed contention that he did not wish to live on in a very dependent state.

CASE DISCUSSION

Although this 12-year illness produced much unhappiness, there was, until less than a year before Mr. Franklin's death, considerable enjoyment by both partners of the relationship, their mutual memories, and the familiarity of their home environment. Had Mrs. Franklin needed to continue working full time and had family and other resources not been available for the multiple costs involved, Mr. Franklin undoubtedly would have needed institutional care earlier in the illness. All could look back on this decade confident that his care had been humane and appropriate.

ANTICIPATORY PLANNING FOR LEGAL AND ETHICAL ISSUES

Relatively early in the illness, the primary care physician should encourage the caregiver to establish a durable power of attorney for health care, a health care proxy, or an advance directive, such as a living will, so that later on profound and difficult decisions about intensity of treatment and investigation can be appropriate to the patient's expressed wishes. Also, a will should be completed while there is still testamentary capacity.

Often such steps have not been taken and legal procedures may be needed to best provide for the needs of an individual who is not competent to decide. Several terms should be understood by health care professionals:

1. A *conservator* is the person appointed to oversee and take care of the property of a person unable to do so, that person being called the *conservatee*. Although appointed by a court, conservatorship is not evidence of competency or incompetency, and the property remains the conservatee's.

2. A *committee* (pronounced with emphasis on the final syllable) is an individual appointed to make personal decisions, including health care, for someone who is impaired. The committee can authorize hospitalization and make other decisions about health care. This individual is likely to be appointed by a

court following a hearing, in which the personal physician may be involved to give evidence of medical and mental status.

Being cognitively intact is good luck not a virtue, and assuming competency is not a compliment. Should individuals with dementia be exposed to harm because of their rights?

3. A *power of attorney* must be appointed by a competent person (the *principal*), and it authorizes an individual (the *attorney-in-fact*) to act on behalf of the principal. Whereas a general power of attorney authorizes decisions on a variety of matters, a special power of attorney gives power to act in only one or more specified areas. This power can be revoked by the principal (i.e., the patient), and unless specified, the power of attorney terminates when the individual becomes incompetent or disabled. A *durable* power of attorney is thus needed in dementias, with the attorney-in-fact retaining authority if the principal becomes disabled or incompetent. Inconsistency about the power of attorney's ability to make health care decisions makes the health care proxy (see below) often the best recommendation.

4. The *health care proxy* is now an almost standardized document and is widely available. It specifically designates an individual and an alternate, chosen by the patient while competent, to have full powers to make future health care decisions affecting the patient. A properly drawn health care proxy is legally recognized as representing the patient's consent to or refusal of treatment; the proxy acts *as* the patient in making decisions.

5. A *living will* is a document drawn up to express an individual's future wishes. There is no standard form, although several prepared ones exist. Unfortunately, the living will is not necessarily recognized as legally binding when decisions actually have to be made. However, any advance directive is better than none.

Clearly, legal advice may be needed, although, increasingly, patient advocacy groups, such as the Alzheimer's Association, Choice in Dying, and the American Association of Retired Persons, give such advice to their members about these issues.

It is not always necessary to resort to formal legal procedures, even when there is no record of the patient's previously expressed wishes. In fact, the above legal proceedings (guardianship etc.) can be reserved for familial disputes, complex situations in which a large estate is involved, or when the patient appears to oppose measures necessary for his or her safety. Generally, reasonable decisions that are clearly in the best interest of the patient can be made if a warm and caring approach is used by the professionals, family members, and other caregivers involved.

> *If the patient cannot make his or her wishes known, family members must remember that they are helping to decide what the patient would have wanted; their own opinion is not being sought.*

LONG-TERM INSTITUTIONAL CARE

The ideal of patients spending their last days in the comfort and familiarity of their own homes can be achieved, but it must not be imposed on caregiving families that lack the considerable capacity and means required for this. Appropriate placement can improve the relationship between caregiver and patient, can make the patient more secure by better meeting multiple needs, and can relieve the caregiver. Unfortunately, many elders resist relocation even when they are lonely and depressed; familiarity easily outweighs the unknown. Since the person in need has to consent to relocation, this produces many management problems for the families and other caregivers. If the patient lacks decision-making capacity, warm, yet firm, persuasion and organizing things so that the move to a different location seems the right thing to do are necessary if the family and others are to act in the patient's best interest.

Placement in a facility should be planned if possible.[86] However, it is often precipitated by an illness leading to hospitalization, with the individual then waiting in the hospital until a place is available. When the situation is deteriorating, the physician and caregiver should openly discuss housing alternatives, including nursing home placement, and attempt a planned placement at an appropriate facility, preferably one close enough to be visited easily and with an acceptable environment for both patient and caregiver.

There are many levels of institutional care. The terminology to describe them varies from state to state. Living in one's own home with a "lifeline" or other emergency contact does not give the social contact, reorienting reminders, and available nutrition of more supervised settings. In an adult home, for example, the individual has his or her own room and privacy and may have some simple food preparation facilities but ordinarily eats communally. Housing specifically designed for older individuals is increasingly available, offering a variable range of (self-pay) services and increasing the amount of supervision and physical care as needs change. Such ar-

rangements can be ideal for patients with Alzheimer's disease, whose needs increase over time. Unfortunately, the more pleasant and modern settings with flexible and enhanceable services are too expensive for many individuals. The highest level of institutional care, a skilled nursing facility (or nursing home), offers nursing services, physical and activity therapy, occupational and speech therapy, and a high level of nurse intensity, often in a setting that is more like a hospital than a home, although there is much local variation.

Given the variety of alternatives, the family if available needs to be highly involved in the placement process. Although it is desirable to make only one relocation, it is sometimes necessary to move to an intermediate level of care and then to skilled care when physical or behavioral needs warrant it. Different states have different terminologies and different systems. In the state of New York, for example, there is a standardized Patient Review Instrument (PRI), which numerically "scores" the patient, categorizing whether or not he or she needs an intermediate (adult home) level of care or skilled care. Whereas a skilled care patient can be cared for at home, the expense is considerable unless family members are providing the hands-on care. Increasingly, especially for patients covered by Medicaid, programs to provide extensive services in the home, thereby postponing expensive institutionalization, are being researched and implemented.

For many elders who live alone, however, the route from independence to the nursing home is frequently that of an acute illness or accident (e.g., pneumonia, hip fracture) that transforms them abruptly from being relatively independent to needing skilled care. Such institutional placement directly from the hospital is to be avoided. The disruption of being hospitalized and never returning home is unkind, and the emergency nature of the situation does not allow planning for the individual's unique needs. When an individual moves directly from the home to the hospital to a long-term care institution (unless it is clear that the long-term care institution's role is as a rehabilitation center concerned with rendering the patient independent enough to return home), it becomes the primary physician's important role to review the situation at intervals, since sometimes the slow recovery of an elder following a period of dependency in the hospital causes the patient to end up at a more dependent level of care than is appropriate. Of course it should be possible for an individual at a skilled level of care to be recategorized and moved to a more independent setting, but this process takes considerable advocacy.

Moving into a facility from home must be carefully planned. Occasionally it is reasonable to "cover" the relocation with tranquilizers, but companionship and familiar things from home, a "buddy system" on arrival at the new location, and early visitation from the caregiver will all help.[45] The primary care physician should encourage the caregiving family to take an active part in the care not only of their own relative, but also of the other residents of the facility. It is frequently hard for caregivers to give up their role to others; they should be encouraged to communicate their own observations to those who will now be caring for the patient. The physician should counsel the family to maintain good relationships with the facility staff, to avoid a contentious approach, and to develop a sense of working together with the professional staff in the care of the patient.

PSYCHOTROPICS IN DEMENTIA

Alzheimer's disease and the other dementias can, at times, mimic almost any psychiatric syndrome: paranoia, psychosis, mania, agitation, hallucinosis, anxiety, depression, melancholia.

Antipsychotics

Antipsychotics have an important place in dementia management although their overuse in the past, sometimes as "chemical restraints," has led to a great deal of confusion and controversy about them. They are sometimes essential to humane management and can wonderfully calm frightened, agitated, hallucinating, or desperately disturbed individuals for whom other measures, such as environmental modification and behavioral handling, are insufficient.

> *Many Alzheimer's patients' lives will be enhanced by psychotropic medications such as antidepressants, antipsychotics, and minor tranquilizers. Use of such medications should not be denied for fear of side effects alone nor forbidden by well-meaning family members.*

Public outcry about the overuse of antipsychotics in nursing homes led in part to federal regulations included in OBRA 1987,[87] which mandated that those prescribing antipsychotics in nursing homes justify their use, document their effectiveness or side effects, and follow-up, discontinuing them as soon as possible. No one likes to be regulated, but all of these are perfectly reasonable approaches to these powerful, useful medications.[88]

The place of antipsychotics is limited to certain specific target symptoms, basically symptoms of psychosis, occurring in patients with dementia: severe mental agitation and fearfulness, agitation with breakthrough aggressiveness or recurrent catastrophic reactions, sundowning syndrome, disturbing hallucinations, actual paranoia, and uncorrectable and disturbing delusional states. Antipsychotics are also useful in rendering an uncooperatively aggressive or dangerously restless (or wandering) patient easier to redirect.

Sometimes antipsychotics are the only answer for patients suffering from meaningless, anxiety-provoking, racing thoughts that they cannot grasp or articulate and that trouble them, causing them to scream or strike out. Such patients sometimes benefit from an antidepressant in addition to or instead of an antipsychotic.

Simple insomnia does not require an antipsychotic, nor does wandering; these medications can be used in combination with behavioral and environmental techniques to calm and comfort these troubled patients.

Many health professionals fear antipsychotics because of the production of parkinsonism and anticholinergic and orthostatic effects. These do indeed limit their usefulness but are fortunately generally reversible on discontinuation of the medication. The less anticholinergic, high-potency medications are preferred (see Table 17-4). The butyrophenone, haloperidol (Haldol), is relatively nonsedating and more of a pure antipsychotic; thioridazine (Mellaril), for which there is much literature, is anticholinergic and orthostatic as well as heavily sedative. Thiothixene (Navane) has a useful place somewhere between these two extremes as a sedative antipsychotic of high potency and low dose. Diphenhydramine (Benadryl), available over the counter as an antihistamine, is often used to tranquilize older individuals at night, but it has a high anticholinergic profile and is more a sedative than an antipsychotic. It comes in many pro-

Table 17-4   Major Tranquilizers Most Frequently Used in Dementia

Drug	Starting Daily Dose (Range)	Starting Night Dose (Range)	Parenteral
Thioridazine (Mellaril): more sedative, more anticholinergic, less extrapyramidal, low potency/high dose	10-30 mg (10-200 mg)	10-25 mg (10-200 mg)	Not recommended
Haloperidol (Haldol): less sedative, less anticholinergic, more extrapyramidal, high potency/low dose	1-3 mg (1-15 mg)	0.5-1 mg (0.5-10 mg)	0.5-2 mg
Thiothixene (Navane): similar to haloperidol, possibly less extrapyramidal	1-3 mg (1-45 mg)	0.5-2 mg (0.5-10 mg)	1-2 mg

prietary preparations along with acetaminophen as a pain-relieving sleep aid (e.g., Tylenol PM). If sedation rather than antipsychotic activity is required or if the patient's symptoms could be better characterized as anxiety than psychotic agitation, a minor tranquilizer such as lorazepam (Ativan) may be preferable.

Titrating the dose of an antipsychotic in a persistently agitated and disturbed patient with dementia must be done slowly and carefully, although in an emergency situation the dose can be increased at intervals of only a few days. However, it is often the development of side effects that defines the optimal dose (i.e., the dose that is just less than the one at which side effects or oversedation occurs). Often the therapeutic window is wide enough that the patient can be calmed without sedation, but sometimes that window is narrow, or the patient is oversedated and still not "calm." Lowering the dose or carefully combining it with low doses of short-acting minor tranquilizers such as lorazepam may then be the answer. The sedating antidepressant trazodone (Desyrel) has been widely used for agitated patients with dementia (some believe that screaming behaviors may be a "depressive equivalent"), but trazodone also has directly tranquilizing properties. Occasionally the calming effect of anticonvulsants such as valproic acid (or devalproex [Depakote]) may be useful for short-term sedation. Each individual's response is unique, so it is necessary to modify the dose carefully and maintain careful observation to find the optimal drug for the individual patient's situation.

> The prescription of any psychoactive drug in an elder is a "therapeutic trial."

Psychiatric consultation can be helpful at times in acutely disturbed situations. Unfortunately, the differentiation at federal level between mental illness and dementia makes mental health services virtually unavailable to patients with dementia of Alzheimer's or other types. The result is that psychiatric situations must be handled in general medical units and in nursing homes. This is why primary care physicians caring for elders must be familiar and comfortable with the use of psychiatrically active drugs.

It is not recommended that antiparkinsonian agents be routinely given with the antipsychotics. Should extrapyramidal symptoms occur and the medication be required, antiparkinsonian medications (e.g., benztropine [Cogentin]) can be considered. There is, however, the possibility that they will increase mental confusion. Extrapyramidal symptoms to watch for include cogwheel rigidity of the extremities (particularly the arms), tremor, stooped posture, flat facies, shuffling gait, drooling, oculogyric crises, and (clinically unimportant but an early sign that extrapyramidal syndrome [EPS] is about to oc-

cur) fine, fibrillatory tongue movements. The latter are to be differentiated from the rhythmic chewing or lip-smacking movements of the lower face, tongue, or mouth that characterize tardive dyskinesia (TD), a dystonic reaction that occasionally persists after the drug is stopped. Akathisia, the irresistible urge to move around, is the other major movement disorder to watch for. Also important is the neuroleptic malignant syndrome (NMS), which is characterized by fever, confusion, and seizures. It can be fatal, although, fortunately, its occurrence is rare. A patient who has had NMS should probably not be allowed exposure to antipsychotics again.

The new antipsychotic risperidone (Risperdal) is developing a significant clinical place, with its better side effect profile. It can be wonderfully effective, with much less chance of EPS than the others.

Where are the data? Much of this section is based on my clinical experiences and the experiences of others.[89] Given the complexity of influences (environment, staff, caregiver experience) and the absolute uniqueness of the individual patient in terms of both response and side effect profile (as well as physical and emotional health), it has been difficult indeed to conduct rigorous therapeutic trials. Some authoritative bodies, including the Alzheimer's Association, merely imply that psychotropics "*may* be useful" but give a heavy warning that they may do harm. Many clinicians believe that excessive conservatism in the prescription of psychotropics leads to unnecessary suffering. Carefully prescribed and followed up, they have a vital clinical function (temporarily) in selected patients. But the prescriber must ensure that every possible environmental and behavioral modification is also made and that the staff and family are well trained. Medications complement, but do not substitute for, the powerful effects that can be achieved by well-trained, warm, and loving individuals who are concerned about calming and redirecting painful and disruptive behaviors.

> Always ensure that everyone involved knows the target symptoms of a psychoactive drug; these are as important as the potential side effects.

In summary:
- Antipsychotics are absolutely essential in the management of a small proportion of patients with dementia, although families and professionals are frequently prejudiced against their use.
- When prescribing any psychoactive drug for an elder, the physician has the important task of specifying the target symptoms so that everyone involved (including family, nurses, and the patient at times) can effectively help in what is always a "therapeutic trial."

- Compliance with medications, particularly psychoactive ones, is enhanced by active follow-up: call the family and see how it is going.

Antidepressants

Antidepressants are also important in the treatment of dementia. Depression occurs with increased frequency in the early phases, leading to worsening of the cognitive and functional impact of early dementia. It is a treatable element that must be sought aggressively and treated with enthusiasm. DSM-IV criteria can be applied, but a trial of antidepressant is reasonable when there is a fairly abrupt onset (occuring over weeks or days) of functional or frank mood deterioration in a patient with early dementia, especially if any vegetative symptoms (sleep disturbance, diurnal variation in mood, appetite change, change in energy level, or actual sadness of mood) are concurrent and persist for 2 weeks or more. Newer agents such as the SSRIs and bupropion are particularly favored rather than older tricyclics with anticholinergic effects.

Depression can occur at any stage during the dementia, and in late dementia persistent sadness of mood or content of speech may also respond to antidepressants. The phenothiazine-like antidepressant amoxapine can be useful in such sometimes deeply melancholic, severely demented individuals. ECT has been successfully used in patients with dementia when depression is severe or persistent or when life-threatening problems such as complete failure of oral intake make treatment urgent. Other measures such as the therapeutic use of light have been tried on a small scale and are reasonable to add as adjunctive therapy. As with other depressed patients, exercise or any activity can be therapeutic.

Anxiolytics and Hypnotics

Short-acting minor tranquilizers, such as the benzodiazepine lorazepam (Ativan), can be useful in the constantly ruminating, anxious-appearing patient with dementia; they can also be useful for acute, short-term tranquilization for procedures. Lorazepam has been used quite effectively as an alternative to antipsychotics in severely disturbed patients, and it can sometimes be given on a regular and continuing basis for weeks or even months if effective. Often the "window" between sleepiness and unsteadiness or the relief of symptoms of anxiety and agitation is narrow, however. Long-acting benzodiazepines like diazepam are generally avoided because of their tendency to cause dysfunction.

The same stricture applies to using hypnotics continuously: the long-acting ones that have more chance of sustaining sleep through the night are associated with dysfunction the following day, and they are generally avoided. There is, however, a place for short-acting hypnotics sometimes: when it is important to initiate sleep and to correct sleep hygiene problems. Chloral hydrate and the more recent short-acting medication zolpidem (Ambien) are occasionally useful for short-term use in attempts to restore sleeping patterns and during relocations and other special circumstances.

CARING FOR THE CAREGIVER

The proactive management implied in this chapter involves establishing close rapport between the physician and the caregivers. Caregivers must be taught the techniques to calm and redirect "their" patient.

Self-help organizations, particularly the Alzheimer's Association through local chapters and its national organization, exist to improve education and support of caregivers.

Many other support services are available in some communities but not in others. Respite programs, day care programs, and senior centers are examples of the range of services that, if well used, can improve caregivers' efficiency and durability and thus lengthen the time that patients with dementia can continue to be managed in their familiar home setting.

ADVICE TO THE CAREGIVER AND FAMILY

1. Be realistic about the nature of the illness and plan accordingly.
2. Recognize your personal need for help and respite. Seek respite, accept it, and pay for it if necessary.
3. Seek a support group, usually through the Alzheimer's Association, for specific advice and psychological support.
4. Make communication within the family optimal so that the caregiving burden is shared among family members.
5. Ensure optimal caregiver health: enough sleep, exercise, and social contacts.
6. Remember that there will be life after the patient is gone.
7. Become informed about the illness to anticipate problems and to plan strategies.
8. Plan financial and legal aspects early, including the will, placement, and intensity of treatment issues.
9. Be aware of the most positive and important work of the caregiver: to continually find and optimize the preserved function of the patient. This not only reduces the burden but increases the quality of life of the patient and the caregiver and increases the quality of their relationship to each other.

POSTTEST

1. Which one of the following is not consistent with the diagnosis of delirium?
   a. Attention wanders during interview
   b. Incoherent speech
   c. Onset over weeks
   d. Onset over days
   e. Hallucinations

2. Which one of the following is not among a feature of the syndrome dementia?
   a. Progression of symptoms over time
   b. Impaired short-term memory
   c. Impaired speech
   d. Personality change
   e. Impaired abstract thinking

3. Which one of the following statements concerning the distinction of delirium from dementia is false?
   a. Delirium may last for weeks.
   b. Consciousness is not clouded in dementia until it is terminal.
   c. Hallucinations are common early in delirium.
   d. Disorientation occurs earlier in dementia.
   e. The onset of delirium can be dated.

4. Which one of the following features would be inconsistent with the diagnosis of dementia of Alzheimer's type (DAT)?
   a. Nonspecific (slow-wave) changes on the electroencephalogram
   b. Normal lumbar puncture results
   c. Onset at age 45 years
   d. Early gait disturbance
   e. Weight loss

5. Which one of the following features is not suggestive of vascular dementia rather than dementia of Alzheimer's type?
   a. Periods of improvement
   b. Associated hypertension
   c. Pseudobulbar palsy
   d. Early gait changes
   e. Late seizures

6. Which one of the following features is not suggestive of depression rather than dementia?
   a. Short duration
   b. Previous psychiatric history
   c. Concealing disabilities
   d. "Don't know" answers
   e. Diurnal variation in mood

7. Which one of the following tests is not recommended in all patients with dementia?
   a. Thyroid-stimulating hormone
   b. Brain imaging
   c. Hemoglobin and hematocrit
   d. Serological test for syphilis

8. Which one of the following antidepressants is least generally recommended in older persons?
   a. Fluoxetine
   b. Amitriptyline
   c. Desipramine
   d. Nortriptyline

9. Which one of the following is not a suitable target symptom for the use of a major tranquilizer in a demented patient?
   a. Aggressiveness
   b. Persistent mental agitation
   c. Wandering
   d. Hallucinations
   e. Sundowning syndrome

10. Which one of the following is not tested in the Folstein Mini–Mental State examination?
    a. Spelling WORLD backwards
    b. Drawing intersecting pentagons
    c. Remembering three names for several minutes
    d. Naming the current president
    e. Performing a three-stage command

11. Which of the following statements, important to caregivers, is false?
    a. Disordered sleep heads the list of patient characteristics stressing caregivers.
    b. There is convincing evidence that patients with dementia have more driving accidents than those without dementia.
    c. Catastrophic reactions can be induced by too much input of any kind.
    d. Hallucinations in Alzheimer's disease are generally not threatening to the patient.

12. Which of the following statements concerning legal issues in dementia is false?
    a. A conservator is appointed by the court only if there is evidence of incompetency.
    b. A durable power of attorney retains authority when the patient becomes incompetent.
    c. A health care proxy is legally recognized as identifying the individual to make health care decisions.
    d. A committee is an individual appointed to make health care decisions for someone who is impaired.

REFERENCES

1. McKhann G, Drackman D, Folstein M: Clinical diagnosis of Alzheimer's disease, *Neurology* 34:939-944, 1984.
2. *Diagnostic and statistical manual of mental disorders* (DSM-IV), ed 4, Washington, DC, 1994, American Psychiatric Association.
3. Inouye SK et al: A predictive model for delirium in hospitalized elderly medical patients based on admission characteristics, *Ann Intern Med* 119:474-481, 1993.
4. Trzepacz PT, Teague GB, Lipowski ZJ: Delirium and other organic mental disorders in a general hospital, *Gen Hosp Psychiatry* 7:101-106, 1985.
5. Dicks R, Besdine RW, Levkoff SE: Delirium. In Ham RJ, ed: *Geriatric medicine annual 1989,* Oradell, NJ, 1989, Medical Economics Books.
6. Lipowski ZJ: Transient cognitive disorders (delirium, acute confusional states) in the elderly, *Am J Psychiatry* 140:1426-1436, 1983.
7. Oppenheim G: The earliest signs of Alzheimer's disease, *J Geriatr Psychiatry Neurol* 7:116-120, 1994.
8. McCormick WC et al: Symptom patterns and comorbidity in the early stages of Alzheimer's disease, *J Am Geriatr Soc* 42:517-521, 1994.
9. Folstein M, Folstein S, McHugh P: Mini mental state, a practical method for grading the cognitive state of patients for the clinician, *J Psychiatry Res* 12:187-198, 1975.
10. Pfeiffer E: A short portable mental status questionnaire for assessment of organic brain deficit in elderly patients, *J Am Geriatr Soc* 23:433-441, 1975.
11. Blessed G, Tomlinson BE, Roth M: The association between quantitative measures of dementia and of senile change in the cerebral gray matter of elderly subjects, *Br J Psychiatry* 114:797-811, 1968.
12. Babikian VL et al: Cognitive changes in patients with multiple cerebral infarcts, *Stroke* 21:1013-1018, 1990.
13. Cummings JL et al: Neuropsychiatric aspects of multi-infarct dementia and the dementia of the Alzheimer type, *Arch Neurol* 44:389-393, 1987.
14. Hachinski VC, Lassen NA, Marshall J: Multi-infarct dementia, a cause of mental deterioration in the elderly, *Lancet* 2:207, 1974.
15. Sultzer DL et al: A comparison of psychiatric symptoms in vascular dementia and Alzheimer's disease, *Am J Psychiatry* 150:1806-1812, 1993.
16. Cooper JK, Mungas D: Risk factor and behavioral differences between vascular and Alzheimer's dementias: the pathway to end-stage disease, *J Geriatr Psychiatry Neurol* 1:29-33, 1993.
17. Hayden MR: *Huntington's chorea,* New York, 1981, Springer-Verlag.
18. Wechsler AF et al: Pick's disease, *Arch Neurol* 39:287-290, 1982.
19. Brown P et al: Creutzfeldt-Jakob disease: clinical analysis of a consecutive series of two-hundred and thirty neuropathologically verified cases, *Ann Neurol* 20:597-602, 1986.
20. Clarfield AM: The reversible dementias: do they reverse? *Ann Intern Med* 109:476-486, 1988.
21. Barry PP, Moskowitz MA: The diagnosis of reversible dementia in the elderly: a critical review, *Arch Intern Med* 148:1914-1918, 1988.
22. Larson EB et al: Dementia in elderly out-patients: a prospective study, *Ann Intern Med* 100:417-423, 1984.
23. Larson EB et al: Diagnostic evaluation of two-hundred elderly out-patients with suspected dementia, *J Gerontol* 40(5):536-543, 1985.
24. Wells CE: Pseudodementia, *Am J Psychiatry* 36:895-900, 1979.
25. Reifler BV, Larson E, Hanley R: Co-existence of cognitive impairment and depression in geriatric out-patients, *Am J Psychiatry* 139:623-626, 1982.
26. Alexopoulos GS et al: The course of geriatric depression with "reversible dementia": a controlled study, *Am J Psychiatry* 150:1693-1699, 1993.
27. Yesavage JA, Brink TL: Development and validation of a geriatric depression screening scale: a preliminary report, *J Psychiatry Res* 17:37-49, 1983.
28. Feher EP, Larrabee GJ, Crook TH III: Factors attenuating the validity of the geriatric depression scale in a dementia population, *J Am Geriatr Soc* 40:906-909, 1992.
29. Wells CE: *Dementia,* Philadelphia, 1977, FA Davis.
30. Cummings JL: Intellectual impairment in Parkinson's disease: clinical, biochemical and pathologic correlates, *J Geriatr Psychiatry Neurol* 1:24-36, 1988.
31. Stern Y et al: Comparison of cognitive changes in patients with Alzheimer's and Parkinson's disease, *Arch Neurol* 50:1040-1045, 1993.
32. Jagust WJ, Eberling JL: MRI, CT, SPECT, PET: their use in diagnosing dementia, *Geriatrics* 46:28-35, 1991.
33. Mortimer JA et al: Head trauma as a risk factor for Alzheimer's disease: a collaborative re-analysis of case-control studies, *Int J Epidemiol* 20:S28-S35, 1991.
34. Facekas F et al: Comparison of CT, MR and PET in Alzheimer's dementia and normal aging, *J Nucl Med* 30:1067-1615, 1989.
35. Johnson KA et al: Comparison of magnetic resonance and roentgen ray computed tomography in dementia, *Arch Neurol* 44:1075-1080, 1987.
36. Holman BL et al: The scintigraphic appearance of Alzheimer's disease: a prospective study using technetium-99-HMPAO SPECT, *J Nucl Med* 33:181-185, 1992.
37. Duara R et al: Positron emission tomography in Alzheimer's disease, *Neurology* 36:879-887, 1986.
38. Chase TN et al: Regional cortical dysfunction in Alzheimer's disease as determined by positron emission tomography, *Ann Neurol* 15:5170-5174, 1984.
39. Schellenberg GD et al: Genetic linkage evidence for a familial Alzheimer's disease locus on chromosome 14, *Science* 258:668-671, 1992.
40. Saunders AM et al: Association of apolipoprotein E allele ε4 with late-onset familial and sporadic Alzheimer's disease, *Neurology* 43:1467-1472, 1993.
41. Yuce et al: The apolipoprotein E/CI/CII gene cluster and late-onset Alzheimer disease, *Am J Hum Genet* 54:631-642, 1994.
42. Corder EH et al: Protective effect of apolipoprotein E type 2 allele for late onset Alzheimer disease, *Nature Genet* 7:180-184, 1994.
43. Small GW et al: Apolipoprotein E type 4 allele and cerebral glucose metabolism in relatives at risk for familial Alzheimer's disease, *JAMA* 273(12):942-947, 1995.
44. Katzman R: Education and the prevalence of dementia and Alzheimer's disease, *Neurology* 43:13-20, 1993.
45. Stern Y et al: Influence of education and occupation on the incidence of Alzheimer's disease, *JAMA* 271:1004-1010, 1994.
46. Strittmatter WJ et al: Apolipoprotein E: high-avidity binding to β-amyloid and increased frequency of type 4 allele in late-onset familial Alzheimer disease, *Proc Natl Acad Sci* 90:1977-1981, 1993.
47. Murrell J et al: A mutation in the amyloid precursor protein associated with hereditary Alzheimer's disease, *Science* 254:97-99, 1991.
48. Joachim CL, Selkoe DJ: The seminal role of β-amyloid in the pathogenesis of Alzheimer disease, *Alzheimer Dis Assoc Disord* 6:7-34, 1992.
49. Olson L: NGF and the treatment of Alzheimer's disease, *Exp Neurol* 124:5-15, 1993.
50. Tuszynski MH et al: Recombinant human nerve growth factor in-

fusions prevent cholinergic neuronal degeneration in the adult primate brain, *Ann Neurol* 30:625-636, 1991.

51. Zandi T, Ham RJ, eds: *New directions in understanding dementia in Alzheimer's disease,* New York, 1990, Plenum Press.

52. Davies: Theoretical treatment possibilities for dementia of the Alzheimer's type: the cholinergic hypothesis. In Crook T, Gershon S, eds: *Strategies for further development of an effective treatment for senile dementia,* New Canaan, Conn, 1981, Mark Powley Associates.

53. Bartus RT et al: The cholinergic hypothesis of geriatric memory dysfunction, *Science* 217:408-417, 1981.

54. Knapp MJ for the Tacrine Study Group: A 30-week randomized controlled trial of high-dose tacrine in patients with Alzheimer's disease, *JAMA* 271:985-991, 1994.

55. Davis KL for the Tacrine Collaborative Study Group: A double-blind, placebo-controlled multicenter study of tacrine for Alzheimer's disease, *N Engl J Med* 327:1253-1259, 1992.

56. Farlow M for the Tacrine Study Group: A controlled trial of tacrine in Alzheimer's disease, *JAMA* 268:2523-2529, 1992.

57. Thompson TL III et al: Lack of efficacy of hydergine in patients with Alzheimer's disease, *N Engl J Med* 323:445-448, 1990.

58. Brenner DE et al: Relationship between cigarette smoking and Alzheimer's disease in a population-based case-control study, *Neurology* 43:293-300, 1993.

59. Sommers WK et al: Use of THA in the treatment of Alzheimer-like dementia: pilot study in twelve patients, *Biol Psychiatry* 16:145-153, 1981.

60. Manning FC: Tacrine therapy for the dementia of Alzheimer's disease, *Am Fam Physician* 50(4):819-823, 1994.

61. Watkins PB et al: Hepatotoxic effects of tacrine administration in patients with Alzheimer's disease, *JAMA* 271:992-998, 1994.

62. Rogers J et al: Clinical trial of indomethacin in Alzheimer's disease, Neurology 43:1609-1611, 1993.

63. Mace NL, Rabins BV: *The thirty-six-hour day: a family guide,* Baltimore, 1981, Johns Hopkins University Press.

64. Cohen D, Eisdorfer C: *The loss of self: a family resource for the care of Alzheimer's disease and related disorders,* New York, 1986, WW Norton.

65. Aronson M, ed: *Understanding Alzheimer's disease,* New York, 1988, Charles Scribner's Sons.

66. Ham RJ: Alzheimer's and the family. In Ham RI, ed: *Geriatric medicine annual 1987,* Oradell, NJ, 1987, Medical Economics Books.

67. Brody EM: The long haul: a family odyssey. In Jarvik L, Winograd CH, eds: *Treatment for the Alzheimer's patient, the long haul,* New York, 1988, Springer-Verlag.

68. Rabins PV, Mace NL, Lucas MJ: The impact of dementia on the family, *JAMA* 248-333, 1982.

69. Chatterjee A et al: Personality changes in Alzheimer's disease, *Arch Neurol* 49:486-491, 1992.

70. Caranasos GJ et al: Caregivers of the demented elderly, *J Fla Med Assoc* 72:266-270, 1985.

71. Gwyther LP, Matteson MA: Care for the caregivers, *J Gerontol Nurse* 9:93-116, 1983.

72. Winograd CH, Jarvik LF: Physician management of the demented patient, *J Am Geriatr Soc* 34:295-308, 1986.

73. Gwyther LP, Blazer DG: Family therapy on the dementia patient, *Am Fam Physician* 29:149-156, 1984.

74. Petersen RC et al: Memory function in normal aging, *Neurology* 42:396-401, 1992.

75. Hunt L et al: Driving performance in person with mild senile dementia of the Alzheimer's type, *J Am Geriatr Soc* 41:747-753, 1993.

76. Donnelly RE, Karlinsky H: The impact of Alzheimer's disease on driving ability: a review, *J Geriatr Psychiatry Neurol* 3:67-72, 1990.

77. Drachman DA for the Collaborative Study Group: Driving and Alzheimer's disease: the risk of crashes, *Neurology* 43:2448-2456, 1993.

78. Hunt L et al: Driving performance in persons with mild senile dementia of the Alzheimer's type, *J Am Geriatr Soc* 41:747-753, 1993.

79. Donnelly RE, Karlinsky H: The impact of Alzheimer's disease on driving ability: a review, *J Geriatr Psychiatry Neurol* 3:67-72, 1990.

80. Bliwise DL et al: Sleep and "sundowning" in nursing home patients with dementia, *Psychiatry Res* 48:277-292, 1993.

81. Satlin A et al: Bright light treatment of behavioral and sleep disturbances in patients with Alzheimer's disease, *Am J Psychiatry* 149:1028-1032, 1992.

82. McCann RM, Hall WJ, Groth-Juncker A: Comfort care for terminally care patients: the appropriate use of nutrition and hydration, *JAMA* 272(16):1263-1266, 1994.

83. Cohen D: Dementia, depression and nutritional status. In Ham RJ, ed: Nutrition in old age, *Primary Care Clinics in Office Practice* 21(1):107-120, 1994, WB Saunders.

84. Romanelli MF et al: Advanced Alzheimer's disease is a risk factor for late-onset seizures, *Arch Neurol* 47:847-850, 1990.

85. Cassel CK, Hays JR, Lynn J: Alzheimer's: decisions in terminal care, *Patient Care* 125-137, 1991.

86. Ham RJ: New Perspectives on long term care. In Reichel W, ed: *Clinical aspects of aging,* ed 2, Baltimore, 1984, Williams & Wilkins.

87. *Omnibus Budget Reconciliation Act 1987,* Washington, DC, 1989, US Government Printing Office.

88. Rovner BW et al: The impact of antipsychotic drug regulations on psychotropic prescribing practices in nursing homes, *Am J Psychiatry* 149:1390-1392, 1992.

89. Ham RJ: Medication and the management of dementia, *NH Practitioner* (1):7-16, 1994.

90. Consultant Dietitians in Health Care Facilities: Dining skills: practical skills for the caregivers of eating-disabled older adults, Chicago, 1992, American Dietetic Association.

PRETEST ANSWERS

1. b
2. c
3. a
4. c

POSTTEST ANSWERS

1. c
2. a
3. d
4. d
5. e
6. c
7. b
8. b
9. c
10. d
11. b
12. a

CHAPTER 18

Depression and Failure to Thrive

J. EUGENE LAMMERS and RICHARD J. HAM

OBJECTIVES

On completion of this chapter, the reader will be able to:

1. Distinguish between major depression, adjustment disorder with depressed mood, bereavement, and dysthymia.

2. Describe differences in presentation of depression in the elderly compared with younger persons.

3. List the physical illnesses associated with depressed mood.

4. List the common medications associated with depression.

5. Understand the importance of history, including the use of screening tools, in the diagnosis of depression.

6. Order appropriate diagnostic tests to evaluate depressed mood.

7. Choose appropriate treatment options for depression, including both pharmacological and nonpharmacological therapy.

8. Recognize urgent cases that need hospitalization or referral to a psychiatrist.

9. Explain the role of electroconvulsive therapy (ECT) to a patient and family and be able to assist a psychiatrist in medical management of it.

PRETEST

1. Which one of the following statements regarding depression is false?
   a. Treatment of depression in the elderly is difficult because the elderly do not respond well to antidepressant medications.
   b. Many depressed elderly patients do not report feelings of dysphoria.
   c. Despite their association with anorexia and weight loss, selective serotonin reuptake inhibitors (SSRIs) are the current antidepressant drugs of choice in the elderly.
   d. Elderly depressed patients respond better to counseling plus antidepressant medication than to medication alone.

2. Which of the following antidepressants cannot be used effectively in elderly patients in a single daily dose?
   a. Nortriptyline
   b. Fluoxetine
   c. Paroxetine
   d. Venlafaxine

3. Referral to a psychiatrist or geriatric medicine specialist should be considered in all of the following situations except for which one?
   a. A depressed patient develops increased nervousness after 3 weeks of fluoxetine therapy.
   b. A depressed elderly white man expresses suicidal thoughts.
   c. A depressed patient continues to have inadequate oral intake despite antidepressant therapy.
   d. A depressed patient fails to respond to an adequate trial of two different classes of antidepressant.

4. Diagnostic evaluation of patients with depressive symptoms should include all of the following except for which one?
   a. TSH
   b. Complete blood count
   c. CT brain scan
   d. Electrolytes

▼ THOMAS XING (Part I)

Mr. Xing is brought to your office with the history that he has not been doing well since the death of his wife 18 months ago. He had cared for her during a long illness, and after her death, shortly before their fifty-second anniversary, he became withdrawn from his family, lost weight, was sleeping poorly, and seemed to have increasing problems with his memory.

▼ CLARA KNIGHTON (Part I)

Clara Knighton is a 78-year-old retired nurse, who is brought to live in your area by her niece. While visiting her aunt, the niece discovered Mrs. Knighton's home to be unkempt, with little food in the house. The niece found that her aunt had lost over 50 pounds in weight. Neighbors confirmed that she had been having a significant downward decline in her physical and mental status for the previous 6 months.

▼ MARTHA JENKINS (Part I)

Martha Jenkins is a 77-year-old woman who has been your patient for over 20 years. She has lived in the assisted living section of a retirement community for 5 years. She comes to you for help with her osteoporosis and compression fractures, which have limited her mobility and cause significant pain.

▼ BETTY POLZINSKI (Part I)

Betty Polzinski is an 84-year-old nursing home patient, newly assigned to you. She is described by staff as a very unpleasant, unrewarding, sarcastic, and manipulative patient, who resists all attempts by the staff to help her out of bed. When the aides lift her out of bed so that she can sit in the chair, although she does not appear to have pain, she screams, yells, and curses at them.

STUDY QUESTIONS

- One diagnosis is a possibility in all four of these cases, but what is the differential diagnosis in each case?
- What information would you seek in order to confirm or exclude the possibility of depression?

"FAILURE TO THRIVE"

The commonly encountered constellation of signs and symptoms that has been characterized as "failure to thrive" in the elderly is one of the most challenging diagnostic dilemmas. Presentations can include fatigue, anorexia, weight loss, functional decline, loss of interest in activities, and medical noncompliance. Other symptoms can include a lack of motivation, unwillingness to participate in activities, unwillingness to eat or be fed, increased dependency, reduced functionality, apparent apathy, or a lack of drive. Sometimes failure to thrive is demonstrated by a previously aggressive patient who becomes benign and accepting instead of feisty and objectionable. In all of these cases a search for reversible causes needs to be diligently and appropriately focused. Depression, with or without accompanying chronic or acute medical diseases, should always be considered as a possible diagnosis.

Depression is so common that it must be sought in all ill elders, especially those who are "failing to thrive."

DEPRESSION

Depression is the most common of the affective disorders seen by primary care physicians.[1] Depending on the diagnostic criteria used, major depression and related disorders affect between 5% and 20% of persons over age 65 living in the community.[2] Depression is even more common in acutely ill hospitalized elderly patients, with a prevalence of 25% noted in some studies. Nursing home residents also have a very high prevalence of 25% to 40%.[3]

Suicide is associated with depression in the elderly, as it is with other age groups. Elderly white men have the highest rate of suicide of the entire adult population.[4-6] Atypical presentation, concomitant acute and chronic diseases, and widely held myths regarding the affect and personality of older persons are among the reasons that depression is often overlooked.[7,8] DSM-IV criteria are useful in distinguishing major depression from other depressive syndromes, such as adjustment reactions, dysthymia, and bereavement.[9] While the stresses found in the life histories of many older adults can lead to sadness and depressed mood, true clinical depression is not a part of the normal aging process. Depression is associated with functional decline and excess mortality, and it should be enthusiastically sought and frequently suspected so that it is both diagnosed and treated whenever possible.

Diagnosis

Diagnosing depression in the elderly is often difficult. Rather than having symptoms of depressed mood or crying spells, older persons are likely to have nonspecific somatic complaints, such as fatigue, abdominal pain, or headache. Family members may bring the patient to the physician with a presentation of "just not doing well." Somatic complaints may be even more prominent in persons with limited education and no previous psychiatric history. The other common syndrome for the presentation of depression in old age is what is now called the "dementia syndrome of depression," in which the patient presents with an apparent dementia but of a generally

more recent and abrupt onset than the more common types of progressive dementia such as Alzheimer's disease; of course, such a presentation with cognitive impairment is often further disguised from the clinician, since families frequently do not notice cognitive impairment but rather notice the effects of it, such as functional decline or an apparent lack of motivation or interest.[6,10,11]

"The dementia syndrome of depression" is now preferred to the term "pseudodementia"; the patient has depression, which can be treated and will resolve, even though it looks like dementia.

As so often occurs in situations with elders, it is frequently a family member who brings the patient to the physician. However, especially if the depression has been persistent and unaddressed, the spouse or other family members may have become depressed themselves or begun to feel hopeless about the situation; this is significant because the physician must frequently rely on family members to assist in compliance with treatment and to observe its effects.

Depression should be regarded as a communicable disease.

The diagnosis of depression should be considered in all older persons who report somatic symptoms, particularly those having chronic symptoms that appear to have no definite organic basis. However, because of the association of depressive symptoms with many medical illnesses, a full medical workup should be performed before saying that it is "just" depression.[12] Patients with nonspecific symptoms such as weight loss, malaise, low energy, and fatigue, should be evaluated for untreated medical causes before the diagnosis of depression is made. Many elders have several concurrent illnesses, some of which may first be discovered during the "depression workup." Major depression and other less specific depressive symptoms are associated with many medical illnesses, including stroke, thyroid disorders, Parkinson's disease, heart disease, and dementia. Stroke is a particularly important factor, with 60% of patients suffering major depression in their first year after a stroke; those with a left-sided cerebrovascular accident (CVA) are particularly predisposed to depression. It is also recognized that major depression occurring in the first 6 months following myocardial infarction actually increases the mortality. (This has been demonstrated to be because of the physical effect of the depression in increasing parasympathetic tone.) Box 18-1 summarizes these illnesses. Screening for underlying malignancy, endocrinopathies, and other metabolic disorders is warranted, and a careful history and physical examination should be performed to detect other medical problems such as clinically silent ischemia or stroke, both of which can lead to depression. Concomitant medical problems can not only contribute to depression but also influence the choice of therapy.[13,14]

> *"Depression without sadness" well expresses what is often seen, but the sadness is usually there, if sought, hidden behind cognitive or somatic symptoms that mask the diagnosis.*

In addition to medical illnesses, certain medications are associated with causing depressive symptoms; such medications include digitalis, propranolol, and the benzodiazepines. An in-depth review of potential side effects of all the patient's prescription and over-the-counter medications must be done, since the list of medications potentially implicated in depression is long[15,16] (Box 18-2).

Assessment and Investigation

Assessment of the patient with failure to thrive or symptoms suggestive of depression includes a complete history and physical examination, with particular emphasis on the history of the present illness, the past history of similar symptoms, and a review of systems. Screening laboratory work should be performed, with more specialized testing performed depending on the particular case. All patients should be screened for malignancy, renal and liver disease, and electrolyte abnormalities; a CBC, chemistry panel, and chest x-ray examination should also be performed. In addition, T_4 and TSH measurements should be ordered for all patients in order to address the possibility of hypothyroidism or hyperthyroidism. Vitamin B_{12} and folate should be evaluated as they would be in patients with cognitive changes, for they are also seen in association with depression. The possibility of rheumatological diseases such as polymyalgia rheumatica or rheumatoid arthritis can be screened

---

BOX 18-1
Medical Illnesses Associated With Depression

Metabolic Disturbances

Dehydration
Azotemia, uremia
Acid-base disturbances
Hypoxia
Hyponatremia and hypernatremia
Hypoglycemia and hyperglycemia
Hypocalcemia and hypercalcemia

Endocrine

Hypothyroidism and hyperthyroidism
Hyperparathyroidism
Diabetes mellitus
Cushing's disease
Addison's disease

Infections

Pneumonia
Encephalitis
Urinary tract infection
Meningitis
Endocarditis
Tuberculosis
Brucellosis
Fungal meningitis
Neurosyphilis

Cardiovascular

Congestive heart failure
Myocardial infarction, angina

Pulmonary

Chronic obstructive lung disease
Malignancy

Gastrointestinal

Malignancy (especially pancreatic)
Irritable bowel
Other (e.g., ulcer, diverticulosis)
Hepatitis

Genitourinary

Urinary incontinence

Musculoskeletal

Degenerative arthritis
Osteoporosis with vertebral compression or hip fractures
Polymyalgia rheumatica
Paget's disease

Neurological

Cerebrovascular disease
Transient ischemic attacks
Strokes
Dementia
Intracranial mass
   Primary or metastatic tumors
Parkinson's disease

Other

Anemia (of any cause)
Vitamin deficiencies
Hematological or other systemic malignancy

Data from Kane RL, Ouslander JG, Abrass IB, eds: *Essentials of clinical geriatrics,* ed 3, New York, 1994, McGraw-Hill; and Levenson AJ, Hall RCW, eds: *Neuropsychiatric manifestations of physical disorders in the elderly,* New York, 1981, Raven Press.

BOX 18-2
Drugs That Can Cause Symptoms of Depression

Antihypertensives

Reserpine
Methyldopa
Propranolol
Clonidine
Hydralazine
Guanethidine

Analgesics

Narcotic
   Morphine
   Codeine
   Meperidine
   Pentazocine
   Propoxyphene
Nonnarcotic
   Indomethacin

Antiparkinsonism Drugs

Levodopa

Antimicrobials

Sulfonamides
Isoniazid

Cardiovascular Preparations

Digitalis
Diuretics
Lidocaine

Hypoglycemic Agents

Psychotropic Agents

Sedatives
   Barbiturates
   Benzodiazepines
   Meprobamate
Antipsychotics
   Chlorpromazine
   Haloperidol
   Thiothixene
Hypnotics
   Chloral hydrate
   Flurazepam

Steroids

Corticosteroids
Estrogens

Other

Cimetidine
Cancer chemotherapeutic agents
Alcohol

Data from Kane RI, Ouslander JG, Abrass IB: *Essentials of clinical geriatrics,* ed 3, New York, 1994, McGraw-Hill; and Levenson AJ, Hall RCW, eds: *Neuropsychiatric manifestations of physical disorders in the elderly,* New York, 1981, Raven Press.

---

with an erythrocyte sedimentation rate (ESR) or other test depending on physical findings. A CT scan of the brain or MRI is indicated if there are neurological or cognitive abnormalities or unusual behavioral manifestations suggestive, for example, of frontal lobe problems. An electrocardiogram is useful as a baseline and may reveal cardiac disease, but it is specifically indicated before initiation of any antidepressants that influence cardiac conduction, such as the tricyclics.

It is always a clinical challenge to know how far to go with the workup of an older patient. Box 18-1 includes many of the conditions to be considered. The differential diagnosis of nonspecific symptoms such as weight loss or fatigue is long, and in many cases a precise medical diagnosis cannot be made if depression is discounted as a possible etiology of the problem. Fortunately, screening tests usually uncover serious occult disease presenting as depressive symptoms. If occult disease is not quickly found to precisely explain symptoms, a trial of antidepressant therapy should be initiated while further medical evaluation is pursued or while the patient's physical symptoms are carefully observed over time, with strict attention to the maintenance of compliance with follow-up.

If obvious causes are not quickly found in the patient whose health is failing, a trial of antidepressants should be initiated while the patient is further investigated and followed up.

The DSM-IV criteria for major depressive episode (MDE),[9] as well as the related disorders of dysthymia and adjustment disorder, would appear to be straightforward and easy to apply to the diagnosis of older persons with depression (Boxes 18-3 to 18-5). The patient and, if appropriate, the family are asked direct questions derived from these criteria. It is usually necessary to ask direct questions, since many of the symptoms are nonspecific or are misattributed by the patient or family. The history of previous depression, as well as any history of mania or hypomania (Box 18-6), should be thoroughly explored. A manic or hypomanic episode would also introduce the possibility of bipolar disorder. Unfortunately, as with many common illnesses, "different" presentations seem to be the rule in the elderly population (Box 18-7). Because of these difficulties, especially when as-

> ## BOX 18-3
> ### Criteria for Major Depressive Episode
>
> A. Five (or more) of the following symptoms have been present during the same 2-week period and represent a change from previous functioning; at least one of the symptoms is either (1) depressed mood or (2) loss of interest or pleasure.
>
> **Note:** Do not include symptoms that are clearly due to a general medical condition or mood-incongruent delusions or hallucinations.
>
> 1. Depressed mood most of the day, nearly every day, as indicated by either subjective report (e.g., feels sad or empty) or observation made by others (e.g., appears tearful)
> 2. Markedly diminished interest or pleasure in all, or almost all, activities most of the day, nearly every day (as indicated by either subjective account or observation made by others)
> 3. Significant weight loss when not dieting or weight gain (e.g., a change of more than 5% of body weight in a month) or decrease or increase in appetite nearly every day
> 4. Insomnia or hypersomnia nearly every day
> 5. Psychomotor agitation or retardation nearly every day (observable by others, not merely subjective feelings of restlessness or being slowed down)
> 6. Fatigue or loss of energy nearly every day
> 7. Feelings of worthlessness or excessive or inappropriate guilt (which may be delusional) nearly every day (not merely self-reproach or guilt about being sick)
> 8. Diminished ability to think or concentrate, or indecisiveness, nearly every day (either by subjective account or as observed by others)
> 9. Recurrent thoughts of death (not just fear of dying), recurrent suicidal ideation without a specific plan, or a suicide attempt or specific plan for committing suicide
>
> B. The symptoms do not meet criteria for a mixed episode. (See related box below.)
> C. The symptoms cause clinically significant distress or impairment in social, occupational, or other important areas of functioning.
> D. The symptoms are not due to the direct physiological effects of a substance (e.g., drug abuse, medication) or a general medical condition (e.g., hypothyroidism).
> E. The symptoms are not better accounted for by bereavement. After the loss of a loved one, the symptoms persist for longer than 2 months or are characterized by marked functional impairment, morbid preoccupation with worthlessness, suicidal ideation, psychotic symptoms, or psychomotor retardation.

From American Psychiatric Association: *Diagnostic and statistical manual of mental disorders* (DSM-IV), ed 4, Washington, DC, 1994, The Association.

> ## BOX 18-4
> ### Abbreviated Criteria for Adjustment Disorders with Depressed Mood
>
> A. Emotional or behavioral symptoms in response to an identifiable stressor within 3 months
> B. Either excessive distress or significant impairment of social or occupational functioning
> C. Do not meet the criteria for another clinical psychiatric disorder
> D. Do not represent bereavement
> E. Do not persist for more than an additional 6 months after the stressor is terminated

Modified from American Psychiatric Association: *Diagnostic and statistical manual of mental disorders* (DSM-IV), ed 4, Washington, DC, 1994, The Association.

sociated with other chronic diseases, a number of screening instruments have been developed and validated for use in elderly patients. These include the Geriatric Depression Scale (GDS; Box 18-8)[17] for outpatients and a scale (Box 18-9) for medically ill elderly inpatients.[18] These can be administered to such patients quickly, are easily reproducible, and correlate well with more traditional diagnostic evaluations such as structured psychiatric interviews. A "positive" score on one of these screening tools can increase the clinical suspicion of major depression as the primary etiology or as an associated finding. However, a "false negative" score can occur in a patient who is denying the symptoms or in somebody with "depression without sadness." These questionnaires do not replace specific questions directed toward uncovering vegetative symptoms of the type implied in the DSM-IV description of a major depressive episode. Use of such structured questionnaires should be strongly considered in primary care practices, since they can help keep the diagnosis of depression in the forefront as a pa-

BOX 18-5
Abbreviated Criteria for Dysthymia

A. Depressed mood for most of the day, for more days than not, for at least 2 years
B. While depressed, has two or more of the following:
   1. Poor appetite or overeating
   2. Insomnia or hypersomnia
   3. Low energy or fatigue
   4. Low self-esteem
   5. Poor concentration or decision-making capability
   6. Feeling of hopelessness
C. Never without the symptoms for more than 2 months at a time
D. No MDE present
E. No manic, mixed, or hypomanic episodes present
F. Does not occur exclusively during a psychotic disorder
G. Not caused by a medication or other drug or medical condition
H. Causes functional deficit

Modified from American Psychiatric Association: *Diagnostic and statistical manual of mental disorders* (DSM-IV), ed 4, Washington, DC, 1994, The Association.

tient is being evaluated for nonspecific signs or symptoms.

Most clinicians use a combination of direct questions and formal questions, asking them intuitively at the appropriate points in the interview, physical examination, or review of systems. The important thing is to ensure that specific questions are asked, with the physician directly inquiring as to the presence or absence of the specific symptoms as described in DSM-IV in the definition of major depressive episode. Clinicians working with the elderly should be thoroughly familiar with the DSM-IV criteria for dysthymia, bereavement, and adjustment disorders, as well as the features of mania or hypomania that would make bipolar illness (manic-depressive disorder) a consideration. These criteria are summarized in Boxes 18-3 to 18-6.

> *Even if major depressive episode is confidently diagnosed, contributory factors and illnesses must be sought and addressed if the treatment is to succeed.*

The usefulness of special diagnostic tests to help with the diagnosis or classification of depression remains unclear. Although some literature suggests a difference in prognosis in patients with abnormalities of biological markers such as dexamethasone suppression tests and platelet monoamine oxidase, the effects of aging alone on these

BOX 18-6
Abbreviated Criteria for Manic and Hypomanic Episodes

A. A distinct period of elevated, expansive, or irritable mood, lasting 4 days (hypomanic) or 1 week (manic)
B. Three or more of the following (four if the mood is irritable only):
   1. Inflated self-esteem or grandiosity
   2. Decreased need for sleep
   3. More talkative than usual or pressure to keep talking
   4. Flight of ideas or subjective experience of racing thoughts
   5. Distractability
   6. Increased goal-directed activity (may be social, sexual, or work related) or psychomotor agitation
   7. Excessive pleasurable activities with potentially painful consequences (e.g., buying sprees, sexual indiscretion, foolish business activities)
C. An unequivocal change in functioning
D. Clearly observable by others (hypomanic) or causing marked impairment in functioning or relationships or requiring hospitalization or with psychotic features (manic)
E. Not caused by substance abuse or a general medical condition nor clearly caused by antidepressant treatment
   NOTE: In a mixed episode the criteria for both a manic episode and major depressive episode are met nearly every day for a week; there is marked impairment, or psychotic features, or a need for hospitalization, and it is not caused by a medication (including an antidepressant or other drug) or a medical condition.

Modified from American Psychiatric Association: *Diagnostic and statistical manual of mental disorders* (DSM-IV), ed 4, Washington, DC, 1994, The Association.

BOX 18-7
How Depression Symptoms Differ in the Older Patient

1. Sadness of mood is usually present but is often masked by other symptoms.
2. Impairment in cognition may be marked and dominate the clinical picture; it may even appear to be dementia.
3. A psychosomatic tendency often dominates, and the patient complains of aches and pains or other physical symptoms. Older depressives are more likely to demonstrate exaggerated and ruminative fears about their physical well-being than younger counterparts.

From Ham RJ, Meyers BS: *Late life depression and suicide potential*, 1993, American Association of Retired Persons.

BOX 18-8
Geriatric Depression Scale (Short Form)

Choose the Best Answer for How you Felt the Past Week.

1. Are you basically satisfied with your life?		Yes	No[a]
2. Have you dropped many of your activities and interests?		Yes[a]	No
3. Do you feel that your life is empty?		Yes[a]	No
4. Do you often get bored?		Yes[a]	No
5. Are you in good spirits most of the time?		Yes	No[a]
6. Are you afraid that something bad is going to happen to you?		Yes[a]	No
7. Do you feel happy most of the time?		Yes	No[a]
8. Do you often feel helpless?		Yes[a]	No
9. Do you prefer to stay at home, rather than going out and doing new things?		Yes[a]	No
10. Do you feel you have more problems with memory than most?		Yes[a]	No
11. Do you think it is wonderful to be alive now?		Yes	No[a]
12. Do you feel pretty worthless the way you are now?		Yes[a]	No
13. Do you feel full of energy?		Yes	No[a]
14. Do you feel that your situation is hopeless?		Yes[a]	No
15. Do you think that most people are better off than you are?		Yes[a]	No

Each answer indicated by [a] counts as one point. Scores between 5 and 9 suggest depression, scores above 9 generally indicate depression.
From Sheikh JL, Yesavage JA: *Clin Gerontol* 5:165-173, 1986.

markers remain poorly understood. In the treatment of depression in the elderly by primary care physicians, these types of biological tests have no place. They have not been found to have sufficient sensitivity or specificity to be useful in clinical management of depression in the elderly.

Suicide Potential. The risk of suicide should always be assessed by direct questioning (Box 18-10).[6] Physicians should directly inquire about suicidal ideation and plans, the availability of companionship and support, and the ability to access the means of suicide (including guns and medications—a high proportion of those who commit suicide use their antidepressants in overdose). It is salutary to note that possibly 80% of those who commit suicide have visited their primary care physician within a month of their death, with 20% doing so within 24 hours.[6,12] Whereas major depression is not necessarily the cause of all suicides, it is likely to be a factor in more than half of the cases and therefore will often be found if it is sought. Those with active suicidal ideation should be considered for referral to a psychiatric unit or an acute care hospital. Even those at relatively low risk should be monitored closely by family or friends and need frequent scheduled follow-up in the physician's office, particularly during the early phase of treatment.

Always ask direct questions of the patient and family about suicide risk; dispose of the guns, dispose of the pills, and don't leave the patient alone if there appears to be any increased risk.

Undernutrition. Change in weight is one of the criteria for major depressive episode, but it must be recognized that weight loss also indicates unmet nutritional need.[19] A significant degree of weight loss (e.g., more than 10% in 6 months, more than 7.5% in 3 months, or more than 5% in 1 month) requires a specific nutritional investigation and approach.[20] Weight loss may be the presenting symptom of depression; depression must always be considered in such circumstances.[21]

Depression must be considered in the differential diagnosis of significant weight loss.

Deconditioning. The interrelationship between physical deconditioning and depression is of interest. Whereas it is always reasonable to introduce activity and physical exercise in an attempt to regain motivation in the depressed patient, the special problem of nonrecognition of this common illness is that it leads to physical deconditioning. After several months of depressive illness an elderly person is likely to be physically as well as emotionally deconditioned; the combination of undernutrition, poor muscle strength relative to mobility, increased dependency for physical functioning, and, especially in the more frail, development of difficult symptoms such as incontinence, loss of confidence for mobility, or even falling can mean that recovery from a depressive episode requires extensive rehabilitative techniques. Prevention is superior to rehabilitation, hence the importance of early detection of depression.

BOX 18-9
Scale for Detecting Major Depression in Hospitalized Patients

Choose the Best Answer for How You Have Felt Over the Past Week.

1.	Do you often get bored?	Yes	No
2.	Do you often get restless and fidgety?	Yes	No
3.	Do you feel in good spirits?	Yes	No
4.	Do you feel you have more problems with memory than most?	Yes	No
5.	Can you concentrate easily when reading the papers?	Yes	No
6.	Do you prefer to avoid social gatherings?	Yes	No
7.	Do you often feel downhearted and blue?	Yes	No
8.	Do you feel happy most of the time?	Yes	No
9.	Do you often feel helpless?	Yes	No
10.	Do you feel worthless and ashamed about yourself?	Yes	No
11.	Do you often wish you were dead?	Yes	No

A score of 3 or more generally indicates depression.
From Koenig HG, Blazer DG: *Clin Geriatr Med* 8(2):235-251, 1992.

Undernutrition and physical deconditioning with all of their consequences are frequently the permanent sequelae of unrecognized depression, continuing as long-term disabilities after the depression resolves.

▼ THOMAS XING (Part II)

Assessment of Thomas Xing in your office reveals a frail man who is tearful at times. The physical examination shows apparent weight loss and a slow, slightly wide-based gait, with slight pitting edema of the lower legs. The GDS and an MMS examination are administered; the GDS score is 7/15 and MMS examination score is 22/30. Screening laboratory work reveals a normochromic normocytic anemia, a T_4 level of 1.9, and TSH level of 98. Because of the patient's past history of

BOX 18-10
Assessing the Potential for Suicide

Ask Direct Questions:

Does the patient volunteer suicidal thoughts?
Has the patient thought through plans for suicide?
Does the patient have access to the means of suicide?
Does the patient have an exaggerated concern about a real or imagined physical illness?
Is there evidence of a sense of hopelessness?
Is the patient extremely depressed and withdrawn?
Is this an elderly white male?
Is there alcohol involved?
Are there social contacts with whom to share emotional thoughts?
Does the patient's cognitive status vary from day to day?
Do you have reason to suspect the patient might not be taking the prescribed medications?
Is someone available at home for companionship until the depressed mood is controlled or resolved?

From Ham RJ, Meyers BS: *Late life depression and suicide potential*, 1993, American Association of Retired Persons.

CAD, T_4 replacement therapy is instituted in a cautious manner; you anticipate that it may take 2 or 3 months to reach an appropriate replacement dose.

CASE DISCUSSION

The death of a spouse often leads to depressive symptoms. However, Mr. Xing's symptoms are clearly beyond normal bereavement. His new physical complaints should be evaluated. The GDS score in combination with the history of the present illness is consistent with major depression. The MMS examination score is consistent with the dementia syndrome of depression, although mild dementia is possible. Medical screening for other illnesses is needed before a diagnosis of depression is made.

▼ CLARA KNIGHTON (Part II)

Examination of Clara Knighton in your office reveals a very thin, frail woman who is slow to answer questions and who sits passively, holding her head in her hands. Blood pressure supine is 120/75 mm Hg, standing 100/70 mmHg. She has cataracts, dry skin, tobacco-stained fingers, and a 2/6 systolic ejection murmur. Her MMS examination score is 24/30, and her GDS score is 11/15. To direct questioning, she admits feelings of hopelessness and worthlessness, loss of appetite, and difficulty sleeping. She feels that life is not worth living, but she denies suicidal ideation. Laboratory test results are BUN level 55, creatinine level 1.8., and albumin level 2.9. The ECG and chest x-ray examination are normal. A diagnosis of major depressive episode and dehydration is made, and you admit her to the local community hospital.

CASE DISCUSSION

Weight loss, functional decline, and mental decline can be associated with many medical illnesses, medication complications, and disorders of mood such as depression and dementia. A full medical evaluation is needed. However, Clara meets the criteria for major depressive episode. Initiation of treatment on an inpatient basis is prudent when there has been such a significant metabolic disturbance as dehydration. In addition, the social situation in this case is unstable, and an inpatient stay allows the treatment team the opportunity to address these issues.

STUDY QUESTIONS

- *Does the hypothyroidism fully explain Mr. Xing's symptoms?*
- *Is specific treatment for depression indicated?*
- *Ms. Knighton is deeply depressed as well as dehydrated; what will the roles of the psychiatrist and family be?*

Treatment

> *However "reasonable" it may appear that an older person should feel depressed, his or her depression may still respond to treatment. Although depression may seem reasonable in the circumstances, that is no reason not to treat it. Depression is disabling and dangerous, and since it may respond to treatment, why not treat it?*

As with the other major syndromes of the elderly, effective treatment of depression generally requires a multidisciplinary approach. It is possible that ongoing stressors are factors in causing depressive illness to persist or relapse. The efficacy of pharmacological therapy appears to be enhanced by simultaneously addressing the social support structure of the patient. This can be as simple as encouraging mildly symptomatic patients to return to previously enjoyable social activities or take up new ones and facilitating such participation. It may be useful to minimize home stressors by organizing appropriate community services such as case management or Meals on Wheels. Many persons with major depression respond well to psychotherapy in combination with antidepressant medications.[22] This can often be arranged through the local mental health association or clinic. However, many patients and families resist such treatment because of the stigma of mental illness. Close follow-up by the primary care physician is imperative in the treatment of depression. Patients need to be seen in the office frequently during the early part of treatment to assess side effects, observe for signs of functional decline or suicidal ideation, and evaluate efficacy of the medical regimen. Asking patients to return "as needed" is not enough.[23]

> *Because depressed patients lack motivation and self-worth, it is essential to follow up aggressively, scheduling the appointment in advance and calling if the patient fails to keep it.*

Early treatment of depression with pharmacological agents is highly recommended in the elderly, particularly for patients with true major depression or depressive symptoms associated with functional decline. The primary physician's knowledge and enthusiasm for the use of these medications are vital; many families and patients associate them with the stigma of mental illness or are aware of the possibility of harm from them. The factors increasing the likelihood of antidepressant response are summarized in Box 18-11. Advances in the development of antidepressants make it even more reasonable now to mount an enthusiastic "therapeutic trial" in a patient in whom depression (i.e., major depressive episode) is present or even highly likely. A reasonably liberal approach to diagnosis and treatment is justified. A therapeutic trial should be started on the basis of marked clinical suspicion, given the prevalence and treatability of these illnesses and their potential for producing both morbidity and mortality.[7,24,25] Even though major depression is theoretically a self-limiting illness, many elders finish their depressive illness in a considerably deteriorated condition, producing chronic morbidity that may never be corrected. It is also beginning to be hinted (although still not proven) that early treatment of the subgroup of elderly individuals with depression who are markedly cognitively impaired may even reduce the proportion of individuals who are left with a residuum of cognitive impairment after the depression resolves.

The broad classes of available medications for the treatment of depression include tricyclic antidepressants, selective serotonin reuptake inhibitors (SSRIs), mono-

Table 18-1   Antidepressants Used in Primary Care for Treatment of the Elderly

Name	Sedation	Excitation	Anticholinergic Effects	Potential for GI Upset	Orthostasis	Therapeutic Dose per Day (mg) Range	Half-life
Nortriptyline	X		XX		X	25-50	Long
Fluoxetine		XX		X		10-30	Very long
Sertraline		X		X		25-150	Very long
Paroxetine		X		X		10-40	Very long
Trazodone	XX				X	100-200	Moderate
Venlafaxine				X		37.5-150	Moderate
Bupropion		X	X	X		150-300	Moderate

amine oxidase inhibitors (MAOIs), and others (Table 18-1). Because of the serious side effects associated with many of these medications and the sensitivity of older patients to such effects, primary care physicians must focus on the safest regimens and defer the more risky modalities for refractory situations. Some regimens should be handled only by practitioners with special skill in dealing with the elderly, such as psychiatrists or geriatricians.[23,25]

Antidepressants are underused in elders; these are not "drugs to avoid." Denying a depressed elder the potential benefit of treatment merely on the basis of the risk of side effects represents medical neglect.

Many family members of older patients, the patients themselves, and a surprising proportion of practicing physicians are filled with doubts and uncertainties about the reasonableness of using a psychoactive medication in an older individual (Box 18-12). Extensive press coverage of the harm caused to the minds of elders by drugs and the overuse of antipsychotics in the past combines with old-fashioned, prejudicial thinking about the nature of "mental illness" to create a high degree of resistance to the use of psychoactive medications. Patients and families willing to undergo all kinds of other therapies hesitate to use these medications. The primary care physician has a central leadership role in clarifying the issues so that the opportunity for useful treatment is not missed.

Families and patients must understand that depression is a physical illness of the brain and that physical treatments (medications or ECT) are thus a reasonable and basic approach; this physical view of depression overcomes the fearful mystique of giving medications that act on the mind.

Many patients and families find a "medical," physical concept of depression easier to accept and understand. A useful explanation that many will recall from high school is that of the chemically induced nature of responses to stress and anxiety; depression is similar in that whatever the initiating cause, it is ultimately produced by a chemical change, which is why a chemical approach with antidepressants can relieve the symptoms. Although circumstances or a depressing environment may have been the obvious precipitant of the depression, the final effect is a biochemical one, which is why a pharmacological approach is logical. Patients and families must be reassured about improvements in antidepressant medications and the relative lack of side effects compared with medications widely used in the past.[14] Unfortunately, many physicians still exclusively use amitriptyline (Elavil) even though because of its unpleasantly sedative and anticholinergic effects, it is the least desirable of all antidepressants to use in older individuals. Recent studies confirm that many physicians tend to use minor tranquilizers rather than antidepressants, which can make the depression worse. Such treatments demonstrate both a lack of knowledge about and a lack of confidence in appropriate treatment for this common illness.[26] Patients and families need to know that the medications are not addictive, that stopping them is easy, and that each person's response is unique so that they may consider it reasonable to try other pharmacological alternatives if a first trial does not work or causes a systemic upset. Lastly, the family in particular must understand exactly what the "target symptoms" are, that is, which of the range of symptoms the physician believes may respond to the drug. Either the family or the patient will be reporting back to the physician, and they need to know what they are supposed to be looking for.

Physicians must enthusiastically initiate treatment for depression and involve the family by having them know and observe the "target symptoms" defined at the outset.

MAOIs have been found effective in the treatment of depression in the elderly and have little cardiotoxic or cholinergic effect. However, the required dietary restrictions
to prevent hypertensive crises and orthostatic hypotension from these drugs make them problematic. Many clinicians, including many psychiatrists, have little personal
experience in the use of them. Therefore this class of
medications probably has little place in the primary physician's care of elderly patients.

The *tricyclic antidepressants* (TCAs) are the most well-
studied therapeutic agents. They have an established and
well-understood side effect profile. For many agents in
this class, blood levels are routinely available and help to
ensure that the patient is not receiving too much or too
little. Undertreatment of depression by underdosage of
antidepressant medications is more of an issue with elderly patients than is generally recognized. Unfortunately, the side effects of TCAs can be difficult for older
patients to tolerate. Of particular concern are the anticholinergic effects such as drowsiness, constipation,
blurred vision, urinary hesitancy, and dry mouth. Orthostatic hypotension can also be a problem. Nortriptyline
is the least sedating of the TCAs and has a lower anticholinergic effect than most other tricyclics; therefore it
should be the TCA of choice in the elderly. Other TCAs
should be considered for use by primary care physicians

only in the case of recurrent depression that has previously responded to one such specific medication. Nortriptyline seems to be especially effective in helping depression associated with or manifested by chronic pain,
insomnia, and psychomotor agitation. It can usually be
taken as a single bedtime dose.

Trazodone has low anticholinergic side effects, but it
is highly sedating and is associated with orthostatic hypotension. In addition, the rare but serious complication
of priapism has caused some practitioners to avoid its use
in men. These side effects can make it difficult to titrate
up to the dosage level needed to achieve reliable antidepressant results. Blood levels can be measured to help
avoid toxicity and ensure that the trial is conducted at
an adequate dose. Therapeutic effect can be seen at levels lower than the recommended therapeutic range. This
medication may have special utility in disruptive, screaming patients with dementia. It can be helpful as a second
medication for SSRI-associated sleep disturbances.[27]

The *SSRIs* (fluoxetine [Prozac], sertraline [Zoloft],
and paroxetine [Paxil]) share a well-tolerated side effect
profile that lends itself to safe usage in the elderly. The
most common side effect is gastrointestinal distress, but
this rarely leads to discontinuation of the medication. Insomnia is a side effect related to the tendency of these
agents to cause activation. They are therefore initially
prescribed to be given in the morning, unlike most other
antidepressants. The single daily dose is convenient and
aids compliance. Occasionally they cause sedation;
should this occur, the dose is switched to bedtime. There
are differences in plasma half-life and the sites of metabolism as well as the degree of "activation" or stimulation
seen with each of these medications; this profile should
be considered in choosing a particular agent for a given
patient. Some patients respond to one SSRI and not to
others. Many practitioners start with a low dose (e.g., 10
mg fluoxetine, 25 mg sertraline, or 10 mg paroxetine)
for a week or so, but an adequate trial is not complete
until the patient has taken the medication at the usual
recommended adult dose for a sufficient period (at least
6 weeks).

Bupropion (Wellbutrin) has many features that favor its
use in the elderly population. Although its mechanism
of action is unclear, it is effective for major depression
and perhaps for bipolar depression (manic depression) as
well. It has energizing properties and therefore rarely
causes sedation, although it can cause nervousness as a
side effect. It has minimal anticholinergic side effects and
no significant cardiac effects. It does reduce the seizure
threshold in patients who are predisposed to them.

Venlafaxine (Effexor) is a new agent with a side effect
profile similar to the SSRIs, but it has the potential advantage of working at the sites of both serotonin activity
and norepinephrine activity. While this may be of theoretical benefit only, there is some evidence that this

mechanism leads to a faster onset of action. The twice-daily dosage is tolerable for patients, and the safety profile appears satisfactory for elderly patients.

With virtually all of the preceding medications, the dose is slowly titrated up until the individual is on a dose that is likely to be therapeutic (Box 18-13). Most experienced clinicians and authorities in this area recommend that a trial of therapy with an antidepressant last for at least 8 weeks at the likely-to-be-therapeutic dose. Establishing this dose for an individual can be difficult. It may be necessary to leave an individual on what may be the therapeutic dose for perhaps a month after which, lacking a definite response, a further increase with a further period of observation might be justified. The patient and family need to realize the principles of dose titration; otherwise their fears of escalating psychiatrically active drugs will appear to be confirmed.

After achieving a remission of the symptoms of depression, it is vital to persist with the medication, continuing the dose that has been effective. Prior recommendations to reduce to a maintenance dose are now outdated. The dose should not be reduced once the patient has responded. Rather, that dose should be continued for a period of at least 6 months, and most physicians would recommend 1 year. This is based on the assumption that the natural history of an episode of major depression is often as long as 1 year, and therefore the episode needs to be "covered" until its natural resolution. The high relapse rate of individuals successfully responding to these medications is leading some physicians to recommend more persistent therapy.[28] It is possible that as many as 20% of individuals require continuing treatment, potentially lifelong, in order to avoid relapse. Many authorities currently recommend that a patient whose depression relapses on withdrawal of the antidepressant be treated again for a period of at least 1 further year before another attempt at reduction, and many consider that even one such relapse would justify continuing the medication for life. Others go further, recommending that a profound antidepressant-responsive depression in old age, especially if there has been a prior episode of depression, should lead to lifelong treatment with antidepressants at the full effective dose.[28,29]

Electroconvulsive therapy (ECT) is an effective treatment for major depression in the elderly, with success rates approaching 90%. Although some experts call ECT the treatment of choice in the elderly, most clinicians reserve ECT for refractory cases or for cases in which a high risk of morbidity or mortality would be associated with waiting as much as 4 to 6 weeks for a significant response to medications. Such high-risk patients include those who are actively suicidal or have significant vegetative signs, including inability or apparent unwillingness to take adequate nutrition and hydration. Psychotic or delusional depression is highly responsive to ECT and much less responsive to pharmacotherapy; ECT should thus be considered as primary treatment in those cases.

Medicolegal concerns, as well as the social stigma attached to ECT, can interfere with the willingness of patients and families to accept ECT as a treatment. In addition, in some parts of the country few psychiatrists perform this procedure because of the lack of training or the cost of medical liability insurance. Reassurance by the personal physician regarding the appropriateness of ECT can be helpful in getting patients and families to have an open mind regarding this treatment. Physicians should be aware of the nearest center available for referral of potential ECT patients, since ECT therapy can be lifesaving in major depression that is refractory to pharmacological therapy.

> ECT should be the primary treatment for patients with psychotic or delusional depression or for patients who are actively suicidal or who will not eat or drink, but societal and legal prejudice limits its use.

The main side effect of ECT, other than the transient tachycardia and elevation in blood pressure seen in the immediate postictal stage, is transient confusion. This seems to be a more serious problem in persons who have both dementia and depression. The use of unilateral electrode placement, as has been standard for years, seems to minimize any cognitive decline associated with ECT.

Referral to a psychiatrist is generally necessary for

BOX 18-13
Titrating the Dose of Antidepressants

Define the target symptoms and ensure that the family (and patient if cognizant) understands them.

Titrate carefully (slowly if possible, quickly if urgent) to the dose that is likely to be effective.

Persist at the "likely-to-be-effective" dose for at least 8 weeks.

Consider increasing after only 4 weeks at the "likely-to-be-effective" dose if there is no response, you feel the patient cannot wait, and the patient is tolerating the medication well.

When the target symptoms respond, you are at the effective dose.

Persist at the effective dose for at least 6 months but generally 1 year (some authorities now recommend 2 years) or longer (possibly lifelong) if this is a recurrent or relapsing depression.

From Ham RJ: Unpublished instructional materials.

ECT, but the primary care physician is in the best position to know whether the person is a medical candidate for it. ECT is performed under brief general anesthesia, so the usual guidelines for preoperative clearance apply. In particular, patients for ECT should not have unstable angina, active CHF, or unstable dysrhythmias. Severe hypertension should be controlled. In addition, persons considered for ECT should have a CT brain scan or MRI to rule out the presence of a significant tumor. A small, benign tumor such as a meningioma is not an absolute contraindication to ECT; it should be discussed with a neurosurgeon if there are any doubts. The previous practice of doing complete spine films before performing ECT to assess for the presence of fractures is no longer necessary because the concurrent use of paralytic anesthesia minimizes the possibility of skeletal injuries. However, this practice persists in some areas of the country because of medicolegal concerns. To disallow ECT for all older persons with osteoporosis and compression fractures would be excessively cautious.

A course of ECT often ranges from 6 to 20 treatments, given 2 to 3 times per week. Response is often noticed within the first week or two.

There are roles for *combination therapy* with more than one antidepressant and for use of augmentation agents such as lithium, thyroid hormone,[30] methylphenidate, and dextroamphetamine.[31] Because of the risk of unfavorable side effects in the elderly population, these therapies, as well as MAO inhibitors, should be reserved for psychiatrists and geriatricians with particular expertise in the treatment of depression in the elderly.

▼ THOMAS XING (Part III)

Mr. Xing has characteristic symptoms of depression; to address this while slowly initiating the thyroid treatment, you decide to start sertraline (Zoloft) 25 mg per day. The patient and family are apprised of potential side effects, the time course for the medication to be effective, and the long-term treatment plan. Mr. Xing is reevaluated in 1 week to reassess suicide potential and to look for medication side effects. Because he has no side effects, the dose is increased to 50 mg per day. At the next scheduled visit, 2 weeks later, he is showing improvement in his mood, affect, and energy level. His symptoms are virtually resolved within 2 months. The patient and family receive counseling from a social worker who helps them deal with the many changes in Mr. Xing's living situation. Three months after his initial visit, Mr. Xing's GDS score is 1/15, his MMS examination score is 26/30, and he is euthyroid. The sertraline is continued for a total of 9 months, at which time Mr. Xing is slowly weaned. Some feelings of low energy and sleep disturbance begin to return within 1 month of stopping the sertraline, and it is restarted, with plans to continue it for a total of 2 years before weaning him again.

CASE DISCUSSION

Simultaneous treatment of depression and intercurrent medical problems is often needed in elderly patients. It was appropriate to initiate sertraline, an SSRI, while the other medical problem was being addressed. Counseling or other patient and family support is helpful as adjunctive therapy, especially when clear social stressors or life-style changes are present.

▼ CLARA KNIGHTON (Part III)

In the hospital you begin treating Clara Knighton with 25 mg of nortriptyline every night, along with IV hydration. After several days, her BUN level is normal and she is sleeping at night, but she refuses to eat and sits in her chair all day. She will not interact at group therapy sessions. A psychiatric consultation is obtained and ECT is recommended. A normal CT scan completes the medical clearance for the ECT. You initiate detailed discussion with the family, involving the psychiatrist in the discussion, and the family agree to ECT. However, the patient refuses, and she also refuses transfer to an inpatient psychiatric unit. The nortriptyline is titrated up to 50 mg per night, causing some constipation, which is controlled with daily lactulose. Five days later the nortriptyline level is therapeutic. She is sleeping better at night but still refuses to eat; IV hydration is maintained. The treatment team thinks that Ms. Knighton lacks the capacity to refuse potentially life-saving treatment and that a guardian is needed. While her niece is arranging to become Ms. Knighton's guardian, the psychiatrist recommends adding a morning dose of dextroamphetamine. No change in the patient's affect is seen, and it is discontinued. After the legal matters are completed, the niece signs for the transfer to the psychiatric unit and for the ECT. The psychiatrist assumes primary responsibility, with you as personal physician managing Ms. Knighton's medical problems and assisting in maintaining the family's support and the patient's compliance. After four treatments the patient's affect begins to brighten and she starts eating. After ten unilateral treatments she is greatly improved, walking well, eating well, and participating in group therapy sessions. She is discharged to the care of her niece with plans to continue nortriptyline for at least 2 years; if any sign of recurrent depression is noted, outpatient "maintenance" ECT will be a consideration.

CASE DISCUSSION

A tricyclic such as nortriptyline was a particularly good choice because of Ms. Knighton's marked vegetative symptoms and her stable cardiac status. However, ECT needs to be considered early in elderly patients who are in medical danger from their depression. Such dangers include weight loss, recurrent dehydration, and suicide. Legal hurdles can be great in cases in which the patient will not agree and there is no guardian to make decisions. Families can be resistant to the idea of ECT, and it is important for the primary physician to be involved in these discussions. Appointing a guardian can be problematic: respect for patients' rights to dictate their own fate, even though depressed, can lead to uncertainty as to what is in the best interest of the patient. Civil libertarians have a hard time acknowledging that persons can be ill enough to be unable to make their own decisions. This patient did receive a therapeutic dose of the nortriptyline, as well as augmentation with dextroamphetamine, under the supervision of the psychiatrist, but she failed to respond. Nonresponders to medical therapy often respond to ECT. This type of depressive episode needs long-term follow-up and treatment. The medication, if tolerated, should probably be continued for life.

▼ MARTHA JENKINS (Part II)

Evaluation of Martha Jenkins in the office reveals a noticeable decrease in energy, depressed mood, and feelings of hopelessness and helplessness. She has a history of a previous episode of depression 4 years ago that responded well to nortriptyline; 35 mg nortriptyline every hour is started. Over the next 6 weeks she begins to sleep better and seemingly has an improved mood, but within 3 months she begins to feel ill again, with increasing pain, weakness, fatigue, and worsening of her mood. Laboratory evaluation reveals a Hct of 28, mean corpuscular volume (MCV) of 91, BUN level of 66, creatinine level of 3.2, total protein is 8.2, albumin level is 2.2, and alkaline phosphatase is 303. Serum protein electrophoresis, x-ray examination, and bone marrow biopsy confirm the diagnosis of multiple myeloma. The patient is referred to an oncologist, and after beginning treatment with oral chemotherapeutic agents, she begins to feel much better.

CASE DISCUSSION

Martha Jenkins has typical features of depression, as well as a past history of depression. Because of her good response in the past and because of the established usefulness of tricyclic antidepressants in the treatment of chronic pain, nortriptyline is a good choice for initial therapy. However, although depression is common in older patients, so are cancer and other chronic illnesses. A complete history, physical, and appropriate screening laboratory work might have discovered this hidden malignancy earlier. The patient still needed treatment for depression, but therapy for the multiple myeloma was also required.

OTHER THERAPEUTIC APPROACHES

Sleep deprivation has been used as a self-treatment for depressed mood for centuries. It has been used and well tolerated in elderly patients, although usually as an inpatient procedure. The patient shows transient improvement after a night deprived of sleep. It is thought that this treatment might be particularly useful for patients with definitely disrupted sleep-wake cycles. Improvements in depression have been reported by advancing the sleep-wake cycle (i.e., having the patient go to sleep 6 hours earlier). The exact place of this in therapy is not yet well defined. It may interrelate to experiments in which depressed patients are woken during REM sleep, with apparent relief of depressive symptoms.

Phototherapy, in which depressed patients are exposed to extra quantities of light, is a further consideration in patients not responding to traditional approaches.[32,33] Whereas data scientific enough to suggest the exact place of light in therapy of depression are unclear, it appears convincing that there are individuals who are depressed by darkness and whose depression is relieved by light. This is probably related to seasonal affective disorder (SAD), one element of which is thought to be light deprivation.[34] More research is needed, but for now it seems reasonable to at least address the gloomy environment in which many dependent elders live, and to increase the quantity and duration of lighting as an adjunctive, inexpensive, and rarely iatrogenic method for helping this prevalent problem.

▼ BETTY POLZINSKI (Part II)

Betty Polzinski had been admitted to the facility for rehabilitation following an episode of pneumonia complicated by congestive heart failure. The nurse tells you that she has lost 4 pounds in the last 30 days. The staff find her to be difficult, grouchy, and aggressive.

STUDY QUESTIONS

- *What should be sought on interview and in your necessarily brief physical examination?*
- *What will you say to the staff who dislike her so much?*
- *What management will you recommend?*

▼ BETTY POLZINSKI (Part III)

Ms. Polzinski is angry and will not talk to you about her feelings. Physical examination reveals a pale, barely cooperative patient without overt signs of CHF. She has stiff lower limbs that can be persuaded to a reasonable range of movement, but there is some restriction of flexion at both hips, although there is good rotation. Ms. Polzinski's mouth is dry and her ears are filled with wax. She is slim and lacks subcutaneous fat. There are pink striae on the abdominal wall. Her abdomen is soft, and the descending colon is somewhat tender with palpable feces. A recent laboratory panel confirms an albumin level of 2.8, BUN level of 27 with a normal creatinine level, and an Hgb of 11.1, with normochromic, normocytic indices.

STUDY QUESTIONS

- *What contributory or causative factors to this patient's decline are suggested by the findings so far?*
- *Which disciplines in the nursing home setting will need to be especially involved and consulted?*
- *What specific questions should be asked of the patient or considered when obtaining the history from the staff or a family member?*

▼ BETTY POLZINSKI (Part IV)

You speak with a nurse on Ms. Polzinski's prior unit, who confirms that when first admitted, Betty was progressing satisfactorily, would get out of bed, and did eat the institutional food. About 2 months ago she began refusing food and declining to get up and go to the activities. The nursing record confirms that her sleep has become interrupted since that time. You ask the staff to note her mood at different times of the day, and it becomes clear that she is grumpiest and most obnoxious in the mornings. Confident of the presence of a depressive illness, you initiate sertraline (Zoloft), starting at 25 mg for a week, then increasing to 50 mg. Routinely following up in the third week of therapy, you find that Mrs. Polzinski is sitting in a chair eating her lunch. She is quiet and calm and no longer irritates the nurses with her passivity and complaining. You speak to the director of nursing and arrange to present an inservice program for the nursing staff aides, using this case as an example of a patient who appeared unlikable and unhelpable, but in whom a simple medication transformed the situation. With the resolution of the depression, the underhydration, undernutrition, and deconditioning with musculoskeletal stiffness all resolve. Ms. Polzinski does not rehabilitate sufficiently to go home, however, and 9 months later becomes acutely diaphoretic, dyspneic, and hypotensive. She is treated with oxygen and intramuscular furosemide (Lasix). At her request she is about to be transferred to the hospital when she dies of an acute myocardial infarction.

CASE DISCUSSION

In the context of this chapter, the diagnosis probably does not seem too difficult in this case. But this scenario was in fact utterly missed both by the previous physician and by all the staff. This one case contributed greatly to increased awareness among staff of the high proportion of persons with potentially treatable depression in the nursing home setting.

SUMMARY

It is the special role of the primary care physician of elderly patients to aggressively and imaginatively seek depression. Although a debilitating and quite frequently a fatal illness, depression is treatable and will respond to antidepressant and other modes of therapy in the vast majority of cases. All the members of the team must take part both in finding the cases and ensuring the patient's adequate treatment. All involved professionals must respond to the great need that exists for better education about depression, using widely available professional and lay resources.[35,36] Family involvement is crucial, not only in identifying the illness and assisting in compliance, but also in reporting back to the physician on whether or not the target symptoms of depression are resolving. Depression is often comingled with many other medical and social problems, so primary care physicians must become expert at initial treatment with antidepressants and knowledgeable about the indications for psychiatric consultation and hospitalization when necessary.

POSTTEST

1. Which of the following statements regarding depression is false?
    a. Electroconvulsive therapy is one of the safest and most effective treatments for depression in the elderly.
    b. Although safer than the older tricyclic antidepressants, the selective serotonin reuptake inhibitors (SSRIs) have the disadvantage of being slower to cause a treatment response.
    c. Depression in the elderly often presents as chronic pain.
    d. Persons who have a good response to an antidepressant should receive continued therapy for 9 to 12 months.

2. Orthostatic hypotension may be a serious side effect of all of the following antidepressants except:
    a. Amitriptyline
    b. Trazodone
    c. Nortriptyline
    d. Bupropion

3. All depressed patients who are to receive ECT should have as part of a pre-ECT medical screen all of the following except:
    a. CT brain scan
    b. Cardiac history
    c. ECG
    d. Spinal film series

4. Symptoms of depression are associated with all of the following medications except:
    a. Benzodiazepines
    b. Digoxin
    c. Codeine
    d. Methylphenidate

5. Which of the following is not correct as a DSM-IV criterion for MDE?
    a. Increase in appetite nearly every day
    b. A sense of being restless or slowed down
    c. Significant impairment of function
    d. Persistence of symptoms for a period of at least 2 weeks
    e. Depressed mood or loss of interest or pleasure

REFERENCES

1. Koenig HG, Blazer DG: Epidemiology of geriatric affective disorders, *Clin Geriatr Med* 8(2):235-251, 1992.
2. Prestidge BR, Lake CR: Prevalence and recognition of depression among primary care outpatients, *J Fam Pract* 25(1):67-72, 1987.
3. Parmelee PA, Katz IR, Lawton MP: Incidence of depression in long-term care settings, *J Gerontol* 47(6):M189-M196, 1992.
4. Rousseau P: Suicide in later life and its risk factors, *Clin Geriatr* 3(7):41-48, 1995.
5. Blazer D: Depression in the elderly, *N Engl J Med* 320(3):164-166, 1989.
6. Ham RJ, Myers B: Late life depression and suicide potential, Monograph, Washington, DC, 1993, American Association of Retired Persons.
7. McCullough PK: Geriatric depression: atypical presentations, hidden meanings, *Geriatrics* 46(10):72-76, 1991.
8. Feightner JW, Worrall G: Early detection of depression by primary care physicians, *Can Med Assoc J* 142(11):1215-1220, 1990.
9. American Psychiatric Association: *Diagnostic and statistical manual of mental disorders,* ed 4, Washington, DC, The Association.
10. Yesavage J: Differential diagnosis between depression and dementia, *Am J Med* 94(supp 5A):23S-28S, 1993.
11. Jones BN, Reifler BV: Depression co-existing with dementia: evaluation and treatment, *Med Clin North Am* 78(4):823-840, 1994.
12. Depression in Late Life—NIH Consensus Conference, *JAMA,* 268(8):1018-1024, August 1992.
13. Drugs for psychiatric disorders, *Med Lett* 36(933), 1994.
14. Yesavage J: Depression in the elderly, *Postgrad Med* 91(1):255-261, 1992.
15. Kane RL, Ouslander JG, Abrass IB, eds: *Essentials of clinical geriatrics,* ed 3, New York, 1994, McGraw-Hill.
16. Levenson AJ, Hall RCW, eds: *Neuropsychiatric manifestations of physical disorders in the elderly,* New York, 1981, Raven Press.
17. Sheikh JL, Yesavage JA: Geriatric Depression Scale (GDS): recent evidence and development of a shorter version, *Clin Gerontol* 5:165-173, 1986.
18. Koenig HG et al: A brief depression scale for use in the medically ill, *Int J Psychiatry Med* 22(2):183-195, 1992.
19. Cohen D: Dementia, depression and nutritional status. In Ham RJ, ed: *Nutrition in old age: primary care clinics in office practice,* 21(1), 1994, WB Saunders.
20. Ham RJ: Indicators of poor nutritional status in older Americans, *Am Fam Physician* 45(1):219-230, 1992.
21. Morley JE, Kraenzle D: Causes of weight loss in a community nursing home, *Am Geriatr Soc* 42(6):583-585, 1994.
22. Shearer SI, Adams GK: Nonpharmacologic aids in the treatment of depression, *Am Fam Physician* 47(2):435-442, 1993.
23. Reynolds CF III: Treatment of depression in late life, *Am J Med* 97(suppl 6A):39S-46S, 1994.
24. Rovner BW: Depression and increased risk of mortality in the nursing home patient, *Am J Med* 95(suppl 5A):19S-22S, 1993.
25. Stewart JT: Diagnosing and treating the hospitalized elderly, *Geriatrics* 46(1):64-66, 71-72, 1991.
26. Wells KB et al: Use of minor tranquillizers and antidepressant medications by depressed out-patients: results from the Medical Outcomes Study, *Am J Psychiatry* 151(5)694-700, 1994.
27. Nierenberg AA et al: Trazodone for antidepressant-associated insomnia, *Am J Psychiatry* 151(7):1069-1072, 1994.
28. Jacoby R for the Old Age Depression Interest Group: How long should the elderly take antidepressants? A double-blind placebo-controlled study of continuation/prophylaxis therapy with dothiepin, *Br J Psychiatry* 162:175-182, 1993.

29. Cadieux RJ: Geriatric psychopharmacology, a primary care challenge, *Postgrad Med* 93(4):281-301, 1993.

30. Joffe RT et al: A placebo-controlled comparison of lithium and triiodothyronine augmentation of tricyclic antidepressants in unipolar refractory depression, *Arch Gen Psychiatry* 50(5):387-393, 1993.

31. Nelson JC: Combined treatment strategies in psychiatry, *J Clin Psychiatry* 54(suppl):42-49, 55-56, 1993.

32. Genhart MJ et al: Effects of bright light on mood in normal elderly women, *Psychiatry Res* 47:87-97, 1993.

33. Kripke DF et al: Controlled trial of bright light for nonseasonal major depressive disorders, *Biol Psychiatry* 31:119-134, 1992.

34. Chung YS, Dhaghestani AN: Seasonal affective disorder, shedding light on a dark subject, *Postgrad Med* 86(5):309-314, 1989.

35. National Institute of Mental Health: If you're over 65 and feeling depressed . . .treatment brings new hope, DHHS publication No (ADM) 90-1653, Washington, DC, 1990, US Department of Health and Human Services.

36. Blazer DG: *Depression in late life*, ed 2, St Louis, 1993, Mosby.

PRETEST ANSWERS

1. a
2. a
3. a
4. d

POSTTEST ANSWERS

1. b
2. d
3. d
4. d
5. b

CHAPTER 19

Dysmobility and Immobility

JOHN B. MURPHY

OBJECTIVES

Upon completion of this chapter, the reader will be able to:

1. Given a community-dwelling older person with osteoarthritis:
   - Perform an appropriate functional screening assessment.
   - Perform an appropriate diagnostic evaluation (history, physical, and laboratory).
   - Develop an appropriate differential diagnosis.
   - Develop a therapeutic plan for the disease and consequent functional limitations.
   - Address the common family issues for the patient.

2. Given a community-dwelling older person with a mobility problem other than osteoarthritis:
   - Develop a differential diagnosis that includes the conditions that most commonly result in mobility limitations for older persons.
   - Understand the principles of therapy for these conditions.

3. Given an older person hospitalized with an immobilizing illness:
   - List the medical complications of immobility or bed rest.
   - Understand the need for a multidisciplinary team approach to the care of a patient with the acute onset of functional decline.
   - Develop a care plan for the prevention of the medical complications of immobility or bed rest.

4. Identify myths related to normal aging and mobility.

PRETEST

1. Which one of the following statements about osteo-arthritis is true?
   a. Prolonged morning stiffness is common.
   b. Osteoarthritis is a symptom of systemic inflammatory illness.
   c. The metacarpophalangeal joints are commonly involved.
   d. Osteoarthritis affects primarily weight-bearing joints.

2. Which one of the following statements about immobility or bed rest is true?
   a. Bed rest should often be part of the therapeutic care plan for hospitalized older persons.
   b. Bed rest or immobility leads to medical complications that may affect the ultimate recovery of an elderly patient.
   c. The major medical complications of immobility occur only after many weeks of bed rest.
   d. Bone loss is decelerated during bed rest.

This chapter is designed to help the reader understand the importance of mobility-related issues in the care of older people, gain insight into the physiological aspects of immobility, appropriately assess and develop therapeutic plans for people with mobility problems (particularly those with osteoarthritis), and prevent the complications of dysmobility and immobility. The importance of functional assessment, interdisciplinary and team care, and the multifactorial nature of mobility problems for older persons are stressed.

DYSMOBILITY

The overwhelming majority of Americans age 65 years and over rate their health as good, very good, or excellent.[1] However, 80% of these individuals have at least one chronic disease, and 45% have some degree of limitation of everyday activities.[2] All too frequently older persons, their families, and health care professionals accept disease and the resultant limitations as normal aspects of aging. Although the incidence and prevalence of chronic illness in older populations is much higher than in younger groups, this does not mean that functional impairment is a normal aspect of aging. To the contrary, chronic conditions and their resultant functional limitations are the result of pathological processes that are often preventable and almost universally treatable. A nihilistic approach to chronic illnesses and functional limitations is wholly unwarranted in the care of older persons.

Although our understanding of the epidemiology of functional limitations in mobility in older populations is limited, certain principles are clear. First, older persons commonly have problems with mobility. In one community-wide epidemiological survey in East Boston, 15.5% of the population age 65 years and older reported difficulty in walking.[3] Second, the prevalence (and incidence) of mobility problems increases with advancing age. In the East Boston study only 9.3% of men and

11.6% of women age 65 to 69 years reported difficulty walking, whereas for those age 85 years and older the figures were 26.1% and 32.7%. Third, the prevalence of mobility problems also varies greatly depending on the setting studied. In the acute hospital setting, 65% of persons age 70 years or older were unable to ambulate independently compared with the roughly 10% figure in community-dwelling settings.[4] Comparable or higher figures have been reported for older persons living in long-term care settings.[5]

The causes of dysmobility problems are numerous and frequently multifactorial. Musculoskeletal and neurological disorders (e.g., osteoarthritis and stroke) are among the most common causes and are discussed in detail in this chapter. Nonetheless, many other conditions can contribute to problems with mobility, including cardiovascular disease, sensory deficits (vision and hearing), foot disorders, environmental conditions, and a host of iatrogenic issues, the most important of which is the use and abuse of medications.

The initial assessment of any patient (regardless of age) should focus on the history. The history provides the most information and should guide the physical examination and the laboratory assessment. For the older patient, the usual history needs to be expanded to include an assessment of functional status.

▼ BEULAH SMITH (Part I)

Mrs. Smith is a 77-year-old woman who comes to your office for her annual examination. You have been her doctor for a number of years, and her only known medical problem is osteoarthritis (OA). She reports that she has no problems, but you note that since her last visit she has started using a straight cane, which she carries in her right hand. She notes that the pain she has had in her right hip for the last 9 years is no worse than a year ago, and she has not increased the use of her only medication, aspirin.

STUDY QUESTION

■ In addition to addressing the usual health maintenance issues, how would you conduct an assessment related to Mrs.
  Smith's only known medical problem, osteoarthritis?

CASE DISCUSSION

The case of Beulah Smith illustrates a number of points characteristic of older persons and of persons with osteoarthritis.
She envisions herself as doing well and, as is the case in the
majority of older adults, has a chronic disease, OA. Although
she has begun using a straight cane recently, she does not
identify this as a problem; she has accepted the mobility limitation as a normal part of aging. Although her OA is the most
likely contributor to her gait abnormality, it is necessary to
conduct a full assessment to ascertain whether or not this is
indeed the case.

*Osteoarthritis is the most common chronic
illness in the world; thus this diagnosis is
often assumed, yet it is often not specifically
addressed.*

Osteoarthritis

Osteoarthritis (OA) will be discussed in detail because of
its high prevalence and significant impact on older people.

Description and Pathogenesis. OA is a chronic progressive disorder that is characterized by pain, deformity,
and frequent limitation of joint motion. It is the third
most common principal diagnosis recorded by family
practitioners for office visits made by older patients.[6]
Population-based studies of OA demonstrate that radiographic OA is much more prevalent than symptomatic
OA and that OA progressively increases in prevalence
with advancing age.[7] An estimated 50 million Americans,
most over age 65 years, have the condition.[8] It has been
estimated that OA is second only to ischemic heart disease as a cause of work-related disability among persons
older than 50 years of age and that 80% of individuals
with OA report some limitation of activity, with 25% of
these individuals being unable to perform a major daily
activity.[8] OA of the lower extremities tends to be more
disabling than OA of the upper extremities, particularly
as it relates to mobility. OA results in more hospitalizations and longer hospital stays than does rheumatoid arthritis; it is the major contributor to the estimated 4 billion dollars spent annually in the United States for total
joint replacements.[9]

Beyond age, there are only a few well-documented risk
factors for OA. Chronic excess body weight is a major
factor in the development of OA. This is particularly the
case with OA of the knee. Heredity is unquestionably a
determinant with certain forms of OA, especially those
types affecting the first carpometacarpal (CMC) joint,
and in women, the distal interphalangeal (DIP) joint. Beyond these presentations and the secondary cases of OA
associated with genetically transmitted disorders, there is
little to support heredity as a factor in the development
of OA.[10] Prior traumatic injury is also a risk factor in the
development of OA.[8]

Although age is closely associated with OA, it is not
thought that OA is an inevitable consequence of aging.
OA is much more common with advancing age, but the
changes seen in osteoarthritic cartilage are distinct from
those of normal aging. There is increasing consensus that
OA is not a single disease entity but that the observed
clinical pattern represents a "final common pathway" for
a number of conditions of diverse etiologies.[10]

History. OA is generally a monoarticular or oligoar-
ticular disease. Commonly affected joints and joints that
are usually spared are listed in Table 19-1. Pain is the
principal symptom of OA. Some joint stiffness can occur
after rest or on arising in the morning, but it is usually
of short duration (less than 30 minutes). Systemic symp-

Table 19-1   Clinical Features of Osteoarthritis

Symptoms	Signs
Monoarticular or oligoar- ticular	Decreased joint range of mo- tion
Joints involved	Joint crepitance
Distal interphalangeal	Joint effusion
(DIP), proximal inter-	Joint instability
phalangeal (PIP), 1st	Muscle atrophy
carpometacarpal (CMC)	Antalgic gait
(thumb)	Heberden's or Bouchard's
Knee, hip, 1st metacarpo-	nodes
phalangeal (MCP)	Gelatinous cysts (dorsal as-
Lumbosacral and cervical	pect of DIP joint)
spine	Marginal bony overgrowth
Acromioclavicular, subtalar	(knees)
Sacroiliac, temporoman-	Varus joint angulation (knee)
dibular	Motor weakness (spine)
Joints spared	Diminished reflexes (spine)
Metacarpophalangeal	
(MCP)	
Wrist, elbow, shoulder	
Pain (primarily with weight	
bearing and motion, rest	
pain is a late finding)	
Stiffness of less than 30 min-	
utes' duration following	
rest	
Paresthesias and weakness	
(secondary to nerve root	
impingement in OA of	
spine)	

toms such as fatigue, weight loss, and fever are generally absent in OA.

Early in the symptomatic phase of OA, pain occurs with motion, particularly with weight-bearing motion, and is relieved by rest. As the disease progresses, pain can occur with minimal motion and even at rest. The pain is often described as a deep aching discomfort that, except in the case of hip OA, is localized to the joint. Pain associated with OA of the hip is often localized to the anterior inguinal region or to the medial or lateral thigh regions. The pain of hip OA may also radiate to, or first be felt in, the buttock, the anterior aspect of the thigh just above the knee, or the knee itself. The pain associated with OA of the spine is usually localized, but radicular symptoms may also occur. The discomfort of cervical spine OA may radiate to the supraclavicular and upper trapezius regions as well as to the occiput and the distal upper extremity. In addition to radicular pain, nerve root compression (caused by osteophytic spurs or by degeneration of intervertebral disks with protrusion of the nucleus pulposus) may cause paresthesias and muscle weakness. Rarely, large anterior osteophytes in the cervical region cause dysphagia.

> *In osteoarthritis always look for the subtle, functional (self-imposed) limitations; these are the "symptoms" although the patient and family may have accepted them as "normal."*

It is not unusual for the symptoms of OA to go unmentioned by an older patient. Patients and families frequently and incorrectly accept pain, stiffness, and disability as normal consequences of aging. Functional assessment can serve as a valuable aid to diagnosis in that it may detect functional impairment (i.e., disability) caused by previously unrecognized OA. A standard functional assessment should include activities of daily living (ADLs), instrumental activities of daily living (IADLs), and some measure of mobility.[11]

▼ BEULAH SMITH (Part II)

Mrs. Smith reports that her pain is unchanged from 1 year ago. However, further history reveals that she has reduced her level of physical function. While still independent in ADLs, she has stopped using public transportation and no longer shops independently because these activities aggravate her hip pain. Her daughter now does her shopping and drives her where she needs to go so that she avoids the pain experienced with these activities. Mrs. Smith notes that in the past few weeks she has become slightly less steady on her feet and,

because of this, bought a cane. She purchased the cane based on aesthetics, receiving no training in its use.

CASE DISCUSSION

Additional useful information was obtained by assessing Mrs. Smith's physical functional status. She has had progression of her osteoarthritis of the right hip, and her symptoms are unchanged only because she has decreased her level of activity. A failure to assess Mrs. Smith's physical functional capacity may have resulted in not recognizing apparent disease progression and the resultant functional decline.

Physical Examination. As with the history, it is important to conduct a thorough and expanded physical examination with the older patient. The "get-up-and-go test" has been recommended to screen for neurological and musculoskeletal problems.[12] This maneuver entails having the patient rise from a chair, walk about 10 feet, return, and sit down. Physical examination of an affected joint may show decreased range of motion, joint deformity, bony hypertrophy, and occasionally an intraarticular effusion. Crepitance, pain on passive and active movement, and mild tenderness may be found. Evidence of inflammation is usually absent. In late stages there may be demonstrable joint instability. Table 19-1 lists the physical findings associated with OA.

Heberden's nodes represent cartilaginous and bony enlargement of the dorsolateral and dorsomedial aspects of the DIP joints. They usually develop gradually with little or no pain or inflammatory signs. Bouchard's nodes are similar findings at the PIP joints. Though usually bony, Heberden's nodes may have a soft consistency and can present acutely with signs of inflammation. Gelatinous cysts sometimes develop over the dorsal aspect of the DIP joints. These cysts, which are often attached to tendon sheaths, may resolve spontaneously or persist indefinitely.

Quadriceps muscle atrophy, marginal bony overgrowth, joint crepitance, effusion, and mediolateral joint instability (in late stages) are all possible physical findings in OA of the knee. Limitation of joint motion, initially with extension, may be found with active and passive motion. Varus angulation can also develop as a result of degenerative cartilage changes that are more prominent in the medial compartment of the knee.

The patient with OA of the hip often holds the hip adducted, flexed, and internally rotated. This may result in functional shortening of the leg and the characteristic limp (antalgic gait). Invariably, some degree of limitation in motion can be found in OA of the hip, usually with loss of full extension and internal rotation.

OA of the spine may be associated with limitation in range of motion and with muscle spasm. Nerve root compression can result in motor weakness and diminution of reflexes in the distribution of the involved root.

▼ BEULAH SMITH (Part III)

Your interest is piqued by Mrs. Smith's comment about her unsteady gait. On further questioning she notes some symmetrical swelling of both legs for the past few weeks. She ascribes this swelling to old age and in her mind the swelling accounts for her unsteady gait. Mrs. Smith denies the use of medications other than aspirin, but when asked about borrowed medications, she admits to the regular use of her neighbor's arthritis medication. This turns out to be ibuprofen, which she started taking about 3 to 4 weeks ago. The physical examination reveals decreased range of motion at the right hip with pain on active and passive range of motion, bony enlargement of multiple distal interphalangeal joints (Heberden's nodes), and bony enlargement of both knees without tenderness or effusion. Mrs. Smith also has edema of both legs to the midcalf.

As part of the neurological examination Mrs. Smith is instructed to rise from a chair, walk 10 feet, turn around, walk back, and sit down again (the get-up-and-go test). In performing this maneuver Mrs. Smith carries the cane in her right hand, attempts to minimize weight bearing on her right hip, and nearly loses her balance as she turns. When standing with her feet together and holding the cane at her side, Mrs. Smith's elbow is bent at 90 degrees. In the past, Mrs. Smith always scored 30/30 on a Folstein Mini–Mental State examination, but today she scores 25/30. The remainder of Mrs. Smith's history and physical examination is unrevealing. Radiographs of her right hip show findings consistent with osteoarthritis.

STUDY QUESTIONS

- *In constructing a problem list for Mrs. Smith, which items would you include aside from those issues related to routine health maintenance?*
- *What would be an appropriate differential diagnosis for her hip pain?*
- *How do you ascertain whether or not her cane is the proper size?*

CASE DISCUSSION

In the case of Mrs. Smith, a number of issues became apparent during formal testing. She has difficulty rising from the chair, suggesting that she may have a diminution in proximal muscle strength. She appears to be experiencing pain in her right hip on weight bearing, is probably using her cane in the wrong hand, and is at risk for a fall given her combination of pain, weakness, and clumsiness related to the edema. Her reduced score on the Mini–Mental State examination suggests the need for further cognitive evaluation. Mrs. Smith has accepted pain and functional decline as normal aspects of aging, and her daughter has fallen into the same trap. Furthermore, Mrs. Smith has embarked on two additional therapeutic programs (a new medication, and an adaptive mobility aid) without professional advice. In fact, it may well be that Mrs. Smith's edema and deterioration in cognitive function are the direct result of her use of her neighbor's ibuprofen.

Laboratory Assessment and Diagnosis. The diagnosis of osteoarthritis is made based on a characteristic history and physical examination, as well as the presence of osteoarthritic changes on radiograph. There are no specific laboratory tests for OA. Unlike the inflammatory arthritides (e.g., rheumatoid arthritis), the erythrocyte sedimentation rate (ESR) and hemogram are normal and autoantibodies are not present. If there is a joint effusion, the synovial fluid is noninflammatory, with less than 2000 white blood cells/mm^3, a predominance of mononuclear white blood cells, and a good mucin clot.

The usual radiographic findings of OA include osteophytes, periarticular sclerosis and cyst formation, and asymmetrical loss of joint space. It should be noted that many older individuals have these findings on radiography and do not have symptomatic osteoarthritis. Furthermore, although the presence of osteophytes is seen with OA, the presence of this feature alone is not thought to be sufficient for the diagnosis of OA, since osteophytes can occur with aging alone (in the absence of OA).

The newer imaging modalities, computed tomography (CT), magnetic resonance imaging (MRI), and ultrasonography, may prove useful in assessing OA, monitoring its progress, and understanding its natural course. However, the diagnosis of OA rarely requires such expensive modalities and their routine use is not justified. Box 19-1 outlines the laboratory and radiological characteristics of OA.

Management. The management of OA should focus on pain relief, prevention of progressive joint damage, and maximization of functional ability. Nonpharmacological, pharmacological, and surgical interventions all play important roles in the management of patients with OA. Ongoing functional assessment is important in the care of the patient with OA, particularly in assessing the effectiveness of treatment interventions and in monitoring the progress of the disease.

Nonpharmacological management strategies for OA (Box 19-2) include limited (1- to 2-hour) periods of rest when symptoms are at their worst, avoidance of repetitive movements or static body positions that aggravate symptoms, joint preservation techniques, heat (or cold) for the control of pain, weight loss if the patient is obese, adaptive mobility aids to diminish the mechanical load on joints, adaptive equipment to assist in ADL skills, range of motion exercises, strengthening exercises, and endurance exercises.[13,14] Immobilization should be

BOX 19-1
Laboratory and Radiological Assessment of OA

Laboratory Tests	Radiological Findings
Normal erythrocyte sedimentation rate	Narrowing of joint space
Normal hemogram	Subchondral bony sclerosis
Negative rheumatoid factor	Subchondral cysts
Negative antinuclear antibody	Marginal osteophyte formation

BOX 19-2
Nonpharmacological Therapies of OA

Weight loss
Rest (during acute exacerbations)
Avoidance of exacerbating activities
Heat (or cold)
Adaptive aids for mobility and ADL skills
Avoidance of immobility
Range of motion exercises
Strengthening
Endurance (aerobic) exercises

Table 19-2   Medications for OA

Drug	Dosage Range/Frequency
Acetaminophen	650 mg q4h or 1000 mg q6h
Salicylates	
Aspirin	650 mg q4h
Aspirin, extended release	1600 mg bid
Nonacetylated Salicylates	
Choline magnesium salicylate (Trilisate)	2-3 g in 1-2 doses/day
Salsalate (Disalcid)	3 g in 2-3 doses/day
NSAIDs	
Acetic acids	
Diclofenac (Voltaren)	150-200 mg in 2 doses/day
Tolmetin (Tolectin)	600-1600 mg in 3-4 doses/day
Anthranilic acids	
Meclofenamate (Meclomen)	200-400 mg in 3-4 doses/day
Indole acetic acids	
Indomethacin (Indocin)	50-200 mg in 3 doses/day
Sulindac (Clinoril)	300-400 mg in 2 doses/day
Propionic acids	
Ibuprofen (Motrin)	1.2-3.2 g in 3-4 doses/day
Naproxen (Naprosyn)	500-750 mg in 2 doses/day
Oxicams	
Piroxicam (Feldene)	20 mg in 1-2 doses/day

avoided because of the deleterious effects on muscle strength, exercise capacity, and joint range of motion with the associated risk of contracture development.

The use of adaptive mobility aids (e.g., canes and walkers) is an important strategy. Care should be taken to ensure that the mobility aid is the correct device, appropriately sized, and in good repair. In addition, the patient should be instructed in the correct use of the adaptive mobility aid. For osteoarthritis of the hip, when a cane is used, it should be carried in the contralateral hand and advanced at the same time as the affected extremity. The heel of the hand, resting on the top of the cane, should be at the level of the greater trochanter, resulting in elbow flexion of roughly 25 degrees. When an adaptive mobility aid is not properly sized and appropriately used, it can actually increase joint stress and pain, as well as become a hazard that precipitates a fall.

Patients and families must understand that pain relief in osteoarthritis is given in order to enable the person to exercise and mobilize more; without pain relief there will be a downward spiral of pain leading to immobility leading to more pain.

Pharmacological approaches to the treatment of OA (Table 19-2) include acetaminophen, salicylates, nonacetylated salicylates, nonsteroidal antiinflammatory drugs (NSAIDs), and intraarticular steroids. Acetaminophen is advocated for use as a first-line therapy by some physicians based on clinical experience and short-term intervention studies.[15] Salicylates and NSAIDs are, however, still the most commonly used first-line medications for the relief of pain related to OA. Intraarticular steroids are generally reserved for the occasional instance when there is a single painful joint or a large effusion in a single joint and the pain is unresponsive to other modalities. Systemic steroids and narcotics should be avoided if possible.

Salicylates and NSAIDs have analgesic and antiinflammatory effects, probably because they act to inhibit prostaglandin synthesis. Toxic side effects, many thought to be related to inhibition of prostaglandin synthesis, involve a number of organ systems. Although these are usually reversible after drug withdrawal, they can be severe. The most common adverse effects encountered with salicylates, NSAIDs, and nonacetylated salicylates are listed in Table 19-3. In addition to the adverse ef-

Table 19-3 Adverse Effects of Drugs for OA

Drug Class	Adverse Effects
Salicylates	Dyspepsia, gastrointestinal toxicity, interference with platelet function, tinnitus, hepatitis and renal damage (both rare), interaction with oral anticoagulants
NSAIDs	Dyspepsia and gastrointestinal toxicity, including bleeding, ulceration, perforation, and diarrhea
	Interference with platelet function
	Decreased renal blood flow, fluid retention, renal failure, renal papillary necrosis, interstitial nephritis, and nephrotic syndrome
	Dizziness, anxiety, drowsiness, tinnitus, and confusion
	Mild hepatic dysfunction, rarely hepatitis
	Aplastic anemia (rare except with phenylbutazone)
Nonacetylated salicylates	Interfere with oral anticoagulants

fects of salicylates, compliance can be a major problem given the short duration of action and the need for frequent doses. This is one reason that NSAIDs are often used rather than salicylates.

Many NSAIDs are available. Most are relatively expensive. Because an individual patient's response to one drug is not predictive of the therapeutic response to other agents, it is often necessary to try several drugs before optimum therapy is obtained. With the exception of phenylbutazone (which should be avoided) and perhaps indomethacin (which has a slightly higher incidence of side effects), there is little compelling evidence for choosing one NSAID over another as initial therapy. Misoprostol (Cytotec), a prostaglandin E analog, has been shown to reduce the incidence of gastric ulceration in some patients taking NSAIDs. However, misoprostol is expensive and is probably not necessary as a routine measure when starting a patient on NSAIDs.

The nonacetylated salicylate preparations are less potent inhibitors of prostaglandins and, as such, are thought to have less gastrointestinal and renal toxicity than do NSAIDs. The nonacetylated salicylates are also thought to have the advantage of not impairing platelet function. Unfortunately, some authorities note that they are not as efficacious in the treatment of osteoarthritic pain as are salicylates and NSAIDs.[16]

Arthroscopic lavage and osteotomy are surgical approaches that have been used to decrease pain in OA of the knee. However, total joint replacement is the primary surgical approach for OA of the knee and the hip. Candidates for arthroplasty are individuals who have experienced severe pain, impairment in joint function, or declines in functional status that do not improve with nonpharmacological and pharmacological measures.

An important preoperative concern for the patient undergoing hip or knee surgery is the risk of deep vein thrombosis (DVT). Low-dose subcutaneous heparin (5000 units every 12 hours) is not maximally effective in preventing DVT in this high-risk group of patients.[17] Better prophylaxis is obtained with the use of low-dose warfarin (Coumadin) sufficient to maintain the prothrombin time at 1.25 to 1.5 times control, adjusted dose subcutaneous heparin (to maintain the partial thromboplastin time in the 30- to 40-second range), or, especially for knee reconstruction, pneumatic compression of the lower extremities.[17] Low molecular weight heparin is now considered by many to be preferable to warfarin (Coumadin) for DVT prevention in patients undergoing total joint replacement.[18] Additional effective preventive measures include elevation of the foot of the bed, graded elastic stockings, and prompt mobilization out of bed. The necessary duration of DVT prophylaxis is not clear, but common sense dictates that the patient be mobile and ambulatory before the discontinuation of therapy.

Postoperatively the orthopedic surgeon, primary care physician, physical therapist, and, as necessary, occupational therapist should work together to develop a rehabilitation program. Physical therapists can also provide valuable assistance in preoperative preparation of the patient with OA through stretching exercises and positioning programs to prevent or reduce contracture and strengthening exercises to prevent or reduce muscle atrophy.

OA should be considered a condition that affects the entire family. OA can result in lost income related to physician and physical therapy visits, disability-related work absences, and absences related to surgery. Sexual intercourse can become difficult and painful, adding to family stress. Sexuality is an often neglected aspect of care and should be discussed openly. Suggestions for adaptive measures to improve sexual function are listed in Box 19-3.[19] Not uncommonly, the pain and functional disability associated with OA can contribute to social isolation and depression that affect the family as well as the patient.

A valuable resource for patients and families is the Arthritis Foundation, which has local chapters throughout the United States. This foundation not only conducts research for the prevention and treatment of arthritis, but more important, provides services and education for patients and families. The importance of educating the patient and family about OA cannot be overemphasized.

Exercise to increase joint mobility
Use heat (e.g., shower or tub) before sexual activity
Avoid positions that prolong pressure on involved joints and experiment with adaptive positions
Premedicate with analgesics or antiinflammatory medications
Use a water bed
Have a period of rest before sexual activity
Explore alternatives to intercourse such as masturbation or oral sex

Osteoarthritis
Paget's disease
Osteomalacia
Osteoporosis
Tumor
Rheumatoid arthritis
Pseudogout
Gout
Trauma

CASE DISCUSSION

In the case of Mrs. Smith, the history, physical examination, and initial laboratory assessment are entirely consistent with the diagnosis of osteoarthritis as her primary problem. Osteoarthritis of her hip has progressed to the point at which she has lost independence in IADLs. This functional decline is exacerbated by fluid retention related to the self-prescribed use of ibuprofen and the improper use of an adaptive mobility aid. It is also quite possible that her diminished cognitive function is a side effect of the NSAID she borrowed from her neighbor. Appropriate and timely recognition of Mrs. Smith's pain and functional decline, which are not normal aspects of aging, could have prevented many of the problems included on Mrs. Smith's problem list. Fortunately, the problems were recognized before an irreversible complication developed (e.g., a fall and resultant hip fracture). Given the reversible nature of Mrs. Smith's complications, an appropriate therapeutic plan has a good chance of success.

The care of the older person with osteoarthritis and resultant functional limitations frequently needs to be interdisciplinary. The physician establishes a diagnosis and treatment plan and educates the patient and family. Using a combination of the physical, pharmacological, and surgical approaches mentioned previously, the physician seeks to maintain treatment of pain and maintenance of mobility. A physical therapist needs to play an integral treatment role, evaluating the patient for the use of adaptive mobility aids and helping the patient learn strengthening and maintenance exercises. A home safety evaluation conducted by a physical or occupational therapist may also be warranted. The therapist can make recommendations regarding adaptive aids for safe use of the toilet and tub as well as identify other environmental risk factors for falls (e.g., poorly lit staircases, loose rugs, exposed electrical cords), thereby preventing injury and further functional decline. A visiting nurse can assess compliance with the therapeutic program and response to treatment.

Other Conditions Causing Bone and Joint Pain

The diagnosis of osteoarthritis is relatively clear when a chronic course, the lack of inflammatory changes, characteristic joint involvement, absence of systemic symptoms, and characteristic x-ray and laboratory findings are present. However, many cases are not as clear cut as this; before a definitive diagnosis is made, other diagnostic possibilities must be considered. Box 19-4 lists some common causes of bone and joint pain in older persons. Each is briefly discussed below.

Rheumatoid Arthritis. Rheumatoid arthritis is a common systemic illness, the major characteristic of which is a symmetrical polyarticular inflammatory arthritis. The cause of rheumatoid arthritis is unknown. Although often presenting at a younger age (peak incidence is in the third and fourth decade), it is not uncommon for rheumatoid arthritis to present de novo in old age. Furthermore, for individuals in whom rheumatoid arthritis develops at a younger age, the chronic and disabling nature of the illness makes it an important factor in later life.

The clinical course of rheumatoid arthritis is highly variable, but the majority of patients have a gradual onset of symmetrical polyarticular arthritis associated with morning stiffness and signs of systemic disease. Prolonged daily morning stiffness is helpful in distinguishing rheumatoid arthritis from osteoarthritis, in which morning stiffness is much less common, and if present, invariably lasts less than 30 minutes. Swelling, tenderness, eventual joint deformity, and decline in functional status are common features. The proximal interphalangeal joints, metacarpals, wrists, elbows, knees, ankles, and metatarsals are commonly involved joints. Extraarticular manifestations are common and include rheumatoid nodules and ocular, pleuropulmonary, cardiac, and neurological complications, as well as vasculitis and Felty's syndrome. The radiographic findings include periarticular osteoporosis, diffuse joint space narrowing, soft tissue swelling, and juxtaarticular erosions. The laboratory evaluation reflects the chronic inflammatory nature of the illness and often reveals a normochromic normocytic anemia, an elevated ESR, thrombocytosis, hypergammaglobulinemia, and a positive rheumatoid factor. However, it should be noted that there is a high prevalence of false-positive tests for rheumatoid factor and other autoantibodies in elderly patients who are otherwise healthy.

> *The length of early morning stiffness is most useful in distinguishing osteoarthritis from inflammatory (rheumatoid) arthritis: in OA, morning stiffness lasts less than 30 minutes.*

The treatment goals in rheumatoid arthritis are similar to those in osteoarthritis: relief of pain, preservation of joint function, and preservation of functional status. Physical approaches to therapy of rheumatoid arthritis include rest, particularly during inflammatory phases, range of motion exercises to prevent disuse atrophy and limit deformity, splints as adjuncts to provide rest (e.g., volar wrist splints and cervical collars), adaptive mobility aids, and heat. Pharmacological approaches to treatment include salicylates, NSAIDs, gold, antimalarial drugs (hydroxychloroquine), penicillamine, immunosuppressive medications, and corticosteroids. Surgery is indicated for persistent severe pain, deformity, restrictive joint motion, and decreased functional ability.[20]

Gout and Chondrocalcinosis. Gout and chondrocalcinosis (pseudogout) are crystal-induced arthropathies. Pseudogout is seldom seen below the age of 50 years, and its incidence increases dramatically with age. Gout, on the other hand, usually has its onset in middle age. Although it can present in old age, it is most commonly seen in older patients who have been inadequately treated and have resultant progressive disease and permanent joint destruction. Pseudogout, more properly known as chondrocalcinosis, is also known as calcium prophosphate dihydrate (CPPD) crystal deposition disease. Chondrocalcinosis shows a broad range of clinical presentation and can mimic the presentations of infectious arthritis, gout, rheumatoid arthritis, and osteoarthritis. The diagnoses of gout and pseudogout are based on the clinical presentation, characteristic x-ray findings, and most important, analysis of the synovial fluid. The inflammatory nature of the synovial fluid and the presence of characteristic crystals establish the diagnosis. NSAIDs are the primary therapy for gout and pseudogout in the management of acute attacks and chronic inflammation. Additionally, in gout, the serum uric acid

must be lowered to the normal range with xanthine oxidase inhibitors or uricosuric agents. Both conditions, if adequately treated, rarely lead to disabling complications. A more extensive discussion is beyond the scope of this chapter but can be found elsewhere.[21]

Trauma. Trauma can obviously result in bone and joint pain. Older persons, particularly those with underlying chronic illnesses (e.g., osteoporosis or malignancy), can suffer fractures from minimally traumatic events. It is not uncommon that simple activities of daily living can result in bony fractures when there is an underlying pathological process. Because of this possibility, fractures should be considered in the differential diagnosis of bone and joint pain even in the absence of any significant traumatic event. Fortunately, in most cases these are easily identified on plain radiographs.

Paget's Disease. Paget's disease of bone (osteitis deformans) is a progressive focal bone disease that rarely occurs before age 30 and is almost exclusively found among older patients. The etiology of Paget's disease is unknown but may be related to a slow viral infection. Paget's disease is characterized by increased bone resorption and increased bone formation. There is an initial osteolytic phase followed by a mixed phase in which new bone formation is accelerated and bone is formed in a chaotic manner. The final phase is osteoblastic in which bone is relatively devoid of cellular activity.

Most patients with Paget's disease are asymptomatic. The predominant symptom, when it occurs, is pain. Neurological manifestations and a number of other complications of bone overgrowth (e.g., cardiovascular, ophthalmological, and gastrointestinal) also occur. As with osteoarthritis and rheumatoid arthritis, the goals for therapy with Paget's disease are to relieve pain and maintain function. Patients without symptoms require no treatment. A full discussion of the treatment of Paget's disease is beyond the scope of this text but can be found elsewhere.[22] However, the three classes of drugs that are used for the treatment of Paget's disease include calcitonin, diphosphonates, and mithramycin. In addition, it is important to avoid immobilization, as this can precipitate hypercalcemia.

Osteoporosis. Osteoporosis refers to a condition in which a reduction in bone mass progresses to the point that fractures occur with minimal trauma. The composition of the remaining bone is essentially normal, and osteoporosis can be classified as either primary or secondary. Osteoporosis is covered in depth elsewhere in this text.

Osteomalacia. Osteomalacia refers to a group of disorders that have a bone mineralization defect in common. The mineralization defect leads to deformities of bone and to pain as a result of fractures. Osteomalacia is relatively uncommon but important to identify because it is reversible. The most common causes of osteomalacia in older populations are conditions that lead to vitamin D deficiency or phosphate deficiency, such as anticonvulsant use, gastrectomy, avoidance of sunlight (e.g., nursing home patients), and malabsorption syndromes.

Post-Polio Syndrome. Before its virtual eradication from the United States during the 1950s, polio affected 1.6 million Americans. Now, many decades after the original illness, approximately 30% (perhaps 500,000 individuals) are reporting new symptoms.[23] This postpolio syndrome (PPS) consists of new muscle weakness, muscle pain, and fatigue in the areas originally affected by the disease. Joint pain caused by muscle imbalance is also common; the back of the knee, the ankle (sometimes with inversion deformity or footdrop), back, and shoulder (often misdiagnosed as a rotator cuff injury) are the joints most commonly affected.[24] The cause of the syndrome is uncertain; the two most popular theories involve nerve cell attrition (the strongest risk factor for PPS is length of time since the original illness) and reactivation of the virus (viral fragments and IGM antibodies have been detected in PPS sufferers).[23-25] Treatment involves life-style changes to avoid overexertion, use of assistive devices, exercise to strengthen weakened muscles, and (in the case of severe muscle contractures) surgery.[24]

Parkinson's Disease. Parkinson's disease is a chronic, progressive illness that most frequently begins between the ages of 50 and 70 years and is rarely seen before age 40. The classic symptoms include tremor, dyskinesias, rigidity, and postural abnormalities. The primary dyskinesias associated with Parkinson's disease inevitably result in dysmobility and immobility, and the condition should be considered in the differential diagnosis of mobility problems for older persons. Parkinson's disease is covered in depth elsewhere in this text.

IMMOBILITY

▼ CLARA WHITE (Part I)

Clara White, a 73-year-old woman, is hospitalized with the sudden onset of right hemiparesis, right facial weakness, and dysarthria. She has a history of hypertension but otherwise has been relatively healthy. Before admission she had been independent in ADLs, IADLs, and mobility and had been living alone in a second-floor apartment. Mrs. White has no family locally but has numerous good friends nearby. She is a retired schoolteacher and hospital volunteer. On admission, Mrs. White's Mini–Mental State examination score is 28/30. Neurological findings are normal except for a mild dysarthria, 3/5 motor weakness proximally and distally in both her right upper and lower extremities, and a positive Babinski on the right. She has no sensory deficits, apraxia, neglect, or aphasia. Aside from a left central seventh nerve palsy and the dysarthria, the cranial nerves are normal. A computed tomography scan and neurological consultation confirm that Mrs. White has had a left brain, nonhemorrhagic stroke. Additional laboratory studies are ordered to ascertain (if possible) the etiology of the patient's stroke. You plan to observe her in the hospital.

STUDY QUESTIONS

- *Does Mrs. White need mobilization orders?*
- *Which complications of immobility is Mrs. White at risk for?*
- *How can these risks be minimized?*

CASE DISCUSSION

Although Mrs. White is at increased risk for another stroke, this risk pales in comparison to the risk she incurs as a consequence of bed rest and immobility.

Risks of Immobility

The bedfast elderly patient is at increased risk for a wide range of complications (Box 19-5). The consequences of immobility are so numerous and grave that bed rest should be reserved for those rare clinical situations in which the risks inherent in maintaining a higher level of physical activity outweigh the very significant risks of immobility. In the case of a new stroke a brief period of bed rest may be warranted, but the emphasis should be placed on mobilization as soon as possible (within 24 hours if the patient is neurologically stable). Furthermore, the need to immobilize one extremity, as in the patient with a fracture or deep vein thrombosis, does not justify immobilizing the rest of the patient. At a minimum the other extremities should receive range of motion and strengthening exercises. In those rare situations when bed rest is clinically necessary or unavoidable, pa-

---

BOX 19-5
Consequences of Immobility and Bed Rest

Pressure ulcers
Constipation
Fecal impaction
Fecal incontinence
Urinary tract infection
Urinary incontinence
Orthostatic hypotension
Deep vein thrombosis
Pulmonary embolus
Atelectasis
Aspiration pneumonia
Osteoporosis
Urinary tract stones
Deconditioning
Contractures
Sensory deprivation syndrome
Depression

tients' families and health care providers need to be hypervigilant to prevent the almost inevitable medical complications that are likely to follow.

> *Only in the hospital does an individual need a specific physician's order to do the natural thing and get out of bed; the consequences of physicians failing to write this order many times over many decades has been death to many elders.*

▼ CLARA WHITE (Part II)

Forty-eight hours after admission, Mrs. White's strength on the affected side is roughly 3.5/5. By 72 hours after admission the patient's condition has stabilized. Initially, Mrs. White is kept at bed rest, during which she has occasional episodes of urinary incontinence and exhibits nighttime confusion. In response to the confusion she receives a standing order for haloperidol, which initially seems to have a beneficial effect. However, by the fourth hospital day, Mrs. White seems more lethargic. On the fifth day, when assisted out of bed for the first time, the patient feels lightheaded and is returned to bed. Because of her lightheadedness, she is toileted on a bedpan rather than a toilet or bedside commode. Her nutritional intake is poor, but she receives no intravenous supplementation because she has pulled out several intravenous lines during her confusional episodes. On the same day Mrs. White is noted to have a minimal amount of skin breakdown over her sacrum.

After a week of hospitalization, Mrs. White exhibits moderate generalized weakness in addition to the focal weakness on her right side. She has not had a formed bowel movement but has developed fecal incontinence of small amounts of liquid stool. Nutritional intake has been minimal, and she has become significantly dehydrated. Her mood is markedly depressed. On the eighth hospital day the patient develops fever, tachypnea, leukocytosis, and a right lower lobe infiltrate on chest radiograph.

Consequences of Immobility

Immobility can affect many physiological functions. These include neuropsychiatric, cardiovascular, musculoskeletal, metabolic, endocrine, integumentary, and excretory systems. The consequences include poor oral intake, overmedication, deep vein thrombosis, pulmonary embolism, constipation, urinary and fecal incontinence, pressure ulcers, urinary tract infection, atelectasis, pneumonia, depression, sensory depression, orthostatic hypotension, deconditioning, contractures, and osteoporosis. These effects can be so profound that even brief periods

of immobility may cause a frail older person to suffer irrevocable functional decline.[26]

Malnutrition can occur quickly in the elderly hospitalized patient. Although total serum albumin levels are maintained in the normal range in healthy older persons, as a group they are less well nourished than younger patients. All too often the older hospitalized patient goes 2, 3, and even 4 days receiving intravenous fluids only. Such relatively brief periods of starvation often result in malnutrition and help to propagate the cascade of deleterious consequences associated with immobility. The older hospitalized stroke patient is at even greater risk of malnutrition because of associated manifestations of the illness, such as dysphagia, motor weakness, and sensory deficits. Failure to maintain adequate nutrition increases the older patient's risk for constipation, pressure ulcers, infection, confusion, dehydration, and fluid and electrolyte abnormalities. To combat malnutrition, the physician, with the assistance of nursing staff, nutritionists, and in some cases speech pathologists and other rehabilitation professionals, should quickly assess the patient's nutritional needs and develop a safe means of providing adequate nutrition. Possible approaches include nurse- or therapist-supervised feedings, intravenous hyperalimentation, and nasogastric tube feedings.

The immobile older patient is susceptible to the adverse effects of *medications*. In particular, the use of medications with central nervous system or anticholinergic side effects should be avoided or minimized. The risks associated with a poor nights' sleep may be far less than those associated with the use of sedative-hypnotic medications for a hospitalized older patient.

Deep vein thrombosis and pulmonary embolus are common complications of immobility that can have disastrous consequences for the older patient. Again, early mobilization and range of motion joint exercises are probably the most effective preventive intervention. However, for the patient with a flaccid hemiparesis, paraparesis, or other truly immobilizing condition, the use of subcutaneous heparin and elastic stockings is thought to be beneficial.[27] For patients who are immobilized because of a hip fracture, it has been demonstrated that pneumatic compression stockings and anticoagulation with adjusted-dose heparin, warfarin, or low molecular weight heparin are effective means of preventing deep vein thrombosis and resultant pulmonary embolus.[17,18]

Immobility, dehydration, and malnutrition together contribute to the high prevalence of *constipation* found in older bedfast patients. Additionally, many elders are chronically constipated or take medications with potential constipating effect. Constipation in the immobile older patient should be considered much more than simply a nuisance. In addition to abdominal discomfort, constipation can lead to decreased oral intake, thereby worsening hydration and nutritional status. *Fecal impaction* (which is a common cause of *fecal incontinence*) and, in extreme cases, bowel obstruction can also occur. Early mobilization, adequate nutrition (including fiber intake), proper hydration, bulk-forming agents (psyllium) or stool softeners, and an established daily toileting regimen are effective preventive approaches.[26]

Pressure ulcers are another common consequence of immobilization. Among hospitalized patients confined to a bed or chair for a week, the prevalence of pressure ulcers, the majority of which develop in the hospital, is as high as 30%.[28] Immobility and malnutrition are leading risk factors for the development of pressure ulcers.[29]

From both time and cost perspectives the best treatment of pressure ulcers is prevention. Again, the most important preventive measure is early mobilization. For the individual who cannot be adequately mobilized, frequent body repositioning, antipressure devices (e.g., pressure-relieving mattress overlays or, in severe cases, special air-fluidized beds), attention to adequate nutrition, avoidance of shearing forces, moisture, and friction over bony prominences, and maintenance of continence are all helpful strategies.[30] The clinician should inspect high-risk skin areas (the sacrum, greater trochanters, ischia, lateral malleoli, and heels) daily for the presence of blanching erythema, which is a sign of tissue ischemia. At this first sign of impending skin breakdown, preventive measures should be intensified and initial treatment begun. Further discussion of pressure ulcers is presented in the chapter on pressure ulcers.

Urinary tract infections occur in the immobilized elderly person for many reasons, including comorbid illnesses (e.g., malnutrition, diabetes mellitus), poor perineal hygiene, altered urogenital flora, underlying bladder retention, and Foley catheter use. *Urinary incontinence* is particularly common in hospitalized elders and occurs frequently in stroke patients. Establishing a functional toileting regimen is a key step in preventing incontinence. The toileting regimen should include prompted voiding on a set schedule and must allow for a patient's limitations. Whenever possible, it should include use of a toilet or commode rather than a bedpan. All too frequently a urinal, for a male stroke patient, or the call button, for a female patient, is placed on the side of the stroke patient's weakness; unilateral neglect or visual field deficit can similarly contribute to functional incontinence.

Besides the functional causes of incontinence noted above, *urinary retention* and consequent overflow incontinence can occur in immobilized patients. For this reason it is important to establish that patients with new incontinence do not have elevated postvoid residual urine volumes (>100 ml). If urinary retention is present, discontinuation of anticholinergic medications, mobiliza-

tion, and intermittent catheterization are the key elements of appropriate management. The use of a Foley catheter should be reserved for cases of urinary retention; urological referral is often needed for these cases.

Bed rest in the supine position impairs clearance of respiratory secretions, lessens the effectiveness of the cough mechanism, and predisposes the older person to *atelectasis* at the lung bases, thereby putting the patient at increased risk for pulmonary infection. Although incentive spirometry may be helpful to prevent atelectasis, the optimum treatment is mobilization to an upright position that improves diaphragmatic movement and increases aeration of basal lung segments. Upright positioning following meals may minimize the risk of aspiration, and a swallowing evaluation by an experienced speech pathologist may also be beneficial.

Depression is prevalent in immobilized patients. As with depression in other settings, therapeutic approaches include medications (antidepressants and psychostimulants), psychotherapy, and in certain cases, electroconvulsive therapy. Undoubtedly, the therapeutic milieu of a rehabilitation program and any associated recovery of functional ability are also powerful therapeutic processes in the treatment of the depressed patient with a stroke or fracture. The side effect profiles of the tricyclic secondary amines (nortriptyline and desipramine) are, in general, less worrisome than that of the tricyclic tertiary amines (doxepin, imipramine, and amitriptyline). For this reason, many physicians recommend the former agents as their first choice. Heterocyclic compounds (trazodone) and serotonin reuptake blockers (fluoxetine, sertraline) are also frequently recommended, although fluoxetine and similar agents are newer drugs that have been less extensively used in elderly populations. With all agents it is advisable to start at a low dose that is increased slowly.

The sterile hospital environment provides little sensory stimulation and social contact for the elderly individual. Immobilization of older patients, combined with social isolation, often leads to the development of neuropsychiatric symptoms. The effects of *sensory deprivation* include anxiety, confusion, noncompliant behavior, perceptual distortions, and depression. These can lead to iatrogenic complications as the physician attempts to treat these behaviors. Sensory deprivation symptoms can be prevented by increasing the patient's interaction with staff and family. Also, the placement of orienting information in the hospital room (calendar, clock) and the provision of necessary glasses and hearing aids are helpful.

Orthostatic hypotension occurs in 20% to 25% of unselected elderly patients.[32] Disease states (e.g., diabetes mellitus, hypothyroidism) and medications (e.g., diuretics, antihypertensives, antidepressants, and major tranquilizers) contribute additional risk. Bed rest and immobility further increase the rate of orthostatic hypotension by slowing normal postural compensatory changes in heart rate, stroke volume, and cardiac output. Measures to prevent the development of orthostatic hypotension include adequate fluid intake, prompt mobilization, and slowly elevating the patient to a sitting position and then pausing before having the patient stand.

Deconditioning, another consequence of immobility, is the loss of muscle strength and exercise tolerance that occurs with inactivity. In conditions that affect neurological function, such as stroke, the superimposed effects of deconditioning may cause further loss of ambulation and ADL skills. To prevent deconditioning, prompt mobilization out of bed is important. Daily range of motion exercises, both passive and (if tolerated) active assistive, done with the patient sitting or standing will maintain muscle strength and prevent the loss of exercise tolerance.

Contractures and disuse osteoporosis may also result from immobility. An immobile joint will develop a *contracture* within 3 to 4 weeks.[32] The resultant joint limitation affects a patient's independence by limiting ADL and mobility skills. The bone loss associated with bed rest and immobility adds to the postmenopausal loss of bone occurring in women and the age-related development of osteoporosis that occurs in both sexes. Early mobilization and weight-bearing exercise (e.g., walking) is thought to prevent both contractures and disuse osteoporosis.

Management of Immobility

Exercise is the specific physiological stimulus that can prevent or reverse many of the adverse medical consequences of immobility. It is for this reason that range of motion and strengthening exercises and a complete rehabilitation plan can and should begin even before the time that a patient with an acute stroke is able to ambulate. Encouraging the patient to perform ADLs is another way to provide joint exercise and foster independence within a patient's limitations.

Although stroke is used as an example of an immobilizing illness, the preventive plan described below is generally applicable to the care of any patient in any health care setting who for any reason has limited mobility or is maintained at bed rest. While mobilization is the most important intervention, the clinician also needs to be vigilant in looking for and preventing the most likely medical complications of immobility. Table 19-4 summarizes interventions designed to prevent the complications of immobility and bed rest. Minimization of physical and chemical restraints is an important element of the management of immobility. In both hospital and nursing home settings, restraints have been associated with an in-

creased incidence of a variety of immobility-related medical complications. In addition, the rate of falling and the occurrence of fall-related injury is not decreased by the use of restraints. All members of the geriatric health care team should be familiar with the assessment of a patient at risk for falls and alternatives to the use of restraints.[33,34]

A rehabilitation approach (addressed elsewhere in this text) is the optimal way to both prevent and treat immobility. Such an approach addresses the medical and functional needs of the patient. Primary care practitioners should be facile in developing a preventive plan for immobility-related problems and key members of a rehabilitation team (physical, occupational, and speech therapists, etc.) should be involved early in the care of an older patient with a potentially disabling condition such as stroke. Such early intervention can greatly assist acute care nurses and physicians in treating the older patient and in preventing the cascade of negative consequences that are likely to occur with bed rest and immobility.

CASE DISCUSSION

Mrs. White's case demonstrates many of the complications that can occur in the immobilized elderly patient. Most of these complications can be prevented. If they are prevented, stroke patients like Mrs. White should be able to return to a relatively independent community living setting following a rehabilitation program. Failure to prevent immobility-related medical complications, as was the case with Mrs. White, will undoubtedly result in a cascade of negative events that may lead to long-term disability, institutionalization, or death. Key principles in the prevention of medical complications in the immobilized elderly patient include early mobilization and an appropriate exercise program; attention to nutrition, bowel, bladder, skin, and mood; and the avoidance of unnecessary medications. A functional approach to care and the early involvement of rehabilitation professionals, as appropriate, will greatly assist this process.

SUMMARY

Mobility problems in older populations are common. Immobility-related medical complications are not normal aspects of aging but are the result of one or more pathological processes. Generally, immobility-related medical complications are preventable. If not prevented, they will likely lead to further functional decline for the elderly patient. Immobility is a grave risk for the older person and should be avoided at all costs. Early interventions designed to address mobility problems and prevent the medical complications of immobility will increase the quantity and quality of life for many older persons.

Table 19-4   Summary of Interventions to Prevent Complications of Immobility or Bed Rest

Medical Complication	Preventive Intervention
Deep vein thrombosis, pulmonary embolus	Prompt mobilization
	Daily range of motion exercises
	Appropriate anticoagulation
	Lower extremity elastic stockings
Constipation, fecal impaction, and fecal incontinence	Prompt mobilization
	Adequate dietary fiber intake
	Adequate hydration
	Bulk agents or stool softeners
	Minimize medication with constipating effect
	Daily toileting routine
	Address environmental impediments to successful toileting
	Disimpaction if necessary
Pressure ulcers	Prompt mobilization
	Frequent body repositioning
	Antipressure mattress devices
	Avoid shearing and frictional forces with patient repositioning and transfers
	Repletion or maintenance of nutritional intake
	Assessment and treatment of incontinence
	Daily skin inspection
Urinary tract infection and urinary incontinence	Prompt mobilization
	Adequate hydration
	Prompted voiding
	Minimize medications that affect bladder function
	Address environmental impediments to successful toileting
	Investigate cause(s) of urinary retention, if present
	Avoid Foley catheter, except in cases of urinary retention
Atelectasis and pneumonia	Prompt mobilization
	Incentive spirometry
	Upright body positioning, as much as possible
Depression and sensory deprivation syndrome	Prompt mobilization
	Provide verbal and environmental cues for orientation
	Establish an effective communication system
	Provide adaptive aids (e.g., glasses and hearing aid)
	Antidepressant medications, as needed
Orthostatic hypotension	Prompt mobilization
	Adequate hydration
	Slow elevation of the patient from supine to sitting and then to standing
	Minimize medications with orthostatic effect
Deconditioning	Prompt mobilization
	Encourage daily performance of ADLs
	Daily range of motion exercises, passive and active assistive, as tolerated, done while sitting and standing
Contractures	Prompt mobilization
	Encourage daily performance of ADLs
	Daily range of motion exercises
Osteoporosis	Prompt mobilization
	Daily weight-bearing exercise

POSTTEST

1. Which one of the following statements about the acute hospital management of the stroke patient is correct?
   a. Rehabilitation of the stroke patient should not begin until 5 to 7 days after hospitalization for the acute event.
   b. The use of tricyclic antidepressants to treat depression in a patient with stroke is contraindicated in the early (1 to 4 weeks) poststroke period.
   c. In the first 72 hours, intravenous fluids alone are inadequate for the nutritional support of the older patient with stroke.
   d. In the immediate poststroke period, a Foley catheter is the appropriate management of urinary incontinence.

2. Which one of the following statements is most true about complications of immobility?
   a. Stroke patients are at relatively low risk of malnutrition.
   b. Range of motion exercises are of little help in the prevention of deep vein thrombosis and pulmonary embolism.
   c. The majority of pressure ulcers develop in nursing homes rather than in hospitals.
   d. A postvoid residual more than 100 ml is considered diagnostic of urinary retention.

REFERENCES

1. Self assessment of health: United States 1983-1988, National Health Interview Survey. In *Health, United States, 1989,* DHHS Publication No (PHS) 90-1232, Hyattsville, Md, 1990, US Department of Health and Human Services.
2. Williams TF: Comprehensive functional assessment, *J Am Geriatr Soc* 31:637-641, 1983.
3. Cornoni-Huntley J et al: Established populations for epidemiologic studies of the elderly. In *Resource data book,* NIH Publication No 86-2443, Hyattsville, Md, National Institute on Aging, US Department of Health and Human Services, Public Health Service, National Institute of Health.
4. Warshaw G et al: Functional disability in the hospitalized elderly, *JAMA* 248:847-850, 1982.
5. Sudarsky L: Geriatrics: gait disorders in the elderly, *N Engl J Med* 322:1441-1446, 1990.
6. American Academy of Family Physicians: *Facts about: family practice,* Kansas City, Mo, 1987, The Academy.
7. Lawrence RC et al: Estimates of the prevalence of selected arthritic and musculoskeletal diseases in the United States, *J Rheumatol* 16:427-441, 1989.
8. Ettinger W, Maradee D: Osteoarthritis. In Hazzard W, Andres R, Bierman E et al, eds: *Principles of geriatric medicine and gerontology,* ed 3, New York, 1990, McGraw-Hill.
9. Felson DT et al: Obesity and knee osteoarthritis: the Framingham Study, *Ann Intern Med* 109:18-24, 1988.
10. Hamerman D: The biology of osteoarthritis, *N Engl J Med* 320:1322-1330, 1989.
11. Applegate W, Glass J, Williams T: Instruments for the functional assessment of older persons, *N Engl J Med* 322:1207-1214, 1990.
12. Lachs M et al: A simple procedure for general screening for functional disability in elderly patients, *Ann Intern Med* 112:699-706, 1990.
13. Kovar PA et al: Supervised fitness walking in patients with osteoarthritis of the knee: a randomized controlled trial, *Ann Intern Med* 116:529-534, 1992.
14. Hicks JE, Gerber LH: Rehabilitation of the patient with arthritis and connective tissue disease. In DeLisa JA et al, eds: *Rehabilitation medicine: principles and practice,* ed 2, Philadelphia, 1988, JB Lippincott.
15. Bradley J et al: Comparison of an inflammatory dose of ibuprofen, an analgesic dose of ibuprofen, and acetaminophen in the treatment of patients with osteoarthritis, *N Engl J Med* 325:87-91, 1991.
16. Drugs for rheumatoid arthritis, *Med Lett* 33:65-70, 1991.
17. King MS: Preventing deep venous thrombosis in hospitalized patients, *Am Fam Phys* 49:1389-1396, 1994.
18. Leizorovicz A et al: Low molecular weight heparin in prevention of perioperative thrombosis, *Br Med J* 305:913-920, 1992.
19. Laflin M: Sexuality and the elderly. In Lewis CB, ed: *Aging: the health care challenge,* Philadelphia, 1985, FA Davis.
20. Calkins E, Reinhard J, Vladutiu A: Rheumatoid arthritis and the autoimmune diseases in the older patient. In Hazzard W et al, eds: *Principles of geriatric medicine and gerontology,* ed 3, New York, 1994, McGraw-Hill.
21. Seegmiller J: Gout and pyrophosphate gout. In Hazzard W et al, eds: *Principles of geriatric medicine and gerontology,* ed 3, New York, 1994, McGraw-Hill.
22. Singer F: Paget's disease of bone. In Hazzard W et al, eds: *Principles of geriatric medicine and gerontology,* ed 3, New York, 1994, McGraw-Hill.
23. Ramlow J et al: Epidemiology of the post-polio syndrome, *Am J Epidemiol* 136:769-786, 1992.
24. Aston JW: Post-polio syndrome: an emerging threat to polio survivors, *Postgrad Med* 92:249-260, 1992.
25. Stone R: Post-polio syndrome: remembrance of viruses past, *Science* 164:909, 1994.
26. Coletta EM, Murphy JB: The complication of immobility in the elderly stroke patient, *J Am Board Fam Pract* 5:389-397, 1992.
27. Prevention of venous thrombosis and pulmonary embolism, NIH Consensus Conference, *JAMA* 256:744-749, 1986.
28. Xakellis GC: Guidelines for the prediction and prevention of pressure ulcers, *J Am Board Fam Pract* 6:269-278, 1993.
29. Berlowitz DR, Wilking SVB: Risk factors for pressure sores: a comparison of cross-sectional and cohort-derived data, *J Am Geriatr Soc* 37:1043-1050, 1989.

30. Panel for Prediction and Prevention of Pressure Ulcers in Adults: *Pressure ulcer in adults: prediction and prevention,* Clinical Practice Guideline, No 3, AHCPR Publication No 92-0047, Rockville, Md, May 1992, Agency for Health Care Policy and Research, Public Health Service, US Department of Health and Human Services.

31. Harper CM, Lyles YM: Physiology and complications of bed rest, *J Am Geriatric Soc* 36:1047-1054, 1988.

32. Kottke FJ: Therapeutic exercise to maintain mobility. In Kottke FJ, Stillwell GK, Lehmann JF, eds: *Krusen's handbook of physical medicine and rehabilitation,* ed 3, Philadelphia, 1982, WB Saunders.

33. Rubenstein LZ, Josephson KR, Robbins AS: Falls in the nursing home, *Ann Intern Med* 121(6):442-451, 1994.

34. Braun JV, Lisson S, eds: Toward a restraint-free environment. In *Reducing the use of physical and chemical restraints in long-term and acute care settings,* Baltimore, 1993, Health Professions Press.

PRETEST ANSWERS

1. d
2. b

POSTTEST ANSWERS

1. c
2. d

CHAPTER 20

Dizziness

PHILIP D. SLOANE

OBJECTIVES

Upon completion of this chapter, the reader will be able to:

1. Describe the physiological mechanisms that give rise to a dizziness complaint, and discuss how these mechanisms relate to specific dizziness symptoms and to the creation of a differential diagnosis.

2. Explain how the epidemiological and clinical features of dizziness in the elderly population differ in comparison to younger adults.

3. Use key historical and physical examination data to create a differential diagnosis, given a patient who reports dizziness on initial examination. These key data include typing of dizziness symptoms, episodic vs. continuous dizziness, duration of episodes, and associated historical features.

4. Identify and describe the presentation, prognosis, and treatment of these common causes of dizziness in the elderly: medications, benign positional vertigo, and cerebrovascular disease.

PRETEST

1. Which of the following is least common as a cause of dizziness in primary care geriatrics?
   a. Anxiety
   b. Vertebrobasilar transient ischemic attacks
   c. Cervical spine disease
   d. An acoustic nerve tumor
   e. Cerumen against the tympanic membrane

2. Which of the following is the commonly accepted definition of postural hypotension?
   a. A postural drop of ≥20 mm Hg systolic or ≥10 mm Hg diastolic
   b. A postural drop of ≥25 mm Hg systolic or ≥10 mm Hg diastolic
   c. A postural drop of ≥25 mm Hg systolic or ≥15 mm Hg diastolic
   d. A postural drop of ≥25 mm Hg systolic or ≥20 mm Hg diastolic
   e. A postural drop of ≥30 mm Hg systolic or ≥20 mm Hg diastolic

3. Mr. K.G. is a 68-year-old retired insurance salesman with a 2-day history of dizziness. He describes a lightheaded sensation as though he is about to pass out that occurs whenever he is standing or walking. He has a milder sensation in the sitting position and is completely relieved when he lies down. There is no sense of spinning accompanying this sensation. What is the likely physiological mechanism underlying Mr. K.G.'s dizziness?
   a. Depression or anxiety
   b. Diminished oxygenation of the cerebral cortex
   c. A cardiac dysrhythmia
   d. Stimulation of the vestibular system when he stands
   e. Irritation of neck proprioceptive fibers

4. Which of the following historical or physical examination details would most effectively argue against benign positional vertigo as a cause of dizziness?
   a. Brief episodes of dizziness, accompanied by nausea
   b. A negative result on Romberg's test
   c. Failure to reproduce the dizziness with Hallpike's maneuver
   d. Episodes lasting 4 to 6 hours, with progressive unilateral hearing loss
   e. Multiple similar episodes over many years

Dizziness ranks with falls, incontinence, and mental confusion as a classic problem in primary care geriatrics. Like other classic geriatric problems, dizziness is not only a diagnostic but also a management challenge. It is a subjective complaint that cannot be measured and reflects a variety of different sensations produced by different mechanisms. Occasionally, two dizziness problems exist in the same patient, representing separate pathophysiological processes. In addition, multiple problems often contribute to creating a sensation that the patient describes as dizziness. To narrow the differential diagnosis from a multitude of possibilities, a thorough clinical history and physical examination are crucial.

The frequency of dizziness as a presenting complaint in primary care increases with patient age. Among patients aged 75 years and older seen by general internists, family physicians, and general practitioners, dizziness is the most common symptom identified as a reason for the visit.[1,2] Epidemiologically, dizziness is less ominous than some other common geriatric symptoms, such as mental confusion or recurrent falls. For this reason primary care physicians have an important role both in reassuring patients with benign dizziness and in identifying those with reversible, serious disease.

▼ CORA GRAVES (Part I)

Mrs. Graves developed severe dizziness while getting ready for church one morning. She reports that everything began to spin around and she felt nauseated, vomited once, and went to bed. She slept for a few hours and woke up still dizzy. Concerned family called the rescue squad and brought her to the emergency room. For 2 weeks beforehand she had noted fullness in her head, possibly with a mild decrease in hearing. She has no history of head trauma, severe exertion, coughing or sneezing, loud noises, flulike symptoms, new medications, twisting or turning activities, emotional stress, or prior similar episodes of dizziness. An 82-year-old grandmother, Mrs. Graves shares her home with another elderly woman for whom she serves as a part-time caregiver. She is generally healthy, does her own shopping, needs some help with housework, has mild bilateral cataracts, and takes a β-blocker daily.

- What anatomical structures generally give rise to the type of dizziness reported by Mrs. Graves?
- What factors related to Mrs. Graves' medical and psychosocial history could contribute to her dizziness?

PATHOPHYSIOLOGY OF DIZZINESS

In general, patients complaining of dizziness are experiencing a sensation of disorientation in relation to the position or movement of their body in space. A classic paper on the topic identified four basic types of dizziness: vertigo, presyncopal lightheadedness, dysequilibrium, and other.[3] For clinicians trying to develop a systematic approach to patients with dizziness, these four categories provide clues to the pathophysiological mechanisms underlying the dizziness complaint (Table 20-1).

Vertigo is an illusion of movement, usually of rotation. Occasionally, vertigo is described as linear displacement or tilt, but usually the patient talks about the environment spinning or whirling about. Vertigo arises from a disturbance of the vestibular system or its connecting pathways. Anatomically, these structures include the saccule, utricle, and semicircular canals within the labyrinth of the inner ear, the eighth cranial nerve, portions of the cerebellum, a number of connecting pathways in the brain stem, and the proprioceptive nerves within facet joints of the cervical spine. Common diseases of the elderly that produce vertigo include benign positional vertigo, neurolabyrinthitis, vascular disease affecting the vertebrobasilar system, and Meniere's disease.

Presyncopal lightheadedness is the sensation that one is about to pass out. It usually is described as a severe lightheaded feeling, often associated with unsteadiness or falling. Such a sensation arises because the cerebral cortex is temporarily not receiving adequate oxygen, usually because of diminished blood flow. Most adults have experienced transient presyncopal lightheadedness after rap-

Table 20-1   Key Points in Taking a Dizziness History

1. Try to Classify the Dizziness Sensation

Sensation	Description	Mechanism
Vertigo	Spinning, movement, or tilting	Impairment of vestibular system
Presyncopal lightheadedness	Feeling one is about to pass out	Global cerebral ischemia
Imbalance (dysequilibrium)	Off balance, especially when on feet	Many mechanisms, including abnormal proprioception, somatosensory, cerebellar, motor, or vestibulospinal function
Lightheadedness, floating, tingling, giddiness	Difficult to describe; vague	Anxiety, depression, or other psychological disorder

Caution: about half of dizziness in older persons cannot be clearly assigned to one type (many have imbalance plus some other sensation)

2. Determine if the Dizziness Is Episodic or Continuous

Temporal nature	Common causes
Episodic	Benign positional vertigo, transient ischemic attack, recurrent vestibulopathy, Meniere's disease
Continuous	Medication, psychological, stroke

3. Ask What Other Symptoms Accompany the Dizziness

Symptom	Possible diagnosis
Stuffy ears	Serous otitis media; Meniere's disease
Unilateral hearing loss	Labyrinthitis, Meniere's disease, acoustic neuroma (rare)
Weakness, diplopia	Transient ischemic attack
Stiff, sore neck	Cervical osteoarthritis

4. Search for Factors that Bring on or Worsen the Dizziness

Factor	Suggested etiology
Nervousness, worry, or emotional stress	Psychological dizziness
Looking up (e.g., to a high shelf)	Neck osteoarthritis with mechanical impingement of vertebral arteries
Using arms vigorously	Subclavian steal syndrome
Cough, sneeze, or strain	Perilymph fistula
Rolling over in bed, bending over, and straightening up	Benign positional vertigo

idly standing from the lying or sitting position. Usually some aggravating factor, such as lying in the hot sun, using medication, or excess alcohol intake, can be implicated in these benign episodes. Severe, persistent, or recurrent presyncopal lightheadedness represents a similar mechanism. Common causes in the elderly are vasovagal episodes, medication, and cardiac dysrhythmia.

Dysequilibrium is a sense of imbalance. Patients with this type of dizziness can usually recognize that they are experiencing a body sensation more than a head sensation. Dysequilibrium can arise from disruption of any of the structures of the balance system (Fig. 20-1). These include the vestibulospinal and proprioceptive pathways, the vestibular system, the cerebellum, the visual system, the cerebral cortex, and the neuromuscular system in the trunk and extremities. Multiple neurosensory impairments commonly contribute to dysequilibrium in the elderly. Consider, for example, a patient with poor vision because of bilateral cataracts, hip weakness caused by an underlying arthritis with deconditioning, and cerebral impairment because of benzodiazepine use for chronic insomnia. Such a patient is likely to have dysequilibrium resulting from the combination of these factors.

Vague, difficult-to-categorize dizziness is often described by patients. In such situations the physician should not rule out the causes of vertigo, presyncopal lightheadedness, or dysequilibrium merely because the patient was not able to articulate the problem adequately. On the other hand, dizziness that is difficult to describe

often accompanies psychological conditions such as anxiety and depression. The mechanism of such symptoms is poorly understood but is thought to arise from biochemical changes in the brain triggered by stress or emotional states. Patients with this psychophysiological dizziness often describe feelings of dissociation, floating, swimming, or giddiness. Associated somatic complaints, such as headache, "nerves," neck pain, insomnia, weakness, and fatigue, are common. Patients who hyperventilate when anxious describe a lightheadedness, often accompanied by tingling of the hands and around the mouth.

UNIQUE FEATURES OF DIZZINESS IN THE ELDERLY

The first factor to remember about dizziness in the elderly is that the complaint is common. During 1 year nearly 20% of community-dwelling individuals aged 60 years and older will experience dizziness severe enough to lead to a physician visit, taking a medication more than once, or interference with daily activities. Overall, these individuals are at no more risk of death and institutionalization than their healthy peers, and only a minority of cases represent a serious or life-threatening condition.[1] However, dizziness can often lead to severe adverse functional consequences, such as reduced physical activity, social isolation, and depression. Furthermore, many common causes of dizziness are curable or treatable; the key is making an accurate diagnosis and knowing the available treatment modalities. Table 20-2 shows some of the more common life-threatening, curable, and treatable problems that should be considered in the differential diagnosis of dizziness in the elderly.

A feature of dizziness complaints in the elderly, in contrast to younger adults, is a greater problem assigning patients to one pathophysiological category. In other words, patients frequently are unable to identify their dizziness as exclusively vertigo, presyncopal lightheadedness, dysequilibrium, or other. Instead, the clinician who takes a careful history is unsure what type of dizziness is present. Of 116 elderly patients with persistent dizziness, for example, only 58% could be classified into a single category.[2] One factor contributing to this observation is the fact that elderly patients frequently identify a balance problem (dysequilibrium) as a component of their dizziness.

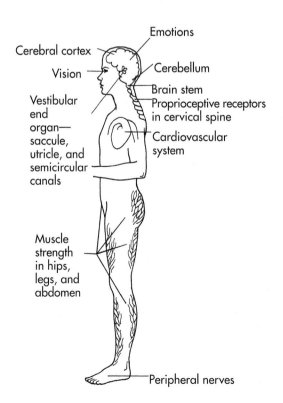

FIG. 20-1   Components of the balance system.

> *Dizziness in old age is a challenging symptom: especially at its first appearance, diagnosis can be difficult, yet accurate diagnosis is essential because of the functional implications.*

A related manner in which dizziness in elderly persons differs from that in younger adults is the frequency with

Table 20-2   Common and/or Curable Causes of Dizziness in Older Patients

Diagnosis	Type of Dizziness	Episodic vs. Continuous	Frequency in Primary Care*	Life Threatening?	Response to Treatment
			Characteristics		
Anemia and/or hypovolemia	Presyncopal lightheadedness	Continuous	M	Y	H
Anxiety (including panic disorder)	Lightheadedness, often vague	Continuous	H	N	M
Benign positional vertigo	Vertigo	Episodes of <1 min	H	N	M
Cardiac dysrhythmia	Presyncopal lightheadedness	Episodic	M	Y	H
Cerebellar atrophy	Dysequilibrium	Continuous	L	N	L
Cervical vertigo	Vertigo, often with headache	Episodic	M	N	H
Cerumen against tympanic membrane	Variable, usually vertigo	Variable	M	N	H
Drug adverse effect	Variable, often postural lightheadedness	Variable	H	Y	H
Depression	Lightheadedness, often vague	Continuous	M	Y	M
Infection, systemic (viral or bacterial)	Presyncopal lightheadedness	Continuous	H	Y	H
Meniere's disease	Vertigo (with hearing loss)	Episodes of 2-12 hr	M	N	M
Middle ear disease (e.g., serous otitis)	Vertigo or lightheadedness	Continuous	M	N	H
Migraine	Vertigo	Episodic	L	N	H
Multiple neurosensory impairments	Dysequilibrium	Continuous	H	N	L
Myocardial infarction (acute)	Presyncopal lightheadedness	Continuous	L	Y	M
Neurolabyrinthitis	Vertigo; later dysequilibrium	Continuous, abrupt onset	H	N	M
Ocular	Lightheadedness and/or imbalance	Continuous	L	N	M
Neurosyphilis	Vertigo (with hearing loss)	Episodic	L	Y	H
Perilymphatic fistula	Vertigo	Episodes associated with Valsalva	L	N	H
Recurrent vestibulopathy	Vertigo	Episodes of hours to days	M	N	L
Transient vertebrobasilar ischemia	Vertigo	Episodes of 5-120 min	H	Y	L
Stroke, vertebrobasilar system	Vertigo, later dysequilibrium	Continuous	L	Y	L
Tumor, acoustic nerve sheath	Unilateral hearing loss, occasionally with lightheadedness or vertigo	Continuous	L	N	M
Vasovagal	Presyncopal lightheadedness	Brief episodes	H	N	M

H, High; *M,* moderate; *L,* low; *Y,* yes, at times; *N,* no.
*Estimated frequency as a cause of dizziness in primary care.

which multiple conditions contribute to the complaint. This is particularly true of dizziness with a component of imbalance (i.e., the majority of chronic dizziness problems in geriatrics).

One expression of the contribution of multiple conditions is diminished capability of elderly patients to overcome new dizziness problems. In young adults, severe dysfunction in one sensory or motor system often fails to produce dizziness or a balance problem because there is compensation by excellent function elsewhere. Young adults with acute neurolabyrinthitis, for example, initially have balance and gait problems. Within days, however, they regain their equilibrium, compensating for vestibular dysfunction through increased use of proprioceptive and visual input, combined with good muscle strength. In contrast, many elderly, given the identical acute problem (neurolabyrinthitis), report persistent dysequilibrium for months or years. Reduced function in other areas of the balance system (see Fig. 20-1) is believed to be responsible.

When no single lesion predominates, multiproblem dizziness is termed multiple neurosensory impairments or, alternatively, dysequilibrium of aging.[4] In these patients, dizziness arises from multiple lesions affecting structures that mediate balance function (see Fig. 20-1). The mechanism is believed to be inability of the central processing structures of the brain to deal with confusing signals from multiple sources. Patients with multisensory dizziness describe continuous dizziness when on their feet. Depending on the structures most severely affected, dysequilibrium of aging may involve sensations of rotation (vertigo), postural lightheadedness, eye discomfort, or vague lightheaded feelings, in addition to a feeling of imbalance. Treatment consists of identifying remediable impairments, such as correcting cataracts, eliminating sedatives, or increasing muscle strength through exercise.

CLINICAL HISTORY

Primary care physicians tend to see dizziness when it first appears, which is when the diagnosis is most difficult. Some diseases, Meniere's disease for example, require observation of a pattern over time to make the diagnosis. Nevertheless, the initial evaluation should create a differential diagnosis, from which a plan for further evaluation, treatment, or observation can be developed.[5]

As previously discussed under pathophysiology, the clinical history provides the cornerstone of effective patient evaluation. The first step is to attempt to identify the primary sensation as vertigo, presyncopal lightheadedness, dysequilibrium, or other. Next, the physician should attempt to identify whether the dizziness is episodic or continuous. If it is episodic, the duration and frequency of the episodes should be identified. Then, associated symptoms should be sought (Table 20-1).

New-Onset Vertigo

Certain factors about the onset, duration, and course of vertigo symptoms will, during the initial evaluation or over time, help differentiate between causes of vertigo (Table 20-2). Features of the major causes of vertigo are discussed here.

Acute Neurolabyrinthitis. Acute neurolabyrinthitis (also called acute labyrinthitis) is caused by viral or vascular destruction of all or part of one vestibular labyrinth. Occasionally preceded by viral symptoms, this disease has a rapid onset of vertigo accompanied by nausea, vomiting, sweating, and horizontal nystagmus. If the auditory as well as the vestibular portion of the labyrinth or the vestibular nerve is affected, hearing loss and tinnitus are reported. Younger patients generally are quite ill for a day or two but rapidly improve as the brain stem learns to overcome loss of information from the damaged labyrinth. Older patients frequently take longer to recover, often reporting vertigo, dysequilibrium, or lightheadedness for months and sometimes even years after the acute attack. Treatment is supportive. Meclizine or promethazine is helpful acutely; low-dose benzodiazepines provide some relief of the more protracted disequilibrium and lightheadedness but must be used with caution.

Transient Ischemic Attacks. Transient ischemic attacks (TIAs) in the posterior circulation often begin with or are accompanied by vertigo. Associated neurological symptoms, such as diplopia, ataxia, dysarthria, weakness or numbness of one side of the body, and perioral numbness, frequently occur concurrently. The absence of other neurological signs and symptoms does not, however, rule out a TIA. Headache is an occasional symptom; syncope is unusual. Isolated vertigo is often the first symptom of vertebrobasilar disease, however. TIAs involving the anterior circulation rarely produce vertigo; in fact, patients with vertigo who have carotid endarterectomies frequently fail to improve because the carotid disease was incidental. The course of TIAs is variable. Fewer than half progress to a completed stroke, and symptoms frequently resolve completely.[6] Therefore, although therapies are limited—confined in the case of vertebrobasilar TIAs largely to aspirin and control of risk factors—the prognosis is by no means hopeless.

Stroke. Symptoms of stroke in the distribution of the vertebrobasilar system are similar to those of TIAs, often initially vertigo or poorly described dizziness. In fact, dizziness is the first symptom in approximately one fourth of basilar artery strokes. Diplopia, ataxia, dysarthria, hemiplegia, sensory deficits, and coma can follow. Thus, an evolving vertebrobasilar TIA or stroke must be considered in patients with new-onset vertigo.

Migraine. Migraine, when it affects blood vessels in the posterior circulation, can produce vascular symptoms similar to vertebrobasilar TIAs. Typical associated symptoms include scotomata, paresthesias, visual and speech disturbances, and paresis. Patients with migraine are difficult to distinguish from those with transient ischemic attacks; a buildup and migration of visual scintillations, the march of paresthesias, and progression from one associated symptom to another are said to be typical of migraine.[7]

Benign Positional Vertigo. Benign positional vertigo, an extremely common cause of dizziness in primary care geriatrics, consists of bouts of vertigo brought on by position change, particularly by rolling over in bed or by bending over and straightening up. Attacks tend to come in flurries lasting a week or two, separated by months to years without symptoms. Neurological and auditory symptoms are absent. Further details are provided later in this chapter.

Meniere's Disease. Meniere's disease consists of a triad of recurrent vertigo, tinnitus, and hearing loss. The hearing loss tends to be low frequency (as also can be the tinnitus). At first, hearing loss is noted only during vertigo attacks, but later a fixed low-frequency loss can be demonstrated. Dizziness attacks typically last between 2 and 12 hours. Disturbances of endolymphatic circulation or transport are thought to cause Meniere's disease; salt restriction and diuretics are the first step in management.

Recurrent Vestibulopathy. Recurrent vestibulopathy is a poorly understood but common entity in which mild to severe attacks of vertigo similar in character to neurolabyrinthitis occur repeatedly, often about once a year. When such patients are followed up for years, the majority of cases resolve. Some continue unchanged; others convert to benign positional vertigo; and still others develop progressive hearing loss and are diagnosed as Meniere's disease. Treatment usually consists of antihistamines such as meclizine.

Cervical Vertigo. Cervical vertigo arises from irritation of proprioceptive receptors in the facet joints of the cervical spine. Osteoarthritis or muscle spasm is usually responsible. Clinically, vertigo or a more vague lightheadedness is reported, accompanied by an occipital headache and neck stiffness or pain. Management involves treating the underlying arthritis or acute neck problem.

Middle Ear Disease. Middle ear disease, such as serous otitis media or cholesteatoma, can give rise to vertigo, vague lightheadedness, and ear stuffiness. Cerumen that touches the tympanic membrane produces vertigo by a similar mechanism. Because cerumen and middle ear disease are curable, evaluation of the vertiginous patient should always seek to rule out these diagnoses.

Neurosyphilis. Neurosyphilis is rare but eminently treatable. Most cases present with hearing loss, often bilateral. Dizziness is less prominent but can occur, usually as positional vertigo or a recurrent vestibulopathy.

Perilymphatic Fistula. Perilymphatic fistula is another diagnosis that, like neurosyphilis, is uncommon but worth thinking about because it can be cured surgically. Patients with perilymphatic fistula have a disruption in the round or oval window, causing perilymph to leak from the inner into the middle ear. A history of head trauma or exposure to loud noise should be present, since most fistulas are traumatic. Persistent dysequilibrium is common. Attacks of vertigo brought on by coughing, sneezing, or straining are more pathognomonic. The majority of patients also have some degree of unilateral hearing loss. Otolaryngologists have devised a variety of clinical tests for a fistula, none of which is specific enough to be considered diagnostic. In the primary care office, pneumatic otoscopy may be a useful screening tool, since it induces a pressure change in the middle ear and may provoke vertigo in these patients.

CASE DISCUSSION

Cora Graves reports the abrupt onset of a rotatory sensation (vertigo) several hours before being brought by rescue squad to an emergency department. Since her dizziness is vertiginous, a lesion somewhere in the vestibular system is implicated. The sudden onset suggests a vascular or traumatic process. Head stuffiness reported several weeks beforehand could indicate a viral process (neurolabyrinthitis) or the first episode of Meniere's disease.

Classically, severe vertigo is said to arise from the peripheral vestibular system and milder vertigo from central structures. In the elderly this rule is not reliable, however; some of the most intense vertigo symptoms of all involve infarction in the brain stem or the cerebellum. Other features of the history that might be important include use of a β-blocker (raising suspicion for dysrhythmia or drug side effect), her living situation (potential stress), and bilateral cataracts (raising concern about the adequacy of compensation for a vestibular problem).

Based on the initial history, Mrs. Graves' physician could construct the following list of most likely diagnoses: benign positional vertigo, a transient ischemic attack, a brain stem or cerebellar infarction, acute neurolabyrinthitis, and the first episode of Meniere's disease. Less likely causes include cerumen against the tympanic membrane, cervical vertigo, and migraine. Other causes of vertigo include neurosyphilis, perilymphatic fistula, or anxiety.

▼ CORA GRAVES (Part II)

Examination reveals a pale, ill-appearing woman with normal vital signs. Fine horizontal nystagmus is noted on physical examination and accentuated during ophthalmoscopy in a fully darkened room. Ears, heart, and lungs are normal. Hearing screening with a tuning fork and watch suggests equal function bilaterally. Mrs. Graves is unable to perform tandem gait, and Romberg's test is positive. The findings for the remainder of the neurological examination, including cranial nerves, fundi, and cerebellar testing, and strength and reflex testing in the extremities, are normal.

PHYSICAL EXAMINATION

The physical examination often provides key diagnostic data. In primary care the physical examination may be individualized based on patient symptoms. However, most examinations of a patient with dizziness should include evaluation for pathological nystagmus; fundoscopy; hearing screening; otoscopic evaluation of both ears; testing for cervical spine motion and tenderness; gait and mobility evaluation; examination of the cranial nerves, peripheral arteries (especially the carotid arteries), and heart; and screening for a peripheral neuropathy.

Several special tests and maneuvers are helpful in certain patients. These include evaluation for postural hypotension, forced hyperventilation, marching in place with closed eyes, and the Hallpike maneuver.

Postural blood pressure measurement is used in the diagnosis of postural hypotension, which is defined as a drop in systolic blood pressure of 20 or more millimeters of mercury, a diastolic drop of 10 or more millimeters of mercury, or both. These values are standardized for patients who arise from the recumbent position. Therefore, to check for postural hypotension, the patient should be asked to lie down in an adequately warm room for several minutes; then the recumbent blood pressure and pulse should be checked. Next, with the patient standing, the blood pressure and pulse should be checked. The examiner should inquire about dizziness symptoms both immediately after the patient arises and after standing for 2 minutes. Classically, postural hypotension is said to be absent if a drop in blood pressure normalizes within 2 minutes.

> *Orthostasis is so common in old age that it should be routine to record blood pressure sitting and standing, especially when the patient is taking medications likely to produce this effect.*

Forced hyperventilation is useful when anxiety is a possible diagnosis. Anxiety and in some cases depression cause a lightheadedness that is probably due to hyperventilation. Having such patients hyperventilate in the examining room can, if it provokes the same dizziness they are concerned about, provide key diagnostic information. Deep breathing at a rate of 20 to 30 breaths per minute for 2 or 3 minutes usually provokes dizziness, often accompanied by finger and perioral numbness. Once dizziness develops, the patient should be asked if his or her dizziness symptoms are similar.

Marching in place with closed eyes is a fairly sensitive test for unilateral vestibular dysfunction. To conduct the test, the patient is asked to stand in a room with closed eyes, and arms extended in front and to march in place for 30 seconds. Care must be taken not to orient the patient with sounds such as the examiner's voice, a radio, or a ticking clock. Patients with absent or reduced vestibular function rotate more than 30 to 45 degrees. A positive test can confirm that unilateral vestibular damage, such as from acute neurolabyrinthitis, has occurred sometime in the past.

The Hallpike maneuver, another useful provocative test, attempts to induce symptoms of benign positional vertigo. It is discussed in detail later in this chapter (under positional vertigo).

▼ CORA GRAVES (Part III)

The initial episode of dizziness is totally resolved by the following morning. During the next 4 months, however, Mrs. Graves experiences several additional episodes of dizziness. Each time the dizziness is rotatory and accompanied by a sensation of the wind blowing in her left ear, with episodes generally resolving within 6 hours. She also complains of progressive hearing loss on the left side, which is now present all of the time. On examination she is an alert, cooperative, vigorous elderly woman who is quite articulate. Folstein Mini–Mental State examination score is 23/30. Visual acuity is 20/30 in the right eye (oculus dexter, or OD) and 20/25 in the left eye (oculus sinister, or OS). Ear examination is normal. Eyes show no spontaneous nystagmus or end-gaze nystagmus. Saccades, smooth pursuit, and extraocular muscles appear normal. Cranial nerves are intact. Neck examination shows excellent stability on extension and turning. Carotid pulses are 2+ on the right and 3+ on the left, with no audible bruits. Her heart rhythm is regular and cardiac examination normal. Blood pressure is 165/80 in the right arm, sitting, and 155/80 in the left arm, sitting. Balance and gait evaluation show good mobility arising from a chair, ambulating, turning, and sitting. The Romberg test is normal for her age: she can maintain the position with considerable swaying with her feet together. She cannot perform tandem gait. Marching in place with her eyes closed for 30 seconds leads to a deviation to the right of 75 degrees.

EVALUATION OF DIZZINESS OCCURRING IN MULTIPLE EPISODES

With multiple episodes of dizziness the diagnosis can often become clearer than it was on initial presentation. Patients who initially cannot differentiate among vertigo, dysequilibrium, presyncopal lightheadedness, and other dizziness symptoms will, after several episodes, be able to distinguish the prominent sensation. Furthermore, episode duration will become clearer, providing helpful additional information. Finally, other associated symptoms, such as hearing loss or anxiety, may become evident.

In recurrent episodic vertigo the duration of the episodes provides an important distinguishing feature. Episodes of benign positional vertigo, while clustered over a period of days to weeks, do not individually last longer than a minute. Transient ischemic attacks (including migraine) generally have a duration of 5 minutes to 2 hours. Meniere's disease episodes are generally longer, about 2 to 12 hours.

Associated symptoms also become more evident with time. In patients with progressive vertebrobasilar insufficiency, vertigo is often the initial symptom. Later, transient ischemic attacks may include facial numbness, dysarthria, motor weakness, diplopia, or imbalance. Similarly, the hearing loss and tinnitus of Meniere's disease become more prominent as the disease progresses. Anxiety and depression may also develop, and over time more prominent associated symptoms, such as sleep disturbance, anhedonia, or overt panic attacks, may occur. In contrast, benign positional vertigo has no associated auditory or neurological symptoms that develop progressively.

CASE DISCUSSION

In the case of Cora Graves an initial vertiginous spell was followed during the next few months by several episodes of vertigo and unilateral tinnitus, generally lasting about 6 hours. In addition, a low-frequency unilateral hearing loss became evident, and marching in place with eyes closed suggested a left-sided vestibular deficit. This combination of factors noted over time establishes a diagnosis of Meniere's disease.

▼ CORA GRAVES (Part IV)

Findings on thyroid function tests, electrolytes, calcium, uric acid, blood urea nitrogen (BUN), creatinine, liver function tests, complete blood cell count, and Venereal Disease Research Laboratory (VDRL) test are normal. Audiometry reveals a unilateral hearing loss in the left ear with accentuation in the low frequencies (250 and 500 cycles per second). Otolaryngology consultation leads to electronystagmography, which reveals right beating spontaneous nystagmus in the left lateral position, normal caloric testing, and generally normal eye movements.

LABORATORY TESTING

The causes of dizziness are so diverse that no laboratory test should be considered either routine or mandatory in primary care. Test selection should be guided by the presentation, duration, and severity of the problem and by the clinician's concern about possible progressive or life-threatening conditions.

Among the laboratory tests useful in certain patients are the following:

1. Hematological and biochemical studies can screen for systemic and metabolic causes of dizziness such as anemia, hyperthyroidism, and syphilis.
2. Audiometry with speech discrimination is the best screening test for acoustic neuroma. It can also identify the progressive low-frequency hearing loss of Meniere's disease.
3. Electrocardiography identifies rhythm disturbances such as atrial fibrillation, ventricular tachycardia, or complete heart block. In episodic dizziness, capturing an episode of the dysrhythmia is often difficult, and prolonged ambulatory cardiac monitoring may be necessary.
4. Brain stem auditory evoked potentials help isolate the anatomical site of a vestibular or auditory deficit as occurring in the inner ear, the eighth cranial nerve, or the brain stem. Evoked potentials are useful in further evaluation of patients with unilateral hearing loss. They also have a role in separating benign positional vertigo from rarer types of positional vertigo.
5. Doppler examination of the cranial blood vessels and cerebral angiography can help diagnose vertebrobasilar disease. The usefulness of such information when the clinical picture already suggests TIA is questionable, however, since treatment of vertebrobasilar TIAs is limited. Probably the greatest use of these tests is in differentiating migraine from vertebrobasilar insufficiency and in identifying subclavian steal, a surgically treatable cause of vertebrobasilar TIAs.
6. Brain imaging procedures frequently are used to identify infarction or to rule out a mass lesion, such as an acoustic neuroma. Since most lesions that cause dizziness arise in the posterior fossa, they can be quite small and still produce significant symptoms. Therefore the enhanced resolution of magnetic resonance imaging makes this procedure preferable to computed tomography in most cases.
7. Electronystagmography (ENG) evaluates vestibular function by measuring the effect of selected stimuli on eye movements, using recordings from electrodes placed over the eye muscles. The test is based on the vestibuloocular reflex, which in many pathological states generates subtle oculomotor abnormalities that can be appreciated only with the eyes closed. The routine ENG can often differentiate between central and peripheral causes of vertigo.
8. Posturography is largely an experimental procedure. Its clinical usefulness is not yet established. It appears less useful in elderly than in younger populations because multiple deficits and, in par-

ticular, limb problems such as arthritis and muscle weakness lower the specificity of test results.

Consultation with an appropriate specialist is often more fruitful than performing multiple laboratory examinations, particularly in patients with chronic dizziness. This is particularly true if the physician suspects a diagnosis within the province of a specific medical subspecialty, such as neurology, otolaryngology, or cardiology. Be aware, however, that consultants tend to arrive at diagnoses within their specialty and to miss diagnoses outside their field. Therefore the generalist's role in integrating consultant opinions with the entire clinical picture cannot be overemphasized.

▼ EMMA SHORT (Part I)

Emma Short, an 81-year-old woman, comes to your office with a 3-day history of dizziness and lightheadedness. She states that she first noticed the room spinning when she tried to get up in the morning to go to the bathroom. The sensation was severe and associated with nausea but abated soon after she lay down, only to recur whenever she rolled over or tried to get up. Finally, she arose slowly, inch by inch, and went to the bathroom. By midafternoon she was able to get up and move about the house, still noting a spinning sensation lasting 10 to 15 seconds when she arose quickly, turned her head, or changed position. She describes no tinnitus, ear stuffiness, or balance or coordination problems. She reports similar episodes occurring periodically since she was about 60 years old, the last attack being about 5 years ago.

STUDY QUESTIONS

- *What mechanisms are most likely responsible for Ms. Short's dizziness?*
- *Over the telephone, how would you assess the urgency of such a complaint?*

POSITIONAL VERTIGO

Many intense dizziness problems worsen during rapid movement. Positional vertigo refers to those special instances when symptoms arise only during or after position changes. One type of positional dizziness, the lightheadedness that occurs on assuming upright posture, is discussed later under presyncope. Positional vertigo implies some disruption of either peripheral or central vestibular function arising because of a change in position.

By far the most common cause of positional vertigo in the elderly is *benign positional vertigo* (sometimes called benign paroxysmal positional vertigo). Most benign positional vertigo (BPV) is caused by small dense calcific particles (otoliths) from the saccule or utricle of the inner ear that break loose and migrate into the posterior semicircular canal. Once positioned in the canal or on its receptor, these particles amplify rotational move-

ments in the plane of the canal. Thus, whenever the patient moves in the plane of the posterior semicircular canal, a short burst of intense vertigo is experienced. With time, particles are either absorbed, scarred down, or otherwise dealt with so that symptoms abate.

Benign positional vertigo (BPV) is the most common positional vertigo in old age: specific management techniques can reduce the impact of the bouts of vertigo.

Clinically, BPV is characterized by episodes of intense vertigo lasting less than a minute. Rolling over in bed, getting in and out of bed, and bending over and straightening up commonly provoke these attacks. Typically, patients have vertigo attacks with even slight rotatory movements for a few hours to days, with a mild lightheadedness noted most of the time. Symptoms improve rapidly and are typically gone within days to weeks. Thus the period during which the patient is susceptible to attacks lasts, on average, a week or two. The disease is recurrent, so the typical patient may have a history of bouts every few years for decades. Unilateral hearing loss, tinnitus, and cranial nerve deficits are generally absent.[8]

The Hallpike maneuver tests for BPV by inducing rotation in the posterior semicircular canals. It is performed as follows: The patient is seated in about the middle of the examining table so that lying back would cause the head and neck to extend beyond the table end. Standing to the patient's right, the physician cradles the patient's head and neck in both hands, advising the patient to hold the physician's upper arm for stability. At the count of three the patient relaxes and the physician quickly lays the patient backward, simultaneously rotating the head about 30 degrees toward the examiner. This places the patient's right posterior semicircular canal in the vertical plane, causing that single canal to experience a rotatory stimulus. The examiner maintains the patient in this head hanging right position for at least 10 seconds or until vertigo subsides. Then the patient is rapidly returned to the initial position, again holding the position for at least 10 seconds. Next, the procedure is repeated with the physician on the patient's left to test the left posterior semicircular canal.

A classic positive response to the Hallpike maneuver includes four components. First, one or more of the positions should induce dizziness (vertigo). Second, the dizziness, which is often signaled by the patient's exhibiting distress and grabbing tightly to the examiner's arm, should be accompanied by a rotatory nystagmus. Third, the dizziness and nystagmus should begin not immediately, but after a few seconds. This latency of onset is the reason that patients should be observed for a full 10 seconds after each positioning. Fourth, repeating the same maneuver that initially caused vertigo and nystagmus should result in reduced symptoms. If three or four repetitions are made, no more symptoms should be noted. This phenomenon is called fatigability. A classic response to the Hallpike maneuver is pathognomonic of BPV. Since BPV is generally unilateral, response is generally either limited to one side or unequal in intensity between sides. Some patients with BPV will not, however, elicit a positive response. Negative Hallpike testing in BPV is most common when an episode is mild or the patient is already recovering.

Vertigo arising in certain body or head positions, such as lying on one side or looking upward, is less common than BPV. Central positional vertigo is not characterized by latency or fatigability; it can be caused by a variety of diagnoses, including tumors, infarction, and multiple sclerosis. When such vertigo occurs in vertebrobasilar insufficiency, it is postulated to involve changes in blood flow from impingement of a vertebral artery by cervical spine osteophytes. Vertigo and nystagmus on lying down characterize acute alcohol intoxication and withdrawal arising as alcohol diffuses into and out of the semicircular canals.

Disabling positional vertigo arises from compression of the inferior or posterior vestibular nerve by tortuous blood vessels near the internal auditory meatus. It consists of a spectrum of symptoms including dysequilibrium and vertigo, which are present every day and worsen over months or years. Characteristically, patients experience more severe symptoms when physically active that are relieved only by bed rest. Brain stem auditory evoked potentials identify the affected side and confirm that the lesion is retrocochlear. Surgery has been reported to relieve the disorder, but the existence and extent of disabling positional vertigo are controversial.[9]

▼ EMMA SHORT (Part II)

The remainder of Ms. Short's history is noncontributory. The patient takes slow-release nifedipine, twice daily ibuprofen, and as needed dicyclomine for abdominal cramps but has had no recent medication change. Cardiovascular and neurological examination findings are normal. Rapid positional testing using the Hallpike maneuver reproduces her dizziness in the right head hanging position. On further questioning, she admits to having greater difficulty rolling over to the right than to the left when in bed. She is given instructions for positional exercises. These consist of reproducing her vertigo by rolling over rapidly to the right. After doing so, she is instructed to wait for her dizziness to resolve and then to roll over rapidly again in the same direction. She is instructed that within five repetitions the dizziness response should be fatigued temporarily, and she can go about her day. As instructed, she performs the exercises every 3 hours while awake. Within 2 weeks she reports no more dizziness.

Management of Benign Positional Vertigo

Medication is generally not helpful in BPV. The dizziness spells, although brief, are so intense that no medication adequately suppresses them. Within a day or two, patients feel fine when not having a vertigo spell. Having a sedating medication in the bloodstream during these times impairs mental alertness and clarity without providing significant relief.

In contrast, physical exercises do appear to help many patients with BPV and should be recommended. There are two forms of exercise particularly suitable for primary care older patients, both of which seek to desensitize the brain by provoking vertigo spells in a safe environment: One authority recommends that patients induce vertigo by falling rapidly to one or the other side from a sitting position on the bed;[9] the other recommends seeking out the exact maneuver that most stimulates the vertigo and instructing the patient to repeat the maneuver several times a day.[10] Exercises should be performed about every 3 hours, being repeated enough times during each session to fatigue the vertigo response (usually three to five repetitions). After being completely symptom free for several days, patients can stop the exercises.[11]

▼ CARL MILLER

A 71-year-old retired accountant, Carl Miller is brought to your office by his concerned wife. At about 2:30 this morning, he got up to go to the bathroom, feeling a little lightheaded. As he prepared to urinate, he felt he was about to pass out, and a wave of nausea came. He sat on the toilet, but even as he did so he could feel himself blacking out. His wife heard a thud and found him unconscious on the bathroom floor, chewing his tongue and moving his legs. She began to drag him into a more open area of the bathroom, and as she was doing so he began to awaken. He did not feel heart palpitations before or after the episode, and he was not incontinent. The whole episode apparently lasted about 10 to 15 seconds. On further questioning, Mr. Miller states that he has had a cold for the past 4 days for which he has taken a combination medication containing pseudoephedrine and chlorpheniramine. Rarely an alcohol drinker, Mr. Miller admits to having a beer last evening while watching Monday night football with his son, who is visiting. He does not have a history of seizures. He had an inferior wall myocardial infarction 6 years ago and has been asymptomatic since. Four months ago, he had a normal cardiac treadmill test performed by his cardiologist as part of a routine evaluation. Other than the cold preparation and one aspirin a day, he is not taking medication.

PRESYNCOPAL LIGHTHEADEDNESS AND SYNCOPE

The presyncopal type of dizziness is distinctive. Caused by diminished cerebral oxygenation, it leads to a feeling of being about to pass out. Patients describe this as the desire to sit or lie down, as the room getting dark, as a shade being pulled over their eyes, or simply as an intense lightheadedness. Nausea and weakness often accompany the dizziness. Presyncopal lightheadedness is often episodic, occurring either on assuming upright posture or in distinct episodes with clear starting and stopping times. Patients who actually lose consciousness are said to experience syncope.

Because its mechanism is diminished oxygen delivery to the brain, the causes of presyncopal lightheadedness tend to be circulatory. Cerebral oxygen delivery is a function of the amount of oxygen carried by the blood and of cerebral blood flow. The determinants of blood oxygen content are the quantity of functioning red blood cells and the pulmonary gas exchange. Determinants of cerebral blood flow include cardiac output, the cerebral vasculature, and reflexes that mediate regional blood flow. Table 20-3 shows the physiological mechanisms and diagnoses that give rise to presyncopal lightheadedness and to syncope.

In primary care geriatrics the most common causes of presyncope and of syncope are probably transient conditions that cause postural hypotension. In addition, a number of situations temporarily increase vagal tone, causing a drop in blood pressure and lightheadedness, sometimes with syncope. These situations include acute stress, blood drawing and other medical procedures, and urination (micturition syncope). Often several physiological factors interact. Fatigue or a missed meal often contributes. Thus a careful history is essential in diagnosing presyncope and syncope.

It should be noted that many older patients with postural lightheadedness do not meet the criteria for postural hypotension yet have for what all practical purposes is postural hypotension. Tilt table studies of persons with syncope and presyncopal lightheadedness have confirmed this; some persons either develop hypotension after a long time (e.g., 20 minutes) or have decreased cerebral perfusion caused by venous pooling in the legs without lowering their blood pressure enough to meet the classic criteria for postural hypotension.[12-14] Treatment with β-blockers, disopyramide, transdermal scopolamine, and hydroflurocortisone has been successful in some such patients[15]; a more conservative approach is the use of fitted elastic stockings.

CASE DISCUSSION

The case of Carl Miller is a typical example of multiple transient conditions leading to syncope. Mr. Miller experienced a fainting spell in the night because of a combination of alcohol intake, use of an antihistamine, and rapidly getting up from lying down. Acute illnesses (often viral) and many drug reactions induce a similar transient postural lightheadedness.

Cardiac dysrhythmias often come to mind when a patient has presyncope or syncope. In a study of 210 elderly with syncope who underwent extensive evaluation, 71 (33.8%) had a cardiovascular cause. Among the more common diagnoses were ventricular tachycardia and sick sinus syndrome. Often, electrocardiographic monitoring for several days was needed to identify the dysrhythmia.[16]

Many patients with presyncopal lightheadedness or with recurrent syncope are not diagnosed even after extensive evaluation. In Kapoor's series of 190 patients aged 14 to 59 years and 210 patients aged 60 to 90, 45% of the younger and 39% of the elderly patients received a final diagnosis of syncope of unknown origin.[16] Among the postulated causes of undiagnosed presyncopal lightheadedness are psychiatric conditions, diffuse cardiovascular disease, and multiple sensory impairments.

Seizures are rarely if ever a cause of dizziness, but they are occasionally the cause of syncope. More commonly, seizurelike movements (eyes rolling back, legs jerking) noted during a syncopal episode are secondary to transient hypoxia, not to an underlying seizure disorder.

▼ ELLEN CARTER (Part I)
Ellen Carter is a 75-year-old woman who complains of gait unsteadiness, dizziness, and persistent nausea. Her symptoms began abruptly 6 weeks ago in the middle of the night and

Table 20-3 Causes of Presyncope and Syncope

Physiological Impairment	Mechanism	Diagnoses Commonly Responsible
Reduced blood oxygen	↓O$_2$ carrying capacity	Anemia, carbon monoxide poisoning
	↓O$_2$ saturation	Chronic or acute pulmonary disease
Reduced cerebral blood flow	Impaired cardiac output	Cardiac dysrhythmias, myocardial infarction, aortic stenosis
	↓Blood pressure reflexes	Vasovagal and situational orthostatic hypotension; drug-induced
	Acute volume depletion	Hemorrhage, third space loss, overdiuresis
	Chronic volume depletion	Adrenal insufficiency, overdiuresis, diabetes mellitus, hypercalcemia, diabetes insipidus
	Other	Subclavian steal, diffuse atherosclerosis
Unconsciousness without presyncope	Abnormal brain electrical discharge	Seizure disorder

have not improved since. She describes her dizziness as a floating, rocking sensation that is worse when she stands but never completely disappears. She has difficulty walking but does not report a tendency to fall to one side. She has almost constant nausea when upright and has vomited several times. She reports some visual blurring but no double vision. Her medical history includes a long-standing problem with nerves, for which she has taken various tranquilizers. Recently, she has been taking 25 mg of amitriptyline at bedtime. She has had mild hypertension for approximately 15 years and has been only intermittently compliant with medications. She is not currently taking medication for hypertension, her last blood pressure having been 160/95 a year ago. She denies drinking alcohol or caffeine. Since developing dizziness 6 weeks ago, she has tried over-the-counter dimenhydrinate (Dramamine) but reports no relief. Living in the country with her husband, who is an alcoholic, she rarely visits a physician and had to be persuaded to come in 6 weeks after the onset of her problem.

CONTINUOUS DIZZINESS

Continuous dizziness implies a physiological or psychological disruption that is present all or most of the time. A wide variety of problems lead to continuous dizziness (see Table 20-2). Diagnostically, the most significant implication of continuous symptoms may be that most peripheral vestibular problems, cardiac dysrhythmias, and vertebrobasilar transient ischemic attacks are ruled out. Among the more common causes of continuous dizziness in older persons are anxiety or depression and multiple neurosensory deficits.

Anxiety and depression are the most common causes of chronic, continuous dizziness in younger populations.[3] These patients tend to report a vague lightheaded or floating sensation. Accompanying signs and symptoms include headache, fatigue, neck soreness, and abdominal pain. When hyperventilation is present, numbness and tingling of the hands and face, and occasionally nausea, are reported. Anxiety and depression appear to be less common causes of dizziness among older persons than among younger persons. Psychological symptoms are more commonly secondary, arising as a response to disabilities caused by dizziness.

Multiple neurosensory deficits (also called dysequilibrium of aging or presbyastasis) lead to dizziness by overwhelming the brain's ability to compensate for impairments in several sensory systems. This mechanism is probably responsible for many of the dizziness symptoms among frail elderly. For example, a patient with old vestibular damage from an acute neurolabyrinthitis years ago, a mild peripheral neuropathy, and bilateral cataracts is likely to have multisensory dizziness. Clinicians must be careful not to overlabel older patients as having multisensory dizziness, however, because in the majority a single lesion is the predominant cause.[17]

A host of other diagnoses produce continuous dizziness. Cerebellar atrophy, which may be idiopathic or secondary to degenerative conditions such as alcoholism, leads to a continuous feeling of dysequilibrium. Anemia, a variety of acute states (including myocardial infarction), and many medications may also produce continuous dizziness. Ocular dizziness is a lightheadedness or a sensation of movement that develops as a result of a change in lens prescription, a large fluctuation in blood sugar, or cataract surgery. Middle ear disease (serous otitis media or cholesteatoma) or sinusitis can produce vertigo or more vague sensations of continuous dizziness. Bilateral vestibular hypofunction, often the result of toxicity from aminoglycoside antibiotics, produces a continuous dysequilibrium that is worse while standing and is accompanied by oscillopsia (a sensation that the eyes bounce up and down) when the patient walks. Acoustic neuroma rarely presents as a vague, mild dizziness; unilateral gradual hearing loss is the more common presentation. Finally, stroke in the vertebrobasilar system frequently presents with vertigo. Within a few days, however, the vertigo often resolves, leaving the patient with a continuous dysequilibrium.

A key element in arriving at a diagnosis is to identify what factors worsen or ameliorate the dizziness. If standing exacerbates the dizziness, a disruption involving the vestibular, cerebellar, or circulatory system is likely. If motion and emotional stress worsen the dizziness, anxiety is suggested.

With continuous dizziness it is important to identify worsening or ameliorating factors.

Physical examination of such patients should concentrate on neurological status. Abnormalities during the neurological examination provide clues to a number of diseases affecting the balance system: bilateral labyrinthine disease (e.g., toxicity from aminoglycosides), cerebellar disease, multiple sclerosis, a severe peripheral neuropathy, and infarction in the vertebrobasilar distribution.

CASE DISCUSSION

The case of Ellen Carter illustrates how historical factors can suggest a number of possible diagnoses in older patients with continuous dizziness. Ms. Carter describes her dizziness as a floating, rocking sense of dysequilibrium. Symptoms are present most of the time, and they are worse while she is standing. A history of psychological problems and an alcoholic husband suggest that anxiety or depression, two common causes of continuous dizziness, may be present. Her antidepressant use supports this diagnostic hypothesis and raises the question of a drug effect. The abrupt onset of her symptoms is more in favor of an acute process such as stroke or neuro-

labyrinthitis; the history of hypertension identifies one risk factor for stroke. Finally, the entity of multiple neurosensory impairments, another common cause of continuous dizziness, should also be considered.

▼ ELLEN CARTER (Part II)

Examination reveals an alert, anxious, elderly woman who is able to give a clear history and appears well oriented. Postural hypotension is absent. Her gait is ataxic, and she walks with a wide-based stance. She is unable to tandem walk or to maintain Romberg's position with eyes open or closed. Visual acuity is 20/50 in the right eye and 20/200 in the left eye, and bilateral cataracts are noted. There is no spontaneous or gaze-evoked nystagmus. Cranial nerves are largely intact, but saccadic eye movements appear to overshoot the target. On neuromuscular examination a fine tremor is noted in the extended hands, but strength and reflexes are normal throughout. There are questionable impairment of finger-nose testing and rapid alternating movements with both sides being equal. Complete blood count, BUN, creatinine, VDRL, electrolytes, glucose, and thyroid function test findings are normal. Audiometry is normal (bilateral mild presbycusis is present). Magnetic resonance imaging of the head shows only some changes consistent with patchy white matter lesions in the periventricular region and some bilateral lacunar infarcts in the basal ganglia. A neurological consultation supports your diagnosis of a posterior circulation infarction and identifies its probable location as the midline cerebellum.

STUDY QUESTION

■ Given that Mrs. Carter has a fixed, irreversible neurological deficit, what measures can you initiate to minimize disability?

MANAGEMENT OF DIZZINESS

Treatment of dizziness depends, obviously, on the diagnosis. Many causes of dizziness are curable: examples include drug adverse effects, cerumen in the ear, anemia, cardiac dysrhythmias, depression, and perilymphatic fistula. In the majority of cases, however, treatment is not curative. Instead it is aimed at reducing disability and minimizing symptoms. Box 20-1 identifies a general approach to treatment of the patient with dizziness.

Antihistamines and sedatives are probably overused in the treatment of dizziness among elderly patients. Sedation, imbalance, and postural hypotension are side effects that may result. Small doses of medication can, however, help in certain circumstances. Meclizine, dimenhydrinate, and other antihistamines provide relief for acute peripheral vestibular problems such as labyrinthitis or attacks of Meniere's disease. Benzodiazepines reduce central sensitivity to some dizziness symptoms but should

---

BOX 20-1
Treatment of Dizziness in Old Age: General Principles

1. Identify the primary diagnosis and use a specific agent, if available.
2. Provide symptomatic relief when needed, but be wary of medications; they can contribute to dizziness and increase the risk of falls.
   - Peripheral vestibular problems respond well to antihistamines or benzodiazepines; central problems often do not.
   - Small doses of promethazine may relieve nausea during acute problems.
   - Low-dose haloperidol may help in refractory cases.
3. Identify contributing sensory deficits and manage them. Vision is a key factor in compensating for vestibular and proprioceptive deficits.
   - Visually dependent individuals benefit from using a night light.
   - Individuals with proprioceptive problems in the legs can gather compensatory information by touching walls or using a cane.
   - Cataract surgery may improve visual compensation.
4. Exercise (physical therapy) can treat benign positional vertigo, reduce balance problems, and lower the risk of falls by improving strength in deconditioned muscle groups.
5. If the patient is at risk for falls, also consider home assessment to reduce hazards and use of a walking aid.

---

be used with extreme caution because they cause sedation and increase the risk of falls; oxazepam and temazepam have short half-lives and are preferable to diazepam in elderly patients.

A variety of nonpharmacological measures can help patients with dizziness and balance problems remain as active and symptom free as possible. Deconditioning plays a considerable role in the persistence of symptoms, so activity generally needs to be encouraged. The most overt example is benign positional vertigo, in which patients do not improve unless they move about. Provoking the dizziness through activity is the key to getting better. Specific exercises provided by a physical therapist can help patients reduce the risk of falls. Localized muscle groups that help stabilize the body and prevent falls are often very deconditioned in patients with dizziness. The abdominal muscles, hip extensors, and back muscles are particularly involved.

Since multiple neurosensory problems contribute to dizziness in many elderly, physicians should search for such problems and seek to ameliorate them. Vision is the key adaptive mechanism for vestibular and proprioceptive deficits; cataract surgery and use of a night light are two examples of ways vision can be enhanced. If loss of proprioception in the ankles and feet contributes to dizziness, the patient can get additional sensory input by touching (not holding onto) the wall or another person; a cane can serve a similar function.

> ⚘ *Improving vision, reconditioning and activity, and psychological approaches should all be considered concurrently with medications in the management of dizziness.*

Finally, the extent to which anxiety and depression contribute to dizziness should not be overlooked. Dizziness is a common symptom of panic disorders, and vertigo is not an unusual description of the symptom. Admittedly, dizziness of purely psychiatric origin is relatively rarer among older patients than among younger adults; in fact, one hesitates to make a psychiatric diagnosis without a long history of similar symptoms. On the other hand, secondary psychiatric problems such as anxiety and depression are extremely common among dizzy older persons. One study of 56 elderly patients with chronic dizziness identified a psychological diagnosis meeting DSM-III criteria in 37.5% of patients. In most cases the diagnosis was a contributing factor to continued disability rather than the primary cause of the dizziness; anxiety disorders, depression, and adjustment reactions predominated.[18] Fearing that a dizziness attack will come on or that they will fall, many older persons with dizziness give up activities crucial to their independence and self-image, such as going to church, shopping, visiting friends, and driving. For these reasons the effective management of dizziness often involves counseling the patient and family about these issues. Occasionally, use of a medication (such as an antidepressant) or referral for more prolonged professional help is indicated.

▼ PAULINE PORTERFIELD

Mrs. Porterfield, an 86-year-old woman, describes two distinct types of dizziness. One type has been present most of the time for approximately 3 years. Its onset was gradual. She describes this dizziness as primarily a feeling that she is losing her balance. It is aggravated by crowds and by movement (such as getting on and off a bus). Her other type of dizziness is a spinning sensation, lasting less than a minute, that occurs when she rolls over in bed, turns her head rapidly, or gets up from a sitting position. That dizziness began acutely 10 days ago and is now much improved. She describes her general health

as fair. She has hypertension, controlled with hydrochlorothiazide, and angina pectoris, for which she takes nifedipine. Four years ago she had a left lumpectomy for breast cancer, without any known recurrence. She has bilateral macular degeneration. While in her 40s, she had an episode of severe vertigo that lasted about 10 days, gradually resolving completely. She has limited her activity over the past couple of years because of her fear of falling, now spending most of her time at home, where she lives with a daughter. On examination she is an alert, cooperative woman who appears younger than her stated age. Blood pressure is 140/60 with a pulse of 78 after lying recumbent for 3 minutes, 135/58 with a pulse of 84 immediately after standing, and 142/65 with a pulse of 82 at 2 minutes after standing. Extraocular movements, pupils, fundi, and cranial nerves are normal for her age. Folstein Mini–Mental State examination score is 29/30. Visual acuity is 20/80 on the right and 20/100 on the left, both corrected with glasses. Considerable cerumen is present in both ears; after cerumen removal the tympanic membranes appear normal. Neck, chest, and cardiovascular findings are normal. Peripheral sensory examination shows inability to sense position of the great toe bilaterally, diminished two-point discrimination bilaterally, moderately impaired light touch, and normal pinprick in the legs and feet. She is unable to perform tandem gait for more than two or three steps. Gait stability is fair and not worsened by head positioning. The Romberg test is positive with her feet together, but negative with feet 8 inches apart. The Hallpike maneuver produces some mild dizziness but fails to demonstrate nystagmus. Hyperventilation for 3 minutes fails to reproduce her symptoms. A physical therapy evaluation identifies extremely slow reaction times; weakness in the abdominal muscles, hip extensors, and hip abductors; poor bed mobility; poor reserve muscle strength; and inability to carry out power movements.

STUDY QUESTION

- Create a differential diagnosis for each of Mrs. Porterfield's two types of dizziness. Include all factors that may be contributing to her dizziness symptoms or to a balance and gait problem. What further evaluation would you recommend? What treatment possibilities are suggested?

CASE DISCUSSION

The case of Pauline Porterfield is complex. Her recent symptoms of brief positional vertigo, which improved over 10 days, support a tentative diagnosis of benign positional vertigo. An equivocal or negative result for the Hallpike maneuver is not inconsistent with resolving BPV. Less clear is the long-standing, progressive equilibrium problem. Among the possible contributing factors identified in the history are atherosclerotic vascular disease, medications, visual impairment, vestibular damage from labyrinthitis during her 40s, moderate impairment of proprioception in the lower extremities, cerumen in the ears, and muscle weakness from deconditioning.

SUMMARY: COMPLEX PROBLEMS

Sometimes, patients have two or more distinct types of dizziness caused by different mechanisms. In addition, multiple contributing factors frequently complicate the diagnosis. In approaching such patients, a comprehensive geriatric assessment is the first step. To the standard geriatric assessment should be added those relevant historical, physical diagnostic, and laboratory tests that have been described earlier in this chapter. Self-imposed restriction of activity or a history of falls should trigger particularly intensive efforts to find remediable conditions. Many such cases are multifactorial. Finding contributing factors that can be ameliorated, while avoiding iatrogenic disease from overtesting or overmedication, provides the key to helping the patient.

POSTTEST

1. Which of the following findings on cardiac monitoring is least likely to explain brief episodes of lightheadedness, as though he were about to pass out, in an 80-year-old man?
   a. Ventricular tachycardia
   b. Left anterior hemiblock
   c. Paroxysmal atrial tachycardia
   d. Complete heart block
   e. None of the above
2. What laboratory test provides the best method of screening for an acoustic neuroma?
   a. Magnetic resonance imaging of the head
   b. Computerized tomography of the head
   c. Brain stem evoked potentials
   d. Electroencephalography
   e. Audiometry with speech discrimination
3. Mrs. E. is a 78-year-old woman who comes to her family's physician's office because she developed dizzy spells while spending a month visiting her daughter. They began about 3 weeks ago and have been occurring more frequently and lasting longer. Normally Mrs. E. lives alone several hundred miles away, in the home she shared for 45 years with her now deceased husband. Her only medications are hydrochlorothiazide 25 mg once daily, a multivitamin, and lorazepam 1 mg at bedtime as needed to help her sleep. Which of the following statements is most correct concerning Mrs. E.'s dizziness history?
   a. Dizziness is less common among patients aged 75 years and older than among younger patients.
   b. Hydrochlorothiazide is unlikely to be the cause of her dizziness unless the prescription has recently changed.
   c. Taking a single nightly dose of lorazepam to help her sleep during the visit should not cause daytime dizziness in this patient.
   d. Stress associated with visiting her daughter could cause episodes of true vertigo.
   e. The timing of her husband's death is not important in determining the role of depression in Mrs. E.'s dizziness.
4. Mrs. D. is an 82-year-old woman who has had episodes of benign positional vertigo several times in the past. Her current episode, typical of past bouts, began 10 days ago. Having broken her hip last year, she is extremely afraid of falling and has remained at home on restricted activity since the attack began. What would be the most appropriate treatment advice for Mrs. D.?
   a. Increased activity with positional exercise
   b. Bed rest with visiting nurse and homemaker services
   c. Meclizine 25 mg 3 times a day and increased activity
   d. A soft cervical collar
   e. Temporary use of a wheelchair

REFERENCES

1. Sloane P, Blazer D, George LK: Dizziness in a community elderly population, *J Am Geriatr Soc* 37:101-108, 1989.
2. Sloane PD, Baloh RW: Persistent dizziness in geriatric patients, *J Am Geriatr Soc* 37:1031-1038, 1989.
3. Drachman DA, Hart CW: An approach to the dizzy patient, *Neurology* 22:323-334, 1972.
4. Jenkins HA et al: Dysequilibrium of aging, *Otolaryngol Head Neck Surg* 100:272-282, 1989.
5. Baloh RW: Dizziness in older people, *J Am Geriatr Soc* 40:713-721, 1992.
6. Fisher CM: Vertigo in cerebrovascular disease, *Arch Otolaryngol* 85:529-534, 1967.
7. Fisher CM: Late-life migraine accompaniments as a cause of unexplained transient ischemic attacks, *Can J Neurol Sci* 7:9-17, 1980.
8. Baloh RW, Honrubia V, Jacobson K: Benign positional vertigo: clinical and oculographic features in 240 cases, *Neurology* 37:371-378, 1987.
9. Brandt T: Positional and positioning vertigo and nystagmus, *J Neurol Sci* 95:3-28, 1990.

10. Norre ME, Beckers A: Vestibular habituation training: exercise treatment for vertigo based on the habituation effect, *Otol Head Neck Surg* 101:9-14, 1989.

11. Herdman SJ: Treatment of benign paroxysmal positional vertigo, *Phys Ther* 70:381-388, 1990.

12. Hackel A et al: Cardiovascular and catecholamine responses to head-up tilt in the diagnosis of recurrent unexplained syncope in elderly patients, *J Am Geriatr Soc* 39:639-663, 1991.

13. Hargreaves AD, Muir AL: Lack of variation in venous tone potentiates vasovagal syncope, *Br Heart J* 486-490, 1992.

14. Streeten DHP, Anderson GH: Delayed orthostatic intolerance, *Arch Intern Med* 152:1066-1072, 1992.

15. Grubb BP et al: Utility of upright tilt-table testing in the evaluation and management of syncope of unknown origin, *Am J Med* 90:6-10, 1991.

16. Kapoor W et al: Syncope in the elderly, *Am J Med* 80:419-428, 1986.

17. Sloane P, Baloh RW, Honrubia V: The vestibular system in the elderly: clinical implications, *Am J Otolaryngol* 10:422-429, 1989.

18. Sloane PD, Hartman M, Mitchell CM: Psychological factors associated with chronic dizziness in patients aged 60 and older, *J Am Geriatr Soc* 42:847-852, 1994.

PRETEST ANSWERS
1. d
2. a
3. b
4. d

POSTTEST ANSWERS
1. b
2. e
3. b
4. a

CHAPTER 21

Falls and Falling

JAKOB ULFARSSON and BRUCE E. ROBINSON

OBJECTIVES

On completion of this chapter, the reader will be able to:

1. Describe the frequency of falls, fall-related injury, and the associated morbidity and mortality for the older population.

2. Understand the major functional components of dynamic balance and the common age- and disease-associated factors that interfere.

3. Enumerate those clinical factors associated with falling in clinical research.

4. Describe the appropriate history of a fall, the pertinent additional medical history, and the physical examination of the faller.

5. For an older patient, attribute falling events and risks to identified clinical factors and recommend a preventive strategy.

6. Develop an exercise prescription for an impaired older person.

7. Develop a strategy for selection of an assistive device for an at risk older patient.

8. List the common hazards in the home of the older person and appropriate corrective actions to reduce falling risk.

PRETEST

1. Which of the following is not a factor more common in fallers than nonfallers?
   a. Dementia
   b. Hypertension
   c. Foot disorders
   d. Depression
2. Which of the following is not a critical component of dynamic balance?
   a. Vision
   b. Muscle strength
   c. Hearing
   d. Speed of central processing

3. Which of the following statements about the epidemiology of falling is correct?
   a. Falls are the leading cause of death in those over 85.
   b. Each year about one nursing home resident in four falls.
   c. One in four hospitalized fallers will enter a nursing home.
   d. One in three hospitalized fallers will die in a year.

DEFINITION

A fall can be defined as an involuntary change in position not explained by an overwhelming separate process such as trauma, syncope, or seizures. Falls are no accident: they are largely explainable by characteristics of the individual and the structure of the environment, which interact to produce the fall and associated injuries. Examining the factors that allow safe mobility and the changes that occur from aging and disease will permit a clear understanding of falls and suggest opportunities for prevention.

▼ FRANCES LAMOND (Part I)

You are asked to assume the inpatient care of Ms. Lamond, a 74-year-old female resident of an assisted living facility. She is to be admitted to your hospital through the emergency room, where she has been brought because back pain has prevented her from getting out of bed. The ER physician reports a fall onto her buttocks occurring early in the evening of the prior night. Evaluation has identified an 80% compression deformity of the second lumbar vertebra, which corresponds to the area of her back pain. She is given the admitting diagnosis of vertebral compression fracture.

STUDY QUESTION

- *What further information will you need to ensure her safe return to the facility?*

EPIDEMIOLOGY OF FALLS

Falls occur in about one in four community-dwelling older persons, and they occur at a rate of one to two per resident per year in institution-dwelling elders.[1] About half of the fallers are recurrent fallers.

If falling is recurrent, it must be on the problem list: plan how to prevent falling and what to do if it happens again.

The consequences of these falls are substantial: nonintentional injury is the sixth leading cause of death in people over 65 in the United States. Mortality associated with falling increases logarithmically with age: 70% of fall-related deaths occur in the over 75 age group. One third to one half of elderly patients hospitalized for a fall do not survive another year.

Falls are potent markers of present disability and future morbidity.[2] About 1 in 40 falls results in hospitalization. Forty percent of hospitalized fallers become long-term care patients. Hip fracture is the most common fracture. With the best care about 25% of these patients die within 6 months of injury, 25% lose significant functional ability, and 50% experience reductions in mobility.

Clinical research has identified a number of clinical factors more common in fallers than in control subjects (Box 21-1). However, in searching for the cause of a fall that will produce the best opportunity for prevention, the practitioner must search not for a single etiology but for a list of contributing factors and other opportunities for intervention. In most fallers, multiple contributors to the impaired postural control (dynamic balance) and falling risk can be identified.[3]

UNDERSTANDING DYNAMIC BALANCE

Dynamic balance requires input from several sensory systems about body position and movement, central integration of this information with selection of response, and adequate musculoskeletal function to permit the necessary reactions. Both aging and age-associated dis-

---

BOX 21-1
Factors Increasing the Falling Risk

Drugs
    Long-acting benzodiazepines
    Other sedative-hypnotics
    Alcohol
Dementia
Depression
Vision impairment
Gait disorder
Foot problems
Lower extremity disability

---

eases often affect these critical systems, increasing the risk of falls and related injury.

> *Do not look for the single cause of falling in an older patient: there will always be multiple factors. Physicians get excited when they find a "medical" cause, but treatment usually involves much more than "just fixing" the dysrhythmia or any other medical problem found.*

Sensory Processes and Falling

The sensory systems responsible for providing information on body position and movement are vision, vestibular function, and proprioception. With aging, vision becomes the predominant method of assessing body position, yet it is diminished by age-related changes including reductions in glare tolerance, nocturnal acuity, peripheral vision, and depth perception. The causes of disease-related visual impairment that increase with age include macular degeneration, cataracts, and glaucoma.

Vestibular function provides information about static head position relative to gravity by means of the maculae and about acceleration via the semicircular canals. Vestibular input is critical for the reflexes of balance that coordinate the response to unexpected body displacements. Peripheral vestibular excitability decreases with aging. Clinical vestibular dysfunction (e.g., acute labyrinthitis, Meniere's disease, benign positional vertigo) increases with age and may contribute to the risk of falling in those affected. Subtle reductions in peripheral nervous system function are recognized with aging. Reduced proprioceptive function also occurs with disorders such as diabetes, alcoholism, nutritional deficiencies, and from cervical and lumbar spondylosis.

Central Processes and Falling

The brain processes sensory inputs and selects the appropriate motor corrections to the various actions that disturb postural stability. Such actions are both in response to the imbalance and in anticipation of the imbalance produced by voluntary motor activities. Both speed and accuracy are required in the selection of these motor responses. One of the most consistent and convincing findings in psychological literature is the general slowing of cognitive-motor responses with age. This is particularly evident when complex choices between responses are available, as occurs with loss of balance. Dementia and Parkinson's disease are common conditions that further slow cognitive responses.

Musculoskeletal Function and Falling

An adequate motor response requires sufficient muscular strength and stability of major joints to be effective. Aging is associated with reductions in muscle strength and tone at least partly related to inactivity. Degenerative arthritis, neurological diseases, and illness-related deconditioning are more common in older persons and add to musculoskeletal disability. The condition of the feet can be particularly important because a stable platform of support is critical to safe mobility. Inadequate footwear, bunions, calluses, and deformities are common.

CLINICAL APPROACH TO THE FALLING PATIENT

▼ *FRANCES LAMOND (Part II)*

In the hospital unit you obtain additional history from Ms. Lamond. She describes a systemic illness of 3 days' duration, with fever, cough, and malaise. The fall occurred 1 hour after retiring, while she was walking to the bathroom. She was feeling particularly unsteady and toppled backward in a short open area where there were no handholds. She did not experience lightheadedness, dizziness, or other symptoms at the time of the fall. She was able to complete her trip to the bathroom and return to her bed despite back pain, but she was unable to get up the next morning.

STUDY QUESTION

■ *What factors predisposing to falling are present?*

History of the Fall

When older people are asked about their fall, common responses include: "My legs just gave way," "I lost my balance," or "I tripped." Additional effort by the interviewer often provides better direction to the diagnostic effort. Specific questions to ask include when, where, and what the subject was doing at the time of the fall; if any premonitory symptoms were present; what was experienced at the time of the fall and immediately afterward;

and whether any environmental factors were involved. The physician should ask the patient if he or she experienced vertigo, lightheadedness, or imbalance and whether there was loss of consciousness. In patients with multiple falls it is often useful to concentrate on the most recent or the best-remembered fall to facilitate recollection of all necessary detail.

Gathering specific information on the location of the fall and the environmental contributors is particularly important in prevention. Often the home has hidden hazards for the elderly, with obstacles and dangerous conditions that are not recognized until after the fall has occurred. The great majority of falls happen at home, mostly in the bedroom, bathroom, living room, and on the stairs. For frail older persons in their homes or in facilities providing for their care, the bathroom is a high-risk location for falls, especially if the patient is unsupervised.

> *Falling is an interaction between a person and the environment; find out everything possible about both aspects.*

▼ FRANCES LAMOND (Part III)

On examination, Ms. Lamond's temperature is 100.2° F, pulse 94 beats per minute, and respiratory rate 24. On prompting, the patient is able to expectorate yellow, obviously purulent sputum. She is unable to sit up because of her back pain. There is tenderness overlying the second lumbar vertebra. The white cell count from the ER is 13,400 per ml, and a chest x-ray examination is then ordered, which shows a left lower lobe pulmonary infiltrate. Sputum gram stain shows many WBCs with mixed gram-positive and gram-negative organisms, and the culture grows Haemophilus influenzae.

STUDY QUESTION

- *How do these findings relate to her presenting injury and fall?*

ACUTE ILLNESS AND FALLING

A *premonitory fall* is a common presentation of illness in older persons, and the fall may dominate the clinical picture. Strokes, transient ischemic attacks, pneumonia, sepsis, anemia, myocardial infarction, gastrointestinal bleeding, spontaneous fracture, and excessive alcohol intake are common conditions that may be associated with falling or fall-related injury. Reduction in cerebral perfusion because of cardiac dysrhythmias or aortic stenosis can lead to falls as well as syncope. These conditions often require prompt action to prevent further problems, so the initial evaluation of a faller must include a careful search for signs and symptoms of other conditions.

> *New-onset falling mandates a search for new-onset medical illness: as a nonspecific sign of illness, falling is as important as confusion.*

▼ FRANCES LAMOND (Part IV)

After 3 days of intravenous antibiotics and bed rest, Ms. Lamond is able to attempt walking. She requires moderate assistance to arise from a chair and shows strong retropulsion when attempting to walk. Romberg's test is positive to the rear.

Gait and Balance Disorders

Most of the strong risk factors for falling produce observable changes in gait and balance. Abnormal gait is the factor most often identified in persons whose falling tendency has many causes. Therefore the evaluation for factors contributing to falls begins with an examination of gait and balance. Gait analysis techniques reveal that changes in gait with aging include a wider base, a slower cadence, a shorter swing phase, and a longer time spent in the stance phase during normal walking.[4] A useful test of gait consists of asking the patient to arise from a chair without using the hands and to walk about 20 feet, turn, and return to the chair, sitting again without using the hands. A Romberg maneuver is then performed, with the addition of a gentle push to allow observation of righting reflexes. The physician observes arising, sitting, step length, step height, symmetry, continuity, path deviation, and trunk sway as well as Romberg stability. The ability to arise without hands and to sit under control without hands provides good information on trunk and lower extremity strength. The older patient who is most likely to fall has a stiff, uncoordinated gait and poor control over posture and body position.[5] Table 21-1 lists some common disorders prominently associated with disturbed gait, with a brief description of the gait produced.

▼ FRANCES LAMOND (Part V)

You ask Ms. Lamond about her activity and walking abilities before this last illness. She reports chronic unsteadiness since the last of two prior small strokes. She has markedly reduced her level of physical activity because, she says, "I am afraid I will fall."

POSTFALL SYNDROME

To an older person the possibility that falls will lead to restricted mobility and therefore impair quality of life is of more significance than issues like death and injury. Restricted mobility produces more long-term immobility than most individual falls do. The fear produced by

Table 21-1 Disorders Commonly Associated with Gait Disturbance

Disorder	Clinical Features
Parkinson's disease	Stooping, shuffling, decreased arm swing, retropulsion
Alzheimer's disease	Physically normal until late, poor safety awareness
Hemiparesis	Unilateral weakness
Hemiparesis with neglect	Leans to involved side, bumps into objects and doorways on involved side
Cervical spondylosis	Stiff-legged, spastic, scissoring
Peripheral neuropathy	Slapping, stumbling
Cerebellar degeneration	Ataxic: wandering path, reaching for support
Normal-pressure hydrocephalus	Irregular steps, "magnetic"
Degenerative arthritis	Antalgic: protecting the painful limb

BOX 21-2
Examination of the Unsteady or Falling Patient

Gait assessment: identify weakness, instability
Blood pressure when standing
Visual: acuity, confrontational fields, cornea, lens
Cervical range of motion and response to head movement
Cognition
Cerebellar (toe tapping, heel to shin)
Peripheral sensation, stretch reflexes
Muscle strength and tone, especially of lower extremities
Joint range of motion, deformity, stability
Feet and footwear

---

recurrent falls and persistent instability even in cognitively intact elders (and in their caregivers) often seems out of proportion to the injuries that have occurred. An extreme example of fall-related restriction in activity is the postfall syndrome.[6] A phobic response to the discordant and inaccurate sensory inputs experienced by the balance-impaired faller may precipitate this syndrome or the lesser degrees of activity restriction found in others who fall.[7] The mobility reductions of the unsteady older person add to physical deconditioning and poor balance, creating a self-perpetuating cycle of increasing weakness and instability. Generalized weakness was the most common factor predisposing to falling in one recent clinical study.[3]

 After the fall comes an equally dangerous syndrome: the fear of falling.

▼ FRANCES LAMOND (Part VI)

You assess cognitive status using the Mini–Mental State examination and discern mild cognitive impairment. An examination finds moderate diffuse cogwheel rigidity, with diminished facial expression suggestive of Parkinson's disease. A physical therapist is consulted and performs a complete neuromuscular evaluation, which confirms these findings and fails to identify muscular or sensory deficits.

ADDITIONAL HISTORY AND PHYSICAL EXAMINATION

In completing the history and physical of the faller the physician should look for contributors to instability that may offer opportunities for intervention. Management of concurrent medical conditions may result in substantial gains in health.[3] Evidence should be sought for medical conditions such as diabetes, hypertension, prior cerebrovascular accident, arthritis, or Parkinson's disease. Medications (prescription and over the counter), alcohol use, diet, living arrangements, and usual level of physical activity should also be determined. Physical examination emphases are listed in Box 21-2. Clinical hypotheses should drive any additional testing: no routine laboratory or other testing is recommended, although liberal use of inexpensive laboratory profiles is often justified, given the broad differential diagnosis.

Postural hypotension is one of the most common medical factors associated with falls.[3] There is growing documentation of an age-associated decline in cardiovascular and neuroendocrine mechanisms responsible for blood pressure homeostasis.[8] The net result of this decline is a tendency to transient falls in blood pressure as a result of such common stressors as position change, defecation, urination, and meals. When coupled with ineffective cerebral autoregulation, these swings in blood pressure may lead to transient interruption of cerebral blood flow to the brain centers that control posture. The frequent clinical coexistence of diseases or drugs linked to orthostatic hypotension and the tendency to fall also supports a causal link.[9] Descriptions of falls that include near syncope and the coexistence of falls with syncopal episodes imply that blood pressure changes are a cause of falling. However, falls that occur when an old person rises from a chair or bed may not be related to hypotension but to weakness or instability exposed by the change in body position.

Dizziness is reported as preceding a fall more often than not, and it can represent diminished cerebral perfusion (type I), labyrinthine dysfunction (type II), or neither. The most common type of dizziness in frail older persons is the uncomfortable sensation that accompanies instability, often caused by a combination of multiple sensory deficits and slow central processing (type III). True vertigo (type II) is clinically defined as an illusion of movement and is associated with dizziness that can be brought on by rolling over in bed. Provocative labyrinthine stimulation (rapidly raising the head from below horizontal position) can sometimes help separate true vertigo from other causes of dizziness.

Drop attacks are defined as sudden, unexpected falls without an identifiable cause. Earlier work on the causes of falling suggested that drop attacks cause as many as one fall in four and proposed vertebrobasilar insufficiency and cervical spondylosis as potential causes. More recent investigations have rarely found falls requiring this label. Body position changes that, because of sensory and processing problems, are undetected by the faller until too late may explain some of these events.

Cognitive dysfunction is strongly associated with falls: in one study it was observed that patients with dementia of Alzheimer's type were three times as likely to suffer a fall as healthy older subjects.[10] Both demented and depressed older persons are prone to undertake activities exceeding their abilities.

Inappropriate drug use, which is also associated with falling, is remediable. Altered pharmacokinetics, polypharmacy, and incorrect use of drugs are all documented factors contributing to the increased risk of falls in the elderly. Mechanisms by which drugs could cause falls include impairment in cerebral blood flow caused by blood pressure change, impairment in central mechanisms responsible for postural reflexes, metabolic changes producing muscular weakness, and alterations in behavioral mechanisms. Alcohol, phenothiazines, benzodiazepines (especially long acting), and tricyclic antidepressants have been shown through clinical research to be associated with falls in the elderly.[11-13] Many other prescription and over the counter drugs could contribute to falls associated with the above mechanisms. Improvement after withdrawal and temporal association of falls with a drug's use would support the drug's being a cause.

▼ FRANCES LAMOND (Part VII)

You decide to treat the parkinsonism with carbidopa-levodopa (Sinemet 25/100), 3 times daily. This results in slight improvement in the speed of movement, but Ms. Lamond remains retropulsive, causing safety concerns. She is moved to a nursing home where ongoing daily physical therapy is provided. Over the next 2 weeks her safety and balance gradually improve and she is taught transfer techniques and the use of a rolling walker, to which she adapts easily. She is returned to the assisted living home from which she came.

CASE DISCUSSION

Ms. Lamond well illustrates the complex background of a seemingly simple incident. The fall was premonitory, precipitated by concurrent acute illness. The darkness, late hour, and rising from recumbency all predisposed the patient to the fall. In addition, her back was vulnerable because she, like many older women, was osteopenic. However, her chronic unsteadiness and fear of falling had not been particularly noticed, since she fit in so well with the other immobilized residents at her facility. Yet careful evaluation revealed not only a reversible fear of falling but also an insidious and chronic condition— Parkinson's disease—for which specific medical and physical therapy treatments and interventions are beneficial. In this case a degree of increased mobility and reduced morbidity is the satisfactory result of the fall. This is an optimistic scenario; the frequent type of fall with devastating hip fracture, for example, and the multiple consequences and factors that are significant in rehabilitation are described elsewhere.

REHABILITATION AND THE PREVENTION OF FALLS

After the underlying problems are addressed and attempts to correct them are made, a program of muscle strengthening and ambulation should be initiated. Exercises to build strength, flexibility, and endurance are added gradually, aiming for as much independence as possible, with good mobility and stability (Box 21-3). Frailty is not necessarily permanent: even the very old can benefit from muscle strengthening.[11] A recent study demonstrated for the first time that muscle strengthening can be achieved even in the oldest persons. A controlled trial conducted over a 10-week period among frail nursing home residents showed that with progressive resistance exercise training, subjects could increase muscle strength more than twofold and improve gait velocity and stair-climbing power.[12] It has been shown that a rehabilitation program can appreciably improve the postural balance of fallers.[13]

BOX 21-3
Interventions to Prevent Falls

Exercise programs with physical conditioning
Environmental modification
    Removal of home hazards
    Improved home lighting
    Safe pathways
Assistive devices—prescription or removal
Reduction of psychotropic drugs
Good nutrition with restricted alcohol
Regular eye examination
Proper shoes and regular foot care
Emergency call system (for after the fall)

> *Balance is a skill learned in infancy; it can be re-learned in middle age and old age, but it is best to maintain balance skills throughout life by staying active.*

The American College of Sports Medicine's recommended guidelines for the development and maintenance of musculoskeletal and cardiorespiratory fitness in healthy adults can be applied to the healthy elderly. The major difference in the exercise prescription (Table 21-2) is that the emphasis is changed from short periods of aerobic exercise to exercising at a lower intensity for a longer duration, avoiding activities that could injure joints.[14] The usual time to complete the exercise prescription is about an hour, and if this produces fatigue, the time may be divided into two half-hour sessions. A stepwise progression of low-impact aerobic and strength training is used for the first 4 to 5 months, after which a maintenance phase is reached and maintained. Exercise should begin at a level similar to that already known to be safe in the patient and increase in duration gradually, with increases in intensity added last. Walking is the most generally applicable aerobic activity. Water is an excellent medium for allowing movement with low impact on diseased joints and bones and recent experience indicates that water exercises are among the most popular and innovative programs offered to older persons.[15] Water exercise provides the smooth engagement of resistance, a full range of motion, and the ability to vary the speed of performance.

A properly chosen assistive device can permit safe mobility; a poor choice may eliminate opportunities for res-

Table 21-2 Exercise Prescription
for the Older Person

Component	Recommended Activities and Times
Warmup	Stretching, gentle movement for 10-15 minutes
Aerobic	Activities that use large muscle groups (walk, swim, stair)
Duration	15-40 minutes
Intensity	50%-85% of calculated maximum heart rate
Frequency	3-5 times weekly
Resistance training	Upper body strengthening
Equipment	1-6 pound barbells, exercise machine
Amount	Begin two sets of 12 repetitions, add 2 reps every 2 weeks up to 24 reps
Types	Curls (wrist, biceps, triceps), lateral raises, presses
Cool down	10-15 minutes of stretching, gentle movement

toration of normal gait and may even predispose to falling. All assistive devices widen the base of support, decrease weight bearing on the lower extremities by transferring a portion of the weight to the upper extremities, and provide extra sensory and proprioceptive feedback. A straight cane can be freely recommended to provide additional stability to those with minor problems of gait and balance. Choosing more substantial equipment such as quad canes and walkers requires more careful assessment and the instruction of the patient in their proper use.

> *Walkers and canes are the symbols of frailty and aging to many, but prescription of either is not saying, "You poor old frail patient, here is a walking cane," but rather "This will keep you active; this will enable you to be more independent."*

Walkers provide more anterior and lateral stability. They are ideal aids for older adults who have balance deficits, weakness of the muscles of the lower extremity, or cognitive impairments that interfere with the ability to follow more complex instructions. Poor technique with these devices can make them hazardous, particularly in those with a tendency to fall backward. Those with a fear of falling may prefer a walker to a cane. Disadvantages of a walker include the inability to use it on stairs and the increased space needed for maneuvering, with the related tendency to put it aside for short trips in tight spaces, such as to the bathroom. The walker also does not provide experience with normal gait and balance, increasing the hazard level to the individual when the walker is not being used.

A glide walker has wheels on either two or four legs and does not provide anterior stability, but it can be useful when imbalance alone is the problem or when cognitive impairment prohibits training with other devices. A hemiwalker is a compromise between a cane and a walker, offering a wide base of support for stability similar to a walker, yet allowing one-handed ease of handling similar to a cane. Proper assessment by a therapist is invaluable in ensuring that appropriate recommendations for assistive devices and proper instruction in their use are achieved.

Often the home has hidden hazards for the elderly. To be safely mobile, an unsteady person with a gait disorder requires a much more supportive environment. Tripping is common and often involves household objects or floor coverings that are not hazardous to the able bodied. Table 21-3 provides a list of common hazards in the home; this list can be reproduced and given to patients and families. Descending stairs is a dangerous activity for

Table 21-3   Environmental Assessment and Home Hazard Preventive Measures

Factor	Preventive Measures
Footwear	Shoes with firm, nonskid, nonfriction soles; low heels; avoid walking in loose slippers or in stocking feet
Entrances, yards	Repair cracks in pavement; fill holes in lawn; remove all tripping hazards; well-lit walkways
Lighting	Light up shadowy areas; reduce glare with evenly distributed light; have light switches at room entrances; night-light in bedroom, hall, bathroom
Floors	Carpet edges tacked down; carpets with shallow pile; nonskid wax on floors; nonskid backing for throw rugs; cords out of walking path; removal of all small objects from floor
Stairs	Lighting adequate, with switches at top and bottom of stairs; securely fastened and well-placed handrails on both sides of stairway; top and bottom steps marked with bright-colored adhesive strips; stair rises of no more than 6 inches; steps in good repair; no object on steps
Bathroom	Raised toilet seat; grab bars for tub, shower, and toilet; nonskid rubber mat or strips in tub or shower; shower chair with handheld shower
Kitchen	Firm nonmoveable kitchen table; rubber mat on floor in sink area; secure step stool if climbing is necessary; shelf and cupboard items at accessible height
Bedroom, living room	Bed at proper height; spills on floor cleaned up promptly; remove unstable tables and chairs; remove clutter in hallways and on floors

many older people, as are slippery or wet surfaces. Overly bright light can interact with opacified ocular lenses to produce incapacitating glare. Darkness caused by inadequate lighting is easily remedied. It is recommended that a visiting nurse or other knowledgeable health worker assess the home for hazards and recommend changes in the home environment.[16] An emergency call system can provide worthwhile security for the unstable ambulator who is often alone.

SUMMARY

Falls are complex clinical phenomena that can suggest present disease or predict future disability. Falls are caused by interactions between the environment and dynamic balance, which is itself determined by the quality of sensory input, central processing, and motor responses. Clinical factors that predispose persons to falling often produce observable disturbances in gait and balance. Observation of gait is critical in falls assessment. Acute illness and drug therapy produce falls that are particularly preventable. The interventions most likely to prevent fall-related injury are therapeutic exercise and environmental modification for safety.

POSTTEST

1. Which one of the following choices is most often implicated as contributing to falls?
   a. Drop attacks
   b. Labyrinthine dysfunction
   c. Generalized weakness
   d. Acute medical illness

2. Clinical research would suggest which of the following drugs as most likely to produce a hip fracture?
   a. Diazepam
   b. Methyldopa
   c. Trazodone
   d. Furosemide

3. Mrs. G is an 86-year-old woman with mild dementia brought in from an assisted living facility for evaluation following a witnessed fall onto her buttocks. She was reportedly in good health the day before but felt nauseated the morning of the fall. Her usual medications are hydrochlorothiazide and conjugated estrogens. She appears lethargic and pale. Vital signs are temperature 38.9° C, pulse 102, blood pressure 115/58 lying, and respirations 24. Examination reveals few left basilar crackles, an S_4 gallop rhythm, and mild abdominal distention. There is mild tenderness over the greater trochanter of the left hip, but free range of motion is possible without pain. Which of the following studies would you expect to be least useful in her evaluation?
   a. MRI of the head
   b. Serum electrolytes
   c. Electrocardiogram
   d. Chest x-ray examination
   e. Abdominal x-ray examination

4. Which of the following factors will be most often found in the evaluation of a falling patient?
   a. Hemiparesis
   b. Abnormality of gait
   c. Foot problems
   d. Dementia
   e. Sedative use

5. Mr. T is a 74-year-old man who presents for routine health care. He is treated with clonidine 0.1 mg twice daily for hypertension, with good control. He suffered a right hemispheric stroke some years ago, and 2 months ago he fell on the way to the bathroom. Since that time he has given up walking outside of his apartment and reports an increased fear of falling. On examination his gait is irregular and unsteady, with a tendency to lean to the left and clutch at available objects. Which of the following choices is most appropriate in helping him regain safe mobility?
   a. Physical therapy evaluation
   b. Discontinuing clonidine
   c. Prescribing an electric cart
   d. CT scan of the head
   e. Straight cane

6. Which of the following is not an appropriate part of an initial exercise prescription for an older adult?
   a. Warmup with 10 minutes of stretching and gentle movement
   b. One hour of aerobic exercise at 85% of MHR
   c. Three to five exercise sessions per week
   d. Swimming as the aerobic exercise component
   e. A 10-minute cooldown of stretching and gentle movement

REFERENCES

1. Sattin RW: Falls among older persons: a public health perspective, *Annu Rev Public Health* 13:489-508, 1992.
2. Dunn JE et al: Mortality, disability, and falls in older persons: the role of underlying disease and disability, *Am J Public Health* 82:395-400, 1992.
3. Rubenstein LZ et al: The value of assessing falls in an elderly population, *Ann Intern Med* 113:308-316, 1990.
4. Imms FJ, Edholm OG: The assessment of gait and mobility in the elderly, *Age Ageing* 8:261-267(S), 1979.
5. Rubenstein LZ et al: Falls and instability in the elderly, *J Am Geriatr Soc* 36:266-278, 1988.
6. Murphy J, Isaacs B: The post-fall syndrome, *Gerontology* 28:265-270, 1982.
7. Brandt T, Daroff R: The multisensory psychological and pathological vertigo syndromes, *Ann Neurol* 7:195-203, 1980.
8. Lipsitz LA: Abnormalities in blood pressure hemostasis that contribute to falls in the elderly, *Clin Geriatr Med* 1(3):637-645, 1985.
9. Robbins AS, Rubenstein LZ: Postural hypotension in the elderly, *J Am Geriatr Soc* 32:769-774, 1984.
10. Morris JC et al: Senile dementia of Alzheimer's type: an important risk factor for serious falls, *J Gerontol* 42:412-417, 1987.
11. Tinetti ME, Speechly M, Ginter SF: Risk factors for falls among elderly persons living in the community, *N Engl J Med* 319:1701-1707, 1988.
12. Ray WA et al: Psychotropic drug use and the risk of hip fracture, *N Engl J Med* 316:363-369, 1987.
13. Woollacott MH: Effects of ethanol and postural adjustments in humans, *Exp Neurol* 80:55-68, 1983.
14. Fiatarone MA et al: High-intensity strength training in nonagenarians: effects on skeletal muscle, *JAMA* 263:3029-3034, 1990.
15. Fiatarone MA et al: Exercise training and nutritional supplementation for physical frailty in very elderly people, *N Engl J Med* 330:1769-1775, 1994.
16. Steinberg FU: Disorders of mobility, balance, and gait. In Felsenthal G, Garison SJ, Steinberg FU, eds: Rehabilitation of the

aging and elderly patient, Baltimore, Md, 1994, Williams and Wilkins.

17. Shephard RJ: The scientific basis of exercise prescribing for the very old, *J Am Geriatr Soc* 38:62-70, 1990.

18. McNeal RL: Aquatic therapy for patients with rheumatic disease, *Rheum Dis Clin North Am* 16:915-929, 1990.

19. Tideiksaar R: Preventing falls: home hazard checklist to help older patients protect themselves, *Geriatrics* 41:26-28, 1986.

20. Waller JA: Injury in aged: clinical and epidemiologic implications, *NY State J Med* 2200-2207, 1974.

21. Tinetti ME, Williams TF, Mayewski R: Fall risks index for elderly patients based on number of chronic disabilities, *Am J Med* 80:429-434, 1986.

22. Wild D, Nayak USL, Isaacs B: How dangerous are falls in old people at home? *Br Med J* 282:266-268, 1981.

23. Tinetti ME: Factors associated with serious injury during falls by ambulatory nursing home residents, *J Am Geriatr Soc* 35:644-648, 1987.

24. Buchner DM, Larson EB: Falls and fractures in patients with Alzheimer's type dementia, *JAMA* 257:1492-1495, 1987.

PRETEST ANSWERS

1. b
2. c
3. d

POSTTEST ANSWERS

1. c
2. a
3. a
4. b
5. a   The physical therapist can lead to improvement in functional capacity, specifically strength, gait, and balance, and assist in proper selection of assistive devices; a straight cane is unlikely to be sufficient support.
6. b

CHAPTER 22

Incontinence

RICHARD J. HAM and DEBORAH A. LEKAN-RUTLEDGE

OBJECTIVES

Upon completion of this chapter, the reader will be able to:

1. Describe the mechanisms of urinary continence and incontinence.

2. Describe the characteristics and clinical presentation of stress, urge, and overflow incontinence.

3. Describe an algorithmic approach to the assessment of urinary incontinence.

4. Discuss iatrogenic, environmental, and functional factors that may precipitate, aggravate, or worsen urinary incontinence.

5. Differentiate approaches for basic assessment and indications for further urodynamic assessment.

6. Describe a framework for bladder health promotion.

7. Describe treatment approaches for stress, urge, and overflow incontinence.

8. Articulate the role of absorbent products, urinary devices, clean intermittent catheterization, and external, urethral, and suprapubic catheters in managing urinary incontinence.

9. Describe the causes and contributing factors to fecal impaction and incontinence.

10. Describe conservative treatment of fecal impaction and incontinence.

1. Which one of the following statements regarding urinary incontinence is false?
   a. Up to 75% of institutionalized individuals are incontinent of urine.
   b. The internal urethral sphincter is under voluntary muscular control.
   c. An α-antagonist will cause the bladder to empty.
   d. The parasympathetic innervation of the bladder arises from sacral nerves S2 to S4.
2. Which one of the following statements concerning urinary incontinence is false?
   a. Bladder training is a specific therapy for stress incontinence.
   b. Double voiding reduces the residual volume.

   c. Stress incontinence following prostatectomy is generally caused by sphincter insufficiency.
   d. Dementia is associated with uninhibited bladder contractions.
3. Which one of the following statements concerning incontinence is false?
   a. Local estrogen has been shown to relieve stress incontinence secondary to atrophic urethritis.
   b. Calcium channel blockers have helped some patients with urgency incontinence.
   c. Intermittent catheterization is associated with more infections than a sterile closed system.
   d. Fecal incontinence is usually caused by constipation.

Urinary incontinence (UI) is a major challenge in the elderly. Perhaps because so many women develop incontinence early in their life and because it is frequent and embarrassing, it is often accepted, underreported, and undertreated. Because of these barriers, careful questioning about urinary incontinence should be part of any comprehensive history in an older person. The incidence and prevalence of urinary incontinence increase with age and are related to cognitive and functional impairments. This chapter addresses the mechanisms of continence and incontinence and the causes and contributing factors to UI; it also presents an algorithmic approach to the assessment of stress, urge, and overflow UI. Clinical strategies for preventing, treating, and managing UI are described. Alterations in bowel elimination, which includes constipation and fecal incontinence, are also addressed.

▼ AGNES TERRILL (Part I)

Miss Terrill has lived in the skilled care facility for over 1 year. She is obese and has mild dementia, and she sits immobilized in her wheelchair, wet in urine most of the time. She is even more wet on standing, but she is unsteady on her feet and generally has to be helped from her wheelchair to the bed and toilet. Her medications include flurazepam 30 mg at night for sleep disturbance, hydrochlorothiazide 50 mg daily for hypertension, digoxin 0.125 mg daily for an apparent history of congestive heart failure, as well as stool softeners, antacids, and as needed pain relievers. She is 73 years old, and her skin is in good condition. Her incontinence prevents her from going on group visits and from attending activities in the facility.

▼ ROSE KRANSTEIN (Part I)

Mrs. Kranstein is an active 73-year-old volunteer at the local library, who has noted during the past month that the slight leakage of urine she has suffered from for more than 20 years has become much worse, with leakage enough for her to need to change her underclothes every 2 hours now whenever she is up and around. She is outraged to be told by friends that it is normal to be losing urine at her age. She has investigated adult diapers at the drugstore, but she comes to see you saying, "Surely something can be done."

▼ HERBERT MARKOVICH (Part I)

Mr. Markovich presents with a history of leaking urine spasmodically from time to time and noticing that the lower part of his abdomen is distended and uncomfortable. He lives with his wife, who is in good health. He has noted a poor urinary stream, and it takes an embarrassingly long time, he says, to initiate urination. He cannot understand how it is so difficult for him to start urination when he wishes to, yet he will leak urine from time to time without any sensation whatsoever. On examination his abdomen is distended and dull suprapubically up to near the umbilicus.

▼ MAUDE SIMPKINS (Part I)

Mrs. Simpkins has become increasingly inactive for the past 3 years because of progressive osteoarthritis in her left hip. An elective hip replacement is planned, and following surgery, she is noted to be consistently wetting the bed. She is a little confused postoperatively. As her primary care physician, you are asked to agree to an indwelling catheter to ease her nursing care and to enable her to be moved out of bed, since the *staff fears that she is becoming immobilized because she would normally be going to physical therapy by now.*

STUDY QUESTIONS

- In these four cases, what is your initial impression or working diagnosis?
- What are the predisposing and precipitating factors already evident?
- In each case, what would be your next step in assessment of UI?
- What treatment or management strategies can you implement now to better manage these patients' UI symptoms?

DEFINITION, PREVALENCE, AND SIGNIFICANCE

Urinary incontinence (UI) is defined as "involuntary loss of urine sufficient to be a problem."[1] Urinary incontinence is common in older persons. Approximately 15% to 30% of noninstitutionalized older persons are affected, including 19% of men and 39% of women. A significant percentage, between 20% and 30%, have frequent UI episodes, usually daily or weekly. As the second leading risk factor for institutionalization, it is of great concern to older persons who may already be experiencing loss of independence because of other health problems or disabilities.[2,3] In nursing facilities between 50% and 70% of the 1.5 million residents are incontinent; 30% of this group also experience fecal incontinence.[4] The high prevalence of UI in nursing facilities is related to functional dependency: most residents require the assistance of others to meet personal care needs, including toileting, and are thus prone to being incontinent. In one study, bowel and bladder dysfunction was significantly associated with dementia.[5] In a study of UI in acute care hospitals, 15% to 35% of inpatients over the age of 65 were incontinent at some time during their hospital stay.[6,7] The majority of these patients had an ongoing problem with UI, and only 5% had "transient" UI (i.e., UI secondary to some acute process).

> *Urinary incontinence is widely accepted as "normal" in old age, although its consequences are devastating; it can often be cured and it can always be relieved by good management.*

Underreporting of often long-standing symptoms is a serious social and public health concern: about 50% of individuals with UI have not reported their symptoms to a physician or nurse. Reasons for this include accepting UI as a normal part of aging or childbirth, not knowing what treatments there are, believing that treatment would not help, fear of surgery,[8-11] and embarrassment (because of the stigma associated with UI). In one survey, individuals who sought treatment for UI reported that their visit to the doctor or nurse was "no help at all" or that the health professional did not seem knowledgeable or sympathetic to the problem.[9] The social and psychological impacts of UI include significant changes in social activities outside of the home, depression, social isolation, anxiety about potential disclosure to friends that UI is a problem, embarrassment about accidents in public, and enforced changes in sexual activity.[12] By necessity, many individuals feel compelled to change their entire life-style—where they go, how long they stay, what they wear—in order to manage their UI. It is not yet widely known that effective treatment can improve or cure the majority of UI nor that, when UI is persistent and severe, effective strategies can prevent sequelae such as skin problems, pressure ulcers, and UTIs.

Conservative estimates of the direct costs of UI in community-dwelling elderly are $7 billion annually and $3.3 billion in long-term care nursing facilities. The use of absorbent products (diapers, pads, briefs) contributes to rising costs, as well as creating ecological and waste concerns. It has been estimated that 52 minutes per day are spent in UI-related care in institutionalized elders, adding $9,771 per year to the cost of each incontinent patient.[13]

Clearly, more needs to be done. The Agency for Health Care Policy and Research (AHCPR) convened an interdisciplinary expert panel, conducted an extensive review of the existing knowledge base for practice, and published the first edition of the *Clinical Practice Guideline on Urinary Incontinence in Adults.*[1] Their *Clinical Practice Guideline* and the *Quick Reference* (both designed for health professionals) and a patient brochure (for consumers) are available free from the AHCPR Clearinghouse, 1-800-358-9295.

NORMAL MECHANISMS FOR MAINTAINING CONTINENCE

Lower urinary tract function has two distinct phases. The first is the bladder filling phase and the storage of urine and the second is the bladder emptying phase. Several mechanisms maintain continence (Box 22-1). Normal function and continence depend on the following:

1. The integrity of the bladder and urethra
2. An intact neurological system that provides voluntary and coordinated control of voiding
3. The pattern of urine production
4. The desire and physical capability of the person to perform the activities associated with normal toileting[14]

Functionally, the bladder and urethra act as a single unit

Mechanisms

Detrusor muscle
Sphincter mechanisms (internal and external)
Vesicourethral angle
Neurological control (local and central)

Filling and Storage

Bladder pressure must be less than urethral pressure
Bladder must be compliant and have sufficient capacity

Emptying

Bladder stretch stimulates sacral reflex
Sacral reflex makes detrusor contract and external
    sphincter relax
Bladder contraction should be strong enough to empty
    bladder completely, with no postvoid residual

in the process of storing and emptying urine. The storage phase depends on a stable detrusor muscle that inhibits contractions as the bladder distends to accommodate increasing volumes of urine. In addition, the storage phase requires a competent "sphincter mechanism" of the urethra.[15] The *internal urethral sphincter* increases urethral pressure when contracted. Two mechanisms accomplish this: the first consists of smooth muscle that extends from the bladder outlet through the pelvic floor, and the second includes striated muscle that surrounds the urethra in circular rings and is separate from the pelvic floor. The *external urethral sphincter,* a striated muscle located at the urogenital diaphragm and part of the pelvic floor muscles, can voluntarily interrupt voiding, and in most individuals it can be used to prevent loss of urine during a rapid increase in intraabdominal pressure.

Spinal reflex contraction impulses are continually generated between the spinal column and the bladder. Continuous inhibitory signals from the brain (in the pons) normally prevent these contraction signals from causing bladder contractions. Voiding is mediated by the sacral micturition center (S2 to S4) and is controlled voluntarily by complex interactions among cortical areas (frontal cortex), subcortical areas (thalamus, hypothalamus, basal ganglia, and limbic system), and the brain stem (mesencephalic-pontine-medullary reticular formation).[16] In older persons suffering progressive brain failure or other cerebral change, the loss of these inhibitory signals can, when combined with other predisposing factors, result in enough of a bladder contraction to provoke leakage.[17] Some apparent

"stress incontinence," in which the individual experiences urine leakage after coughing or some other sharp increase in intraabdominal pressure, is in fact caused by uninhibited bladder contractions. These spinal arc reflex signals are also stimulated by bladder fullness and sometimes by intravesical pathological states. This can lead to an unstable bladder.

> *In many elders the bladder contracts spontaneously, uninhibitedly, and unpredictably; the sphincters lack strength and are uncoordinated; and the urge to void occurs only when the bladder is full. No wonder urinary incontinence is common in old age!*

During bladder filling, there is little or no increase in intravesicular pressure as smooth muscle and connective tissue in the bladder wall stretch and accommodate increased urine volume. Detrusor muscle contractility is probably inhibited by activation of a spinal sympathetic reflex, which results in bladder relaxation. Approximately 150 to 250 ml of urine can be stored before bladder pressure begins to increase and the urge to void is felt.[15] As bladder filling approaches functional bladder capacity (the volume at which one would usually become uncomfortable and seek toileting facilities), mechanoreceptors in the bladder wall are stimulated and an urge to void is felt. Bladder outlet resistance increases by reflex stimulation of α-adrenergic receptors within the smooth muscle of the bladder neck and proximal urethra. As long as the urethral pressure is greater than the intravesical pressure, continence is maintained.

An important factor in women is loss of the vesicourethral angle (the angle at the juncture of the bladder and the urethra) as a result of overstretching of pelvic muscles during childbirth and relaxation of pelvic muscles after menopause related to estrogen deficiency. The vesicourethral angle helps to maintain the anatomical integrity of the bladder neck to prevent leakage of urine during physical activity or rapid increases in intraabdominal pressure.

Normal voiding is a voluntary act coordinated through central and autonomic nervous systems to first facilitate relaxation of the urethra and decrease urethral pressure, followed several seconds later by a rise in intravesicular pressure secondary to sustained contraction of the bladder. The bladder neck descends and funnels to allow urine to flow until the bladder is completely emptied. With termination of voiding, the striated muscles of the urethra and pelvic floor contract to elevate the bladder base and increase intraurethral pressure and inhibit further detrusor contractions.[16]

Increased residual urine
Diminished bladder capacity
Decreased bladder sensitivity
Detrusor instability
Prostatic hypertrophy
Increased nocturnal urinary output
Prior childbirth
Obesity
Smoking
Estrogen withdrawal and menopause
Brain failure
Dysmobility

PREDISPOSING AND AGE-RELATED FACTORS IN URINARY INCONTINENCE

These underlying factors explain the proneness of elders to UI (Box 22-2).

Increased Residual Urine

Any postvoid residual urine volume predisposes to both infection and incontinence. More than 100 ml is regarded as abnormal. Residual urine may be due to poor bladder contractility or outlet resistance. In men, a common cause is obstruction from benign prostatic hyperplasia. Other causes of outlet resistance include stricture, cystocele, and fecal impaction.

Diminished Bladder Capacity

Normal aging contributes to a reduction in muscle mass of the bladder wall, decreased elasticity and compliance of the bladder wall, and increased tone. Bladder capacity may decrease from 500 to 600 ml in younger adults to 250 to 300 ml in older adults. Decreased bladder capacity may contribute to frequency and nocturia.

Decreased Bladder Sensitivity

With increasing age the desire to void may occur only when the bladder is near its functional capacity. Bladder filling sensations may not be perceived. One explanation is that there is a reduced number and deterioration of the sensory nerves and sensory receptors, which do not provide sufficiently strong enough signals about bladder filling. This may be one reason that many older persons often lack the classic symptoms of urinary tract infection such as dysuria or burning.

Detrusor Instability

Normal age-related changes in the cerebral cortex and spinal reflex arc predispose to uninhibited bladder con-

tractions. These contractions often occur at small bladder volumes and may be inappropriately strong, given the small urine volume. These contractions can be produced not only in response to very slight bladder distention but also to increased intraabdominal pressure from coughing and sneezing. Older persons often report decreased "holding time," the time between when a strong urge is felt and when they absolutely must void at the risk of losing urine (thus the saying, "When you've got to go, you've got to go!"). Many older persons with detrusor instability have no other obvious neurological disorders typically associated with uninhibited bladder contractions. Neurological disorders associated with uninhibited bladder contractions include brain tumors, cerebrovascular accidents, multiple sclerosis, Parkinson's disease, and spinal cord injury.

Benign Prostatic Hyperplasia

Benign prostatic hyperplasia (BPH), noncancerous enlargement of the prostate gland, is a normal age-related development in men, with a prevalence of greater than 50% in men older than 60 years of age. By age 85 the prevalence is approximately 90%.[18] It increases urethral resistance and contributes to increased residual urine volume. Over time, prolonged obstruction can lead to marked loss of bladder tone, secondary to chronic bladder overdistension. Prolonged bladder distension is both insidious and surprisingly painless. As urethral resistance increases, however, the strength of bladder contractions also increases to effectively empty the bladder. Uninhibited bladder contractions and bladder urgency may also result, leading to frequency, urgency, and incontinence. Symptoms of outlet obstruction caused by prostatic hyperplasia include difficulty starting the urine stream, weak urine stream, hesitancy, intermittent stream, prolonged voiding, postvoid dribbling, and a sensation of incomplete emptying. Chronic bladder overdistention ultimately leads to hydronephrosis as a result of retrograde pressure and tissue damage. Clinical practice guidelines for BPH are available free from the AHCPR.[18]

Excessive Nocturnal Urine Excretion

With increasing age the kidneys become less efficient in concentrating and excreting urine and may produce more urine at night than during the day. Excessive urine production at night may be related to diabetes mellitus or insipidus, congestive heart failure, venous stasis, or deficits in antidiuretic hormone production. Nocturia greater than twice per night is considered abnormal.

Childbirth

A significant association has been drawn between a number of factors associated with childbirth and the onset of UI; these factors include parity, high birth weight, difficult delivery with prolonged stage 2, use of forceps during delivery, and childbirth injury related to severe lacerations or tears. Vaginal delivery may lead to weakened, damaged, or denervated pelvic muscles and pelvic fascial supports. Although, during the postpartum period, pelvic muscle supports may be restored in the normal course of events or with a program of pelvic muscle exercises, in some women pelvic muscle strength and function may be impaired, with urinary incontinence becoming manifest postmenopause. In a prospective study of the effect of vaginal delivery on the pelvic floor, neurophysiological evidence of enervation of pelvic floor muscles with pudendal neuropathy was demonstrated, and the data suggest that the injury may persist and worsen over time.[19] In a study of pelvic floor function in nulliparous and parous women, sphincter weakness appeared to result from a number of alterations related to childbirth, including loss of motor units, altered activation patterns, and other neurophysiological abnormalities that affect continence mechanisms.[20]

Obesity

Obesity, defined as greater than 20% over the average or desirable body weight for height and age, is associated with increased risk for UI and is a common cause of incontinence in women.[21] Excessive body weight may weaken pelvic muscle supports. In incontinent, morbidly obese women who underwent surgically induced weight loss, significant improvement in lower urinary tract function and resolution of incontinence were noted in most of the women, obviating the need for further incontinence intervention.[22]

Smoking

Smoking has been associated with urinary incontinence, and it is the number one risk factor for bladder cancer. Active ingredients in cigarettes, including tars, are bladder irritants, which may contribute to urgency, frequency, and urge incontinence. Smokers tend to develop chronic coughs, which may put undue strain on pelvic muscles thus provoking stress incontinence. In a case-control study of smokers and nonsmokers, it was found that stress UI develops in smokers, even when urethral support is stronger and risk factors are fewer than in nonsmokers.[23]

Estrogen Withdrawal and Menopause

The vagina, urethra, and trigonal area of the bladder have similar epithelial linings, rich in estrogen receptors. Normal urethral function, involving urethral pressure, closure, length, and vascularity, is influenced by estrogen. When supplied with estrogen, the intraurethral walls are soft, moist, and interdigitated to form a watertight seal. With declining hormone levels the walls of the urethra become harder, the folds become less pronounced, and mucus production decreases, resulting in less efficient closure. Decline in circulating estrogen levels in postmenopausal women contributes to atrophic urethritis, trigonitis, atrophic vaginitis, and thinning and weakening of endopelvic fascia and pelvic muscles.[24] Irritative voiding symptoms, including frequency, urgency, dysuria, and urge incontinence, are often associated with estrogen deficiency. These irritative symptoms may improve with estrogen therapy. However, estrogen may have little effect on urethral or pelvic muscle function.[25] Estrogen therapy may be taken orally, transdermally, or intravaginally. Nonhormonal intravaginal moisturizers used daily may also reduce irritative symptoms.

Brain Failure

Reduced cognition in the older person with dementia or transient or acute confusion reduces awareness of the sensation of bladder filling and the need to void. Difficulties adapting to a new situation and inability to find the toilet cause incontinence to be a frequent problem in the relocated individual with acute or chronic cognitive impairment. As so often occurs in geriatric care, the environment, the physical state, and the predisposing aging changes all interact. This multiplicity of factors gives the clinician an opportunity to intervene and prevent or treat the incontinence. In situations with a frail, cognitively impaired older person the physical and social environments take on greater significance in the person's care.

Dysmobility

Factors that inhibit mobility, including musculoskeletal problems (stiffness, pain, rigidity, decreased range, instability, etc.), neurological problems (weakness, paralysis, reduced sensation), easy fatigability and poor endurance, exertional dyspnea, frailty, and apathy, predispose to UI.

FACTORS PRECIPITATING URINARY INCONTINENCE

With the above predisposing factors as the background or health history of the patient, incontinence may be exacerbated or aggravated by one or more precipitating factors (Box 22-3).

Relocation and Environment

The interaction of changed environment and decreased compensatory reserve may be enough to precipitate UI. Hospitalization often involves enforced immobility, medications that affect cognition or cause hypotension, blurred vision, or gait unsteadiness, and tubes and devices that impede access to the bathroom. The lack of privacy may inhibit voiding. Restraints (physical or chemical) and bedside rails are further inhibition; many hospital rooms have little space for patient transfers, wheelchairs, and mobility. Urinary incontinence may ensue as a result of physical deconditioning and the immo-

---

BOX 22-3
Factors Precipitating Urinary Incontinence

Relocation
Inappropriate environment
Urinary tract infection
Other acute illness
Intravesical lesions
Medications
Urinary obstruction
Neurological lesions
    Atonic bladder
    Reflex neurogenic bladder
    Uninhibited neurogenic bladder
    Detrusor-sphincter dyssynergia

---

bility inflicted on the patient during the hospital stay. Attitudes of the nursing and medical staff about maintaining continence, or assessing and treating incontinence, affect the patient's motivation and optimism.

Urinary Tract Infection

A lack of characteristic urinary tract infection symptoms should not inhibit the clinician from ordering urinalysis and culture. Often extensive bacteriuria is found, and it will not be certain whether this represents a new infection or chronic bacteriuria. Symptoms of bacteriuria may include frequency, urgency, or a worsening of incontinence, whereas dysuria and fever may not be manifested. In general, chronic asymptomatic bacteriuria is not treated with antibiotics. Nonpharmacological measures such as increased fluids, especially water, urine acidification with vitamin C, cranberry juice daily, and good hygiene practices may be helpful.[26] It is recommended that symptomatic bacteriuria or bacteriuria associated with definite or probable new onset of UI be treated with the appropriate antibiotic. Recurrent urinary tract infections may warrant referral to a urologist.

Acute Illness

Any acute illness in an older person can precipitate transient incontinence, in part because of the common cerebral effects of illness on function and in part because of the consequences of other treatment, hospitalization, or the acute illness itself.

Intravesical Lesions

Debris, calculi, sludgelike deposits from retained urine, as well as polyps, carcinomata, and previously unsuspected bladder diverticula, can precipitate urinary incontinence. New-onset UI with urgency and frequency symptoms should be further evaluated with cystoscopy after a therapeutic trial of behavioral treatment has not

significantly improved or resolved the UI. Hematuria, whether associated with urinary tract infection or not, should be further evaluated with cystoscopy.

Medications

Multiple drug use is common in older persons. Diuretics obviously can precipitate incontinence, but the more briskly potent diuretics such as furosemide can also precipitate retention in men with prostatic enlargement, and many other drugs produce a degree of diuresis, especially if renally excreted. The depressing effects of tranquilizers and hypnotics (many medications are unintended tranquilizers and hypnotics) on the central nervous system precipitate incontinence by diminishing awareness or deepening sleep. Frequently these same medications have anticholinergic effects, which can cause partial or complete retention or overflow. α-Adrenergic drugs, such as clonidine and calcium channel blockers, have also been implicated as medications potentially causing UI; ironically, the latter have also been used to treat certain types of incontinence (Table 22-1).

Urinary Obstruction

Obstruction of the bladder outlet can be precipitated by anticholinergic drug side effects, fecal impaction, and cystocele. Obstruction with overflow incontinence may also be the presenting clinical picture in the atonic bladder.

Neurological Lesions

Voiding dysfunction in old age is now being systematically studied.[27] Frankly neurological lesions as precipitants can be classified into four types: atonic bladder, reflex neurogenic, uninhibited neurogenic, and detrusor-sphincter dyssynergia.

The *atonic bladder* is most often associated with diabetic autonomic neuropathy. Either bladder sensation or the ability to maintain coordinated contractions is lost, leading to bladder distention. This picture can also be caused by lesions low in the spinal cord or in the cauda equina: not only metastatic but also local thrombotic conditions.

In the *reflex neurogenic bladder*, sometimes called the reflex bladder, the bladder suffers sensory loss but continues to empty and fill. This is caused by a lesion above the sacral area but below the brain and is thus often seen in paraplegics. Tumors in the spinal cord, disk lesions, osteophytes (associated with the osteoarthritis of many older persons), and multiple sclerosis may be other etiologies.

In the *uninhibited neurogenic bladder* the picture of the reflex neurogenic bladder is compounded with loss of bladder inhibition and recurrent emptying. The terms uninhibited neurogenic bladder, neurogenic bladder, unstable bladder, and dystonic bladder are used inter-

Table 22-1 Drugs Associated with Lower Urinary Tract Dysfunction

Type	Action	Effect
Diuretics	Polyuria, frequency, urgency	Urgency and urge UI
CNS depressants (sedatives, hypnotics, tranquilizers, narcotics)	Diminished awareness of bladder filling and need to void	Urge and functional incontinence
	Decreased ability to inhibit bladder contractions and to control voiding	
	Decreased outlet resistance	
α-Sympathetic antagonists	Decreased bladder outlet and urethral resistance	Stress UI
Anticholinergics (psychotropics, antiparkinsonians, antispasmodics, antihistamines)	Decreased bladder contraction strength	Acute or chronic retention
	Decreased urge signal	Overflow incontinence
	Diminished sensorium and awareness of need to void	
α-Antagonist/α-adrenergic blockers	Decreased outlet resistance	Stress UI
β-Adrenergic agonists	Decreased bladder contraction	Urinary retention
Calcium channel blockers	Decreased bladder contraction	Urinary retention
Caffeine	Bladder irritability, diuresis	Urgency and urge UI
Nicotine	Bladder irritability, smoker's cough	Urgency and stress UI
Alcohol	Sedation, impaired mobility, diuresis	Functional UI

changeably. Although dementia is a common predisposing factor, other acute events in the brain should also be considered (such as tumor or infarct). Incontinence is usually a relatively late feature of dementia, and its onset should be thoroughly assessed.

Detrusor-sphincter dyssynergia occurs when the urethral sphincter contracts simultaneously when the bladder contracts to expel urine. This may be caused by a spinal cord lesion between the pons and the bladder and is diagnosed by urodynamic studies.

TRANSIENT AND PERSISTENT INCONTINENCE

Determining the timing and circumstances associated with the onset of UI helps to focus diagnostic and treatment interventions. One of the first questions usually asked in geriatrics is "How long has this been going on?"

Transient incontinence is characterized by a fairly sudden or recent onset of symptoms. Appropriate treatment of transient causes of UI will result in cure or significant improvement.[28] It is believed that approximately 30% of all cases of urinary incontinence in older people are transient. If not appropriately treated, transient UI will not reverse itself and will persist. Transient causes of UI are summarized in Box 22-4.

CASE DISCUSSION

Mrs. Simpkins has become suddenly incontinent following elective hip replacement; because of this, she is catheterized. This may precipitate many problems, possibly permanent, in what is essentially a transient situation. She has become somewhat confused as a result of the impact and anxiety of the surgery, the immobility, the pain-relieving medications, the

relative postoperative anemia, and an incidental urinary tract infection.

STUDY QUESTION

■ *What adjustments can be made in Mrs. Simpkins' situation to improve her transient incontinence?*

▼ MAUDE SIMPKINS (Part II)

When directly questioned, Mrs. Simpkins says she seems to get little warning of the need to urinate, but it has always been like that for her; however, there is no possibility of responding in time, given her situation. Adjustments to her medication, instructions for frequent offering of the bedpan at regular intervals, and a program of rapid mobilization, using diapering at first to give her confidence that she will not leak urine, results in her being back on schedule for her physical therapy in less than 2 weeks.

Persistent UI is present when transient causes are ruled out or therapeutic trials of treatment have not successfully reversed the UI; it compels more in-depth evaluation. In evaluating, look carefully at both the storage and emptying phase, including symptom profile and history, physical examination, bladder function studies and, in some, urodynamic studies. Problems associated with the *filling and storage* of urine are described in terms of the bladder function, including detrusor activity and contractility, sensation, compliance, and capacity. Urethral competence is also necessary to maintain closure except under conditions of normal voiding. Alterations in ure-

From Resnick NM, Yalla SV: *N Engl J Med* 313:800-805, 1985.

BOX 22-4
Common Causes of Transient Incontinence

Delirium or confusional state
Infection, urinary (symptomatic)
Atrophic urethritis or vaginitis
Drugs
  Sedatives or hypnotics, especially long-acting agents
  Loop diuretics
  Anticholinergic agents (antipsychotics, antidepressants, antihistamines, antiparkinsonian agents, antiarrhythmics, antispasmodics, opiates, and antidiarrheals)
  α-Adrenoceptor agonists and antagonists
  Calcium channel blockers
Psychological problems, including depression
Endocrine disorders (hypercalcemia, hyperglycemia)
Restricted mobility
Stool impaction

BOX 22-5
Types of Persistent Urinary Incontinence

Stress incontinence (leakage with physical activity or increased intraabdominal pressure; small to moderate volume leaks)
Urge incontinence (detrusor instability; leakage following a strong uncontrollable urge to void, or inability to delay voiding; moderate to large volume—a "gush")
Mixed incontinence (stress and urge together)
Overflow incontinence (leakage without the urge to void, from a distended or obstructed bladder; intermittent or continuous; volume varies)
Functional incontinence (factors outside the urinary tract cause the loss of urine: mobility problems, cognitive deficit, sedatives, environmental barriers, etc.)
Enuresis (leakage without awareness occurring during sleep)

Table 22-2   Characteristics and Causes of Four Types of Persistent Urinary Incontinence

Type	Associated Characteristics	Pathophysiology	Common Causes
Stress	Usually in daytime only; infrequently nocturnal	Sphincter incompetence; urethral instability	Pelvic prolapse (women); sphincter weakness or damage (e.g., following prostatectomy)
Urge	Urinary frequency, nocturia, possible suprapubic discomfort	Detrusor overactivity (instability or hyperreflexia)	Central nervous system damage (stroke, Alzheimer's, brain tumor, Parkinson's disease); interference with spinal inhibitory pathways (spondylosis or metastasis); local bladder disorder (bladder cancer, radiation effects, interstitial cystitis, or outlet obstruction)
Overflow	Hesitancy, straining to void, weak or interrupted urine stream; occurs day or night	Outlet obstruction or underactive detrusor	Obstruction (prostatic hypertrophy, bladder neck obstruction, urethral stricture); underactive detrusor (myogenic or neurogenic factors, e.g., herniated disk, or diabetic neuropathy); anticholinergic/antispasmodic drugs
Functional	Other medical problems; iatrogenic illnesses associated	Normal bladder and urethral function	Impaired mobility or cognitive status; inaccessible toilets; depression, anger, hostility, psychosis

From Wyman JF: *Nurs Clin North Am* 22:169-187, 1988.

thral competence allow for leakage of urine in the absence of a bladder contraction and may be related to poor periurethral muscle supports or intrinsic sphincter damage.

Problems associated with bladder *emptying* are described in terms of bladder contractility and urethral function. A poorly contracting bladder may be related to neurological, musculoskeletal disorders, or psychological disorders that contribute to abnormal voiding patterns and chronic holding of urine. In some cases the etiology of a poorly contracting bladder is idiopathic. A disorder described as "detrusor instability with impaired contractility" (DHIC) has been identified in elderly in the ab-

sence of other identifiable etiologies. This disorder is manifested by detrusor instability with urgency and urge incontinence and a poorly contracting bladder so that voiding and incontinence episodes do not fully empty the bladder.[29] Urethral disorders may also affect bladder emptying.

TYPES OF URINARY INCONTINENCE

It is clinically useful to differentiate four types of UI: stress, urge, mixed, and overflow. To these should be added functional incontinence (also called nongenitourinary) and enuresis, in which urinary leakage occurs during sleep (Table 22-2 and Box 22-5).

Stress UI is characterized by leakage of urine during physical activity (such as walking, exercising, bending, or lifting) or periods of increased intrabdominal pressure (such as coughing, laughing, or sneezing). Urine loss is usually in small amounts, a few drops to a teaspoon or so, and nocturia or UI at night is usually not reported. True stress UI implies that a urodynamic study has determined that there is decreased urethral resistance and leakage of urine not associated with a bladder contraction. Clinically, this may be demonstrated by having the patient cough vigorously in both lying and standing positions with a full bladder to confirm leakage that occurs without bladder contraction. Stress UI is most commonly caused by hypermobility or significant displacement of the urethra and bladder neck during physical activity. This type of UI is noted frequently in women because of factors related to childbirth and hormone status, and it may occasionally be documented in men with a history of prostate surgery.

> *Urge incontinence is the most common type of urinary incontinence in elders: "When you've got to go, you've got to go!"*

Urge UI, or detrusor instability, involves leakage of urine that is associated with a sudden, strong, uncontrollable urge to void and the inability to delay voiding. This condition is due to an abnormal bladder storage, detrusor overactivity, or uncontrolled bladder contractions. Characteristics include urgency, frequency, and usually nocturia. Detrusor overactivity that has neurological origins, as from Parkinson's disease, cerebrovascular accident, multiple sclerosis, or spinal cord injury, is termed detrusor hyperreflexia. Urine loss is usually in large amounts and may be described as a "gush." In patients without neurological disease, detrusor instability and urge UI are idiopathic. This is the most common type of UI in older adults. In one study of patients with detrusor instability the majority had normal coordinated reflex micturition at normal bladder volumes but an abnormal perception of bladder fullness and lack of voluntary inhibitory controls.[30] In another study a subset of older persons with detrusor instability also had documented urine retention resulting from ineffective or poor bladder contractility (i.e., detrusor instability with impaired contractility, or DHIC) as mentioned before.[29] Such patients may experience recurrent urinary tract infection or acute urinary retention secondary to anticholinergic drugs.

Mixed UI is characterized by the presentation of stress and urge UI simultaneously. Often, mixed symptoms of stress UI and urge UI (detrusor instability) are reported; however, mixed UI may not be confirmed on examination. Clinical presentation may reveal primary and secondary symptoms; that is, leakage is associated with physical activity and with strong uncontrollable bladder urges. Since bladder activity and urethral sphincter function are interrelated in the mechanisms of maintaining continence, mixed UI probably involves a continuum of interrelationships contributing to a mixed symptom pattern.[31]

Overflow UI is leakage of urine without the urge to void, resulting from a distended bladder. Bladder retention may be due to outlet obstruction or impaired contractility. Overflow UI may present as stress UI in patients with poor bladder contractility, since urine loss is often provoked by physical activity, which increases intrabdominal pressure thus causing urine to be expelled. The bladder may be underactive because of drugs, fecal impaction, neurological conditions such as lower spinal cord injury or diabetic neuropathy, or recent pelvic surgery. Obstruction may be due to prostatic hyperplasia in men and cystocele or pelvic prolapse in women; patients with multiple sclerosis may have detrusor-sphincter dyssynergia, since the sphincter inappropriately contracts simultaneously with detrusor contractions during voiding.

Functional UI is urine loss caused by factors outside of the lower urinary tract, such as physical immobility (the ability to disrobe and maneuver oneself) or cognitive deficits that impair the ability to perceive the need to toilet and be motivated to do so or to behave in a manner that is socially appropriate. Medications that adversely affect cognitive function and sensorium particularly contribute to functional UI. Environmental barriers that impede access to toilets, or the simple unavailability of toilets, also cause functional UI.

Enuresis is incontinence without awareness occurring during sleep. Enuresis is considered primary if the condition has persisted since childhood and nighttime continence has never been achieved, and it is secondary if it develops later in life. Enuresis may be associated with abnormal antidiuretic hormone production, resulting in an inappropriate increase in urine production at night.

ASSESSMENT AND INVESTIGATION OF URINARY INCONTINENCE

The purpose of the basic evaluation of UI is to detect and confirm UI objectively, recognize factors that may be contributing to or precipitating UI or that result from UI, and identify patients who need further specialized evaluation before any therapeutic interventions are initiated.[1] Health professionals, particularly physicians and nurses, conduct initial screening and basic evaluation in patients who present with UI and other voiding symptoms. Complex patients with neurological, urogynecological, or urological disorders should be referred to a specialist for more comprehensive evaluation and possibly for advanced urodynamic testing.

The basic evaluation includes history, including a bladder diary and medication review, physical examination with additional tests such as urinalysis, and when indicated, simple tests of lower urinary tract function. In older persons with physical or cognitive impairments, mental status testing, functional status testing, and environmental assessment are also considered.

History

Screening for UI poses challenges to the clinician. The patient's main concern about bladder symptoms should be explored with questions such as "Do you leak urine when you don't want to?" or "Do you have trouble holding your urine?" Such seemingly straightforward questions, however, may not yield accurate information or acknowledgment of the problem. Embarrassment, modesty, acceptance of the problem, or misunderstood terminology may inhibit the older person from accurately describing the symptoms. Some individuals accept mild degrees of urine loss if it can be adequately contained and managed with absorbent products and if there is no odor or hygiene problem. In such instances it is helpful to follow up with questions about whether pads or absorbent products are worn for protection.

> *It is vital to ask direct questions about urinary incontinence, since so many patients accept this symptom as "normal."*

It is important to determine the onset, timing, and frequency of UI. Symptoms of frequency, urgency, nocturia, dysuria, bedwetting (nocturnal enuresis), or voiding dysfunction (hesitancy, straining, postvoid dribbling, intermittency) should be elicited. Fluid intake pattern, bowel function, sexual function, and use of pads or devices should be assessed. Previous treatment and outcomes should be noted.

A *bladder diary* is vital in recording the day to day voiding and incontinence pattern and associated symptoms. Bladder diaries are usually more reliable than self-report of symptoms because people may overestimate or underestimate the magnitude of the problem. Patients should be given a urine collection receptacle that may be fitted over the toilet seat so that urine volumes may be easily measured. Men can use a urinal if preferred. Accurate measurement of voided volumes can provide a good estimate of functional bladder capacity. Often, the first voided volume of the day is the largest void. Different types of bladder diaries exist, and one may be more appropriate than another. Some bladder diaries are simply designed with blank columns for the patient to fill in the exact time of voids and incontinent episodes. Other diaries are more detailed with columns for recording voided volumes, incontinent episodes, whether a bladder urge was present, food and fluid intake, bowel function, circumstances associated with leakage, and pad usage. Usually, a bladder diary is recorded for 3 to 7 days.

It is important to ask how UI symptoms have affected life-style and quality of life. Alterations in daily routines, self-management, financial cost, effect on sexual function, and exercise and activity patterns should be elicited.

Medication review identifies and determines the extent to which medications may adversely affect continence and bladder function. Categories of drugs that are associated with lower urinary tract dysfunction include diuretics, anticholinergics, α-adrenergic agonists, β-adrenergic agonists, α-agonists, calcium channel blockers, and CNS depressants (sedatives, hypnotics, tranquilizers, narcotics). Caffeine, nicotine, and alcohol are also important to consider when obtaining a drug history. Medication review should carefully account for both prescription and over-the-counter medicines (Table 22-1).

Physical Examination

The physical examination begins with a general assessment of the older person's overall health, wellness, mobility, and function. Body size, grooming, movements, gait, speech, communication ability, and comprehension provide information about potential predisposing or precipitating factors.

The neurological examination focuses on the lumbosacral and pelvic areas. Tone, movement, and strength of the lower extremities are evaluated, including deep tendon reflexes. Neurological assessment of S2-S4 spinal roots is accomplished via several maneuvers. Examination of perineal sensation for symmetrical perception of light touch and pinprick determines intact perineal sensation and S2-S4 spinal roots; if the ankle jerk can be elicited, this also confirms S2-S4 integrity. Light stroking of the skin near the anus should cause the anal sphincter to contract reflexively (anal wink). The bulbocavernosus reflex is evaluated by tugging the glans penis or clitoris (or pulling on the indwelling catheter if present), and checking for the production of an anal sphincter contraction (the finger of the examiner's other hand being concurrently in the rectum). A strong cough should provoke a reflex contraction of the pelvic floor. Although these tests offer clinical value, sacral reflexes may be difficult to elicit even in neurologically intact patients, and their absence may be nonconfirmatory.

In older patients an assessment of mental status and motivation is critical; an individual with memory difficulty may not do well with behavioral treatment approaches. However, if there is a willing and able caregiver to assist, bladder training or pelvic muscle exercises are more feasible.

In women a gynecological exam is of great importance. Vulvar and vaginal atrophy, pallor, or irritation may suggest estrogen deficiency. Elasticity of the vaginal vault should be assessed; in many older women, the vault is narrowed and atrophied. Vaginal redness and irritation may suggest inappropriate use of absorbent products or infection. Pelvic support abnormalities such as urethrocele, cystocele, rectocele, uterine descent and prolapse, or urethral mobility should be assessed. If the woman has a full bladder (at least 200 ml volume), the stress maneuver may be performed with the woman exerting a strong cough or bearing down. This may be performed in the lying position and, if negative, repeated in the standing position with a pad or tissues placed at the urinary meatus. Loss of urine is usually associated with downward displacement of the bladder neck and urethra; a small spurt of urine suggests stress UI. Delayed urine loss, particularly of large volume (unless the bladder is not full), is associated with unstable bladder activity or urge UI.

The pelvic muscle body may be assessed for mass (thin, moderate, thick), ribbing (smooth or ribbed), symmetry, and strength and duration of contraction.

The rectal examination evaluates anal sphincter tone, sensation, and contraction. Fecal impaction may be detected. In males the genitalia are inspected to detect abnormalities of the foreskin, glans penis, and perineal skin. Rectal examination also evaluates the contour, consistency, and size of the prostate gland.

Functional assessment of the ability to access a toilet or toilet substitute, the time it takes to toilet, and the skills needed is essential. Clothing may unnecessarily complicate toileting (use Velcro, minimize buckles). Cognitive ability should be considered; lost visuospatial skills inhibit undressing and toileting.

Environmental assessment identifies the location and accessibility of toilets, availability of toilet substitutes, distance to the toilet, cleanliness and safety in the toileting area, and adaptive toilet equipment such as grab bars and raised seats.

▼ *AGNES TERRILL (Part II)*

The nursing record of Miss Terrill's urinary incontinence reveals that she leaks at any time of the day or night and that association with movement is absent. The nurses avoid moving her around, but the incontinence is not especially precipitated by being moved; rather, she is almost always to be found sitting in urine. On examination, Miss Terrill does not have a palpable bladder. However, examining her standing and encouraging her to cough and stress, even with a full bladder, does not consistently produce incontinence of urination. She becomes agitated on attempts at a pelvic examination, but the uterovaginal descent can be seen even without a full pelvic examination. A rectal examination is achieved, confirming quite severe constipation, despite her regular bowel habits. There is no fecal incontinence. She is not fully cooperative in these examinations and is clearly unaware that she has a urinary in-

continence problem. She is not in congestive failure, but she is in sinus rhythm, and she has a normal blood pressure.

STUDY QUESTIONS

- *What initial steps should be taken to improve Miss Terrill's incontinence?*
- *To which broad category of incontinence does Miss Terrill belong?*
- *Is a specific incontinence management indicated?*

▼ *HERBERT MARKOVICH (Part II)*

There is no clinical doubt that Mr. Markovich has urinary retention. His rectal examination confirms, as his history suggests, marked prostatic hypertrophy.

STUDY QUESTIONS

- *What investigations are indicated?*
- *Should Mr. Markovich be hospitalized?*
- *Is surgical treatment likely to be indicated soon?*

Diagnostic Tests

Diagnostic tests for UI are summarized in Box 22-6.

Urinalysis. Urinalysis, with culture and sensitivity if infection is suspected, should be carried out in all patients. A simple bedside approach uses chemical reagent dipsticks for rapid assessment of pH, specific gravity, bacteria, white blood cells, hematuria, glucose, and nitrite. A positive nitrite measure is highly suggestive of urinary tract infection, warranting culture and sensitivity. Hematuria should always be further evaluated. Urine cytology should be obtained in patients reporting recent onset of UI.

BOX 22-6
Primary Care Diagnostic Tests in Urinary Incontinence

Urinalysis, with culture and sensitivity if infection is suspected

Postvoid residual measurement (three measurements between 50 and 200 ml is normal, but consistently above 100 ml should be closely monitored) either by straight catheterization or by noninvasive bladder ultrasound

Simply cystometry (first desire to void at less than 100 ml, pain or incontinence during filling, or capacity less than 400 ml or more than 650 ml)

Uroflowmetry (listen while the patient voids)

Urodynamic studies (reserved for those unresponsive to a trial of treatment for the type of UI diagnosed or where surgery is anticipated)

Postvoid Residual Urine Measurement. Postvoid residual urine measurement (PVR) is recommended in the basic evaluation of UI, particularly in individuals with suspected bladder-emptying problems. Individuals with diabetes mellitus, Parkinson's disease, multiple sclerosis, and prostatic hyperplasia, to name a few, should be assessed for bladder emptying. Although the "normal" PVR is zero, most would consider that three PVR measurements between 50 and 200 ml are within normal limits in older persons; however, volumes between 100 and 200 ml warrant close monitoring for upper and lower urinary tract disorders.[31] This is useful diagnostic information even if a definitive diagnosis is not confirmed, since treatment for patients with poor bladder emptying function is limited to management methods such as intermittent catheterization, voiding maneuvers, urine collection devices, and fluid monitoring. Behavioral approaches such as bladder training and pelvic muscle retraining would not be indicated.

A noninvasive approach to postvoid residual measurement uses bladder ultrasound. This is particularly useful in frail individuals who are at higher risk for bladder infection from urethral catheterization or in whom catheterization would be psychologically distressing or uncomfortable. Portable bladder ultrasound units are becoming more widely used in geriatric and rehabilitation settings because they are noninvasive, easy to use, and reasonably accurate in approximating bladder volume when operated by skilled users.

Simple Cystometry. Simple cystometry evaluates bladder filling, storage, and emptying (Table 22-3). After the patient voids, the bladder is filled in a retrograde manner to assess bladder sensation during filling, ability to control a detrusor contraction, functional and maximal bladder capacity, bladder wall compliance, and the presence and strength of detrusor contractions. The descriptor "simple" is used because this is an approach that relies on a limited range of equipment to monitor bladder function. Complex cystometry involves measuring a number of parameters of bladder function via intrabladder, rectal, and vaginal pressure by way of electronic transducer pressure catheters, electromyographic assessment of pelvic muscles or anal and urethral sphincters, and dynamic videography of voiding. For the health professional in primary care practice, simple cystometry can yield important information necessary to increase diagnostic accuracy. Simple cystometry may be useful in differentiating urge and stress UI and detecting impaired bladder sensation and reduced bladder capacity that may be present without UI. Simple cystometry is conducted using a urethral catheter through which sterile water or normal saline is slowly instilled. To do this, an intravenous bag of fluid may be connected by a Y-adapter to the catheter, or a bulb syringe without the plunger may be connected to the end of the catheter for the bladder instillation. Abnormal findings include the first desire to void at less than 100 ml, pain or incontinence during filling, a bladder capacity of less than 400 ml or greater than 650 ml.[31]

Simple cystometry may not be indicated in the basic evaluation of all patients in primary care practice. However, in patients with urge UI or to further confirm stress UI, this test can offer additional information necessary in determining a clinical diagnosis and can narrow the treatment options. The reliability of simple cystometry in cognitively impaired or uncooperative patients is limited, however.[32]

Especially if simple cystometry is carried out in the office, the majority of incontinent elders can be completely managed in the primary care setting.

Uroflowmetry. Measurement of bladder emptying function can be simply accomplished by listening while the patient voids. The flow of urine should be smooth, uninterrupted, and initially strong. Intermittency, audible sounds of straining or grunting, prolonged voiding, or a weak, dribbling stream suggests voiding abnormalities. However, accurate urinary flow measurement can be made (uroflowmetry) using a special container to assess the rate of flow; the graphic curve so produced is normally bell shaped. In BPH, for example, the curve is flattened, with increased time taken to empty and a reduced peak flow rate. Uroflowmetry can be a valuable, noninvasive, primary care test.

Specialized Studies. Cystometry (bladder pressure measurement), profilometry (urethral pressure during the voiding cycle), pressure/flow studies (uroflowmetry combined with cystometry), pelvic floor electromyography, and video-urodynamic studies are reserved for selected patients who are unresponsive to a trial of treatment suitable for the type of UI diagnosed or for whom surgery is the most appropriate, or desired, option. They are generally organized in consultation with a urologist or gyne-urologist. Cystoscopy is indicated in some to rule out intravesical problems. Endoscopic and urinary tract imaging tests may sometimes be necessary. Thus referral to specialists in urology or urogynecology is indicated for the following:

- Those who have previously undergone pelvic surgery
- Those with microscopic hematuria or any other symptom suggestive of an intravesical problem (cystoscopy would be the indicated procedure)
- Those with an uncertain diagnosis and for whom a reasonable management plan based on the basic diagnostic evaluation cannot be developed
- Those who fail to respond to an adequate therapeutic trial and are thus candidates for further therapy

Table 22-3   Simple Cystometry

Maneuver	Observation/Data	Interpretation/Implication
I. Void		
Have patient void into urinal or commode. Observe and listen to urine stream. Ideally this is done when patient has full bladder.	A. Observe quality of urine stream: is it normal/continuous, multiple peaked/continuous, interrupted, hesitant, strained? B. Observe urine flow rate.* C. Measure amount voided. D. Observe urine character, color. E. Observe toileting skills, dexterity, time needed to disrobe and initiate voiding, holding time.	Slow, interrupted urine stream suggests obstruction, hypocontractility, or dyssynergy. Low voided volume (<200 ml) suggests small bladder capacity or incomplete bladder emptying. Deficits in toileting skills and dexterity suggest functional incontinence. Prolonged disrobing time and shortened holding time suggests need for environmental adaptations.
II. Catheterization		
Within 10 minutes of bladder emptying, insert a 12-14 French single-lumen catheter using sterile technique.† Use a coudé catheter for men. Place fracture bedpan under women, have urinal available for men.	A. Measure postvoid residual volume. B. Is catheter difficult to pass? C. Collect specimen for urinalysis, culture, and sensitivity. D. Use dipstick to check urine for leukocytes, hemoglobin, nitrites, glucose, pH.	Difficulty passing catheter suggests obstruction. Residual volume >100 ml is abnormal and may indicate obstruction, hypocontractility, or dyssynergy. Negative dipstick readings may negate need for costly urine culture.
III. Bladder Filling		
Attach 40 ml catheter-tip syringe without the plunger to the catheter and hold about 15 cm (about 6 inches) above the pubis. Encourage patient to relax, take slow deep breaths, and not tighten abdominal muscles. Pour sterile water into syringe in 50 ml increments. Instruct patient to report first urge to void, when the bladder feels so full that the patient would normally void, and the maximal volume "must go now" urge. Do not fill beyond 500-600 ml. When patient experiences bladder contraction (detected by the column of water rising in syringe or leakage from around the catheter), stop instillation. Remove catheter and instruct patient to hold fluid in bladder, observe for leakage.	A. Observe volume at which first urge is felt. B. Observe volume at which patient feels full and would normally void. C. Observe maximum volume retained. D. Observe volume at which bladder contraction occurs. E. Observe volume of leakage after catheter removal.	Difficulty filling at 15 cm pressure suggests poor bladder compliance. Upward movement of fluid column or leakage around catheter, in the presence of an urge to void that the patient is unable to suppress, suggests urge incontinence. Severe urgency without a bladder contraction at low volume (<300 ml) suggests sensory urgency or intrinsic bladder disease. Instillation of 600 ml without feeling of fullness suggests abnormal sensation.

From Lekan-Rutledge D: *J Urol Nurse* 11:267-276, 1992.

*Calculated as follows: divide the amount of urine voided by the total time required to pass it (normal, 20 to 25 ml/s); not valid if total bladder volume is less than 200 ml.

†Consider using 2% lidocaine topical lubricant, and inject into meatus.

- Those who have hematuria without infection
- Those with other conditions, such as UI associated with recurrent UTI, severe symptoms of difficult bladder emptying, severe and symptomatic pelvic prolapse, prostate nodule, abnormal postvoid residual urine, and neurological conditions except for patients for whom further investigation is not feasible[1]

APPROACH TO THE PATIENT: AN ALGORITHMIC METHOD

In the context of the traditional model of the history, physical examination, investigation, and a trial of management, it is possible to broadly categorize the patient's symptoms into the three categories of stress, urge, and overflow UI, bearing in mind the contributing iatrogenic, functional, and predisposing factors. A detailed

Table 22-3   Simple Cystometry—cont'd

Maneuver	Observation/Data	Interpretation/Implication
IV. Provocative Maneuvers		
Place preweighed pad below meatus; while patient is supine, instruct to cough vigorously three times or strain to precipitate leakage. If there is no leakage, have patient stand; observe for leakage. After 15-30 seconds and no leakage, repeat cough maneuver.	A. Measure leakage amount: weigh pad, subtract dry pad from wet pad = volume in ml, or estimate (drops/moderate volume/large volume). B. Observe timing of leakage: is it coincident with coughing or following coughing?	Leakage with stress maneuvers suggests *stress* incontinence when leakage occurs during the maneuver or *urge* incontinence when leakage occurs shortly *after* the maneuver. Leakage of large volumes suggests stress-induced bladder instability in which both sphincter weakness and bladder instability are present.
V. Bladder Emptying		
Remove catheter and have patient void into commode. Measure voided volume.	A. Calculate postvoid residual by subtracting voided volume from total amount of fluid instilled. B. Observe/listen to urine stream as in section I.	See section I above. Repeating this part provides opportunity to evaluate bladder emptying with a known maximum bladder volume if fluid loss has not already occurred. Inability to empty fully suggests problems with contractility, obstruction.

history and bladder diary combined with a focused physical examination and selected bedside tests such as the postvoid residual urine measurement and simple cystometry will suffice in many instances to provide a reasonable first-line diagnostic approach. An algorithmic methodology can guide the diagnostic reasoning process.[17,33] Detailed algorithms for male, female, and frail elderly patients have been developed for clinicians.[1] A general basic algorithmic approach is described below:

1. Is there UI? Is the patient aware of the UI?
2. How long has UI been a problem? Was onset sudden and recent or insidious and long term?
3. How often does UI occur in the day and how often at night? What is the volume of urine loss?
4. Do certain circumstances precipitate the UI? Does the patient do anything to avoid or prevent UI? How is UI currently being managed?
5. Does the patient lose urine with coughing, sneezing, laughing, lifting, walking, exercising?
6. Is there dysuria, urgency, nocturia, trigone, or bladder pain?
7. Are there obstructive voiding symptoms?
8. Is there evidence of incomplete bladder emptying?
9. Is the bathroom or commode accessible?
10. Are there manual dexterity problems or excessive or inappropriate clothing?
11. List all medications and identify whether drugs affect lower urinary tract. (Consider removing offending drugs or changing to drug with less lower urinary tract effects.)
12. What other illnesses are present? Do any of the illnesses predispose to bladder contractility or obstructive disorders?
13. Has there been any pelvic or urinary tract surgery?
14. Is there any history of back injury or other injury?
15. Perform a physical examination for general state of health, including mental status assessment.
16. Perform an abdominal examination and palpate for full bladder.
17. In women, examine the genitalia and perform a vaginal examination to detect atrophy, pelvic floor laxity, pelvic descent, or pelvic masses. Perform a stress maneuver lying and standing with full bladder. Treat atrophic vaginitis if found. For mild pelvic descent, consider a pessary. For severe pelvic descent, refer to specialist for surgical consideration.
18. Have patient void and perform a urinalysis with culture and sensitivity if microscopy is suggestive. Refer for cystoscopy if hematuria is found. Treat for urinary tract infection if found.
19. Perform measurement of postvoid residual volume if a bladder-emptying problem is suspected.
20. If the postvoid residual is greater than 100 ml, repeat measurement on two other occasions.

21. Consider performing simple cystometry if bladder dysfunction is suspected (urge or overflow UI symptoms or voiding dysfunction); perform uroflowmetry if the patient retains a full bladder without detrusor instability.

22. Perform a rectal examination to check tone, sensation, and control of anal sphincter, and to check for fecal impaction; perform a complete prostatic examination in men. Treat for impaction and constipation if found; refer to urologist if prostate is enlarged.

23. Complete a neurological examination, assess sacral reflexes and perineal sensation, and observe gait and posture.

24. If findings suggest stress or urge UI, initiate a trial of behavioral therapy (pelvic muscle strengthening, biofeedback, bladder training, dietary measures, supportive measures); if a reasonable effort of behavioral therapy fails (at least 8 weeks), consider referral for urodynamics.

25. For stress UI, if a therapeutic trial of behavioral therapy fails to satisfy the patient, consider surgical referral.

26. If findings suggest impaired bladder emptying or contractility, obstructive symptoms or obstruction, or voiding dysfunction, refer for urodynamics or surgical evaluation or both. If urodynamics is not feasible or appropriate, consider intermittent catheterization, long-term urethral catheterization, or pharmacological treatment.

PROMOTING HEALTHY BLADDER FUNCTION

Promote bladder health by promoting fluid intake: many patients deliberately restrict their intake to reduce "accidents."

A number of simple strategies can help older persons maintain good bladder function (Table 22-4). Learning positive ways of managing age-related changes in the bladder can go a long way to offset potentially negative habits or behaviors that may develop in response to bladder symptoms. For example, self-restriction of fluids and frequent voiding are counterproductive behaviors intended to deal with urgency and UI; concentrated urine can produce debris or in itself can be a bladder irritant. The technique of "double voiding" in which the patient empties the bladder, relaxes, and then attempts to empty again can sometimes be helpful in both men and women to reduce the residual volume. Undoubtedly, generally increased physical fitness, in particular improved perineal tone as may occur in general reconditioning, should be encouraged and may encourage healthy bladder function.

"Double voiding" can reduce residual volume, decreasing the reservoir for infection and the constant presence of urine available for leakage.

Most elderly men should sit down to urinate; it is safer, and it ensures the bladder is more fully emptied each time.

TREATMENT FOR URINARY INCONTINENCE

Treatments for UI can be categorized as behavioral, pharmacological, surgical, and the use of equipment and devices (Box 22-7).

Behavioral Treatment

Behavioral treatment involves educating the patient about UI to change the individual's response to UI symptoms. It is noninvasive and low risk and has no known side effects; it is recommended in the treatment of urge and stress UI. The UI Guideline Panel[1] recommends a model for the staging of treatment, whereby behavioral therapy be offered as first-line treatment for UI unless obstruction, poor bladder emptying, and overflow UI are suspected or confirmed. Behavioral interventions include toileting schedules, pelvic muscle exercises, and dietary modifications.

Toileting schedules can reduce bladder symptoms and UI through regular and consistent bladder emptying. Toileting schedules are the backbone of a continence restoration program. Four types of toileting schedules are described below.

Scheduled toileting, also known as timed voiding, is a fixed pattern of voiding (usually every 2 or 3 hours). Scheduled toileting is indicated when individuals tend to wait long periods between voids or when physical or cognitive impairments necessitate caregiver assistance for toileting.

Bladder training is a voiding schedule that incorporates progressively longer intervals between voids; it involves educating the patient about maintaining the voiding pattern as closely as possible, instructing the patient in control of urgency in order to stay on schedule, and providing positive reinforcement. It requires that the patient be motivated and capable of maintaining a bladder diary. The goal of bladder training is to increase voiding volumes, increase voiding intervals to every 2 to 3 hours, and change the way in which a bladder urge is handled from that of rushing to the bathroom to that of being able to successfully delay voiding until a time of convenience or the next scheduled void. Initial voiding intervals are determined from the voiding diary, starting with the time interval that

Table 22-4   Bladder Health Promotion in the Elderly

Behavior	Rationale	Strategy
Drink water.	Drinking enough liquids, especially water, keeps urine from becoming too concentrated. Concentrated urine irritates the bladder, increases urgency, has a foul odor, and can lead to urinary tract infection and skin irritation.	In general drink 6-8 cups of liquid each day. To determine a more accurate fluid goal, take the person's body weight and divide by 2 to get the total number of ounces needed per day. Add extra liquid for febrile states, during exercises, or hot weather. If nocturia is a problem, fluids may be limited after 7 PM but should not be limited during the day. Sipping liquids in small amounts throughout the day avoids rapid bladder filling.
Avoid bladder irritants.	Bladder irritants, especially caffeine, may cause frequency, urgency, nocturia, and increased urine production.	Limit caffeinated beverages such as coffee, tea, carbonated drinks, and chocolate. Some over-the-counter cold and allergy medicines also contain caffeine. Caffeine elimination will reduce bladder urges.
Promote bowel regularity.	Constipation makes bladder symptoms worse when pressure from the overfilled rectum pushes on the bladder, causing urgency, frequency, and incomplete bladder emptying. Straining to defecate weakens pelvic muscles and contributes to stress incontinence and fecal incontinence.	To promote bowel function, drink adequate liquids, especially water and fruit juices, eat plenty of high-fiber foods, get daily exercise (especially walking), and develop a bowel evacuation schedule. Add unprocessed wheat bran to the diet. Bran may be added directly to food (like pudding or yogurt) or consumed in a mixture (1 cup unprocessed wheat bran, 1 cup applesauce, ½ cup prune juice) taken 1-6 tablespoons a day to maintain regularity. Avoid laxatives and enemas.
Maintain a bladder schedule.	A regular schedule for bladder emptying can improve urgency and frequency of urination. Voiding too often or too little can cause deconditioning of the bladder.	Empty the bladder every 2-4 hours when possible. Frequent holding of urine for more than 5-6 hours can increase the risk for urinary tract infection and decreased bladder contractility. Bladder training can help gradually increase the bladder capacity, decrease bladder urgency, and increase time between voids.
Practice urge control.	Urges are signals that are felt as the bladder stretches to hold urine. Urges are perceived even if the bladder is not completely filled. Urges are not a command to void, just a reminder that the bladder is filling.	Practice urge control so that voiding can occur when it is convenient, not when the urge strikes. To control the urge: (1) stop what you are doing and stand still or sit down, (2) breathe slowly and relax, (3) tighten and contract pelvic muscles 5-10 times, (4) concentrate on pushing away the urge. Practice a mental exercise by counting back from 100 by 7 to provide distraction from the discomfort of the urge. When the urge passes, wait a few minutes before going to the bathroom.
Do pelvic muscle exercise.	Pelvic muscles help support the bladder neck and keep pelvic organs in correct position. Weakened muscles allow urine to leak with physical activity, coughing, or sneezing.	Pelvic muscle exercises are helpful for both stress and urge incontinence and for bowel incontinence. Doing 30-80 exercises a day helps to maintain good muscle tone and to facilitate urge control.

the patient has been able to manage comfortably. On a weekly basis, this interval is increased by 15 to 30 minutes. The patient should void according to the schedule, whether or not a desire to void is felt. Frequent follow-up is necessary, either with weekly or biweekly visits or with telephone contact, to attain compliance. A controlled study of bladder training in community-dwelling women reported that 12% of those who completed bladder training became continent, and 75% improved by at least a 50% reduction in the number of incontinent episodes.[34] Both women with stress and those with urge incontinence (continence diagnoses determined urodynamically) benefitted equally from bladder training. A detailed guide for implementing the bladder training protocol is available.[35]

Habit training is a toileting schedule that is individualized according to the patient's voiding and incontinence

---

BOX 22-7
Treatments for Urinary Incontinence

---

1. Behavioral Techniques

Scheduled toileting (fixed interval, e.g., every 2-3 hours)
Bladder training (progressively longer intervals)
Habit training (where urine volume varies over time, e.g., with diuretics)
Prompted voiding (schedule toileting with positive reinforcement, praise, and encouragement to be assisted and to stay dry)
Kegel exercises (levator ani and pelvic floor muscle contractions, with or without electromyographic biofeedback or vaginal cones)
Electrical stimulation treatment (with implants)
Avoidance of bladder irritants (caffeine, tomatoes, citrus fruits)
Rehydration (half the body weight in pounds is the number of ounces of liquid needed per day)

2. Pharmacological Treatment

Bladder wall: anticholinergics (propantheline, dicyclomine, oxybutynin), tricyclics (imipramine), calcium channel blockers (nifedipine, terodiline), cholinergics for retention (rather unsuccessful)
Urethra: α-adrenergics (phenylpropanolamine, pseudoephedrine), estrogen, α-blockers (prazosin, terazosin), central relaxants (baclofen, dantrolene, diazepam)

3. Surgical

Artificial urinary sphincters to improve sphincteric function (with pump, requires competent patient)
Prostatectomy or TURP (for prostatic obstruction)
Dilation of urethral stricture
Circumcision (for phimosis or balanitis)
Penile reconstruction (in trauma and cancer cases)
Urinary diversion
Suprapubic catheter (the better long-term indwelling catheter)

4. Equipment and Devices

Absorbent products (diapers, gels, pads, cone-shaped absorbents for men, reinforced-fit undergarments for high volume)
Skin care (nonalcohol cleansers, waterproof barriers)
Devices and urinals (male and female for the immobilized or skin compromised)
External catheters (condom type for men)
Indwelling urethral catheters (only if surgery and intermittent catheterization have failed or there is skin breakdown or frailty of the patient such that even movement is painful)
Intermittent catheterization (the better alternative for obstruction with overflow)

---

pattern. This type of schedule can be helpful in preventing UI in patients taking diuretics when there is increased urine production over a number of hours. A 7-day bladder diary is kept, and patterns of voiding and UI are noted. The patient voids at times that are consistently noted on the bladder diary and also 30 minutes before the time UI episodes can be expected based on the diary.

> *Toileting schedules are the essential first step in reducing urinary incontinence for many elders.*

Prompted voiding is a scheduled toileting program with a communication protocol guiding caregivers in their interaction with the patient. The protocol engages the patient in increasing awareness about bladder status, successful toileting, and expectations for staying as dry as possible. Prompted voiding has been successfully used in long-term care nursing facilities and may improve UI in approximately 35% of incontinent nursing home residents.[36-38] The patient is given positive reinforcement and praise for staying dry and is encouraged to accept toileting assistance. In frail nursing home residents, prompted voiding is a primary treatment for UI, and medication may offer additional benefit. Interestingly, one study that documented the effectiveness of prompted voiding found that when anticholinergic drug therapy (oxybutynin hydrochloride) was added to the prompted voiding treatment protocol, continence status worsened and further drug therapy was abandoned because of adverse side effects including lethargy and delirium.[39]

Pelvic muscle exercises, also known as Kegel exercises, improve UI by increasing urethral resistance with contraction of pelvic floor muscles, primarily the levator ani muscle complex. The contraction exerts a closing force on the urethra and increases muscle support of pelvic organs.[1] Pelvic muscle exercises are indicated for stress UI to strengthen and improve muscle responsiveness during increased intraabdominal pressure and as a mechanism to control bladder urges and urge UI. Pelvic muscle contractions exert closure of the urethra and also reflexively inhibit bladder contractions.

> *Strengthening the pelvic muscles is the basic treatment for stress incontinence and can help in urge incontinence, too.*

Pelvic muscle exercise instruction includes both physical examination and verbal instructions to coach the patient in correct contraction. Traditional instruction tends to rely on written and verbal instructions; this is in contrast to Kegel's teaching approach, which relied on the use of a perineometer (a pneumatic cone-shaped device attached to a hand-held manometer with a dial much like a nonelectronic blood pressure dial) to show the strength and effectiveness of a pelvic muscle contraction. A recent study comparing the effectiveness of verbal instruction alone or verbal instruction combined with physical examination (coaching the patient during digital vaginal examination)[40] found that over 50% of those receiving verbal instruction alone did not correctly perform a pelvic muscle exercise, even when they thought they were.

Initial pelvic muscle instruction involves palpation of the pelvic muscle body for tone and mass and instructing the patient to breath in a relaxed and normal manner, concentrating on keeping abdominal, gluteal, and adductor muscles completely relaxed. To locate the muscle, the patient can initially tighten the anus as if holding back gas, then gradually ascend and tighten the muscles around the vagina, and then the urethra. Visualization of climbing stairs or riding an elevator may be helpful. The patient is coached to tighten the muscle and draw it upward and inward and hold for a count of three, then relax, repeat, and hold for a count of five, then relax, repeat, and hold for a full count of ten, then relax. An individualized pelvic muscle retraining is developed based on the muscle strength and duration of the contraction, with weekly adjustments in the exercise schedule designed to challenge and fatigue the muscle. Older women may have limited pelvic sensation and difficulty perceiving the muscle contraction. Between 30 and 80 pelvic muscle exercises per day are recommended. Results from a trial of a pelvic floor training program in women with stress UI determined that the majority of women experienced improvement or cure (45% and 23%, respectively) and 29% remained unchanged.[41] In addition, long-term follow-up in this group of patients found that improvements were not maintained in some patients primarily because the exercise program was not continued as prescribed. This suggests that periodic monitoring, pelvic muscle assessment, and encouragement from the clinician are necessary in some patients to maintain outcomes.

Electromyographic (EMG) biofeedback is helpful in teaching the correct pelvic muscle exercise performance. Biofeedback is a technique for teaching the patient how to recognize and control psychophysiological processes; it requires special equipment to monitor physiological signals and provides visual or auditory feedback. It assists the patient to recognize physiological sensations associated with pelvic muscle contraction and helps minimize inappropriate physiological responses. Biofeedback is particularly useful in patients with limited sensation or difficulty isolating pelvic muscle and inhibiting involvement of abdominal, gluteal, and adductor muscles.[42,43]

Vaginal cones (Dacomed) are tampon-shaped plastic devices of the same size in graduated weights. The cone is placed intravaginally, and the woman is instructed to retain the cone by contracting pelvic muscles intermittently. Only correct contraction of the pelvic muscles will retain the cone in the vagina. A cone that can be retained for 2 minutes is selected, and the woman tries to retain the cone for longer intervals until 15 minutes twice per day is attained. When cone retention is successful for two consecutive times, the next size cone is initiated. The sensation of the cone slipping out of the vagina provides feedback about placement, muscle contraction, and retention of the cone. In older women with atrophied vaginal vaults or poor pelvic support, retaining even the lightest cone may be difficult. An interesting idea, the urethral plug, has been shown to help certain women with stress incontinence,[44] but is not yet widely available.

Electrical stimulation has been in practice for the treatment of UI since the early 1960s. Newer systems offer anal and intravaginal probes connected to independent units or to portable battery-operated devices. A number of electrical stimulation treatment systems are available. Electrical stimulation can be helpful in patients with weak pelvic muscles or with limited sensation of pelvic muscle contractions as a way to promote awareness and build strength sufficient to enable more effective voluntary pelvic muscle contractions. Once effective pelvic muscle contractions can be voluntarily generated, the muscle training program may continue without electrical stimulation. Long-term electrical stimulation of the pelvic floor passively exercises the pelvic muscles to facilitate muscle strengthening, reinnervate injured muscle, enhance axonal sprouting, and improve reflex activation of muscles.[31]

Dietary modifications can alleviate irritative bladder symptoms including frequency, urgency, and dysuria. Caffeine-containing products including coffee and tea (even decaffeinated), soft drinks, chocolate, and some cold or allergy medications can worsen irritative symptoms. In patients with particularly sensitive bladders, certain foods may be irritating to the bladder, including tomato-based and highly sweetened foods, spicy foods, citrus fruits and juice, milk and milk products, and artificial sweeteners. Underhydration can be addressed with a fluid hydration protocol that gradually increases the daily ingestion of fluid by small amounts. Individual fluid goals are determined by taking the patient's body weight in pounds and dividing by 2 to calculate the total number of ounces of liquids needed per day.[45] Individuals who exercise, have respiratory disorders, or have diarrhea, fever, or other conditions that increase fluid needs would accordingly increase their intake. Over a 4- to 6-week period, daily fluid intake may be increased by 2 to 4 ounces each week, thus allowing for gradual accommodation and less likelihood for excessive diuresis. Fluid intake increases are also helpful for patients with chronic constipation. Adding fiber and bran to the diet also effectively restores regular bowel action even in long-term laxative and enema users.

There are limitations to behavioral therapy in older persons. First, it requires significant changes in life-style, habits, and diet. Such changes may be difficult for some to accommodate. Behavioral treatment takes time before results are seen, so keeping the patient's level of motivation and compliance requires a high degree of involvement from the clinician and in some cases a caregiver as well. Behavioral interventions are considered first-line treatment because they are effective, are relatively simple to implement, are inexpensive, are noninvasive, may be used in combination with other treatment, and do not limit other treatment options.[46]

Pharmacological Treatment

Medication may be used to treat stress, urge, and overflow UI, although unwanted or unintended actions and side effects restrict their use. However, an effective medication regimen can be designed and initiated in conjunction with behavioral treatment. The regimen should always start with the lowest possibly effective therapeutic dose, and side effects should be monitored.

Drugs Affecting the Bladder Wall. *Anticholinergic drugs* are often used for detrusor instability and urge UI to increase the urine volume associated with the first contraction, reduce the magnitude of the bladder contraction, increase the bladder capacity before bladder urges are perceived, and reduce overall symptoms. Propantheline bromide is commonly used to produce an antimuscarinic effect in the lower urinary tract. Dicyclomine hydrochloride has smooth muscle relaxant properties in ad-

dition to anticholinergic and local analgesic effects. It has a short half-life and is used in doses of 10 to 30 mg tid or qid. Oxybutynin chloride is described as a moderately potent anticholinergic agent with strong musculotropic relaxant and local anesthetic activity.[28,47] Dosage in the elderly is 2.5 mg to 5 mg PO bid, increasing slowly to tid and qid. Oxybutynin in liquid form makes dosage titration easier. Doses may also be episodic (for trips or social outings), since the medication has a short half-life. Side effects such as blurred vision and decreased alertness should be anticipated, especially if the patient is driving or engaged in other activities. Mental confusion, blurred vision, dry mouth, drowsiness, and constipation are particular hazards. A constipation prevention program should be initiated because constipation is common. Increased intraocular pressure (and acute intraocular crisis in patients with narrow angle glaucoma) and acute urinary retention may be precipitated. Anticholinergics should be avoided in patients with detrusor instability with impaired contractility and chronic urinary retention.

> *Medications can be effective in urinary incontinence, especially in combination with behavioral methods.*

Tricyclics, imipramine hydrochloride in particular, increase urethral and bladder outlet resistance in addition to decreasing bladder contractility. Imipramine is used primarily for treating detrusor instability but offers added benefit if the patient also has some degree of urethral sphincter weakness. An hs dose of 25 mg is increased every third night until the patient becomes continent, has side effects, or reaches 150 mg. Another dosing regime utilizes 10 mg PO tid with gradual increases in dosage. Side effects in the elderly include postural hypotension, cardiac dysrhythmias, fatigue, and weakness.[47]

Calcium channel blockers, such as nifedipine and terodiline, limit the availability of calcium ions required for bladder contractility and suppress detrusor instability.[48] Terodiline has mixed anticholinergic and calcium channel blocking activity. One multicenter study determined terodiline to be highly effective in reducing urge UI in older, noninstitutionalized patients; however, its potential association with ventricular tachycardia warrants further testing.[49]

Pharmacological therapy for chronic urinary retention resulting from an underactive or atonic bladder has produced mixed results and in general has not been deemed helpful. Cholinergic agents such as bethanechol chloride, prostaglandin, α-adrenergic blockers such as phenoxybenzamine, and anticholinesterase inhibitor agents such as distigmine bromide have generally not been successful in treating patients with neuropathic bladders.[50] Management of chronic urinary retention is best achieved with intermittent catheterization.

Drugs Affecting the Urethra. α-*Adrenergic agonists* increase bladder neck and proximal urethral smooth muscle contraction. Phenylpropanolamine and pseudoephedrine both have α-adrenergic agonist properties and are available by prescription or over the counter in drug combinations, marketed as nasal and sinus remedies and appetite suppressants. These drugs should be used with caution in patients with hypertension, cardiovascular disease, or hyperthyroidism. Side effects should be closely monitored, including blood pressure elevation, anxiety, insomnia, cardiac dysrhythmias, palpitations, headache, tremor, and respiratory difficulties.[28,47] There may be a synergistic beneficial effect on urethral smooth muscle with α-adrenergic agonists and estrogen replacement therapy.

Estrogen replacement therapy can be beneficial in elderly women and should always be considered. Hormone replacement therapy often improves irritative voiding symptoms associated with urge UI and may play a role in increasing urethral resistance in stress UI. If the woman is considering surgery, estrogen may improve the thickness and vascularity of the vaginal tissue and endopelvic fascia, thus decreasing the fragility of these tissues during surgery and improving postoperative healing.[31] Contraindications include active gallbladder or liver disease, hormonally dependent cancers (breast, endometrium), active thromboembolic disease or acute deep venous thrombophlebitis, and undiagnosed vaginal bleeding. Administration of estrogen may be oral, transdermal, or intravaginal. Women without a uterus may use a continuous daily dose regimen. If the woman has a uterus, estrogen is used in combination with a progestin to avoid the development of endometrial hyperplasia or carcinoma. Progestin may be given continuously or on a cyclic schedule. Continuous doses of both drugs may help the patient avoid endometrial hypertrophy and bleeding or spotting. Patients on a cyclic regimen may experience some withdrawal bleeding on days progestin is not taken.

α-*Sympathetic antagonists,* such as prazosin and terazosin, can effect relaxation of the external striated sphincter, and centrally acting muscle relaxants, such as baclofen, dantrolene, or diazepam, relax the pelvic floor musculature.[50] These drugs may provoke stress UI symptoms in some patients without urethral obstruction.

▼ ROSE KRANSTEIN (Part II)

Mrs. Kranstein is active, athletic, and used to walking several miles a day. She is enthusiastic when the possibility that specific exercises might help her is mentioned. On examination, stress incontinence is demonstrated, with rapid leakage of a significant volume of urine on coughing or sneezing when she is in the upright position. (This is not observed when she is lying flat.) There is some uterovaginal laxity and uterine descent, but it is not marked; there are no atrophic changes. A urinary infection is ruled out; the rectal examination shows some laxity of the external sphincter, but it does not present a problem to her; and the neurological findings are normal. A program of Kegel exercises is started. Mrs. Kranstein is very cooperative in being taught by the physical therapist (who normally assists postpartum mothers) to identify which muscle she is to work on, and she enthusiastically exercises the external sphincter 100 times a day for ten contractions. This initially relieves her symptoms.

▼ AGNES TERRILL (Part III)

A urinary culture reveals many bacteria, but this has been found previously on several occasions, and Ms. Terrill has had multiple courses of antibiotics. One last attempt is made, with a full 2-week course of an antibiotic to which the bacterium is fully sensitive, but there is no effect on the intermittent incontinence. The bowel is cleared by a series of enemas, with again no impact on the urinary incontinence. The indications for digoxin and thiazide diuretic that she is taking are not at all clear, and they are withdrawn with no adverse effect on the patient whatsoever and a subjective improvement, some of her nurses feel, in her urinary incontinence. The benzodiazepine sleeping medication is also withdrawn, resulting in her becoming less somnolent and inactive, but it does not noticeably improve her incontinence. Since she is unable to articulate whether she is having warning of her incontinence, it is not certain whether she fits into the category of urge incontinence. However, since this is the most common cause and since she does not appear to be suffering clinical overflow or stress incontinence, the staff enthusiastically start a program of bladder retraining. She is taken to the toilet initially every 30 minutes, and it is found that at those intervals she is generally still dry. After a week of these very frequent toileting trips, the interval is progressively extended over a period of several weeks until she can manage 2½ hours of dryness. This appears to be her maximum, but within the context of the facility, this represents a great improvement.

▼ HERBERT MARKOVICH (Part III)

Slow decompression over several hours is deemed advisable, and this is carried out at your office. It is physically quite difficult to catheterize him. He is decatheterized but is unable to urinate, and the catheter has to be reinserted and left indwelling. A urine specimen is obtained, and analysis reveals no infection. A BUN and creatinine are obtained and are within normal levels. You schedule an intravenous pyelogram, which shows no evidence of hydronephrosis. A prostate-specific anti-

gen test (PSA) is carried out and is normal. It is thought to be advisable to proceed directly to surgical management in view of the marked obstruction. He undergoes a transurethral resection of the prostate (TURP). A few weeks later, Mr. Markovich is extremely disappointed that when he coughs and sneezes or if he allows his bladder to become full, he finds himself wet with urine. There is no dysuria, and a urinalysis is negative. He is treated for a time with prazosin for these symptoms, with some relief; fortunately, the neuronal damage is not permanent, and ultimately he is continent without medication.

CASE DISCUSSION

Had Mr. Markovich's obstructive symptoms been less marked, he would have been a candidate for a trial of medical treatment of his BPH before consideration of surgery. Such treatment, which has an important place in the management of urinary incontinence, is detailed elsewhere in this book.

Surgery

The algorithmic approach outlined above will at times reveal situations in which surgical treatments are indicated. Rarely, previously undetected anatomical abnormalities, such as fistulae, phimosis, or urethral abnormalities, that could have been corrected in earlier life will be found. Sometimes carcinomatous changes or trauma to the area may warrant extensive surgery, and these and lesser indications sometimes require the provision of urinary diversions (e.g., to the colon) or other extensive plastic and reconstruction procedures. It will become clear during the workup if specialized help is required.

More commonly, surgery is considered for persistent obstruction, especially in BPH and urethral stricture. This is organized through the urologist or, in some situations, a general surgeon. However, medical treatment of BPH should generally be considered before initiating prostatectomy.

Provided a reasonable trial of pelvic floor exercises has been carried out, patients with marked uterine descent, or even those with only mild to moderate descent, may be considered for one of a variety of bladder neck suspension procedures to correct the vesicourethral angle. These are sometimes combined, using a vaginal approach, with vaginal hysterectomy, and they can be very effective. Obviously, in the more fragile patient, careful preoperative evaluation is necessary. Of greatest importance in this situation, and indeed in any surgical approach to the urological tract, is a careful workup (as previously detailed) to detect and suitably manage any other factors contributing to the symptoms. In the past, disappointment following gynecological repair of uterine descent may often have been because the patient's symptoms were caused largely by, for example, an unrecognized, unstable bladder.

Suprapubic catheterization should be mentioned here, although it is discussed in detail below in relation to other aspects of catheterization; this, too, is a surgical procedure and is the preferred permanent catheterization when this is deemed necessary.

Different types of artificial urinary sphincters are available for treatment of urethral sphincter deficiency caused by surgical interventions (posttransurethral resection), pelvic radiation injury, or neurological conditions. Artificial sphincters are composed of three components: the urethral cuff, an implantable pump, and a reservoir, all connected by tubing. The cuff surrounds the urethra and is filled with fluid to exert pressure on the urethra. To initiate bladder emptying, the pump, which is located in the scrotum in males or the labia in females, is squeezed several times, which transfers the fluid out of the cuff and into the abdominally placed reservoir. Urine empties from the bladder and the cuff automatically reinflates within a few minutes.[51] Clinical outcomes with artificial sphincters seem positive in measures of improvement in continence and patient satisfaction.[52]

Periurethral bulking agents, such as collagen and Teflon implants, are becoming more readily available. The injectable material increases urethral pressure and closure with improvement in continence. Injections may need to be repeated over time. Potential complications include urethritis, retention, abscess formation, and migration of bulking material.

Equipment and Devices

Complete resolution of UI may not be feasible in some older patients. Management strategies to prevent and manage the morbidity associated with persistent UI should not be overlooked. An excellent review of products and devices is published and made available by Help for Incontinent People (HIP, Inc., 1-800-BLADDER), which provides useful source information about sources of incontinence products.

Absorbent Products. There is no "one-size-fits-all" solution in absorbent products. It is estimated that approximately 30% of purchases of menstrual products, which are not designed for urine containment, are used for UI. Product selection should be guided by the amount and frequency of UI, size of the patient, mobility and daily activities, absorbent capacity, size, comfort of different products, and cost.[53,54] A wide array of disposable and reusable absorbent products are now available. Absorbent products differ from menstrual products because they have highly absorbent polymers or gels, which can absorb large volumes of urine and prevent it from leaking out of the product when sitting. They also have a layer of material on the surface of the product that wicks away moisture from the skin, and some have constituents that counteract odor and bacterial growth.

∞ *Improved absorbent products technology has revolutionized diapering, but it must not substitute for a full investigation for other potential solutions to the problem.*

Determining the frequency and volume of the leakage is the first step in product selection. For mild leakage there are thin inserts or panty liners that are self-sticking or that fit in specially designed cotton underpants. For men with dribbling, cone-shaped absorbent material can effectively contain approximately 100 ml of urine. For moderate leakage there are thicker pads, stretchable mesh briefs with contoured pad inserts, pads that are buttoned to an elastic belt, and diaper-style full-fit undergarments. For large volume UI there are full undergarments that attach with Velcro or self-adhesive strips or with snaps. For both men and women, cloth undergarments with reinforced absorbent fabric in the crotch are available. For high-volume incontinence, highly absorbent cloth or disposable liners can be used with a full absorbent undergarment to prolong the life of the undergarment. Technology for absorbency and skin protection has contributed to the higher quality of products currently available, but each product has advantages and disadvantages that must be considered in the individual patient's situation. Absorbent products are also expensive. Some patients may shoulder a financial burden of up to $100 a month for absorbent products. Ecological and public health concerns in some states have led to the banning of disposable absorbent products in public landfills.

Skin Care Protocols. Meticulous skin care is necessary when UI is moderate or severe. Urine that is left on the skin is irritating, promotes bacterial colonization, and facilitates maceration and skin breakdown. Skin care protocols require an agent for cleansing the skin and returning it to normal pH. Cleansing agents should not contain alcohol as this can dry and irritate the skin, and if skin is already broken, cause irritation and stinging. Moisturizing the skin helps to prevent dryness caused by frequent washings and friction. A waterproof barrier cream protects the skin from prolonged contact with urine, adding extra protection when incontinence is severe. Some barrier creams have antifungal and antibacterial agents to prevent infection.

Urinary Devices. Male urinals are readily available for male incontinent patients; female urinals are also available and are helpful when immobility is a problem. They can be used while the patient is in a wheelchair or bed. A female external urinary device by Hollister, Inc., fits around the urethral and vaginal meatus, connects via a tube to a urine collection bag, and is held in place by a stretchable brief. Providing the patient has an adequately functioning bladder, this device can be helpful when the patient is immobile, lacks a caregiver to provide appropriate incontinence care, or has skin breakdown. A male external collecting device consists of a cotton or vinyl pouch that holds absorbent pads. It is held in place by an elastic belt. External collecting devices in which a collecting pouch adhere to the perineum are available for women. A special procedure for prepping the skin is necessary. A retracted penis pouch is also available for men.

External Catheters. Male condom-type catheters can be self-adhesive, nonadhesive with self-adhering strips, or made with an inflatable ring in order to be reusable. Correct sizing is necessary, and some brands are available in a wide range of sizes. Skin care is vital when using external catheters, and regular changes with a breathing period are helpful to prevent skin maceration and ulceration. One brand is made of clear silicone to allow skin observation; this is helpful because skin reactions may occur to the materials.

External condom catheters carry risks of urinary tract infection, penile necrosis and ulceration, dermatitis, encrustations, and infection. The incidence of bacteriuria and urinary tract infection is less than with indwelling urethral catheters but greater than if no device is used at all.[55,56] Bacterial colonization and migration are facilitated when urine pools in the tip of the condom sheath and when skin care is poor. Prevention of complications includes avoiding constriction, choosing the correct size, applying it carefully, changing it every 24 hours, and inspecting the skin and tubing position to avoid kinking. The catheter should be removed several hours each day to prevent maceration. It should fit well enough that urine does not dwell in the tip of the shaft, which can become a reservoir for bacterial growth.

Urethral Catheters. Long-term urethral catheterization is not indicated in the management of UI. Accepted indications for long-term catheterization include bladder outlet obstruction not correctable by surgery and not manageable with intermittent catheterization, skin breakdown, and some cases of neurogenic bladder. Severe pain or terminal illness in which patient movement would provoke undue suffering could warrant catheterization as a comfort measure.

∞ *Long-term urethral catheterization should always be avoided and must be used in only extremely exceptional cases of urinary incontinence.*

Long-term catheterization is associated with a myriad of complications from bacterial colonization and infection, including upper tract damage (pyelonephritis, nephritis), acute and chronic cystitis, bladder cancer, stones, periurethral damage (epididymitis, scrotal abscesses, urethral fistula, and stricture), and urethritis.[57] In a large trial, nonprescribed removal of the catheter, usually by the patient because of the discomfort associated with long-term catheterization, was the most frequent cause of catheter replacements.[58] Catheter management problems are debilitating to the patient and time consuming for the clinician. The prime objectives are to prevent bacterial entry and urethral and bladder irritation.

Preventing bacterial entry has become easier because new technology uses a closed catheter system that reduces the rate of bacterial colonization. The catheter system should never be opened, and routine bladder irrigations are not recommended. Strict technique when handling catheter tubing and emptying urine is observed, using gloves and good handwashing. In institutions, catheterized patients should not be placed in a room together. Although polymicrobial urine is common, systemic antibiotic suppressive therapy is discouraged, since sensitive organisms are eradicated and replaced with resistant bacteria. Fluid intake greater than 2000 ml helps keep the urine diluted and accomplishes "bladder irrigation from above." Urine acidification with vitamin C inhibits bacterial overgrowth. One to three grams of vitamin C per day taken in divided doses, including a dose at night, is suggested to acidify urine pH.[31] Gentle cleansing of the urinary meatus and perineum with soap and water, avoiding vigorous rubbing, is essential. To further avoid manipulation of the catheter around the meatus, the catheter should be securely taped to the thigh (in women) or abdomen (in men) to maintain gravity drainage. New catheter tubing designs include a valve that prevents backflow of urine from the drainage bag into the tubing, which prevents bacterial ascent. Stretchable leg bands are also available for the ambulatory patient.

Preventing irritation is another prime objective in catheter management. Minimizing trauma to the urethra and bladder helps avoid leakage, spasm, and pain. Selecting the correct size catheter is vital. It is important to use the smallest lumen catheter that is retained (usually a 12F, 14F, or 16F). Larger catheters do not solve the problem of leakage; in fact they make leakage worse by distending and irritating the urethra. Larger lumens also block mucus-secreting glands in the urethra, leading to urethritis and infection. Large catheters (18F and up) have no clinical utility in long-term catheterization and are indicated mainly for postoperative care to manage hematuria and clotting. Large catheters have been misused in clinical practice. The balloon size is another important decision in catheter selection. The smallest balloon (5 ml) should be used and inflated to the fullest volume (10 ml). Larger (30 ml) balloons are indicated for hematuria (and for short-term use) but do not decrease the problem of leakage of urine. The larger balloon sits on the trigone muscle at the base of the bladder, causing bladder spasms that expel urine. Also, balloons that are not filled to the prescribed volume have an uneven distribution of liquid that sits asymmetrically on the trigone muscle, contributing to irritation and bladder spasm. Catheter material is important, too: latex, silicone, Teflon, and lubricous materials or coatings are available. For long-term use, latex catheters promote the most bacterial ascent (and are thus discouraged for long-term use), and lubricous polymer-coated catheters promote very little bacterial ascent. The lubricous coating interacts with moisture in the urethra, forming a gel-like material that decreases friction against the wall of the urethra as well as decreasing the formation of encrustations and blockage. Catheter changes are not recommended on a routine basis. However, patients who have problems with encrustations and blockage should have catheter changes scheduled before blockage is likely to occur, which may be every 10 days to 2 weeks; others may go several months without changes. It is recommended that catheters be left in place until problems develop.[59]

> *Suprapubic catheterization is now the preferred route for long-term indwelling catheterization of the bladder if it is necessary; in patients with obstruction and overflow, intermittent catheterization is the preferred technique.*

Suprapubic catheters are being used more often now for long-term catheterization because they are associated with fewer complications of bacteriuria, urethral trauma, and bladder spasm.[60] The urethral defense mechanism is left intact, and the suprapubic site is easy to keep clean.[61] A small catheter is introduced percutaneously through the abdominal wall into the bladder while the patient is under general or local anesthesia; it is secured with a suture, a retention disk, or a balloon. A Foley catheter may also be used. Once the catheter entry tract has been established, the catheter may be changed by medical or nursing staff through the original tract. If the catheter is removed or discontinued, the openings of the abdominal and bladder walls normally close spontaneously.[61]

Clean intermittent catheterization is an alternative to chronic indwelling catheterization in patients with obstruction and overflow UI. This procedure allows the periodic, regular emptying of the bladder while the bladder maintains normal filling function. Risk for upper and lower urinary tract infection and sepsis is lower than with urethral indwelling catheterization when good technique and hydration guidelines are followed. Upper urinary tract function is preserved in the majority of patients, although regular screening for hydronephrosis or reflux may be indicated in patients with recurrent or chronic infection.[62] Catheterizations are administered every 4 to 6 hours to maintain a urine volume below 400 to 500 ml. If the patient is able to void, catheterization is performed after voiding. Preventing bladder overdistention helps prevent UTI, and adequate fluid intake keeps the urine diluted and effectively "washes out" the bladder. Urethral complications in males should be prevented by adequate lubrication, using topical anesthetic gel if available, and coudé-tipped catheters. In the home, clean technique is recommended; in institutions, sterile or aseptic technique with gloves is usually performed.

Treatment Summarized

The application of the differing treatment techniques to the four main clinical categories of UI is summarized in Table 22-5.

▼ *ROSE KRANSTEIN (Part III)*

Two years after beginning Kegel exercises, Mrs. Kranstein finds that problems are redeveloping. She has been less able to exercise recently, and there have been one or two episodes when a cough, a sneeze, or lifting a pile of books has caused more leakage than usual. She finds that wearing a tampon when she volunteers at the library helps. She undergoes urodynamic testing, which confirms that her uterovaginal prolapse

Table 22-5   Treatment of Urinary Incontinence

UI Type	Goal of Treatment	Treatment
Stress	Restore continence by strengthening periurethral and pelvic muscles, correcting anatomical defects, and preventing pelvic muscle straining.	Bladder training, scheduled toileting Pelvic muscle exercise Biofeedback training for pelvic muscle exercises Vaginal cones Bowel program, avoid straining Electrical stimulation Pessary or diaphragm Estrogen replacement therapy α-Adrenergic therapy Urethral bulking agents Artificial urinary sphincter Urethral plug Bladder neck suspension surgery
Urge	Reduce bladder instability and leakage by reducing irritating factors and increasing bladder capacity.	Bladder training, prompted voiding, habit training Urge inhibition techniques Fluid hydration Eliminate bladder irritants (caffeine, alcohol, etc.) Bowel program Estrogen replacement therapy Nonhormonal vaginal moisturizers Anticholinergic therapy Electrical stimulation
Overflow	Promote complete bladder emptying and prevent bladder overdistention.	Voiding maneuvers Double voiding Scheduled toileting Bowel program Intermittent catheterization
Functional	Optimize functional status by minimizing factors that impair mobility and cognition and correcting environmental barriers to successful toileting.	Scheduled toileting, prompted voiding Assistive devices: bedside commode, urinal, bedpan Clothing modifications Fluid hydration Bowel program Avoidance of drugs with adverse effects on lower urinary tract or cognition

is the main contributor to this apparent stress incontinence. She elects to undergo a bladder suspension operation, and the results are good.

▼ AGNES TERRILL (Part IV)

To allow Miss Terrill to take more part in activities, diapers are used in addition to the retraining techniques when she goes out on trips and at night. After nearly 2 months of the bladder retraining, it is evident that her pattern is now of nocturnal incontinence. Since her skin becomes raw by morning from the wetness of the diaper, a small dose of imipramine is added at night; this appears to enable her to go through most nights without wetness. Ultimately, she rarely requires diapering, and although she is still dependent, her incontinence is much less of a management problem in the facility.

FECAL INCONTINENCE

Fecal incontinence, the involuntary leakage of stool, is an extremely distressing symptom associated with considerable stigma and embarrassment. Symptoms may range from staining of the underclothes to uncontrollable frank passage of flatus and stool. The prevalence in nursing homes may be as high as 10% to 17% of residents.

Neurological control of anorectal continence is, in general, parallel to neurological control of urinary continence. Pelvic muscle structures, in particular the levator ani muscles, play as integral a role in maintenance of bowel continence as they do in urinary continence. Normal continence depends on intact mental function, stool volume and consistency, colonic transit, rectal distensibility, anal sphincter function, anorectal sensation, and anorectal reflexes. Abnormalities in any of these factors can lead to incontinence.[4]

Causes of fecal incontinence are listed in Box 22-8. Abnormal pelvic floor innervation or injury from childbearing in females predisposes to rectal prolapse and pelvic descent. Neurological or neuropathic conditions, common in institutionalized older patients, contribute to a high prevalence of both urinary and fecal incontinence. Fecal impaction is a primary cause of fecal incontinence in frail older patients. It is a type of overflow incontinence and is also called the "terminal reservoir syndrome." Fecal impaction is preventable when a consistent bowel program is in place, including adequate fluids, dietary fiber supplementation, and activity. In comparison to continent elderly persons, incontinent older patients have abnormal rectal sensation and decreased resting sphincter pressure, a situation that is aggravated by diarrhea.[4]

BOX 22-8
Causes of Fecal Incontinence

Normal Pelvic Floor
Diarrhea states

Infectious diarrhea
Inflammatory bowel disease
Short-gut syndrome
Laxative abuse
Radiation enteritis

Overflow

Impaction
Encopresis
Rectal neoplasms

Neurological conditions

Congenital anomalies (e.g., myelomeningocele)
Multiple sclerosis
Dementia, strokes, tabes dorsalis
Neuropathy (e.g., diabetes)
Neoplasms of brain, spinal cord, cauda equina
Injuries to brain, spinal cord, cauda equina

Abnormal Pelvic Floor
Congenital anorectal malformation

Trauma

Accidental injury (e.g., impalement, pelvic fracture)
Anorectal surgery
Obstetrical injury

Aging

Pelvic floor enervation (idiopathic neurogenic incontinence)
Vaginal delivery
Chronic straining at stool
Rectal prolapse
Descending perineum syndrome

From Madoff RD, Williams JG, Caushaj PF: *N Engl J Med* 326:1002-1007, 1992.

 Fecal impaction, a type of overflow incontinence, is the prime cause of fecal incontinence in old age.

Normal bowel function is dependent on intact neuromuscular activity in the colon, rectum, and anus. Feces and gas are propelled along the gastrointestinal tract, and on reaching the cecum the bolus is emptied into the colon, stimulating the gastrocolic reflex.[63] When feces enter the rectum, sensory nerve endings are stimulated as the rectum distends to accommodate the bolus. When the rectum is distended by about 150 ml of feces, the internal anal sphincter relaxes and allows the feces to enter the anal canal. If defecation is not voluntarily initiated, the external anal sphincter contracts and the defecation reflex is inhibited and passage of stool is withheld. The anal canal is lined with sensitive epithelium that allows the distinction among gas, liquid, and solid matter. When defecation is activated, the external anal sphincter relaxes and with rectal contractions, gravity, and minimal abdominal effort, the stool is evacuated.[63]

Evaluation of fecal incontinence relies heavily on a careful history. Fecal incontinence must be differentiated from frequency and urgency without incontinence that may be associated with inflammatory bowel syndrome, pelvic radiation, irritable bowel syndrome, and low anterior resection of the rectum. A simple test to confirm true fecal incontinence is to administer an enema with a volume of at least 150 ml. The ability to retain the enema suggests intact function. Severity of incontinence is determined by the patient's ability to retain gas, liquid, and solid feces. The inability to retain solid feces suggests severe incontinence, whereas leakage of gas alone indicates minimal loss of function.[4] The history should address onset, frequency and amount of incontinence, stool consistency, duration, associated medical problems that may be contributory, dietary and medication regimen (especially laxative or stool softener use), and psychosocial and environmental issues.

> *Leakage of gas alone indicates minimal loss of fecal retentive function.*

Physical examination focuses on inspection of the anal area and digital examination. Inspection notes soiling, excoriations, scarring, deformities, abnormal tissues, prolapse with or without straining, and perineal descent. Digital examination notes the resting tone of the sphincter muscle, the intensity of voluntary sphincter contraction, inappropriate use of accessory muscles during the contraction, sphincter defects (imperforate anus), hemorrhoids, masses, and impaction. Further tests include anoscopy, sigmoidoscopy, anal manometry, radiological studies (anal defecography), and EMG neuromuscular testing.

Conservative treatment of fecal incontinence includes dietary measures, biofeedback training, and medication. Dietary measures are intended to bulk up liquid stool until it is easier to control and retain. These include a high-fiber diet, fiber supplementation with unprocessed wheat bran or stool-bulking agents, and avoidance of foods that cause loose stools. Bowel management with regular tap water enemas helps induce bowel action and leaves the rectum empty between evacuations. Antidiarrheal or constipating agents may also be helpful in managing stool consistency. Biofeedback training involves passing a special balloon catheter into the rectum and gradually distending the balloon to fill the rectal vault and facilitate sensory awareness of rectal filling and fullness. The patient is trained to perceive decreasing volumes of air in the balloon and to simultaneously contract the external anal sphincter.[4] Visual displays of sphincter pressure encourage the patient to perform the contraction correctly and increase the strength of the contraction. Treatment requires a number of sessions before results are seen. EMG biofeedback using perianal skin sensors or rectal electrodes may also be used as a biofeedback modality. Biofeedback can significantly improve fecal incontinence in more than half of patients.[64] The severity of incontinence influences the viability of treatment options. Minor degrees of incontinence may be responsive to dietary strategies, sphincter exercises, biofeedback, and antidiarrheal medication. More severe incontinence may require surgical correction. Management approaches to contain or prevent incontinence include the fecal incontinence pouch and the anal plug.[65]

Preventing constipation and fecal impaction is a primary concern to the clinician. If an impaction is confirmed, several manual disimpactions will be necessary as the hard feces move down nearer the anal margin. Following this, a bowel retraining program is necessary, with bran and other fiber, extra liquids, stool softeners, and daily suppositories. Bowel movement for most people may be timed for 30 to 60 minutes following breakfast. Increasing intraabdominal pressure to stimulate and assist defecation may be accomplished by assisting the patient to put their feet on a footstool while seated on the toilet and to lean forward slightly. For some a hot drink promotes relaxation and aids in the process. Temporarily reduced mobility or acute illness with dehydration should receive anticipatory treatment to reduce the likelihood of constipation and impaction.

SUMMARY

Urinary and fecal incontinence are treatable problems in the elderly. While these conditions may be difficult to cure, symptoms can always be effectively managed to prevent adverse sequelae and promote quality of life. Focused assessment and treatment strategies can be individualized to address the unique presentation and characteristics of older patients.

POSTTEST

1. Which one of the following statements is false regarding neuropathic bladder conditions?
   a. The reflex bladder is characteristically seen in paraplegia.
   b. Diabetic autonomic neuropathy is characteristically associated with an atonic bladder.
   c. Detrusor-sphincter dyssynergia is caused by loss of cerebral inhibition.
   d. Osteophytes can cause a reflex neurogenic bladder.

2. Which one of the following statements is false regarding urgency incontinence?
   a. Biofeedback is helpful in some patients.
   b. Bladder training is not helpful in cerebrally impaired patients.
   c. Drug-induced outlet obstruction can cause urgency UI.
   d. Both imipramine and oxybutynin are useful in management.

3. Which one of the following statements regarding stress incontinence is false?
   a. Urethral hypermobility is worsened by obesity.
   b. Local estrogens relieve the incontinence when there is atrophic vaginitis.
   c. Pelvic floor exercises should be repeated ten times daily for at least a month.
   d. Bladder neck suspension has been successful in the majority of older patients so managed.

4. Which one of the following statements is false regarding overflow incontinence?
   a. Antihistamines can cause overflow UI.
   b. A spinal tumor above T12 can cause it.
   c. Intermittent catheterization is preferred to a sterile closed system.
   d. Detrusor insufficiency can cause overflow UI.

5. Which one of the following statements is false regarding aspects of incontinence?
   a. Bacteriuria is inevitable with chronic catheterization.
   b. In reestablishing fecal continence, a bowel movement should be attempted just before meals.
   c. The external urethral sphincter can be retrained through voluntary control.
   d. β-Adrenergic fibers cause the bladder to relax and fill.

REFERENCES

1. Urinary Incontinence (UI) Guideline Panel: *Urinary incontinence in adults: clinical practice guideline,* AHCPR Pub No 92-0038, Rockville, Md, March 1992, US Department of Health and Human Services.
2. Ouslander JA, Kane RL, Abrass IB: Urinary incontinence in elderly nursing home patients, *JAMA* 248:1194-1198, 1982.
3. McDowell BJ et al: An interdisciplinary approach to the assessment and behavioral treatment of urinary incontinence in geriatric outpatients, *J Am Geriatr Soc* 40:370-374, 1992.
4. Madoff RD, Williams JG, Caushaj PF: Fecal incontinence, *N Engl J Med* 326:1002-1007, 1992.
5. Seidel GK et al: Predicting bowel and bladder continence from cognitive status in geriatric rehabilitation patients, *Arch Phys Med Rehabil* 75:590-593, 1994.
6. Urinary incontinence among hospitalized persons aged 65 years and older—United States, 1984-1987, *MMWR* 40:433-436, 1991.
7. Sier H, Ouslander JG, Orzeck S: Urinary incontinence among geriatric patients in an acute care hospital, *JAMA* 257:1767-1771, 1987.
8. Mitteness LS: Knowledge and beliefs about urinary incontinence in adulthood and old age, *J Am Geriatr Soc* 38:374-378, 1990.
9. Jeter KF, Wagner DB: Incontinence in the American home: a survey of 36,500 people, *J Am Geriatr Soc* 38:379-383, 1990.
10. Goldstein M et al: Urinary incontinence: why people do not seek help, *J Geront Nurs* 18:15-20, 1992.
11. Burgio KL et al: Treatment seeking for urinary incontinence in older adults, *J Am Geriatr Soc* 42:208-212, 1994.
12. Clark A, Romm J: Effect of urinary incontinence on sexual activity in women, *J Reprod Med* 38:679-683, 1993.
13. Borrie MJ, Davidson HA: Incontinence in institutions: costs and contributing factors, *Can Med Assoc J* 147:322-328, 1992.
14. Staskin DR: Age-related physiologic and pathologic changes affecting lower urinary tract function, *Clin Geriatr Med* 2:701-710, 1986.
15. Wyman JF: Incontinence and related problems. In Chenitz WC, Stone JT, Salisbury SA, eds: *Clinical gerontological nursing: a guide to advanced practice,* Philadelphia, 1991, WB Saunders.
16. Benson JT, Walter MD: Neurophysiology of the lower urinary tract. In Walters MD, Karram MM, eds: *Clinical urogynecology,* St Louis, 1993, Mosby.
17. Brocklehurst JC: Incontinence. In Ham RJ, ed: *Geriatric medicine annual 1986,* Oradell, NJ, 1986, Medical Economics Books.
18. McConnell JD et al: *Benign prostatic hyperplasia: diagnosis and treatment. Clinical practice guideline, No 8,* AHCPR Pub No 94-0582, Rockville, Md, February 1994, US Department of Health and Human Services.
19. Snooks SJ et al: Effect of vaginal delivery on the pelvic floor: a 5 year follow-up, *Br J Surg* 77:1358-1360, 1990.
20. Deindl FM et al: Pelvic floor activity patterns: comparisons of nulliparous continent and parous urinary stress incontinent women; a kinesiological EMG study, *Br J Urol* 73:413-417, 1994.
21. Dwyer PL, Lee ETC, Hay DM: Obesity and urinary incontinence in women, *Br J Obstet Gynaecol* 95:91-94, 1988.
22. Bump RC et al: Obesity and lower urinary tract function in

women: effect of surgically induced weight loss, *Am J Obstet Gynecol* 167:392-397, 1992.

23. Bump RC, McClish DM: Cigarette smoking and pure genuine stress incontinence of urine: a comparison of risk factors and determinants between smokers and nonsmokers, *Am J Obstet Gynecol* 170:579-582, 1994.

24. Fantl JA et al: Postmenopausal urinary incontinence: comparison between non-estrogen-supplemented and estrogen-supplemented women, *Obstet Gynecol* 71:823-826, 1988.

25. Molander U: Urinary incontinence and related urogenital symptoms in the elderly, *Acta Obstet Gynecol Scand Suppl* 158:1-22, 1993.

26. Avorn J et al: Reduction of bacteriuria and pyuria with cranberry beverage: a randomized trial, *J Am Geriatr Soc* 41:A51, 1994.

27. Elbadawi A, Yalla SV, Resnick NM: Structural basis of geriatric voiding dysfunction. 1. Methods of a prospective ultrastructal/urodynamic study and an overview of the findings, *J Urol* 150:1650-1656, 1993.

28. Resnick NM, Yalla SV: Management of urinary incontinence in the elderly, *N Engl J Med* 313:800-805, 1985.

29. Resnick NM, Yalla SV: Detrusor hyperactivity with impaired contractile function: an unrecognized but common cause of incontinence in elderly patients, *JAMA* 257:3076-3081, 1987.

30. Geirsson G, Fall M, Lindstrom S: Subtypes of overactive bladder in old age, *Age Ageing* 22:125-131, 1993.

31. Wall LL, Norton PA, DeLancey JO: *Practical urogynecology,* Baltimore, 1993, Williams & Wilkins.

32. Lekan-Rutledge DA: Simple cystometry in the evaluation of urinary incontinence, *J Urol Nurs* 11:267-276, 1992.

33. Hilton T, Stanton SL: Algorithmic method for assessing urinary incontinence in elderly women, *Br Med J* 282:940-942, 1981.

34. Fantl JA et al: Efficacy of bladder training in older women with urinary incontinence, *JAMA* 265:609-613, 1991.

35. Wyman JF: Managing urinary incontinence with bladder training: a case study, *J ET Nurs* 20(3):121-126, 1993.

36. Schnelle JF: Treatment of urinary incontinence in nursing home patients by prompted voiding, *J Am Geriatr Soc* 38:356-360, 1990.

37. Colling JC et al: The effects of patterned urge response toileting on urinary incontinence among nursing home residents, *J Am Geriatr Soc* 40:135-141, 1992.

38. Burgio LD et al: The effects of changing prompted voiding schedule in the treatment of incontinence in nursing home residents, *J Am Geriatr Soc* 42:315-320, 1994.

39. Smith DA et al: Reduction of incontinence among elderly in a long-term care setting. In Funk SG et al, eds: *Key aspects of elder care: managing falls, incontinence, and cognitive impairment,* New York, 1992, Springer.

40. Bump RC et al: Assessment of Kegel pelvic muscle exercise performance after brief verbal instruction, *Am J Obstet Gynecol* 165:322-329, 1991.

41. Hahn I et al: Long term results of pelvic floor training in female stress urinary incontinence, *Br J Urol* 72:421-427, 1993.

42. Wells M: A tangible means of assessing progress: biofeedback in the management of urinary incontinence, *Prof Nurse* 6:396-399, 1991.

43. Burgio KL, Whitehead WE, Engel BT: Urinary incontinence in the elderly: bladder-sphincter biofeedback and toileting skills training, *Ann Intern Med* 103:507-515, 1985.

44. Nielsen KK et al: The urethral plug. II. An alternative treatment in women with general urinary stress incontinence, *Br J Urol* 72:428-432, 1993.

45. Pearson BD, Larson JM: Urine control by elders: noninvasive strategies. In Funk SG et al, eds: *Key aspects of elder care: managing falls, incontinence and cognitive impairment,* New York, 1992, Springer.

46. Colling JC et al: Behavioral management strategies for urinary incontinence, *J ET Nurs* 20(1):9-13, 1993.

47. Wein AJ: Pharmacologic treatment of incontinence, *J Am Geriatr Soc* 38:317-325, 1990.

48. Sourander LB: Treatment of urinary incontinence: the place of drugs, *Gerontology* 36(suppl 2):19-26, 1990.

49. Terodiline in the Elderly American Multicenter Study Group: Effects of terodiline on urinary incontinence among older non-institutionalized women, *J Am Geriatr Soc* 41:915-922, 1993.

50. Partoll LM: Voiding dysfunction and retention. In Walters MD, Karram MM, eds: *Clinical urogynecology,* St Louis, 1993, Mosby.

51. Duffy LM: Male incontinence. In Jeter K, Faller N, Norton C, eds: *Nursing for continence,* Philadelphia, 1990, WB Saunders.

52. Gundian JC, Barrett DM, Parulkar BG: Mayo Clinic experience with AS800 artificial urinary sphincter for urinary incontinence after transurethral resection of prostate or open prostatectomy, *Urology* 41:318-321, 1993.

53. Bierwirth WW: Which pad is for you? *Urol Nursing* 12:75-77, 1992.

54. Jeter KF: The use of incontinence products. In Jeter K, Faller N, Norton C, eds: *Nursing for continence,* Philadelphia, 1990, WB Saunders.

55. Ragi G, Kalb RE, Klaus MV: Penile encrustation due to a condom catheter, *J Am Geriatr Soc* 37:160-162, 1989.

56. Ouslander JG, Greengold B, Chen S: External catheter use and urinary tract infections among incontinent male nursing home patients, *J Am Geriatr Soc* 35:1063-1070, 1987.

57. Kunin CN et al: Association between the use of urinary catheters and morbidity and mortality among elder patients in nursing homes, *Am J Epidemiol* 135:291-301, 1992.

58. Muncie H, Warren JW: Reasons for replacement of long-term urethral catheters: implications for randomized trials, *J Urol* 507-509, 1990.

59. Wong ES: Guidelines for prevention of catheter-associated urinary tract infections, *Am J Infect Control* 11:28-32, 1983.

60. Warren JW: Urine-collection devices for use in adults with urinary incontinence, *J Am Geriatr Soc* 38:364-367, 1990.

61. Constantino G: Catheterization. In Jeter K, Faller N, Norton C, eds: *Nursing for continence,* Philadelphia, 1990, WB Saunders.

62. Wyndale JJ, Maes D: Clean intermittent self-catheterization: a 12-year follow-up, *J Urol* 143:906-908, 1990.

63. Jensen LL: Fecal incontinence. In Jeter K, Faller N, Norton C, eds: *Nursing for continence,* Philadelphia, 1990, WB Saunders.

64. Jorge JM, Wexner SD: Etiology and management of fecal incontinence, *Dis Colon Rectum* 36:77-97, 1993.

65. Christiansen J, Roed-Petersen K: Clinical assessment of the anal incontinence plug, *Dis Colon Rectum* 36:740-742, 1993.

PRETEST ANSWERS
1. b
2. a
3. c

POSTTEST ANSWERS
1. c
2. b
3. c
4. b
5. b

UNIT III
CLINICAL PROBLEMS

So we'll go no more a-roving
So late into the night,
Though the heart be still as loving,
And the moon be still as bright.
For the sword outwears its sheath,
And the soul wears out the breast,
And the heart must pause to breathe,
And Love itself have rest.
Though the night was made for loving,
And the day returns too soon,
Yet we'll go no more a-roving
By the light of the moon.
—George Gordon, Lord Byron, "So We'll Go No More A-Roving"

Old people, on the whole, have fewer complaints than young; but those chronic diseases which do befall them generally never leave them.
—Hippocrates, *Aphorisms*

Sleep and watchfulness: both of these when immoderate constitute disease.
—Hippocrates

The older we grow, the greater become the ordeals.
—Goethe

Is it not strange that desire should by so many years outlive performance?
—Shakespeare, *Henry IV*

Sickness comes on horseback and departs on foot.
—Dutch proverb

Wine is only sweet to happy men.
—John Keats, "To——(Fanny Brawne)"

CHAPTER 23

Perioperative Care

PATRICIA P. BARRY

OBJECTIVES

On completion of this chapter, the reader will be able to:

1. Understand the effects of advanced age on surgical risk.
2. Identify disease-related factors that affect surgical risk.
3. Perform preoperative assessment of the older surgical patient.
4. When possible, modify operative risk.
5. Manage perioperative care of the older surgical patient.

PRETEST

1. The most significant risk factor for perioperative mortality in the elderly is:
   a. Advanced age
   b. Urgency of the procedure
   c. Chronic disease
   d. Type of anesthesia

2. Cardiac risk associated with noncardiac surgery is primarily due to:
   a. Untreated cardiac dysrhythmia
   b. Undiagnosed coronary artery disease
   c. Early congestive heart failure
   d. Unsuspected aortic valve stenosis

BOX 23-1
Important Considerations in Preoperative Assessment

Diagnosis and prognosis of the underlying problem
Therapeutic options, risks, and benefits
General health of the patient; life expectancy
Patient's values and desires
Experience of the surgical team and facility
Availability of appropriate postoperative care

SURGERY IN ELDERLY PATIENTS

Since the rate of surgical procedures in adults increases with chronological age, aging of the population has resulted in a greater number of older surgical patients.[1] Decisions regarding surgery in the elderly person involve several important considerations (Box 23-1). Age is likely to be a "marker" rather than an independent risk factor for serious underlying disease and should not be used to make decisions regarding the appropriateness of surgical procedures.[2]

Critical review of current literature on the subject is not always helpful in determining optimal clinical management of the elderly surgical patient. Surgical studies frequently do not include adequate numbers of elderly subjects, and the definition of "elderly" may vary from over 65 to over 85. Comorbid conditions are not well described, and age is often the only risk factor considered. Cross-sectional studies comparing older with younger patients are confounded by cohort effects, while historical comparison may not take into account the improvements in surgical techniques over the years.[2] In addition, few studies have actually evaluated the validity of preoperative assessment and recommendations or their effect on outcomes of surgery.[3]

Improved surgical techniques, support, monitoring, and better anesthesia have resulted in more appropriate surgical treatment and declining risk for the older patient in recent years. Recent studies suggest that well-prepared elderly persons can undergo major surgery without un-

reasonable mortality.[4] The primary care physician's participation is critical in assessment of the patient's medical risk factor, preoperative preparation, and postoperative management, including discharge planning. The primary care physician may also have the best understanding of the patient's values, and may have previously discussed and determined the patient's wishes for end-of-life care.

▼ KATHLEEN O'CONNOR (Part I)

Mrs. O'Connor is an 85-year-old widow who has been followed by you for 5 years. She is brought to the emergency room for a fall at her home, where she lives independently. She has a past medical history of hypertension, diabetes, and cigarette smoking that she discontinued 5 years ago. Medications include hydrochlorothiazide 25 mg daily, lisinopril 10 mg daily, and glipizide 10 mg daily. On examination, she is alert, with normal vital signs: pulse 78 beats/min, blood pressure 150/85, respirations 14 breaths/min, and she is afebrile. Physical examination reveals an externally rotated and shortened left leg. Electrolytes and complete blood count are normal, random glucose level is 190, urea level is 25, and creatinine level is 1.2. Chest x-ray examination findings are clear, with hyperinflated lungs, and electrocardiogram shows nonspecific ST-T wave abnormalities. On x-ray film of the left hip, she is found to have an intertrochanteric fracture. She is admitted to the orthopedic service, and the primary care physician is requested to "clear for surgery."

STUDY QUESTIONS

- *What further evaluation is needed before surgery?*
- *What risk factors are present for perioperative care?*

▼ GEORGE ROBERTSON (Part I)

Mr. Robertson is a 72-year-old man who lives with his daughter and her family. He has not seen any physician for several years, until he is brought to the emergency room with increasing confusion and worsening abdominal pain, which began 2 days ago. According to his daughter he takes no medi-

cations, has smoked a pack of cigarettes a day for 55 years, and drinks "several bottles" of beer every evening. Lately he has complained of vague chest discomfort and a persistent morning cough productive of clear sputum, and she has noted some "problems with his memory." On examination he is thin, somewhat lethargic, and oriented to person only. His vital signs are pulse 95 beats/min, blood pressure 120/60, respiration 18 breaths/min, and temperature 100.2° F. His lungs are clear but with prolonged expiration and decreased breath sounds. Cardiac examination is unremarkable. Bowel sounds are hyperactive; his abdomen is tense, with guarding and tenderness to palpation. Rectal examination is negative for blood and reveals no masses; his prostate is enlarged. Laboratory evaluation is normal except for a hemoglobin of 9 g/ml and a hematocrit of 28 (hypochromic, microcytic), with a white blood cell count of 15,000. Chest x-ray examination shows hyperinflation with a left upper lobe mass; electrocardiogram shows right axis deviation. Abdominal x-ray examinations and CT scan are consistent with obstruction and a right colonic mass. You are the physician on call for unassigned admissions, and you take over his care.

STUDY QUESTION

- Is Mr. Robertson ready for surgery if indicated?

SURGICAL RISK IN ELDERLY PATIENTS

The increased prevalence of disease frequently (but not always) associated with aging is an important risk factor for postoperative morbidity and mortality in the elderly surgical patient. In addition, physiological changes of aging, especially the cardiac, pulmonary, and renal responses to stress, interact with many diseases to affect homeostatic mechanisms. Atypical presentation of common illness may complicate the identification and diagnosis of disease in the perioperative period. For example, vague symptoms such as decreased appetite, fatigue, "taking to bed," or confusion (delirium) may represent the "nonspecific" presentation of pneumonia, heart failure, or electrolyte imbalance. Individual variations are common, and the heterogeneity may be due to the effects of comorbid conditions. Altered pharmacokinetics, resulting in the slowed clearance and changes in distribution of many drugs, increases the risk of adverse drug reactions in the perioperative period, especially in elderly patients taking numerous medications.

> *Elective surgery has no extra mortality in the old; emergency surgery is the hazard.*

Surgical Risk Factors

In many studies comparing older with younger surgical patients, mortality of elective surgery is not appreciably different. However, emergency surgery is considerably more hazardous for elderly patients in all studies and appears to be the greatest risk factor for high morbidity and mortality.[2,5] The site of surgery also affects risk: thoracic and cranial procedures have the most complications, and risk decreases from upper abdominal to the lower abdominal to the extremities as operative sites. The increased risk of vascular surgery appears to be due to associated cardiovascular disease. Increased duration of surgery, especially procedures lasting longer than 3 hours, is also associated with an increased risk of complications.

Anesthetic Risk Factors

Available data do not indicate that spinal anesthesia is safer than general anesthesia. Decisions regarding anesthesia are best made by an experienced anesthesiologist after a careful preoperative assessment.[3]

Disease-Related Risk Factors

Preexisting conditions, especially heart disease and pulmonary disease, appear to increase surgical risk in the elderly patient. In addition, malnutrition and dementia contribute to postoperative morbidity.

Cardiovascular Disease. Heart disease is the most common cause of perioperative mortality and a leading cause of morbidity; preexisting heart disease is a major risk factor for postoperative problems.

Pulmonary Disease. Postoperative pulmonary diseases are the *most common cause* of morbidity and a significant cause of mortality. Cigarette smoking is a major risk factor, as is a history of respiratory disease.

Malnutrition and Digestive Diseases. Poor nutritional status appears to be a major risk factor for postoperative morbidity and mortality. Protein deficiency is especially problematic for appropriate management of fluids and for postoperative healing. Hepatic insufficiency may require special consideration regarding anesthesia. In several studies patients with cirrhosis have had poor surgical outcomes. Active peptic ulcer disease is a serious risk factor for postoperative complications.

Endocrine Diseases. In most studies, diabetes does *not* appear to be a major risk factor for postoperative morbidity, but it does require careful management throughout the perioperative period. Adrenal insufficiency has a high mortality rate, and hypothyroidism may lead to the complications of hypotension and myxedema coma.

Cognitive Impairment. Dementia is prevalent in the elderly and has been associated with increased postoperative mortality. Acute confusional state (delirium) must be evaluated as a symptom of drug toxicity, infection, metabolic abnormality, or other acute medical problem and often occurs in the absence of preexisting dementia.

Other Conditions. Dehydration (e.g., patients taking diuretics) may decrease blood pressure intraoperatively.

Anemia (hemoglobin less than 10 g/ml) may complicate concurrent ischemic heart disease. Previously undiagnosed malignancy may influence the decision to operate. Recent stroke appears to confer an increased risk of surgical complications.

PREOPERATIVE EVALUATION

The purpose of preoperative evaluation is to identify conditions that may affect surgical outcome. Some conditions may need to be treated preoperatively to reduce risk. Others may not be alterable but still need to be identified in order to reconsider surgical decisions or plan for appropriate postoperative management. Preoperative information may be useful in three ways:

1. As a "case finder" for previously undetected conditions that increase surgical risk and may require perioperative intervention
2. As a "predictor" that identifies patients at particular risk of postoperative complications
3. As a "baseline" that may be used for comparison purposes in the postoperative period

Routine preoperative evaluation provides all three types of information and is clearly necessary for all elderly surgical patients. The components of such an evaluation should be a standard examination appropriate for all patients, consisting of a thorough history, physical examination, mental and functional status assessments, and a review of medications, including over-the-counter drugs. The patient's advance directive should be obtained. Although few studies have evaluated the usefulness of laboratory tests in the elderly, the high prevalence of disease justifies a reasonable number of routine tests including a complete blood count, electrolytes, glucose, urea, and creatinine.[6] Serum albumin is a nutritional parameter.[7] Hepatic function tests are usually required for anesthesia, and a urinalysis should be performed. Specific tests are indicated for patients with other identified risk factors.

 For acute surgery the general physician must work quickly to stabilize all systems.

Cardiac Risk

A preoperative electrocardiogram is recommended for all patients over 65, and it is useful to detect abnormalities that may modify the surgical plan as well as provide a baseline for comparison.[8] ECG abnormalities are common in the elderly and therefore are not particularly helpful as predictors of postoperative complications. Clinical information can predict the likelihood of a coronary event.[9] Older men with chest pain and older persons with a number of cardiac risk factors may be at *moderate risk*. Patients at *high risk* of unexpected coronary events include those with angina, previous myocardial in-

farction, or symptoms or signs of left ventricular dysfunction (history of congestive heart failure, rales, S_3 gallop, or jugular venous distention), even though they appear clinically stable. Patients at *very high risk* include those with overt congestive heart failure, recent myocardial infarction, or New York Heart Association class III or IV angina. In a recent study, five major preoperative predictors of postoperative myocardial ischemia included left ventricular hypertrophy, history of hypertension, diabetes mellitus, definite coronary artery disease, and use of digoxin.[10]

Certain types of surgery—vascular, aortic, orthopedic, intrathoracic, or intraperitoneal—impart a higher risk of postoperative coronary events. Patients at moderate or high risk undergoing such surgery need evaluation to define the severity of underlying heart disease. Ambulatory electrocardiographic (Holter) monitoring of the ST segment and dipyridamole-thallium imaging are suitable tests for further evaluation of elderly patients at moderate to high risk who may be unable to undergo a standard exercise test. Abnormalities on dipyridamole-thallium imaging have been shown in several studies to correlate with postoperative cardiac events. Ambulatory monitoring, which is cheaper and more widely available, can identify episodes of preoperative myocardial ischemia that predict postoperative ischemia. In addition, the absence of preoperative ischemia indicates a low risk of postoperative ischemia.[9]

Recent myocardial infarction should delay surgery for 3 to 6 months, if possible. Unstable angina may be as serious as recent myocardial infarction and mandates evaluation and treatment, including invasive procedures, if necessary, before elective surgery. Unstable dysrhythmias are "markers" for underlying severe heart disease and may require pacemaker or pharmacological therapy in consultation with a cardiologist. Decompensated congestive heart failure has a grave prognosis with significant mortality. Uncontrolled hypertension has been noted to negatively affect morbidity; in most studies it is defined as a diastolic pressure of greater than 110. Patients identified as high risk may need aggressive monitoring and antiischemic therapy or even more invasive treatment such as angiography and revascularization. Cancellation of elective surgery may be necessary if the risk is unacceptable.

STUDY QUESTION

- *Given the available information, what are the cardiovascular risks for Mrs. O'Connor as she faces orthopedic surgery for her intertrochantic fracture?*

Pulmonary Risk

The incidence of major postoperative respiratory complications is significantly higher in patients over age 70;

however, the benefit of routine preoperative chest radiographs in patients without known pulmonary disease is not established. An abnormal chest x-ray examination finding in a patient with known disease does not increase the already high risk of postoperative complications. The preoperative chest x-ray examination may thus be most useful as a baseline for comparison.[11] The value of preoperative spirometry is unclear and in several studies has not been helpful in identifying patients at increased risk. Clinical information, especially a history of asthma or chronic bronchitis, may be a better predictor.[12] Arterial blood gases may be useful as a baseline, especially in patients with known pulmonary disease, but have not been adequately evaluated as predictors of complications. The exception is hypercapnia, which is an important indicator of high risk.

In contrast to cardiac complications, in which preexisting cardiac disease is the most important risk factor, postoperative pulmonary complications are also associated with other risk factors. The most important of these is the site of surgery: the closer the procedure is to the diaphragm, the greater is the risk. Duration of surgery (over 3½ hours) appears to be an important risk factor as well. No difference between spinal and general anesthesia has been determined. The role of increased age and obesity as independent risk factors is less clear.[13]

Infection, such as bronchitis or pneumonia, must be treated before surgery. Smokers should stop smoking *2 months* before elective surgery. Decompensated bronchospasm, with or without pulmonic insufficiency, requires aggressive management before surgery. Preoperative education should teach the need for, and techniques of, postoperative pulmonary toilet (deep breathing, coughing, incentive spirometry). Preoperative institution of respiratory therapy, antibiotics, and bronchodilators is of benefit in patients with pulmonary disease.[13]

STUDY QUESTION

- Mr. Robertson has a persistent, productive morning cough; what steps should be taken to prepare him for potential surgery?

▼ KATHLEEN O'CONNOR (Part II)

Mrs. O'Connor is further evaluated before surgery. Formal mental status testing is within normal limits, and her preinjury functional status was independent in all activities of daily living. Because of her moderate preoperative risk of cardiac disease, she is evaluated with dipyridamole-thallium imaging, which does not reveal evidence of ischemia. Her history of cigarette smoking confers an increased risk of pulmonary complications; an arterial blood gas measurement is obtained as a baseline.

▼ GEORGE ROBERTSON (Part II)

Mr. Robertson is quickly evaluated for urgent surgery. His mental status examination reveals impaired attention, orientation, memory, language, and level of consciousness consistent with delirium. Cardiac risk is moderate, and intraperitoneal surgery confers increased risk of postoperative coronary events, but the urgency of his surgery precludes further evaluation. His pulmonary risk is high because of his active smoking history and chronic bronchitis, and his abnormal chest radiograph raises suspicion of malignancy. Arterial blood gases reveal a P_{O_2} of 60 and P_{CO_2} of 40; spirometry is consistent with moderately severe obstructive lung disease. He is transfused with 2 units of packed red cells for his anemia.

STUDY QUESTION

- How should both of these patients be managed in the perioperative period?

PERIOPERATIVE MANAGEMENT

Hypertension should be well controlled before surgery, but hypotension should be avoided. For patients with insulin-dependent *diabetes,* half the usual dose may be given the day of surgery and small doses of regular insulin given in a glucose infusion based on blood glucose determinations. For non–insulin-dependent diabetics undergoing major surgery, the insulin-glucose infusion may be used. For minor surgery the blood glucose level should be monitored, with regular insulin given if needed. In patients with *steroid dependence* or suspected *adrenal insufficiency,* intravenous hydrocortisone should be instituted preoperatively and continued postoperatively. Patients undergoing orthopedic procedures have the highest risk of *postoperative deep vein thrombosis,* which can, however, occur after any major surgical procedure. Early ambulation, compressive stockings, and antithrombotic prophylaxis are important preventive measures.[14]

General measures of particular importance in the postoperative care of elderly surgical patients are noted in Box 23-2. Careful fluid management is necessary to pre-

---

BOX 23-2
Important Considerations in Postoperative Care

Careful fluid management
Adequate pain relief
Cautious use of medications
Removal of tubes and restraints
Early mobilization
Monitoring of cardiopulmonary status
Early and liberal nutrition
Early discharge planning

vent overload and possible precipitation of congestive heart failure. However, too little fluid may cause prerenal azotemia and hypotension. Adequate pain relief is necessary to encourage mobilization and pulmonary toilet, but medications with depressant and sedative effects must be used with special care, since they may have greater toxicity in the elderly. Removal of tubes, including intravenous lines and Foley catheters, promotes greater comfort and mobility. Restraints should be used as little as possible and only for important indications. Early mobilization, with assistance if needed, is critical to pulmonary function and ambulation. Attention to cardiopulmonary status, with careful monitoring of symptoms and physical findings, is important for the early diagnosis of complications. Adequate nutrition should be encouraged with a liberal diet and use of supplements if necessary. Timely discharge planning, initiated before surgery if possible, is needed for continuity of care in the current health care milieu, which emphasizes early hospital discharge.

> *Fluid management, pain relief, and early mobilization are the three essentials to efficient postoperative recovery in elders.*

▼ KATHLEEN O'CONNOR (Part III)

Mrs. O'Connor's hydrochlorothiazide is discontinued before surgery; her lisinopril is continued throughout the perioperative period. Glipizide is discontinued and her diabetes is managed with blood glucose determinations and an insulin/glucose infusion. Warfarin prophylaxis is initiated. She receives preoperative teaching regarding her postoperative pulmonary exercises. Planning for her posthospital rehabilitation is initiated, and her advance directive is reviewed.

On the second hospital day, Mrs. O'Connor undergoes uncomplicated open reduction and internal fixation of her left intertrochanteric fracture. This is followed by early mobilization, resumption of her usual medications, and aggressive pulmonary toilet. On her fourth postoperative day, she is transferred to a rehabilitation facility, from which she eventually returns home.

▼ GEORGE ROBERTSON (Part III)

Mr. Robertson undergoes urgent surgery under cardiac monitoring to relieve his obstruction, which is found to be caused by a carcinoma (Duke's stage C) of the right part of the colon; bowel resection is performed. He tolerates the procedure without immediate complications; he is extubated in the recovery room, and aggressive pulmonary toilet is instituted. Despite this, his postoperative course is complicated by worsening confusion and development of dyspnea on the second postoperative day. Examination reveals rales and consolidation in the left base of the lung; chest x-ray examination shows an infiltrate consistent with left lower lobe pneumonia. Intravenous antibiotic therapy is instituted. Medications are reviewed, and Mr. Robertson's meperidol dose is reduced from 100 to 75 mg every 4 hours. His Foley catheter is removed, but he is unable to void. Intermittent catheterization is ordered every 6 hours with good response. He is mobilized to a chair and ambulates with assistance.

Over the next 2 days, Mr. Robertson's mental status becomes more alert and attentive, but formal testing reveals persistent impairment of short-term memory and language skills throughout his hospital course. Intermittent catheterization is discontinued before discharge. Mr. Robertson's diagnosis and prognosis are discussed with the patient and his daughter; both decline further evaluation of his pulmonary mass or treatment of his carcinoma, and his daughter expresses her desire to take him home. They are counseled regarding an advance directive consistent with Mr. Robertson's wishes for end-of-life care. Home nursing and social services are arranged, and Mr. Robertson is discharged home on the tenth postoperative day.

CONCLUSION

The elderly patient presents a challenge to the primary care physician when surgery is indicated, but older patients are generally able to tolerate necessary surgical procedures. Careful preoperative evaluation, with special attention to prophylaxis and to cardiopulmonary status and appropriate consultation as needed, enables the physician to minimize risk. Urgent surgery remains a challenging and more threatening situation. The malnourished are at particular risk. Conscientious evaluation during the postoperative period and attention to early rehabilitation and discharge planning promote recovery and the resumption of previous life-style as quickly as possible.

POSTTEST

1. Which of the following is *not* associated with high risk of perioperative cardiac complications?
   a. Obesity
   b. S$_3$ gallop
   c. Previous myocardial infarction
   d. Rales

2. In elderly patients, routine preoperative chest x-ray examination is probably most useful as which of the following?
   a. A "case finder" for previously undetected conditions
   b. A "predictor" of postoperative complications
   c. A "baseline" for comparison in the postoperative period

3. Impaired cognitive function in the postoperative period may be due to any of the following except:
   a. Adverse drug reaction
   b. Respiratory infection
   c. Age over 90 years
   d. Urinary retention

REFERENCES

1. Keating HJ: Preoperative considerations in the geriatric patient, *Med Clin North Am* 71:569-583, 1987.
2. Sandler RS et al: Biliary tract surgery in the elderly, *J Gen Intern Med* 2:149-154, 1987.
3. Goldman L: The art and science of perioperative consultation: where we are and where we should be going, *J Gen Intern Med* 2:284-285, 1987.
4. Keller SM et al: Emergency and elective surgery in patients over age 70, *Am Surg* 53:636-640, 1987.
5. Keating HJ, Lubin MF: Perioperative responsibilities of the physician/geriatrician, *Clin Geriatr Med* 6:459-468, 1990.
6. McKee RF, Scott EM: The value of routine pre-operative investigations, *Ann Royal Coll Surg* 69:160-162, 1987.
7. Leite JFMS et al: Value of nutritional parameters in the prediction of postoperative complications in elective gastrointestinal surgery, *Br J Surg* 74:426-429, 1987.
8. Seymour DG, Pringle R, Maclennan WJ: The role of the routine preoperative electrocardiogram in the elderly surgical patient, *Age Ageing* 12:97-104, 1983.
9. Eagle KA, Boucher CA: Cardiac risk of noncardiac surgery, *N Engl J Med* 321:1330-1332, 1989.
10. Hollenbert M et al: Predictors of postoperative myocardial ischemia in patients undergoing noncardiac surgery, *JAMA* 268:205-209, 1992.
11. Boghosian SG, Mooradian AD: Usefulness of routine preoperative chest roentgenograms in elderly patients, *J Am Geriatr Soc* 35:142-146, 1987.
12. Williams-Russo P et al: Predicting postoperative pulmonary complications: is it a real problem? *Arch Intern Med* 152:1209-1213, 1992.
13. Jackson CV: Preoperative pulmonary evaluation, *Arch Intern Med* 148:2120-2127, 1988.
14. Merli GJ: Prophylaxis for deep vein thrombosis and pulmonary embolism in the geriatric patient undergoing surgery, *Clin Geriatr Med* 6:531-542, 1990.

PRETEST ANSWERS
1. b
2. b

POSTTEST ANSWERS
1. a
2. c
3. c

CHAPTER 24

Elder Abuse

JAMES G. O'BRIEN

OBJECTIVES

Having completed this chapter, the reader will be able to:

1. Understand the phenomenon of abuse from an epidemiological perspective.

2. Describe factors associated with increased risk of abuse.

3. Describe the different types of abuse.

4. Outline how the victim and the perpetrator should be approached.

5. Describe aspects of the history and physical examination useful in detecting abuse.

6. Suggest initial intervention and management strategies.

PRETEST

1. Which one of the following statements is true?
   a. Most elderly victims do not know their abusers.
   b. Elder abuse is more likely to be reported than child abuse.
   c. Substance abuse is associated with elder abuse.
   d. Informal caregivers are the most frequent perpetrators of abuse.

Elder abuse is encountered by primary care physicians in most practice settings. The least intimidating approach to identification and intervention, and the most likely to be accepted by victim and family, is from the personal clinician. There are dilemmas that a clinician has to cope with and questions that are raised when a potential abuse victim is encountered. What really constitutes abuse? What biases will influence whether it is identified?

There is evidence that abuse has occurred since antiquity, even during the idealized family times of the nineteenth century when three-generation families commonly lived together. Sermons and court documents affirm that elders were victimized, usually by family members; often the incentive for keeping grandparents at home was to ensure the transfer of property.

In 1981 the House Select Committee on Aging convened experts who gave testimony verifying the occurrence of abuse.[2] It was thought that approximately 4% of the elderly population in the United States were victims and that typically family members, not strangers, were the perpetrators.

Physician involvement in elder abuse has been much less than in child abuse. The primary care physician is in an ideal position to detect it, but evidence suggests that elderly victims may be relatively isolated. Abuse is also difficult to detect and is typically not considered in the differential diagnosis.

Older individuals have an increased tendency to fall, to bruise, and to fracture, so the manifestations of abuse can be misattributed. In addition, less credence may be given to an older adult's statements. An accompanying family member may dominate the physician's assessment and reduce suspicion of abuse, especially if the older adult is perceived as difficult and the family member communicates well.

Elder abuse is defined as an act or omission that leads to harm, or that threatens harm, to the health or welfare of an older person.[4] Generally, five different types are identified (Box 24-1).

The problem of self-neglect is common and poses ethical dilemmas to physicians.

BOX 24-1
Types of Abuse

1. **Physical abuse:** slapping, burning, beating, sexually assaulting
2. **Physical neglect:** withholding necessities of life such as food, medications, and nourishment
3. **Psychological abuse:** threatening, demeaning, denigrating, or isolating
4. **Material or financial abuse:** stealing or misappropriating money or property
5. **Violation of rights:** evicting, inhibiting autonomy, placing in a nursing home against the individual's will

---

▼ ROBERTA ROBERTS (Part I)

Your patient, Mrs. Roberts, is 80 years old and has lived for the past 3 years with her 75-year-old sister, Florence Lusty. Florence had moved in because of her sister's problems with diabetes and her memory. Florence requests medication for Roberta "to make her sleep at night" and "to control her kidneys." Roberta appears disheveled and smells of urine; her gait appears unsteady. This represents a marked change from her usual neat demeanor; she complains to you of being left alone for long periods. Florence interrupts and claims that Roberta is very demanding, doesn't sleep well at night, and needs constant attention, leaving her with no free time.

ASSESSMENT

Patient abuse is underreported, so physicians need to be proactive and to consider the possibility more frequently. It is important to ask direct questions such as, "Is anyone hurting you or harming you?" or "Have you been confined against your will?" or "Has anyone stolen from you?" These questions must be asked privately, separate from family members, so the potential victim can be secure and open. The victim often hides abuse because of fear or embarrassment. It may be easier for the patient to be open with other office staff than with the physician. Accusations should be corroborated if the victim is cognitively impaired, unless the evidence is so flagrant that there is no other reasonable explanation. All medical problems, medications, home situation, and available support systems must be identified. Describing a typical day may help to provide the context in which the abuse occurs.

 To detect elder abuse, it is vital to ask direct questions.

▼ ROBERTA ROBERTS (Part II)

You interview the sisters separately. Roberta claims that her sister, before going out for the evening, puts her to bed and puts restraints on her so she can't get out of bed. She usually eats twice a day, and she frequently receives her evening insulin dose late at night. She is disoriented to time, has trouble with abstract thinking, and remembers one of three items at 3 minutes. She seems to understand her situation. She admits feeling worried about being placed in a nursing home. You note that she appears weak and needs assistance with transferring and undressing. Her clothes are soiled, and she smells of urine.

STUDY QUESTIONS

- What aspects of this case cause suspicion of abuse?
- What should be sought on physical examination and laboratory investigation?

Physical examination needs to be detailed and comprehensive. It should include a review of general appearance, which may indicate poor hygiene, emaciation, fractures, incontinence, and weight loss, and an observation of gait, transfer capability (e.g., the ability to get from chair to examining table), mobility, and the ability to undress.

Cognitive status should be established by using an objective questionnaire if possible, and mood noted.[5,6] The response of the patient to the examiner (fearful or frightened) should be noted. Careful inspection of the skin is vital, with a particular emphasis on inspection of hidden areas such as the axillae, inner thighs, soles of the feet, palms, and abdomen, looking for bruising, burns, abrasions, or tenderness. Bruising on the extensor surfaces of the arms is common and generally benign; bruising at different stages of resolution and located on the *inner* surfaces of extremities is more likely to indicate abuse. Sexual abuse should always be considered, as age does not confer immunity. All external injuries or abnormalities should be carefully documented and photographed if possible. (Use a coin in the photograph to reference

size.) Diagrams may be useful to depict trauma accurately. The color and dimensions of any traumatic lesions should be noted.

 Suspect abuse if there is bruising on the inner surfaces of extremities.

Laboratory and other investigations may yield supportive data. Anemia, hypoalbuminemia, and lymphocytopenia may indicate malnutrition or neglect. Radiographs may show new or old, previously unrecognized fractures. Note especially fractures associated with direct trauma, such as midshaft fractures of the humerus or femur, or spiral fracture of the humerus. Brain CT scan may show subdural hematoma from trauma. Serum levels of psychotropic or other drugs may reveal toxic or subtherapeutic drug levels, supporting inappropriate treatment.

In summary, the assessment should enable the physician to have a sense of the nature and severity of the abuse, the vulnerability of the victim, the functional and cognitive abilities, and the social support systems available to the patient. Box 24-2 summarizes factors associated with abuse.

▼ ROBERTA ROBERTS (Part III)

Mrs. Roberts' weight is 130 lb, a 30-lb weight loss since her last visit, 7 months ago. Her mucous membranes appear dry, and her tongue is red and smooth. Blood pressure is 150/88 sitting and 120/78 standing. She is unsteady standing, but her skin shows no bruising, except purpuric lesions on the extensor surfaces of her hands. You note no other abnormalities. On your instructions the medications are brought to the office: insulin zinc suspension (Lente Insulin U-100) 30 U in the AM and 10 U in the PM, verapamil SR 240 mg daily, temazepam 15 mg at bedtime, furosemide 40 mg daily, as

---

BOX 24-2
Factors Associated with Abuse

1. Mental illness, alcoholism, substance abuse in caregiver or victim
2. Financial dependence of caregiver on victim
3. Functional impairment of caregiver
4. Past history of abuse
5. Social isolation and single caregiver
6. Delay or neglect in treating medical problems
7. Multiple visits to emergency or urgent care clinics
8. Unexplained trauma
9. Sex of the victim (abuse is more common in women)
10. Prolonged caregiving with heavy burden of care

needed for leg swelling, and diphenhydramine (Benadryl) 25 mg as needed for anxiety. Laboratory analyses have the following results: hemoglobin, 9.9 g/dl; hematocrit, 27%; mean corpuscular volume, 72 μm³; blood sugar, 84 mg/dl; albumin, 2.8 g/dl; and cholesterol, 160 mg/dl. No x-ray examinations are indicated.

STUDY QUESTIONS

- What should be done now?
- What statutory action must you take?

MANAGEMENT

In many states, health care providers are mandated by law to report actual or suspected abuse; this specifically takes precedence over privileged communication with the patient. Unfortunately, many states lack the facilities and resources to provide the services needed in abuse situations.[6] The primary goal is to ensure the victim's safety and then to intervene in ways that cause the least disruption for both victim and family.[7-9]

Often, abuse occurs where there is a dependent patient and an overwhelmed caregiver. In such situations assistance and help in the home, with possibly some counseling, is the type of intervention required.

Adult Protective Services (APS) is a statutory agency available in all communities and specifically mandated to protect the interests of individuals at risk for harm, especially if they are potentially unable to help themselves. Such agencies are generally staffed by social workers and vary in degree of aggressive intervention, depending on the resources available to them and on state law. However, it is clearly the duty of the physician faced with possible abuse, danger, or harm to the patient to inform and involve this agency. Prior contact from other health-related sources, or even simply reports from neighbors, may (unknown to the personal physician) already have been collated by the agency. Extra professional help and services, and perhaps legal counsel, may be made available through this source.

▼ ROBERTA ROBERTS (Part IV)

You inform the sisters that many services are available to help them, including visiting nurses to assist with diabetic management, Meals on Wheels, adult day care to provide respite for Florence and a therapeutic milieu for Roberta, and a caregiver support group for Florence. You tell them that, because of Roberta's problems, Adult Protective Services (APS) needs to be informed, and you explain the function of APS. You explain that, given the nature of the case, APS will probably help with mobilizing the support services and no punitive action will take place. You will see Roberta regularly for follow-up.

▼ DOLORES BROWN (Part I)

Mrs. Brown is a 72-year-old independent patient of yours, who lives with her 49-year-old son. He has recently divorced and moved back home; his marriage broke up because of his drinking and abusive behavior. Mrs. Brown comes to the emergency room with a black eye, multiple bruises, a fractured humerus, and cigarette burns. She tells the ER physician that her son has beaten her up. The ER physician calls the police, Adult Protective Services, and you, Mrs. Brown's primary physician.

STUDY QUESTIONS

- What needs to be done to effect acute protection of this patient?
- What action should be taken against the potential abuser?

When the victim is independent and the caregiver is psychopathic or a substance or alcohol abuser, the emphasis must be on protection and often requires legal action. In such situations the abuse will escalate or recur unless there is intervention. A restraining order on the abuser should be discussed with APS. The abuser, rather than the victim, should be removed from the home if possible.

If the injuries are severe enough, hospitalization affords instant protection, respite, and time to make plans. Since elder abuse is generally a family problem, interventions need to be focused. A team approach emphasizing accurately defining the problem and providing services such as counseling, social work, nursing, respite care, or day care is appropriate. The physician is often the only professional who will continue to see the victim over time, and thus should remain aware of the home situation and continue communication with agencies whose representatives visit the home. If the situation deteriorates, interventions can be promptly planned.

An ethical dilemma may arise when a victim who is competent to make a decision exercises the right to refuse any intervention. In this situation the physician clearly has a duty to ensure that there is no coercion and that the individual's ability to make a sound judgment is not compromised (e.g., no cognitive deficits, no true depression of mood, no irrational fearfulness). Technically, the victim has the right to decide to stay in an abusive situation, although the personal physician clearly has a duty to stay informed about the situation, even if this follow-up has to be informal.

SUMMARY

Elder abuse is frequently overlooked. Detecting and managing what is often an ongoing family situation exercises all of the skills of the primary care physician. Good management requires efficient collaboration with community services, where available, for support and respite.

POSTTEST

1. All of the following statements regarding elder abuse are true except which one?
   a. Elder abuse is seldom reported by the victim.
   b. Bruises on the extensor surfaces of arms usually indicate abuse.
   c. Neglect is the most frequent type of abuse seen by practitioners.
   d. Abuse tends to escalate over time.

REFERENCES

1. Callahan J: Elder abuse: some questions for policymakers, *Gerontologist* 28:453-458, 1988.
2. Pepper C, Oaker R: Elder abuse: an examination of a hidden problem, House Select Committee on Aging, Ninety-Seventh Congress Pub No 97-277, San Francisco, US Government Printing Office.
3. Phillips L, Rempussheski V: Making decisions about elder abuse, *Soc Casework* 67:131-140, 1986.
4. Council on Scientific Affairs, AMA: Elder abuse and neglect, *JAMA* 257:966-971, 1987.
5. Fulmer T: Clinical assessment of elder abuse. In Fillinson R, Ingman S, eds: *Elder abuse: practice and policy*, New York, 1989, Human Sciences Press.
6. Wolf R: Elder abuse: ten years later, *J Am Geriatr Soc* 36(8):758-762, 1988.
7. Quinn M, Tomita S, eds: *Elder abuse and neglect: causes, diagnosis and intervention strategies*, New York, 1986, Springer Publishing.
8. O'Malley T et al: Identifying and preventing family-mediated abuse and neglect of elderly persons, *Ann Intern Med* 98:988-1005, 1983.
9. Taler G, Ansello E: Elder abuse, *Am Fam Physician* 32:107-114, 1985.
10. American Medical Association: *Elder abuse and neglect: diagnostic and treatment guidelines,* Oct 1992.

PRETEST ANSWER

1. c

POSTTEST ANSWER

1. b

CHAPTER 25

Alcoholism

JAMES W. CAMPBELL

OBJECTIVES

On completion of this chapter, the reader will be able to:

1. Identify risk factors and diagnostic criteria for alcoholism in older persons.

2. Discuss screening instruments and laboratory tests used in the diagnosis of alcoholism and the effects of aging on their clinical utility.

3. Describe the mechanisms of initiating treatment and the types of treatment available.

4. Discuss the relationship of alcohol dependency to other common syndromes of old age: dementia, depression, suicide, polypharmacy, falls, and multiple medical illnesses.

PRETEST

Select the single best answer:
1. Which of the following are possible presentations of alcoholism?
   a. Cognitive impairment
   b. Incontinence
   c. Hip fracture
   d. Depression
   e. All of the above

2. The most effective mechanism to screen for early alcoholism is:
   a. Blood level of gamma glutamyl transferase
   b. Measurement of red cell mean corpuscular volume
   c. Physical examination for spider angiomas
   d. Physical examination for asterixis
   e. Questionnaire and family history

Alcoholism is often missed in older patients. Many of the classic clues are mistaken for age-related changes or diseases. The psychosocial factors that are often pivotal in moving younger alcoholics into treatment (spouse, job, and legal pressures such as being charged with driving while intoxicated) are less likely to occur in elders. Pharmacokinetic changes make the quantity of ethanol used a less reliable indicator of problems, falsely reassuring the health care professional. Physicians must be alert to the significance of features such as falling, incontinence, poor social support, cognitive decline, depression, noncompliance, and others.

Alcoholism is difficult to diagnose, and yet it is one of the most remediable ailments of the elderly. Treatment modalities developed over the past 50 years are particularly effective in older patients.

▼ JACKIE DANIELS (Part I)

Mrs. Daniels is a 79-year-old retired nurse who comes to you for a complete "checkup." She was last seen by a physician 3 years ago. She reports feeling a little depressed in the last 3 months. There is no reported weight change. She generally sleeps from 11 PM to 7 AM with one episode of awakening for urination. She seems to enjoy some activities, and she does not show suicidal ideation. She has a 20-year history of hypertension, intermittently medicated. She reports urinary incontinence since 1987. She had a postpartum depression after the birth of her son, 51 years ago. She had a cholecystectomy in 1982 and a hysterectomy in 1967. She is currently taking hydrochlorothiazide 25 mg every day and follows a no-added-salt diet. On examination, she is thin, blood pressure is 180/98, and vital signs are normal.

STUDY QUESTIONS

- *What are the risk factors for alcoholism here?*
- *How should you proceed to investigate, and what physical signs should be sought on examination?*

DEFINITION

It is important that alcohol dependency be defined as a medical syndrome. This determines the types of treatment and the profession responsible for care.

Evidence of alcohol production dates back to 4000 to 6000 BC. Restrictions of consumption have been documented as far back as 1700 BC. Regarding habitual drunkenness as a disease was first proposed in 276 AD by Domitius Ulpinus in Rome.

Early in the twentieth century, alcoholism was defined in moralistic terms; treatment involved condemnation and punishment and was in the scope of the religious and criminal justice systems. Although Benjamin Rush seriously reintroduced the concept of alcoholism as a disease in the early 1800s, it was not until the rise of Alcoholics Anonymous (AA) in the 1930s and the recognition of AA in 1956 by the American Medical Association (AMA) that alcohol dependency became clearly categorized as a disease.[1] Alcoholism was thus moved from the legal system and placed in the purview of public health. The medical community then developed diagnostic criteria, prevalence and natural history data, and screening and treatment modalities were defined.

In the early 1950s the World Health Organization's (WHO) definition of alcoholism was paraphrased as "having problems from drinking and drinking anyway."[2] In 1975 the WHO redefined the drinking behaviors characteristic of alcohol-dependence syndrome: drink-seeking behaviors; increased tolerance to alcohol; repeated withdrawal symptoms; repeated relief, or avoidance, of withdrawal symptoms by further drinking; subjective awareness of a compulsion to drink; and reinstatement of the syndrome after abstinence.

In this chapter the terms "alcoholism," "alcohol dependence," and "alcohol addiction" are used synonymously. These terms imply development of tolerance, withdrawal reactions, loss of control of alcohol use, and psychosocial decline.[3] A practical classification scheme for elderly alcoholics identifies four patterns: (1) chronic,

BOX 25-1
Age-Related Factors Affecting Rate and Impact of Alcoholism

Factors Contributing to Low Reported Rates	Factors Increasing Impact
Increased biological sensitivity	Increased biological sensitivity
Underdiagnosis by health care providers	Underdiagnosis by health care providers
Cohort values and underreporting	Cohort values and underreporting
Institutionalized persons not in community surveys	Institutionalized persons not being diagnosed and treated
Less socialization and less awareness by peers of drinking behaviors	Less socialization and less awareness by peers of drinking behaviors
Less job or legal pressure to initiate treatment	Less job or legal pressure to initiate treatment
Family unwillingness to report	Family unwillingness to report
Less overall driving, so less while intoxicated	Coexisting conditions limiting sensory input while driving
Spontaneous remission	Increased concomitant disease
Selective survival	Increased prescription drug use
Ill health	High nonprescription drug use
Financial constraints	

(2) intermittent, (3) reactive (after a significant psychosocial stress), and (4) late onset.

 Alcoholism is one of the most remediable ailments of the elderly.

Prior studies must be interpreted carefully. While some studies simply distinguish late from early onset, in terms of the four-part classification, chronic and intermittent are almost always early onset and reactive may be either late or early onset, since the drinking is in response to a biopsychosocial stress. Two thirds of older alcoholics fall in the chronic or intermittent class, and one third are either reactive or true late onset.[4]

PREVALENCE

Five to ten percent of the elderly are heavy alcohol users. It is estimated that there are a half million elderly alcoholics.[5] Alcoholism is the third most prevalent psychiatric disorder among elderly men, surpassed only by dementia and anxiety disorders.[6] Older persons hospitalized for general medical and surgical procedures and institutionalized elderly demonstrate a prevalence of approximately 18% alcohol abuse.[4] One third of older alcoholics are estimated to have begun their alcohol abuse *after* the age of 65.[3]

Patterns of alcohol use are affected by such experiences as the Industrial Revolution, the Temperance Movement, Prohibition, the Depression, and the two world wars. Alcohol use should be understood to be a habit, whereas alcoholism is a separate disease entity. This explains the apparent contradiction of elderly persons' decreased alcohol use with no decline in alcohol abuse.

Box 25-1 summarizes the factors contributing to the low reported rates of alcoholism and to the increased impact of drinking in old age. Many of these factors arise from society's unwillingness to label older persons as alcoholic because of the continued stigma. The mistaken thought that older alcoholics are untreatable is prevalent and reduces detection.

▼ JACKIE DANIELS (Part II)

Mrs. Daniels smoked one pack per day for 32 years. She quit in 1979. She reports no prescription drug use. She occasionally takes 2 mg diazepam. She states that she is a social drinker. She agrees that her alcohol intake was slightly increased during her postpartum depression.

STUDY QUESTIONS

▪ *How should you establish her current alcohol use?*
▪ *What questions would establish if she has a problem?*

DIAGNOSIS

The older alcoholic is likely to drink only five to six times per week and only four to five drinks per occasion,[7] yet ethanol has greater pharmacological impact as we age. Ethanol absorption is no different with increasing age. However, using a constant rate of ethanol infusion, peak concentration is higher in the elderly. This is a result of the smaller volume of distribution, since ethanol is distributed in body water, which is decreased in elderly persons.[4] The elderly patient is unlikely to be cross-addicted to other nonprescription drugs; however, the possibility of misuse of prescription drugs must be considered because it has been estimated to occur in over 10% of elders.

An important psychosocial change is the shrinking support network. In one study, concern of a family member or friend was the most common factor motivating patients for admission to a treatment program.[8]

▼ JACKIE DANIELS (Part III)

Mrs. Daniels reports that she drinks two drinks (each 4 oz) weeknights and occasionally more on weekends or when under stress. She is elusive and annoyed at specific questions. She has been married for 53 years; her husband is alive and well, and they have two daughters and one son. Her main social activity is a bridge club twice a week. She is very much involved in her church. On direct questioning, she admits to a dramatic decline in these activities over the last 6 months.

STUDY QUESTIONS

- *What specific questions can be asked to better define her alcohol problem or discover whether she actually has an alcohol problem?*

SCREENING AND DETECTION

Screening questionnaires have been shown to differentiate alcoholics from nonalcoholics, although these screening tests are less sensitive in the elderly population. They cover the level of consumption, alcohol-related social or legal difficulties, alcohol-related health problems, symptoms of drunkenness or dependence, and self-recognition.[9] Certain questions on the CAGE[10] and the Michigan Alcoholism Screening Test (MAST)[11,12] are significantly less likely to be answered in the affirmative if the subjects are elderly. Nonetheless, the CAGE is a useful brief clinical screen (Box 25-2).[10] The 24-item MAST-G (Geriatric MAST), developed at the University of Michigan, is age appropriate and therefore useful (Box 25-3).[13]

Laboratory tests including a complete blood count (CBC), blood chemistries, liver function, gamma glutamyl transferase (GGT), and blood alcohol level usually

---

BOX 25-2
The CAGE Questionnaire

1. Have you ever felt you ought to *C*ut down?
2. Have you ever been *A*nnoyed by criticism of your drinking?
3. Have you ever felt *G*uilty about your drinking?
4. Have you ever felt the need for an *E*ye opener?

---

demonstrate some abnormality that can be attributed to alcohol use. These tests are likely to be abnormal in an older individual. Such tests can help reinforce the reality of the diagnosis, especially in resistant patients.

A number of clinical clues to alcoholism that are often misinterpreted in elders are summarized in Box 25-4.

The medical problems associated with alcoholism must be specifically sought: diseases of the esophagus, stomach, pancreas, or liver, as well as cognitive impairment, blackouts, and cerebellar dysfunction.

 An alcoholic child or grandchild is the most helpful clinical clue to the presence of alcoholism in an elderly patient.

It is important to review the family history, since alcoholism is frequently familial. The most helpful clinical clue to the presence of alcoholism in an elderly patient is often the presence of the disease in a child or grandchild. Patterns of family behavior and rituals merit examination. Families whose rituals and behaviors became distorted as a result of alcoholism are more likely to transmit the disease familially.[14]

▼ JACKIE DANIELS (Part IV)

You ask Mrs. Daniels the CAGE questions. She has been able to cut down her alcohol intake on a number of occasions, but she becomes annoyed at the questions and denies feeling guilty. Review of symptoms reveals that incontinence has been a concern for 5 months. Her family reports increased memory difficulty for 3 months. You ask her daughter about the family and alcohol, and she reveals that she herself regularly attends AA. She reports that often dinnertime and the holidays are disrupted by her mother's drinking, especially during Mrs. Daniels' depressions.

ALCOHOLISM AND OTHER ILLNESSES

Alcoholism is distinctly related to *dementia;* it is estimated that 10% of the instances of dementia in older persons are alcohol related. Cognition usually improves after treatment, but at the very least, progression can be aborted. *Depression* is commonly the medical illness precipitating to alcohol abuse; alcohol is an easily available, nonprescription psychotropic. Although in moderate doses alcohol has mood elevating effects,[4] it is primarily a central nervous system depressant. Ten to fifteen percent of depressed people use it for self-medication.[15] One study found that over 50% of patients admitted for alcoholism treatment had symptoms of depression that persisted for at least 1 year after alcohol treatment.[16] Alcohol is also associated with suicide.

Alcoholism has a definite relationship to *falling*. Although there is a significant association of hip fracture with heavy alcohol consumption in younger persons, after age 65 the association is less strong.[17]

▼ *JACKIE DANIELS (Part V)*

With encouragement from the family, Mrs. Daniels is persuaded to enter a 14-day inpatient unit. Delirium tremens do not develop. The follow-up treatment plan is 90 AA meetings in 90 days. Her incontinence resolves and her memory improves. Her depression remains unchanged 4 months after treatment.

STUDY QUESTIONS

- How would you have proceeded if she had refused to comply with this plan?
- Should the depression be treated with an antidepressant?

TREATMENT

The family not only is helpful in making the diagnosis but is the key element of treatment. In fact, use of the family is the most significant advance in treatment and rehabilitation of the alcoholic. The key principles of treatment are summarized in Box 25-5.

The approach to the patient and family must avoid being judgmental and emphasize the disease model and the need for further evaluation. It is important to initiate the treatment plan the same day the patient is confronted with the diagnosis. The physician can facilitate this by maintaining relationships with AA members who can be called on to help. AA is appropriate for older patients; one third of AA members are over 50. The treatment plan must use family and friends. Legal commitment is occasionally necessary; recovery rates for such patients approximate those for persons who seek help voluntarily.[18]

Three significant barriers to management of elderly alcoholics have been defined: physicians are less likely to

---

BOX 25-3
Michigan Alcoholism Screening Test-Geriatric Version (MAST-G)

	Yes (1)	No (0)
1. After drinking have you ever noticed an increase in your heart rate or beating in your chest?	1. __	__
2. When talking with others do you ever underestimate how much you actually drink?	2. __	__
3. Does alcohol make you sleepy so that you often fall asleep in your chair?	3. __	__
4. After a few drinks have you sometimes not eaten or been able to skip a meal because you didn't feel hungry?	4. __	__
5. Does having a few drinks help decrease your shakiness or tremors?	5. __	__
6. Does alcohol sometimes make it hard for you to remember parts of the day or night?	6. __	__
7. Do you have rules for yourself that you won't drink before a certain time of the day?	7. __	__
8. Have you lost interest in hobbies or activities you used to enjoy?	8. __	__
9. When you wake up in the morning do you ever have trouble remembering part of the night before?	9. __	__
10. Does having a drink help you sleep?	10. __	__
11. Do you hide your alcohol bottles from family members?	11. __	__
12. After a social gathering have you ever felt embarrassed because you drank too much?	12. __	__
13. Have you ever been concerned that drinking might be harmful to your health?	13. __	__
14. Do you like to end an evening with a night cap?	14. __	__
15. Did you find your drinking increased after someone close to you died?	15. __	__
16. In general, would you prefer to have a few drinks at home rather than go out to social events?	16. __	__
17. Are you drinking more now than in the past?	17. __	__
18. Do you usually take a drink to relax or calm your nerves?	18. __	__
19. Do you drink to take your mind off your problems?	19. __	__
20. Have you ever increased your drinking after experiencing a loss in your life?	20. __	__
21. Do you sometimes drive when you have had too much to drink?	21. __	__
22. Has a doctor or nurse ever said they were worried or concerned about your drinking?	22. __	__
23. Have you ever made rules to manage your drinking?	23. __	__
24. When you feel lonely does having a drink help?	24. __	__

Scoring: 5 or more "yes" responses is indicative of alcohol problem.

From Blow et al: *Alcohol Clin Exp Res* 16(2):372, 1992.

BOX 25-4
Alcoholism Clinical Clues Misattributed to Other Causes

Clues Attributed to Geriatric Syndromes

Dementia
 Confusion
 Memory loss
 Disorientation
Falls
 Bruises
 Fractures
Malnutrition
Polypharmacy
 Sedative use
 Anxiolytic use
 Analgesics
Incontinence

Clues Attributed to Age-Biased Views of Elderly Persons

Treatment resistance
Self-neglect
Functional decline
Sleep impairment
Anxiety
Postsurgical recovery
 difficulties

Clues Attributed to Coexisting Diseases with High Prevalence in Older Persons

Depression
Hypertension
Malnutrition
Sleep disturbances
Chronic fatigue
Peripheral neuropathy
Cerebellar degeneration
Seizures
Sexual dysfunction
Repeated infections
Cardiomyopathy

BOX 25-5
Principles of Treatment for Elderly Alcoholics

The Family is the Key to Management

Nonjudgmental, medical/disease approach
Initiate plan same day as patient is confronted
Use Alcoholics Anonymous membership
Abstinence is the principle: controlled drinking is not
 recommended
Replace drinking with people
Group therapy
Hospitalization may be needed for detoxification and
 in case of delirium tremens

---

identify elderly alcoholics; if identified, the elderly patient is less likely to be referred; the elderly are less likely to be accepted into treatment programs.[19] The first step in treatment is recognition. One study found that the diagnosis may be missed in three out of four elderly hospital patients with alcohol dependence.[3] The essential principle of treatment is abstinence; controlled drinking is not recommended. Many successful modalities redirect the dependency from the alcohol onto others: "Replace drinking with people." Group therapy is the choice in most situations, including situations involving the elderly. Therapy may require more time in elders. Late- and early-onset alcoholism do not appear to differ substantially in terms of treatment. Disulfiram (Antabuse, aversion therapy) is limited in the elderly because of cardiovascular complications.

> *First detect the alcoholism; then "replace drinking with people" and look for reversible factors.*

Initial treatment may require hospitalization for drinking control or detoxification. Delirium tremens is a significant disease with known mortality. Alcohol withdrawal states are just as common in the elderly; some evidence exists that they exhibit more severe initial withdrawal.

Self-help groups for family members (Alanon for spouses; Alateen for children; and ACOA for adult children of alcoholics) are important, since a family-centered approach is universally recommended.

Studies on the efficacy of alcohol treatment include data from alcoholism treatment facilities that indicate that clients who seek, or achieve, reduced or moderate drinking tend to have consumed less alcohol, have fewer lifetime alcohol problems, and be more socially stable. Successful community-dwelling abstainers reported more drink-related problems and higher consumption. Community quitters were more likely to drink to reduce negative effects, whereas other drinkers drank for salutary reasons during evenings out and in family settings.[17]

> *Frail old alcoholics often have a friend or family member supplying the alcohol: they must be stopped.*

It is often thought that older alcoholics are more resistant to treatment, yet, using 6 months of sobriety as the definition of success, subjects over 60 do at least as well as 20- to 60-year-old subjects.[14] Early- and late-onset alcoholism treatment compliance was similarly high in elders.[8]

Current debate focuses on the value of an elderly-specific milieu. Advantages could include the management of associated medical problems. Management of alcoholism involves effective treatment of individuals, controlled availability and advertising, and control by price and tax, as well as health and safety warning labels.[21]

SUMMARY

Although alcoholism is common and impairing in elders and underrecognized and undertreated by the health care system, elderly alcoholics are at least as treatable, probably more so, as younger alcoholics.[22]

POSTTEST

Select the single best answer:
1. The diagnosis and treatment of alcohol dependency is best facilitated by using the model that defines alcoholism as a:
   a. Moral issue
   b. Psychological issue
   c. Disease
   d. Habit
   e. Response to social stresses

2. All of the following are patterns of alcoholism except:
   a. Resolved
   b. Chronic
   c. Late onset
   d. Reactive
   e. Intermittent

REFERENCES

1. Chafetz M: Alcoholism criteria: an important step, *Am J Psychiatry* 129:214-215, 1972.
2. Goodwin D: Commentary on defining alcoholism and taking stands, *J Clin Psychiatry* 43:394-395, 1982.
3. Beresford T et al: Alcoholism and aging in the general hospital, *Psychosomatics* 29:61-72, 1988.
4. Scott R, Mitchell M: Aging, alcohol and the liver, *J Am Geriatr Soc* 36:255-265, 1988.
5. Blose I: The relationship of alcohol to aging and the elderly, *Alcohol Clin Exp Res* 2:17-21, 1978.
6. Myers J, Weismann M, Tishler G et al: Six month prevalence of psychiatric disorders in three communities: 1980 to 1982, *Arch Gen Psychiatry* 41:955-967, 1984.
7. Schuckit M: A clinical review of alcohol, alcoholism, and the elderly patient, *J Clin Psychiatry* 43:396-399, 1982.
8. Hurt R et al: Alcoholism in elderly persons: medical aspects and prognosis of 216 inpatients, *Mayo Clin Proc* 63:753-760, 1988.
9. Graham K: Identifying and measuring alcohol abuse among the elderly: serious problems with existing instrumentation, *J Stud Alcohol* 47:322-326, 1986.
10. Ewing J: Detecting alcoholism: the CAGE questionnaire, *JAMA* 252:510-516, 1989.
11. Moran M, Naughton B, Hughes S: Screening elderly veterans for alcoholism, *J Gen Intern Med* 5:361-364, 1990.
12. Willibring M et al: Alcoholism screening in the elderly, *J Am Geriatr Soc* 35:864-869, 1987.
13. Blow FC et al: The Michigan Alcoholism Screening Test—Geriatric Version (MAST-G): a new elderly-specific screening instrument, *Alcohol Clin Exp Res* 16(2):372, 1992.
14. Wolin S, Bennett L, Noonan D: Family rituals and the recurrence of alcoholism over generations, *Am J Psychiatry* 136:589-593, 1979.
15. Tobias C et al: Alcoholism in the elderly, *Postgrad Med* 86:67-79, 1989.
16. Pottenger M et al: The frequency and prevalence of depressive symptoms in the alcohol abuser, *J Nerv Ment Dis* 166:562-570, 1978.
17. Felson D et al: Alcohol consumption and hip fracture, the Framingham study, *Am J Epidemiol* 128:1102-1110, 1988.
18. Haugland S: Alcoholism and other dependencies, *Primary Care* 16:411-429, 1989.
19. Curtis J et al: Characteristics, diagnosis and treatment of alcoholism in elderly patients, *J Am Geriatr Soc* 37:310-316, 1989.
20. Hermos J et al: Predictors of reduction and cessation of drinking in community dwelling men; results from the normative aging study, *J Stud Alcohol* 49:363-368, 1989.
21. Prevention in perspective: a statement of the National Association of State Alcohol and Drug Abuse, Directors and the National Prevention Network, Washington, DC, 1989.
22. Council on Scientific Affairs, American Medical Association: Alcoholism in the elderly, *JAMA* 275(10):797-801, 1996.

PRETEST ANSWERS
1. e
2. e

POSTTEST ANSWERS
1. c
2. a

CHAPTER 26

Driving

J. CHRISTOPHER HOUGH and JEAN M. THIELE

OBJECTIVES

On completion of this chapter, the reader will be able to:

1. Describe those components of the medical evaluation that are applicable to assessing driving capacity.

2. Understand the resources and roles of other professionals who can assist in evaluating driving abilities of older patients.

PRETEST

1. The reason that older drivers tend to have fewer absolute numbers of accidents than younger drivers is:
   a. They drive more miles than do younger drivers.
   b. They are always slower and safer than younger drivers.
   c. They drink and drive less than younger drivers.
   d. They often limit their driving.

2. The factor that most influences driving abilities with advancing age is:
   a. Visual acuity
   b. Knowledge of the rules of the road
   c. Coordination of steering or transmission
   d. Reaction time

Questions about the driving ability of elderly patients are frequently presented to primary health care providers. The goal is to screen elderly drivers, determine which drivers are at high risk for motor vehicle accidents, and make recommendations for preserving the independence of the older driver, while protecting others in society.

▼ ANNA FORD (Part I)

Anna Ford's daughter calls your office about her 85-year-old mother's declining health. Just recently she has noticed that her mother's vision and memory are deteriorating. Mrs. Ford can't read the street signs as well, and she became lost one time driving to her daughter's home, which is approximately 2 miles away, on familiar roads. About 2 weeks ago, she fell at night on her way to the bathroom, aggravating the arthritis in her hands, shoulders, hips, and knees. Up until this time she had fairly good pain relief from the NSAID that her physician prescribed for her over a year ago. She also has a history of hypertension, arteriosclerotic heart disease (ASHD), and osteoporosis. You suggest that she come in for a visit.

STUDY QUESTIONS

- How can driving capability be assessed?
- How should you respond to both the patient's and the family's needs?

In 1988 the 16.5 million drivers aged 65 and older accounted for 10% of all drivers in the United States. The percentage of older drivers is expected to increase substantially over the next six decades, approximately 28% by the year 2000 and 39% by the year 2050.[1]

The increase in elderly drivers is related to the increase in the elderly population. By the year 2020, 17% of the population will be elderly; there will be over 50 million elderly persons eligible to drive.[2]

Along with the increase of elderly drivers there is an increase in the number of motor vehicle accidents because driving skills deteriorate as the population ages. This increase is related to the prevalence of dementia, loss of vision, number of drivers who have not received formal driver's education, psychomotor slowing, decrease in musculoskeletal stability, endurance, coordination, polypharmacy, and multiple chronic medical conditions affecting attention. These changes, coupled with the desire to maintain driving skills for continued independence, cause the elderly to adapt by driving fewer miles, driving during daylight hours, and avoiding rush hour traffic. Unfortunately, motor vehicle accidents continue to be an important cause of injuries in the elderly population. The percent of accidents increases in the elderly population after age 60. Although older drivers drive fewer miles compared with younger drivers, the number of crash-related injuries and deaths per million drivers increases after age 60.[6] Crashes and violations in the elderly population seem to reflect errors of inattention, failure to yield, difficulty maneuvering, and driving too slowly.[5] Data from 1986 indicate that crashes were the leading cause of accidental death in older persons up to age 78 and second only to falls in persons aged 79 and older.[6]

Understanding an elderly individual's potential driving difficulties involves understanding the skills involved in driving and how they can be affected by normal aging changes. Requirements for driving include: (1) cognitive capacity, with knowledge of road regulations, how to operate a motor vehicle, and how to arrive at a certain destination; (2) sensory capacity, with visual acuity and hearing ability; (3) motor function, with an intact musculoskeletal system and manual dexterity; (4) neuromuscular capacity, with strength, coordination, and reaction time; and (5) skills to integrate the above activities simultaneously in order to drive safely.[7]

Changes of aging that affect driving ability include changes in vision and hearing, mental capacity, musculoskeletal conditions, and reaction time. Normal vision changes that occur with aging are categorized into physical, optical, and neuroanatomical changes. The physical changes include cataracts, macular degeneration, glaucoma, and diabetic retinopathy. The above conditions affect both central and peripheral vision. Central vision determines acuity, contrast, sensitivity, and color discriminations, and peripheral vision determines light sensitivity in certain areas of visual fields. It is estimated that 19% of adults ages 65 to 75 have at least one of the changes, and 50% of adults over the age of 75 have one of these changes.[8]

> *The primary care physician has a duty to society to consider driving ability when any potential impairment to driving skills is defined.*

Optical changes include a decrease in the retinal illumination. For example, in darkness the pupil in a young adult dilates to allow more light in, but in old age the pupil remains relatively constricted. Therefore the elderly have difficulty with night driving. In addition, there is increased light scattering in the elderly eye that causes a reduction in the contrast of a retinal image, making the elderly more susceptible to glare problems in driving. Finally, the elderly have a reduced ability to accommodate. Corrective lenses prescribed for near vision are usually targeted to improve vision for the usual reading distance, about 40 cm.[8] Unfortunately, the dashboard in most motor vehicles is greater than 40 cm from the eye, so that the instruments on the dashboard appear to be out of focus. Neuroanatomical changes also occur, but further research is needed to determine how loss of photoreceptors and retinal ganglion cells affects driving in the elderly.

Older adults may have problems with tasks involving peripheral vision or useful field of vision. Useful field of vision is defined as a spatial area where an individual can be rapidly alert to visual stimuli.[9] Sensory function as it pertains to driving can be evaluated by objective measurement of depth perception, color vision, dynamic visual acuity, night vision, glare recovery, ability to change from near to far vision, and awareness of the entire visual field. Further research is needed to determine if deterioration in one or all of the above visual functions places an individual at greater risk for a motor vehicle accident.

Several studies sponsored by state and federal agencies have examined the relationship between vision and crashes in older adults.[8] Statistical differences in the relationship between vision and the number of crashes were found, but correlations were weak. Such studies provide limited information because of their use of the number of crashes as a measure of driving performance; crash data are subjectively reported. Also, most drivers self-impose driving restrictions, which decreases the number of accidents, and not all sensory functions used in safe driving are included in such studies, since only static and peripheral vision are tested.

The second component of sensory function is the ability to hear. Research is limited as to how hearing impairment can increase an individual's risk for motor crashes. Clinically, hearing should be evaluated to determine if a driver can detect a malfunction in the motor vehicle and if the driver is able to hear directions accurately from a passenger who is assisting with navigation.

Motor capacity includes four key components: (1) muscle strength, (2) range of motion of extremities, (3) trunk and neck mobility, and (4) proprioception.[9] All of these can be affected by the common changes of aging of the musculoskeletal system. Arthritis is present in 50% of the elderly population and can affect the driving ability when pain produces hesitancy in movement and restrictions in the range of motion of joints used in driving. Motor functions necessary for turning a steering wheel include cervical spine rotation, shoulder range of motion, and grip. Muscle strength is rarely a major influence in driving because of availability of automatic transmissions and power steering. Arthritis affecting grip strength and the wrist is an important factor in an older person's ability to turn the steering wheel.

Cognitive function is defined as a higher level of cortical functioning that involves short-term and long-term memory, the capacity to cope with day-to-day living situations, the correct use of social skills, and the control of emotional reactions. The normal changes of aging include delayed memory and decrease in reaction time when making multiple decisions. These have little effect on the increased risk of motor vehicle crashes: elderly without dementia continue to have fewer crashes than elderly with moderate and severe dementia. Dementia, however, poses a great threat to society in that the prevalence of dementia increases with age.[10] Cognitive function as it relates to driving includes memory and attention, systematic scanning of the environment, other visuospatial skills, verbal processing, decision making, and problem solving. Memory related to driving includes knowledge of vehicle operation and knowledge of how to get to a destination. Attentional demands include monitoring traffic, the road, weather conditions, and pedestrians. Visuospatial skills include systematically scanning the environment both inside and outside of the vehicle, judging distances and speed, and locating appropriate controls to maneuver the vehicle.

> *Patients with mild dementia may be able to drive quite safely, but only if they do not have visuospatial impairments (which can easily be tested). If the dementia becomes more severe, they must give up driving.*

Some studies regarding the effects of dementia on driving safety conclude that driving privileges should not be revoked on the evidence of dementia alone. Patients with mild dementia did not have higher motor vehicle accident rates than drivers without cognitive impairment. But as the dementia becomes more severe, the number of motor vehicle accidents increases dramatically. However, data from caregivers are subjective and further research is needed on the incidence of motor vehicle accidents.[11-13]

Reaction time is defined as the time from the presentation of the stimulus until the initiation of a motor response. Thus there is an afferent sensory component and a central processing component. The afferent sensory component includes stimulus detection, encoding, and transmission. The central processing component includes initiation and completion of a response movement. In the elderly, complex reaction time—defined as two or more stimuli at a time and two or more responses—compared to simple reaction time—one stimulus and one response—is increased. This has a negative effect on an elderly person's ability to drive safely because decisions and judgments take longer to process; for example, a decision about turning to avoid another car needs to be made without delay. Fortunately, the elderly usually make adaptations to their driving times by avoiding rush hour and highway driving.

In summary, the decision to restrict an individual's driving involves a comprehensive sensory, mental, functional, and psychomotor assessment and the decision to restrict driving privileges cannot be made because of a deficit in only one area. The goal of the evaluation should be, if possible, to maintain or improve the mobility and independence of the older driver, thus continuing the ability to socialize and conduct basic activities such as shopping and physician appointments.

When evaluating an elderly driver, assessment is ideally done by a team of health care providers such as a physician, nurse practitioner, physician's assistant, occupational and physical therapist, and social worker in combination with government officials, including the State Legislative Board and Department of Motor Vehicles. The goal is to identify the medical conditions that impair driving, determine the need for continued driving, explain alternatives to driving, and explain the treatment of medical and functional conditions that pose a threat to driving capability.[14] The goals of government agencies are to establish rules governing licensure to operate a motor vehicle, issue a license under these rules, and determine if the elderly driver is safe.

ROLES AND RESPONSIBILITIES OF THE PHYSICIAN

The responsibility of the physician is to assess, diagnose, and if possible, treat the conditions that are a threat to the patient's driving. Medical conditions that may increase the risk of safe driving can be classified into two groups: (1) the physiological changes associated with

normal aging, and (2) the changes that can occur with diseases and conditions that are common in the elderly (Box 26-1).[14] Another role of the physician is to be aware of the state regulations regarding medical conditions and their affect on driving (e.g., individuals with seizure disorders cannot drive for 6 months) and, if necessary, report the medical condition to the motor vehicle department. The state is then responsible for determining whether the risk is high enough to warrant revoking the driving privilege.

In a primary care practice the physician can obtain pertinent information from the history and physical examination. Before beginning, steps should be taken to reassure patients that the information collected is only for the purposes of the patient's health and safety. The patient should also be aware that the physician is required by state law to comply with respect to specific requirements. These reassurances are in accord with the principle of confidentiality in the physician-patient relationship and should not be violated except as specified by law or when the danger is so overwhelming that the safety of others is imminently jeopardized. In addition to the history and physical examination, the interview should include a driving questionnaire (Box 26-2).[14]

BOX 26-1
Medical Conditions That May Increase the Risk of Unsafe Driving

Age-Related Physiological Changes
Decreased vision
  Static visual acuity
  Dynamic visual acuity
  Temporal fields
  Resistance to glare
  Low luminescence vision
Decreased reaction time
Hearing loss

Diseases and Disorders Common in Older Persons
Cardiovascular and pulmonary diseases
Ischemic heart disease
Arrhythmias
Sleep apnea
Chronic lung disease with hypoxia
Diabetes mellitus
Neurological diseases
  Alzheimer's disease and other cognitive impairment
  Parkinson's disease
  Stroke
  Neuropathies
  Seizures
Polypharmacy
Arthritis
Alcohol use

> **BOX 26-2**
> *Items From the Patient History Relevant to the Older Driver*
>
> 1. How many days did you drive last week?
> 2. Do you drive at night?
> 3. Do you drive on the freeway?
> 4. What essential errands do you drive for?
> 5. Have you changed your driving habits in the past year?
> 6. Have you had accidents or "near-misses" in the past year? _____ If so, how many?
> 7. Do you have any of the following:
>   _____ Visual loss
>   _____ Hearing loss
>   _____ Memory problems
>   _____ Arthritis
>   _____ History of falling
> 8. What medications do you take?
> 9. How many alcoholic drinks did you take in the last week?

The physical examination should include conditions identified during the health history. In particular it should include assessment of vision using Snellen's eye chart. A hearing test can be done by using the whisper test or an audioscope to test for loss of high and low pitches. Memory, attention, visuospatial skills, verbal processing, decision making, and problem solving can be screened by using, for example, the Mini-Mental Status Exam, which objectively screens for deficits in orientation, short-term and long-term memory, attention, visuospatial skills, verbal processing, and ability to follow simple commands. Examination of the musculoskeletal system should include range of motion in the neck, shoulders, wrist, hips, trunk, knees, ankles, and feet. Grip strength should be tested. Gait should be assessed for a hesitancy in step that may cause difficulty when braking and for coordination and balance to assess possibility of driving. Family, friends, or community resources available should be identified if the elderly driver can no longer drive safely. Because giving up driving is difficult, the social worker may be asked to counsel the patient through this loss of independence. An ophthalmologist

may be able to provide a detailed assessment of specific visual problems. Aspects of vision other than static visual acuity can then be tested. Static visual acuity is not a complete measurement of how driving is affected by vision. Other useful tests include acuity under reduced illumination, dynamic visual acuity, visual fields contrast sensitivity, and glare resistance.

The occupational therapist is useful in determining the driving capabilities of patients who have had strokes, visual impairments, and arthritis; and the therapist can also assess strength, range of motion, and sitting balance. Once a complete assessment has been conducted and a road test has been taken, ways for disabled drivers to compensate for their impairment or modify their vehicles can be recommended. Computer-simulated road tests have been used, but research has shown that the best way to identify safe driving skills is by testing actual driving. A neuropsychologist may be used for detailed testing of cognition in some cases.

Once recommendations have been received from other professionals, the physician should meet with the patient and family to talk openly about driving skills and available alternatives.

▼ ANNA FORD (Part II)

Mrs. Ford reluctantly arrives at your office with her daughter for her visit. She does not know why she needs this examination and states that her vision and memory are perfectly fine. She does admit having some difficulty driving because her joints are more painful since her recent fall. A history of medical conditions that may reduce the safety of driving is identified: arthritis and mild dementia. Mrs. Ford has no evidence of cardiovascular impairment, diabetes, stroke, polypharmacy, or alcohol use. Her driving history reveals difficulty driving at night, in the rain, and in fog. She drives about four times a week and denies having any accidents in the past year. Her medications include hydrochlorothiazide-triamterene (Dyazide) for hypertension, salsalate (Disalcid) for arthritis, and conjugated estrogens (Premarin) and calcium for osteoporosis. Physical examination reveals mild dementia and decreasing visual acuity. Finally, referrals are made to the Secretary of State's office to have a road test and to an occupational therapist to recommend any adaptive devices for Mrs. Ford's car until her arthritic pain is decreased.

POSTTEST

1. Which of the following changes has *not* been shown to reduce driving capability?
   a. Abnormalities of the feet
   b. Mild dementia
   c. Inability to walk several blocks
   d. Poor design copying or mental status tests

2. Which one of the following professionals does not have a role in determining a patient's ability to drive?
   a. Occupational therapist
   b. Ophthalmologist
   c. Neuropsychologist
   d. Physical therapist
   e. Dietitian

REFERENCES

1. Malfetti J, ed: Drivers 55 plus, Falls Church, Va, 1985, AAA Foundation for Traffic Safety. In Persson FD: The elderly driver: deciding when to stop, *Gerontologist* 33(1):88-91.
2. Retchin SM, Anapolle J: An overview of the older drivers, *Clin Geriatr Med* 9(2):279-296, 1993.
3. Katz S et al: Active life expectancy, *N Engl J Med* 309(20):1218-1224, 1983.
4. Reuben DB, Silliman RA, Traines M: The aging driver: medicine policy and ethics, *J Am Geriatr Soc* 36:1135-1142, 1988.
5. Graca J: Driving and aging, *Clin Geriatr Med* 2:583, 1986.
6. National Safety Council: *Accident facts, 1989,* Chicago, 1989, The Council.
7. Koepsell TD et al: Medical conditions and motor vehicle collision injuries in older adults, *JAGS* 42:695-700, 1994.
8. Owsley C, Bill K: Assessing visual function in the older driver, *Clin Geriatr Med* 9(2):389-401, 1993.
9. Marottoli RA, Drickamor MA: Psychomotor mobility and the elderly driver, *Clin Geriatr Med* 9(2):403-411, May 1993.
10. US Congress, Office of Technology Assessment: *Losing a million minds: confronting the tragedy of Alzheimer's disease and other dementias,* Washington, DC, 1987, US Government Printing Office.
11. Hunt L et al: Driving performance in persons with mild senile dementia of the Alzheimer type, *JAGS* 47(7):747-753, 1993.
12. Dubinsky RM et al: Driving in Alzheimer's disease, *JAGS* 40:1112-1116, 1992.
13. Drachman DA, Sweaner JM: Driving & Alzheimer's disease: the risk of crashes, *Neurology* 43:2448-2456, 1993.
14. Reuben DB: Assessment of older drivers, *Clin Geriatr Med* 9(2):449-459, 1993.
15. Marottoili RA et al: Predictors of automobile crashes and moving violations among elderly drivers, *Ann Intern Med* 121:842-846, 1994.

PRETEST ANSWERS

1. d
2. a

POSTTEST ANSWERS

1. b
2. e

CHAPTER 27

Vision

JOHN M. HEATH and JOHN A. HOEPNER

OBJECTIVES

On completion of this chapter, the reader will be able to:

1. Understand the physiological factors of ocular aging that affect visual acuity.

2. Describe the three leading ocular diseases and the visual effects of systemic illnesses that lead to decreased visual function in the elderly.

3. Appreciate the curative and rehabilitative strategies applicable by health care professionals that can improve and preserve visual function.

PRETEST

1. The functional visual changes seen with glaucoma can include:
   a. Increased volume of tears
   b. Increased glare and blurring with bright light
   c. Decreased peripheral visual fields
   d. Localized visual field defects in central vision

2. Strategies to improve the reading ability of patients with macular degeneration may include:
   a. Eye drops that reduce intraocular pressure
   b. Magnification of printed materials
   c. Use of systemic corticosteroids in high doses
   d. Tinting the corrective lenses

Changes in visual function with aging go beyond the need for eyeglass prescription. Frequently the physiological ocular changes that accompany aging interact with environmental or disease factors to cause visual impairment. Three eye diseases have high prevalence in the elderly: glaucoma, cataracts, and macular degeneration. In addition, the effects of systemic disease on the eye can cause visual impairment. Opportunities for the primary care physician to recognize such conditions and offer interventions and referrals that can improve visual function can significantly contribute to the overall health of older patients.

▼ BRENDA RUSSELL (Part I)

Brenda Russell, a 72-year-old widow, mentions to you during a routine follow-up appointment for hypertension that she has noted increasing problems reading the label on the bottle of antihypertensive pills. On further questioning she reports a fuzziness in her vision when driving at night and facing headlights or when walking in bright sunlight. She does not have double vision, headache, or pain on either blinking or eye movement. She has not recently changed her glasses, which she uses because of long-standing nearsightedness. The reading problem seems to be primarily in the right eye, although some blurring is present when either eye is used in bright light.

STUDY QUESTIONS

- *What factors should be assessed in the office before referral for professional ophthalmologic assessment?*
- *Are the two complaints of fuzzy bright light vision and monocular reading difficulties likely to be related to the same cause?*

VISUAL IMPAIRMENT IN AGING

Visual impairment is the most common sensory problem faced by the elderly. Prevalence data accumulated from the National Health Interview study reveals that 12.8% of the elderly reported some vision problems, and this number increased to over 25% for those aged 85 years

---

> **BOX 27-1**
> *Physiological Changes in the Aging Eye*
>
> Decreased tear viscosity
> Increasing eyelid laxity
> Decreased color sensitivity
> Decreased light sensitivity
> Impaired lens accommodation

and older, 12% of whom were legally blind.[1] Perhaps the most common problem with aging and visual acuity is refraction. Almost 95% of those surveyed over age 65 years either wore glasses or reported needing glasses or some form of corrective lenses to improve acuity. However, only 45% of those over age 85 years reported that their glasses corrected all of their visual problems.

AGING CHANGES IN OCULAR FUNCTION

The aging process itself has a number of effects on the eye, some of which have variable effects on vision.[2] Most of these factors are considered physiological changes of the aging eye and are presented in Box 27-1.

The almost universal impairment in the accommodation capability of older persons is caused primarily by an increase in the density and inelasticity of the lens. Decreased contrast sensitivity and increased susceptibility to glare also occur frequently and impair reading, driving, and detailed near vision. Color vision is generally well preserved, although the progressive yellowing of the lens over time may interfere with blue-green vision.

Interaction of such normal aging changes with medication effects or with ocular manifestations of systemic illness results in a net decrease in visual function. For example, an older individual with mild eyelid laxity and decreased tear production and viscosity may have relatively intact vision until the drying effects of anticholinergic medication impair blinking. When combined with the decreased eyelid contact and traumatic periorbital soft tissue swelling from a fall, for example, this could result in significant corneal drying and abrasions. Interventions to improve vision in such cases can include supplementing tear production and ensuring complete eyelid closure during sleep or at times of exposure to dust or foreign particles.[3] If lid laxity is marked, surgical tightening may be necessary to protect the cornea.

Because of the progressive narrowing of the pupil's diameter and reduced translucency of the lens with advancing age, increasing the quantity of light striking the retina by increasing lighting intensity in the living environment can improve acuity.[4] This is especially important in areas of the home where clear vision is required, such as on stairs, on uneven flooring, near reading chairs, and in the bathroom. Enhancing the visual contrast between objects of different depths within a single visual field may also help. This is best accomplished by establishing marked color differences between an object and its background. Examples might include putting bright adhesive tape on the top of a stair railing to enhance the contrast between it and the wall behind, or making a table edge or doorknob appear in dramatic visual contrast to the surrounding furnishings if it is used frequently for support during transfers.

> *Improving the intensity of lighting will improve visual acuity; enhancing light-dark contrast can help depth perception.*

OCULAR DISEASE IN OLD AGE

The primary care physician must be familiar with three principal ocular diseases because of their incidence in the elderly and their interaction with other medical problems: glaucoma, macular degeneration, and cataracts.

Glaucoma

Glaucoma is formally defined as a progressive optic neuropathy frequently associated with elevated intraocular pressure. The characteristic cupping on ophthalmoscopic examination is accompanied by progressive abnormalities of the visual field and is generally related to elevated eye pressure. The vast majority of cases of glaucoma develop slowly and are associated with a normal-appearing outflow track for the fluid, which is called simple or open-angle glaucoma. Abrupt increases in intraocular pressure can occur with obstruction of the vitreous outflow track through either a foreign body or obstruction during dilation of the pupil. Such closed-angle glaucoma attacks are painful and can be precipitated by the use of mydriatic eye drops or systemic anticholinergic medications; this requires urgent ophthalmological evaluation for possible iridectomy.

Therapeutic efforts for open-angle glaucoma focus primarily on reducing intraocular pressure to a level at which no further optic nerve damage occurs. This may vary from 12 to 25 mm Hg. The pressure is decreased by lowering the production of aqueous fluid or by increasing its outflow. Primary treatment is with eye drops. Major categories of myotic eye drops are β-blockers, parasympathomimetic drops (pilocarpine), epinephrine, and α-agonists. Systemic medications such as acetazolamide (Diamox) are occasionally indicated. If none of the above is effective in controlling intraocular pressure, surgical procedures can enhance the outflow of aqueous humor.

The visual loss associated with glaucoma is primarily a loss of peripheral visual field. Because the location of the field loss is somewhat variable, primary assistance is given by retraining the patient in common everyday activities. The most common visual defect of glaucoma results from a combination of myotics (usually pilocarpine) with early cataracts. The decreased size of the pupil combined with the cataract decreases the amount of light coming into the eye. Increased lighting is the most effective way of dealing with this decrease in available light. With early diagnosis and prompt treatment, the extent of visual loss can be reduced.

Cataracts

Cataracts are the most common ocular disease that occurs with aging. About 50% of persons over the age of 40 years show developing signs of lens clouding on detailed examination. The cause of most cases of acquired lens opacification is thought to be cumulative UV-B light exposure.[3] The degree to which the opacification distorts light or impedes it from striking the retina determines the extent of resultant visual impairment. Antioxidant therapy has been proposed as a means to help reduce or prevent some lens opacification, but no medical therapies for cataracts have been established. As excessive bending of light passing through the cataract occurs, the blue wavelength light frequencies are most distorted. Thus some improvement in vision can occur through the use of yellow-tinted filters, which reduce the blue components of light entering the eye, applied to corrective lenses.

The need for surgery should be based on function rather than the density, location, or type of cataract. When cataracts interfere with function to a degree that it bothers the patient, cataract surgery is indicated. The indications for surgery vary depending on the patient's age, physical and mental well-being, and daily activities.

Macular Degeneration

Macular degeneration is perhaps the least understood of these ocular diseases.[5] The overall prevalence of the condition is thought to be about 30% at age 75 years or older, although only 10% of individuals with macular degeneration have significant functional visual loss. Since the macula is the area for central vision and provides the highest degree of visual resolution, deterioration of this portion of the retina leads to the loss of central vision. Deficits in form recognition and light sensitivity result.

Macular degeneration is divided into two groups, wet and dry. Dry macular degeneration is the most common. It is manifested by a progressive loss of retinal and pigment epithelium and a gradually increasing central blind spot. This form is not treatable. Wet macular degeneration occurs because of the accumulation of subretinal blood or exudate. This usually results because of subretinal neovascularization. If the condition is detected early and does not occur in the fovea, laser photocoagulation therapy is possible.

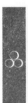

Laser photocoagulation can treat "wet" macular degeneration and diabetic neovascularization, providing opportunities to treat situations that were previously untreatable.

Patients with macular degeneration are often taught to self-monitor their central vision. One common method involves use of Amsler's chart, a small printed grid of straight, intersecting lines with a central focus point. A monocular appearance of increasing waves or curves in sections of the grid can indicate possible deteriorating macular vision. If exudative or wet macular degeneration is identified, laser photocoagulation can reduce the chances of retinal detachment. Unfortunately, 80% to 90% of cases are dry macular degeneration and thus are not surgically treatable. Some recent literature suggests that zinc supplementation combined with other antioxidants may be helpful.[6]

Visual rehabilitative efforts in macular degeneration generally involve attempts to magnify the area of central vision so that the impact of the actual field defect can be minimized. Instead of inability to see an entire word, the defect can be reduced by magnification to only the middle letter or two. Central visual field magnification can be accomplished with both hand-held ocular lenses and video enlargement or microfilm reading systems. Another method is increased field illumination. (See Box 27-2.)

DIABETES MELLITUS AND THE EYE

Diabetic eye changes are the leading cause of blindness in the adult population and almost always occur after the diagnosis of diabetes mellitus has been long established. Changes are generally found in the retina and are grouped into initial microvasculature degenerative changes (small hemorrhages and aneurysms) and the subsequent proliferative changes of neovascularization. These latter changes can often result in greater hemorrhage from fragile new blood vessels and can be treated with laser photocoagulation; this also results in ablation of the underlying retina. Close monitoring of diabetics is critical to further decrease the visual loss resulting from

BOX 27-2
Components of Low Vision Rehabilitation

Educate the patient (and family) about visual loss and compensation.
Refract for optimal near and far vision acuity.
Decrease the impact of peripheral visual field losses through prisms, mirrors, and reorientation of materials into the functional visual field.
Decrease the impact of central visual field loss through magnification systems.
Optimize lighting intensity and contrast sensitivity.
Organize reading aids.
Enhance use of nonoptical sources of information.

diabetic retinopathy. In some instances, decreased central vision is indicative of progression of diabetic retinopathy; however, in the majority of cases macular edema and neovascular change outside the macula can occur without causing any visual symptoms. Routine evaluation is the only way of detecting this at an early, treatable stage.

VASCULAR DISEASE AND THE EYE

Vascular changes in the eye are of two types. Of the typical atherosclerotic changes that affect all parts of the body, the most common ocular manifestation is transient monocular decreased acuity, or amaurosis fugax. This is often indicative of carotid disease. If an isolated carotid lesion is diagnosed based on visual symptoms, it is often surgically treatable.

The other type of vascular change and the most common treatable form of ocular vascular disease in the elderly is temporal arteritis. This occurs in individuals over age 50 and is often associated with symptoms of polymyalgia rheumatica. Temporal artery tenderness, jaw claudication, muscle soreness, and malaise often occur before visual loss. An elevated erythrocyte sedimentation rate is the most consistent laboratory finding. Once visual loss occurs, therapy is usually not effective in treating the involved eye. Diagnosis is made by noting typical signs and symptoms, high sedimentation rate, and positive temporal artery biopsy. Treatment with high dose-corticosteroids is essential to prevent bilateral visual loss. A high degree of suspicion is necessary to avoid missing this diagnosis.

▼ *BRENDA RUSSELL (Part II)*
Eye examination of Mrs. Russell in your office identifies small but equally reactive pupils and intact extraocular motions. Funduscopic examination is limited by small undilated pupils and seemingly poor light transmission through the lenses, but no gross retinal hemorrhages or large exudates are identified

in either fundus. While Mrs. Russell's reading and distant visual acuity is 20/40 OU (each eye) with her corrective lenses in place, she does have some difficulty identifying letters on near vision testing with the central vision of the right eye. Informal assessment of depth perception shows that she is able to consistently touch the closer of two objects in the same visual field. Referral for formal ophthalmological assessment is made. Ophthalmological examination with pupil dilatation reveals bilateral lens clouding from early cataract development, without focal areas of density. Surgical cataract removal is not recommended at present. Visual acuity is slightly improved by a slight change in refraction. Dry macular degeneration of the right eye is also identified. Intraocular pressures are normal bilaterally and a small central visual field defect is noted in the right eye, corresponding to the diagnosis of macular degeneration.

CASE DISCUSSION

A small change in refraction in Mrs. Russell's lenses may improve her complaint of blurring in bright lights. She needs to be instructed about self-monitoring for changes in the right eye central visual defect that could indicate progression of the macular degeneration. If the progression were found to be of the wet variety, immediate referral for possible laser therapy would be essential. Mrs. Russell may also benefit from a low vision assessment, which might lead to recommendations for magnification of reading materials and enhanced home lighting. She should limit her nighttime driving. Her blood pressure medication instructions can be printed in large type on a separate sheet by her pharmacist.

POSTTEST

1. The need for increased lighting intensity for patients with glaucoma is because:
   a. Intraocular pressure decreases with age.
   b. There is increased laxity of the eyelid with age.
   c. Myotic eye drops decrease the amount of light entering the eye.
   d. Wet macular degeneration occurs symmetrically in both eyes.

2. Vision rehabilitation in old age can include all except:
   a. Magnification systems for macular degeneration
   b. Increased lighting for glaucoma patients taking myotics
   c. Anticholinergic medication to decrease the excess tear formation associated with normal aging
   d. Implantation of intraocular lenses after cataract extraction

REFERENCES

1. Kovar MG: Aging in the eighties, Preliminary data from the supplement on aging to the National Health Interview Survey, United States, Jan-June 1984, *Advance data from vital and health statistics,* No 115, DHHS Publication No (PHS) 86-1250, Hyattsville, Md, 1986, Public Health Service.
2. Adams AJ et al: Visual acuity changes with age: some new perspectives, *Am J Optom Physiol Ophthalmol* 65:403-406, 1988.
3. West SK: Daylight, diet, and age-related cataract, *Optom Vis Sci* 70(11):869-872, 1993.
4. Wasson JH et al: The prescription of assistive devices for the elderly, *J Gen Intern Med* 5:46-54, 1990.
5. Kashani AA: Pathogenesis of age-related macular degeneration: embryologic concept, *Ann Ophthalmol* 22:246-248, 1990.

PRETEST ANSWERS
1. c
2. b

POSTTEST ANSWERS
1. c
2. c

CHAPTER 28

Hearing

JOHN M. HEATH and HELEN M. WATERS

OBJECTIVES

Upon completion of this chapter, the reader will be able to:

1. Define the common causes of conductive and sensorineural hearing loss and the metabolic causes of hearing loss in older age.

2. Initiate a hearing assessment screening in preparation for formal audiometric referral.

3. Describe the distinctions among common methods of amplification.

PRETEST

1. Presbycusis, the leading form of hearing impairment in old age, is characterized by:
   a. Sensory nerve damage of cranial nerve VIII
   b. External ear wax impaction
   c. Progressive, high-frequency symmetrical sensorineural hearing loss
   d. Otosclerosis of the middle ear bony structures

2. Age-related hearing impairment is best improved through:
   a. Using a higher frequency in spoken communication
   b. Using a hearing aid alone
   c. A combined amplification and nonverbal approach
   d. Teaching sign language early

Hearing loss is extremely common in old age; it is socially isolating and can make the patient appear and feel cognitively impaired. It is the most unrecognized, yet correctable, sensory impairment in geriatric medicine. Many elderly patients seen in primary care are not aware of their hearing loss or are reluctant to report their impairment. Hearing difficulty can impede both the delivery of medical care and the overall quality of life. Early recognition, efficient efforts to improve hearing, and other steps to improve communication are essential. Specialized help is often indicated.

▼ ED AUSTIN (Part I)

Mr. Austin is a 68-year-old man referred to your office for authorization of an audiology evaluation by the occupational health office at his workplace. His health insurance coverage required a preauthorization from his primary care physician before seeking audiological services. He has been preparing for retirement by gradually working fewer hours. He is employed as a maintenance specialist for the printing presses of a small newspaper and is spending more time providing child care for his grandchildren. His decreased hearing was first noted at home by family members who then encouraged him to speak with the occupational health officer at the job site. He reports that his hearing is worst with the grandchildren and that the hearing in his right ear seems more impaired than the hearing in his left ear. There has been no dizziness, ringing, or vertigo, although hearing sensitivity does worsen at the end of his workday. His overall medical history is otherwise good, and his only regular medication use is 1 g of aspirin taken after work because of chronic backache.

STUDY QUESTIONS

- *What factors may be contributing to hearing problems in this case?*
- *How can you assist with both the work and home concerns of his hearing problems?*

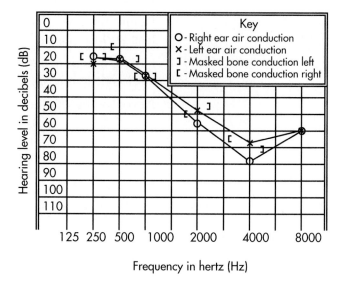

FIG. 28-1 Audiogram typical of presbycusis.

HEARING LOSS IN NORMAL AGING

The prevalence of self-reported hearing problems among community-dwelling elderly is 30%, with about 12% reporting either unilateral or bilateral deafness.[1] However, unlike visual impairment, which frequently becomes recognized when simple adaptive equipment such as glasses are addressed, hearing impairment frequently remains an unaddressed problem for many older persons. While approximately 65% of those aged 85 years report some hearing problem, only 16% have a hearing aid or other assistive listening device and only 8% actually use their aid or device. Evidence for pure age-associated effects on hearing comes from longitudinal studies, which follow the same individuals with various levels of hearing abilities over time. There appears to be a 10 dB reduction in hearing sensitivity per decade of life after age 60.

The best known overall age-associated change in hearing is described by the term presbycusis, literally meaning old man's hearing. The most characteristic feature is a decrease in perception of higher frequency tones. While this loss of high-frequency hearing can initially be improved with amplification, presbycusis generally progresses over time, regardless of the amplification. A lesser known but equally important characteristic of presbycusis is a decreased ability to focus on a desired sound by internally masking competing sounds (e.g., conversation in a restaurant). This feature of hearing sensitivity is sometimes termed "cocktail party hearing": the ability to pick out and follow one desired voice amid other sounds at equal or even greater volume. In presbycusis a disabling distortion of multiple sounds is heard, without an isolation of the desired voice or sound intended to be heard[2] (Fig. 28-1).

> *In presbycusis, there is both a reduced selectivity of hearing (the patient cannot pick out a conversation in a crowded room) and a loss of high frequencies (consonants are less audible, so words become only vowels).*

Strategies to assist the elderly patient with presbycusis have often been limited to amplification. But background noise should also be eliminated or decreased when direct verbal communication is attempted. Since lower frequency hearing is often better preserved than higher frequency hearing, the lowest comfortable tone should be used. This is often in conflict with the tendency to raise vocal pitch along with volume of speech. Shouting at persons with presbycusis instead of trying to talk with them incorporates a number of the worst communication features: higher pitch, vocal and facial distortion, and removing the context of the communicated message.

EAR DISEASES AND HEARING LOSS

Other types of hearing loss have been traditionally classified into conductive, sensorineural, and metabolic. In pure conductive hearing loss, air conduction is worse than bone conduction on audiometric testing. Causes of conduction loss can arise in both the external and middle ear. Cerumen impaction represents the most common external ear cause of conductive hearing loss and is a frequently overlooked problem in elderly people with hearing impairment (Fig. 28-2).

The most common middle ear conductive hearing loss in old age is related to otosclerosis, an idiopathic stiffening of the bone surrounding the cochlea. While amplification can assist with this hearing loss to a limited degree, surgical approaches that improve ossicle mobility have resulted in significant improvement.

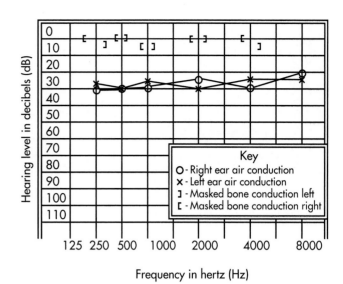

FIG. 28-2   Audiogram typical of mild conductive hearing loss.

Sensorineural hearing loss causes both air and bone conduction to be decreased, especially toward the higher frequencies. Gradual progressive sensorineural hearing loss, usually accompanied by tinnitus, is characteristic of neoplasms of the brainstem or the eighth cranial nerve and of long-term exposure to high-intensity noise. Sensorineural hearing loss may occur suddenly as a result of a vascular event within the inner ear or of medication effects. Sudden sensorineural hearing loss is also often accompanied by vestibular symptoms of vertigo, dizziness, and nystagmus.

Metabolic causes of hearing impairment can be from toxic medication effects or from endocrine diseases: thyroid, pancreatic, and adrenal. The prevalence of renal disease, diabetes mellitus, and hypertension is high in the elderly. Fig. 28-3 is an example of hearing loss secondary to high-intensity noise exposure.

A further type of hearing impairment is seen with auditory processing problems, reflecting higher brain level dysfunction. In these disorders, grouped under the term "central auditory processing disorders (CAPD)," speech discrimination rather than frequency perception seems to be the principal problem. Assessment for CAPD includes speech audiometry and pure-tone audiometry.

ASSESSMENT OF HEARING IMPAIRMENT

The first step in evaluating hearing impairment, after obtaining the history related to factors previously described, involves examination of the external ear canal. The importance of seeking and removing cerumen impactions cannot be overemphasized; it is by far the most common and most cost-effective means for improving hearing im-

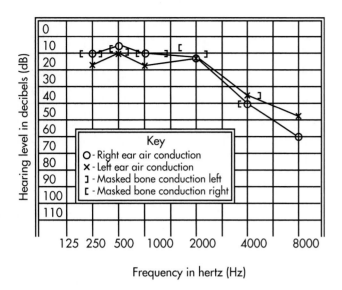

Key
O - Right ear air conduction
X - Left ear air conduction
] - Masked bone conduction left
[- Masked bone conduction right

FIG. 28-3 Audiogram typical of ototoxicity or noise induced hearing loss.

Table 28-1 Amplification Devices

	Hearing Aids	Listening Devices
Advantages	Discreet	Directional
	Adaptable for phone use or for specific frequencies	Loud amplification possible
	Cosmetically appealing	Relatively inexpensive
	Relatively low battery drain	
Disadvantages	Considerable manual dexterity required	Bulky
	Expensive	Rapid battery drain
	Custom fitting required	Visible in use

pairment in old age. Cerumen removal with either ear canal irrigation, often preceded by use of cerumen-dissolving drops, or manual (instrumental) removal is easily accomplished. Subsequent inspection of the anatomical landmarks of the tympanic membrane should be accompanied by screening assessment of hearing sensitivity to the spoken word. One means proposed to do this in a reproducible manner is through whisper testing.[5] After occluding the opposite ear and standing behind the patient to ensure that lipreading is not possible, the examiner says two series of numbers in both normal and whispered voice toward the tested ear both at close range and at arm's length distance. The patient is asked to repeat the numbers with each testing and with each ear. Past published work with such screening techniques has indicated that patients unable to repeat the number series whispered at about 2 feet may benefit from formal audiometric evaluation. An additional screening tool is the hand-held otoscope combined with a builtin audiometer that has a four-tone, three-frequency sound generator. Such screening tools can be used to recognize patients who need formal audiological evaluation.

> ✂ *Always look for wax, and always try a "whisper test" (or screen with an audiometric otoscope).*

HEARING REHABILITATION

Rehabilitative efforts directed at the hearing-impaired elderly have been grouped into two complementary strategies: amplification devices and nonverbal communication enhancement. Both are important for adequate communication between primary care physicians and their hearing-impaired patients. Hearing aids are the most commonly recognized means of amplification. A controlled study looking at the impact of providing hearing aids for hearing impaired elderly demonstrated significant improvement not only in the expected communication function but also in cognition and mood.[2] Hearing aids obviously require manual dexterity for correct use, and they also have limits as to their amplification capabilities. Table 28-1 presents some features and limitations of hearing aids.

Another method for amplification is provided through assistive listening devices, sometimes called pocket talkers. Unlike hearing aids, which are generally worn by hearing-impaired individuals (requiring their own control and manual dexterity to operate), assistive listening devices are set up by the person wishing to communicate. They may involve hard-wired systems with wireless FM-band, low-frequency radio transmitters at a sound source (e.g., a speaker's podium in a church or auditorium) broadcasting to an earpiece receiver-amplifier unit, or portable, hand-held units with attached microphone and earpiece. These latter audio amplifier units are particularly well suited for health care professionals' communication with the hearing-impaired elderly. Often it is in the setting of acute health care delivery that older patients have misplaced or forgotten their own hearing aids. These devices can save the voice and patience of the health care provider and allow respectful and private interactions to take place. Cochlear implantation of electrode systems, the latest form of surgical intervention systems, may benefit selected patients.

> ✂ *Some patients hear better with their teeth in or their glasses on.*

Nonverbal communication strategies rely on the motivation of the person attempting communication. Lipreading is an effective tool for many hearing-impaired individuals but is useful only if what is being spoken is pronounced in a normal manner and if the person attempting to lipread has good eyesight. Often the shouting that is initially used to communicate only distorts the ability to lipread so that both parties are frustrated. The emotional content of what is being communicated is also a factor important to interactions. If gestures, smiles, and periodic physical contact can be maintained during an interaction, the interest of both parties in trying to complete a successful interaction will remain high. Sometimes unexpected interactions of associated conditions result in either improved or worsened hearing. For example, some patients with both upper and lower full-plate dentures report that their hearing is significantly impaired with their teeth out. The improved bone conduction that can be achieved through having the dentures in place against the mandible and maxilla is a valuable adjunct for assistance with hearing in such cases. Other assistive tools include telecommunication devices for the deaf (TDD) phone systems and closed captioned television or video presentations.

These technologies can provide emotional and intellectual encouragement to the hearing-impaired elderly, meaningfully improving their quality of life through music, conversation, and fuller appreciation of the world around them.

▼ ED AUSTIN (Part II)

On physical examination, Mr. Austin seems to be able to conduct adequate conversation with the male receptionist but has difficulty hearing the female nurse's voice except when he can see her face directly, suggesting some compensation by lipreading. Further history reveals that his hearing problems seem better on weekends when he does not use aspirin. Examination of the ear canals revealed bilateral cerumen deposits that are successfully removed through irrigation and instrumentation. External ear examination is unremarkable, although he cannot repeat whispered number sequences into his right ear consistently. He is referred for formal audiological assessment. Audiological testing reveals evidence of a mild sensorineural hearing loss in the right ear. Review of Mr. Austin's work habits identifies this side of his face as always closest to the printing presses at his job site. Speech discrimination is well preserved, and Mr. Austin demonstrates good lipreading skills. Only mild amplification is required to improve his bilateral high-frequency hearing loss, and a trial of a hearing aid in the right ear is prescribed. Mr. Austin demonstrates good skills in managing the aid but elects to use it only in the home environment. He continues to rely on lipreading at work, with the use of ear protective equipment for the time remaining before his retirement.

CASE DISCUSSION

It is not surprising that Mr. Austin is reluctant to use a hearing aid in the workplace; many patients are reluctant to wear a hearing aid because of the high levels of noise to which they are exposed. Use of ear protection is often recommended. The complaint that Mr. Austin's hearing is worse at home is probably related to the higher vocal frequency of his grandchildren. In contrast, his work noise environment is more familiar and direct conversation with primarily lower-pitched male voices is more common. Aspirin may also be contributing to his hearing difficulties. To determine the possible contribution of this metabolic cause of hearing impairment to his overall problem, you should suggest that he use a nonsalicylate analgesic after work. Other appropriate hearing rehabilitative suggestions included reducing background noises of higher pitched sound sources such as the electric motor whine of kitchen utensils in the home environment when providing child care and positioning himself to lipread when making direct contact with his grandchildren. Routine ear canal examination and periodic use of cerumen-dissolving drops should be accompanied by follow-up audiological assessments for monitoring his hearing aid performance and the progression of the presbycusis.

SUMMARY

Hearing loss could be regarded as a normal accompaniment of old age. Yet many specific steps can be taken to overcome the potentially devastating effects on the individual. Early recognition and intervention are optimal, and responsibility for this lies squarely with the primary care team.

POSTTEST

1. The best strategy to facilitate spoken communication with an individual who has presbycusis is by:
   a. Normal vocal tone and inflections with direct eye contact
   b. Higher vocal pitch at softer volume
   c. Directing conversation into the affected ear, without direct eye contact
   d. Louder voice amplification and exaggerating vocal inflections and expressions for emphasis

2. Audio assistive devices ("pocket talkers") can be helpful in situations:
   a. When the patient is embarrassed by the need to wear amplification
   b. When the patient is unable to manage the controls of a traditional hearing aid because of arthritis
   c. When pure nerve deafness has been documented
   d. When the need for amplification is minimal

REFERENCES

1. LaVisso-Mourey RJ, Siegler EL: Hearing impairment in the elderly, *J Gen Intern Med* 191-198, March/April 1992.
2. Kenney RA: *Physiology of aging,* ed 2, Chicago, 1989, Year Book Medical Publishing.
3. Mulrow CD et al: Quality of life changes and hearing impairment: a randomized trial, *Ann Intern Med* 113:188-194, 1990.
4. Lichtenstein, MD: Hearing and visual impairments, *Clin Geriatr Med* 8(1):173-182, 1992.
5. Macphee GJ, Crowther JA, McAlpine CH: A simple screening test for hearing impairment in elderly patients, *Age Aging* 17:347-351, 1988.

PRETEST ANSWERS
1. c
2. c

POSTTEST ANSWERS
1. a
2. b

CHAPTER 29

Sexuality

RICHARD J. HAM

OBJECTIVES

On completion of this chapter, the reader will be able to:

1. Describe the usual male genital changes that affect sexual function in the elderly.

2. Describe the usual female genital changes that affect sexual function in the elderly.

3. List the common drugs that can adversely affect sexual function.

4. Describe the sexual implications of several common illnesses and syndromes, such as osteoarthritis, dyspnea, diabetes mellitus, prostatectomy, stroke, and myocardial infarction rehabilitation, and some approaches to the prevention and management of sexual problems associated with them.

5. Understand the principles of sexual counseling suitable for the primary care office setting.

6. Understand the place and potential of mechanical and prosthetic devices.

PRETEST

1. Sexual changes noted in average aging men and women include all except which one of the following?
   a. Weaker erection in the man
   b. Shorter, less intense orgasm in the woman
   c. Reduced secretions in the woman
   d. Increased penile sensitivity in the man

Societal prejudice and professional ignorance lead many health care professionals to avoid the subject of sexuality in old people. Simple advice can relieve much potential suffering from sexual dysfunction in both men and women. It is clear that age alone is not a barrier to sexual fulfillment in men or women. However, physical changes in both sexes can be inhibitory, and health professionals need to understand them. The sexual aspects of several illnesses, many prescriptions for medication, and a number of procedures commonly occurring during hospitalization, rehabilitation, and surgery mandate discussion and specific recommendations concerning sexuality.

▼ JAMES DAVEY (Part I)

James Davey comes to you for a follow-up check on his blood pressure. He has been taking a thiazide diuretic for several years. When you ask about sexual function, he unexpectedly becomes tearful while describing with great sadness the cessation of all sexual activity a year ago after several unsuccessful attempts at intercourse over a period of about 1 month. He is 70 years old and had a myocardial infarction 2 years previously. He is retired. As a full-time hobby he makes furniture in his basement, and his wife is well, aside from some low back pain attributed to osteoporosis.

▼ FRANK AND HARRIET JOHNSON (Part I)

Frank and Harriet Johnson, aged 71 and 65 years, respectively, see you for the first time 2 months after their marriage. Mr. Johnson is preoccupied with their sexual difficulties. Both had been married previously; Mr. Johnson has recently been divorced and Mrs. Johnson has been widowed for 15 years. As he describes, and as is found when you complete a pelvic examination, her introitus is tiny and narrow, with a great deal of vaginal spasm on examination; even a single-digit examination is painful.

▼ THOMAS MCNAMARA (Part I)

On visiting the nursing home, you are confronted by several staff members who are disturbed about behavioral problems in Tom McNamara. Mr. McNamara has lived in the facility for less than a year, since his separation 1 year ago from his 70-year-old wife following a stormy marriage of 40 years. His personal hygiene leaves much to be desired, and he frequently leaves the bathroom unclean. He has never been regarded as demented, but he is overactive and paces around the facility, although he does not take part in group activities. He spends most of his time with his roommate, a quiet elderly man of 83 years. The new problem is that he has exposed himself to several (uninterested) elderly women residents. This behavior was seen by one of the family members, who have complained and insisted that something be done to control these behaviors.

STUDY QUESTIONS

- What is the next step in each of these cases?
- What is the likely source of Mr. Davey's problems?
- Is sexual activity an unrealistic aim for the Johnsons?
- Will medications help control these behaviors in Mr. McNamara?

Increasing attention is now paid to sexuality in old age.[1-3] Whereas for centuries sexuality in old age was regarded almost as an aberration, it is now clear and accepted that sexual satisfaction and function are both desirable and possible for the majority of older persons. Yet much sexual unhappiness is unreported and untreated.[4,5] Physical problems in women, many of which are related to estrogen withdrawal, cause dyspareunia. What appear to be the average changes of aging in male sexual function can easily be misinterpreted as impotence and become self-fulfilling.[6] Inappropriate sexual behaviors, particularly in men in long-term care facilities, are an important problem in nursing home care.[7,8]

LOST OPPORTUNITIES

Widowhood, a state much more common in women than men, deprives women in particular of the opportunity for social and sexual contact. Masters and Johnson[2] have defined the "widow's and widower's" syndromes to describe the difficulties of reestablishing sexual function when elderly persons remarry. Placement in the hospital, which is occasionally prolonged during old age, or placement in long-term care institutions may deprive older couples of the necessary privacy, as can living with family members who may have limited views about what is appropriate sexual behavior of the older woman in particular. Health professionals must recognize that they often contribute to the invasion of privacy that deprives older individuals of the sensual and sexual contact they desire; this includes appropriate privacy for masturbation as well as interaction with a partner of the same or opposite sex. Older couples are sometimes separated simply because they need different levels of care.

▼ THOMAS McNAMARA (Part II)

When you interview Mr. McNamara, he is angry, in part about being placed with "all these old people." You interview him in his room, and his roommate takes his part, saying, "I will always stand by him." The social worker at the facility knew Mr. McNamara from before and informs you that he had always been a "man's man" and in fact was an alcoholic, gambler, and petty criminal. His placement in the facility had been a probationary requirement following the separation from his wife. Thus he is in an environment that he specifically would not have chosen for himself. His angry and unreasonable behavior in the bathroom is one manifestation of this behavior; exposing himself to other residents may be another.

STUDY QUESTIONS

- *How should you proceed?*
- *If he cannot be relocated, how can this be handled in the facility setting?*

PSYCHOLOGICAL PROBLEMS

As previously mentioned, male changes can look like impotence, and female changes can produce pain. However, the effect of such misinterpretation of physical changes can be exacerbated by anhedonia, the withdrawal from pleasurable activities, sometimes because of boredom with a partner or with life itself, or as a result of major depression.

 The changes in male sexual response with age generally look like impotence; female sexual changes with age generally produce pain.

It has been proposed that in women fear of rejection and poor self-image cause some elderly women to give up the challenge of sexual relations with relief.[9] Whereas aging men are often regarded as more sexually attractive than aging women, such considerations must not blind us to the increasing literature on the sexual response of elderly women[10] who have their own needs for fulfillment of sexual feelings.

Problems with sexual function around the time of retirement may be related to the castrating loss of role for the previously busy professional of either sex, or these problems may be secondary to increased expectations on retirement, especially sexually and socially. If these are unfulfilled, difficulties may arise in a couple's relationship, highlighted by the extra time available.

 "I married him for better or for worse but not for lunch." (Anon.)

An important psychological disincentive is the fear of illness or even death during intercourse. This is often a problem following stroke and myocardial infarction. The addition of specific sexual counseling following myocardial infarction has been shown to improve well-being and various other psychological parameters.[11]

 In terms of physical exertion, sexual activity with a familiar partner is equivalent to climbing a flight of stairs.

Manifestations of sexual dissatisfaction include inappropriate sexual activity, sometimes disastrous extramarital relationships, and sexual behaviors such as exposure and molestation.

Some of the psychological factors of sexuality in old age are positive. Freedom from the fear of pregnancy may greatly enhance sexual activity and satisfaction. The freedom of being able to schedule one's own time so that sexual activity can occur when both partners are feeling their best is clearly a positive factor to be used in counseling.

▼ JAMES DAVEY (Part II)

You establish that fear of harming Mr. Davey's health during intercourse had inhibited both Mr. Davey and his wife. He felt anxious when the first attempt at sexual intercourse failed. Both he and his wife had a highball on subsequent occasions but state, "It didn't seem to relax us enough." Before his heart attack they were both satisfied with sexual activity about every 2 weeks. During the first few occasions of sexual activity after the 3-month hiatus following Mr. Davey's heart attack, Mrs. Davey experienced more discomfort than usual. Her low back pain had become worse during the time he had been ill, and she found it uncomfortable to lie flat. Mr. Davey's blood pressure at this visit is 115/75.

STUDY QUESTION

- *What factors are already evident that made this initial failure become a persistent problem?*

BOX 29-1
Genital Changes in the Average Elderly Male

Reduced penile sensitivity
Slower, weaker erection
Reduced ejaculatory volume
Anejaculatory orgasm
Reduced forewarning of ejaculation
Speedier detumescence
Increased refractory period

MALE GENITAL TRACT SEXUAL CHANGES

Some men are especially anxious about potency, and Masters and Johnson have described the phenomenon of "first-time failure," when one failed sexual experience leads to long-term sexual breakdown because of misinterpretation and anxiety.[2,4] A transient problem, for example, being tired or taking more alcohol or caffeine than usual, can produce poor sexual activity. This failed activity then becomes a long-term or even permanent dysfunction unless appropriately handled by both partners. Forcing sexual activity (rather like forcing sleep) can produce more anxiety and reduce performance.

"First-time failure" can easily lead, through performance anxiety, to self-fulfilling and persistent failure.

The changes that take place in male sexual response in the average aging man often look like impotence.[2,3,6,12] It appears that athletic elderly men may not suffer these same changes, but many patients have to live with the changes described in this chapter. All phases of the sexual response can be affected. With proper interpretation and adaptation the changes can in fact improve sexual activity. These changes are summarized in Box 29-1.

Erection is, on average, both slower and weaker, with the maximal erection sometimes only just before ejaculation. The sensation of ejaculatory inevitability is often reduced, which reduces pleasure and control. The ejaculatory volume is generally decreased. However, it is the frequency of an ejaculatory orgasm that should be particularly noted; the sense of sexual completeness and satisfaction still takes place, and the only barrier to fulfillment is psychological: the tolerance of not having ejaculated fluid. Both partners should be aware of this. Detumescence is usually quicker after ejaculation, and the refractory period, which is the time before ejaculation can be achieved again, is often prolonged (up to 12 or 24 hours in some). As with other sensations in old age,

penile sensitivity itself tends to be reduced. If there is also vaginal laxity in the partner, this can be a problem and may require manual stimulation by either partner. In summary, average male changes can include a brief orgasm that causes little sensation and is sometimes without actual ejaculation and the speedier loss of the erection, with increased time before ejaculation can once again be achieved.

Male genital changes in sexual function permit a degree of self-control that can improve sexual performance.

However, the reduced sensitivity and extra control and experience of an older man, especially with a familiar partner, can significantly improve sexual function with increasing age (at least, so it is related by many elderly men and recorded in the *Kama Sutra*).

CHANGES IN FEMALE SEXUALITY

For women, it is physically more difficult to readapt to regular sexual activity after a period of abstinence. Sometimes marked physical changes take place, which may require plastic surgery. Often the painfulness associated with estrogen deficiency adds to this problem, and it takes little in the way of extra anxiety to produce vaginismus, a common problem and part of the "widow's syndrome."[2]

Most of the "normal" sexual changes of older women are related to estrogen deficiency and produce pain; thus they may also be remediable or preventable.

The physical changes associated with aging in the female genital tract[2,5,10,13] are related mostly to estrogen loss (Box 29-2). This may be a factor in recommending estrogen supplementation in many older individuals. In the average older woman, vascularity and fat content in the walls of the vulva are reduced, and both vulva and vagina are smaller, smoother, and thinner. The walls of the vagina are more lax, yet the vagina itself is narrower. Variation in vaginal size during intercourse is reduced, and in fact it appears that all four phases of the sexual response (excitement, plateau, orgasm, and resolution) are modified, with reduction in length and intensity. Orgasm itself can be painful in some women, which is thought to be related to progesterone deficiency. Atrophic vaginitis, although common, should not be considered normal; these patients experience tenderness and friability of the vaginal walls, with bleeding, rawness, and

> **BOX 29-2**
> *Genital Changes in the Average Elderly Female*
>
> Reduced vascularity and fat content of vaginal walls
> Reduced size of vulva and vagina
> Stickier, reduced secretions
> Thinner, more lax vaginal walls
> Less variability of vaginal size during intercourse
> Shorter, less intense orgasms
> Reduced sexual response in all four phases
> Painful orgasms in some
> Atrophic vaginitis, with bleeding, infection, and dyspareunia in some

the danger of infection. The relative dryness of the vagina in older age, which parallels the drying up of many other secretions, is a special problem. Lubrication alone, as at other ages, is an important and simple sexual aid.

 Stimulation and lubrication remain the essential sexual aids for older couples.

▼ FRANK AND HARRIET JOHNSON (Part II)

At the initial examination and interview, you describe the physical barrier and discuss the pain and anxiety it is producing in Mrs. Johnson. Privately, she confides that she is desperate that her new husband be able to have intercourse, although it matters little to her. She feels insecure, since he had remained sexually active after his own divorce. Following discussion about potential treatment, including surgical treatment (to which she agrees if it is necessary), you carefully explain the physical problem to Mr. Johnson. You explain that if simple dilation, combined with lubrication and care on his behalf, does not work, surgery for her may be indicated.

PHYSICAL ILLNESSES

There are certain common medical situations in which the physician should specifically mention the sexual aspects to the patient.[14]

Dyspnea, from whatever cause, interferes with sexual activity and may require some adjustment of sexual positioning.

Osteoarthritis and the many other causes of musculoskeletal stiffness alter body movement as a means of sexual expression and require modified sexual technique, especially modification of sexual positioning; for example, the traditional dorsal sexual position ("missionary position") involves external rotation of the hips, which may be especially difficult in osteoarthritis.

All health professionals should be comfortable discussing specific sexual positions to accommodate the needs of their older patients.

Diabetes mellitus is immediately associated in health professionals' minds with neurogenic impotence. However, psychological factors are important here, and in one study individuals thought to be suffering permanent neurogenic impotence could be cured by counseling.[15] However, in certain of these patients such impotence ultimately requires a male prosthesis or the new tumescence techniques.[16,17]

Gynecological surgery always has sexual implications. Sexual activity may have to be limited, but specific instruction must be given about when to resume and what to expect, both when surgery is planned and afterward.

Prostatectomy can also affect sexual function. Although the periurethral approach (TURP) is less likely to cause nerve damage than the traditional perineal approach, patients must be counseled concerning sexual function. As with gynecological surgery, operating on a sexual organ, whether the prostate gland, the scrotum, the penis, the vagina, the uterus, or the ovaries (or even if the surgery is close to the genital area, e.g., herniorrhaphy), must include counseling about sexuality.

Mastectomy has generally had sexual implications, but these have been lessened by the recognition that lumpectomy is frequently as effective as more radical and mutilating surgery.

Colostomy can also have sexual implications. Ostomy nurses and therapists realize the likely effect of an ostomy, and include sexual counseling in their perioperative advice. Such specific support is generally not available for other major surgeries, and the primary care physician should consider the sexual implications of any major procedure, especially if abdominal or inguinal surgery is anticipated.

Urinary incontinence is a common phenomenon that clearly has sexual implications. Frank discussion of perineal hygiene, sexual positioning, and the need to have the bladder empty before intercourse is potentially helpful.[18]

MEDICATIONS AND OTHER DRUGS

Alcohol, the easily available psychotropic, generally diminishes sexual performance. Its role in first-time failure has been described. Other available "psychotropics," such as caffeine, can diminish sexual performance rather than enhance it.

Many prescribed and over-the-counter drugs alter the sexual response. This includes all minor and major tranquilizers, virtually all antihypertensive drugs (including thiazide, but probably excluding calcium channel blockers), many antidepressant drugs, antihistamines, analgesics of the narcotic and near-narcotic variety, digoxin (this medication comes up frequently), cimetidine, anticancer medications, phenytoin, levodopa (although it increases sexual activity in some), and naproxen.[19]

> *Many drugs effect the sexual response, although many patients will not tell the physician unless he or she asks.*

▼ JAMES DAVEY (Part III)

Mrs. Davey willingly comes to a follow-up appointment. She confirms that Mr. Davey's sexual performance has diminished and says it has now been nearly 2 years since any attempt at sexual intercourse. Surprisingly, they have not discussed this between themselves. Mrs. Davey has felt that James is happier without the challenge of sexuality; she on the other hand feels frustrated and distanced from him. On examination, she is obese, with some vaginal atrophy, narrowing of the vagina, and a degree of uterovaginal prolapse without urinary incontinence. Mrs. Davey asks whether it could just be the medications, and you decide to attempt discontinuing the thiazide in view of Mr. Davey's normal blood pressure. You emphasize that they will need to take some time to readjust to sexual activity.

At subsequent visits over a 6-month period, both partners seem to be relieved to have discussed the subject. Local estrogen and lubrication improve the vaginal atrophy problem, Mr. Davey's thiazide is discontinued, and intermittent sexual activity becomes possible. Sexual activity is never fully established with the frequency and satisfaction they had before the myocardial infarction.

CASE DISCUSSION

Further deterioration in their relationship may have been prevented by this frank discussion, even though a completely satisfactory outcome for sexual activity was not achieved. For that to have worked fully, counseling (as recommended in this chapter) following Mr. Davey's myocardial infarction might have prevented this problem. It is important also to address the physical barriers to intercourse (i.e., the atrophy and the thiazide).

▼ FRANK AND HARRIET JOHNSON (Part III)

You prescribe vaginal dilators, obtainable through the drugstore, and permit petting but not full intercourse until a subsequent examination reveals physical improvement. At the 1-month follow-up there is no change in the vaginismus and narrowing, and thus a plastic surgical operation on the introitus is necessary, combined with professional sexual counseling for both partners. The result is that satisfactory sexual relations are achieved, and the marriage, which had become distinctly threatened by the difficulties, survives.

▼ THOMAS MCNAMARA (Part III)

You leave the facility that day considering if Mr. McNamara should move. A psychiatrist (assigned to Mr. McNamara as a probationary requirement) visits the following week and prescribes thioridazine (Mellaril) 25 mg three times a day to calm him. You are told by staff that this does calm Mr. McNamara and helps him to sleep. But when he awakes, a refreshed, new man, he continues his previous behavior. Although it is not possible to relocate Mr. McNamara, the staff approach the situation with good humor and positiveness. Specific programming and social activities for the relatively small group of men in the facility are gently nurtured by the facility's social worker. Mr. McNamara becomes happy and settled into the environment, and the behaviors lessen. Two years later, much against his daughter's wishes, he marries a new resident in the facility.

CASE DISCUSSION

The autonomy and independence of this free spirit are never in doubt. Humor and imagination are needed. Medication has no place. Consideration of whether the sexual behaviors are a manifestation of depression or dementia is important, but once such medical factors have been excluded, it is behavioral and social interventions that correct the problems.

These three cases demonstrate the range of interventions on which primary care physicians should draw in optimally managing sexual problems. A practical and positive approach worked for the Johnsons, a case in which the marriage could easily have failed. A less than fully satisfactory result in the Daveys is unfortunately attributable to the delay in sexual counseling. This was a situation in which sexual counseling should have taken place at the time of the infarction. Mr. McNamara is just one example of the range of problems that come up in the nursing home setting, ranging from embarrassing incidents involving language and touching to exhibitionism (like Mr. McNamara's) to, much more rarely, sexual incidents between staff and patients (initiated by either party). Such incidents require careful judgment and candid, warm staff interrelations.

THERAPY

As with other concerns, a preventive approach to sexual problems is advised. Individuals facing the physical illnesses and investigations mentioned above or anticipating beginning or continuing on any of the medications described must be made aware of the sexual implications.

Physicians should explain that they are available to discuss sexual issues, since many older patients feel inhibited. On the other hand, physicians need to be ready; older people increasingly expect their health professional to be informed about such matters!

> *Include sexual matters in your preappointment questionnaire and in your "review of systems."*

Limited history taking and brief discussion have considerable value, at least for couples.[20] Much can be done in a short time, provided the health professional is frank and specific and both partners can share the information.

The average changes can be quickly communicated. Simple advice that is applicable to many couples includes the following:

1. Mornings are generally best for physical and therefore sexual activities.
2. Lubrication with petroleum jelly or water-soluble lubricants (these wash off and can be heated) helps.
3. There is often a need for increased physical stimulation of each other by both partners.
4. Often one partner is much more concerned than the other about changing sexuality.
5. Our human needs for sensual closeness and warmth (e.g., a hug) may be somewhat separate from sexual needs; it is wrong for the former (emotional) needs to suffer from the (physical) problems of the latter.
6. Elderly women, especially if there are atrophic changes, often benefit from short-term or sometimes long-term use of estrogens (vaginally or orally).

> *The intimacy and affection of the relationship must not be destroyed because of a physical, sexual problem.*

All health professionals should be prepared to discuss sexual positions. Female superior or sitting upright positions may be unfamiliar yet may be necessary for medical reasons. Lateral positioning, where both partners lie on their sides, or the male superior position with the female face down and the male entering from behind may be medically better for some. A useful position for many elderly persons involves the couple both lying on one side and facing one another, with torsos at 90 degrees and legs intertwined; this allows the partners to face one an-

other and to be lying down during foreplay or even actual intercourse, and neither partner is stressed by having to support weight on the arms.

The management of sexual problems must be imaginative and handled with tact and good humor. In all cases a brief history involving both partners, if possible, and counseling about normal physical changes, their relationship, the individual's particular problems, or medications is a good start. Physical examination of both partners should be completed, since remediable physical problems must be found and corrected in the woman (narrow introitus, atrophic vaginitis, other pelvic problems, urinary incontinence, and prolapse) as well as the man (phimosis, balanitis, etc.).

Not all physicians wish to be adept at counseling on the principles of managing vaginismus, premature ejaculation, and orgasmic dysfunction. A useful principle of sexual counseling is to separate out the four different phases of the sexual response; this helps establish a diagnosis, clarifying where the problem lies, and it is also useful in therapy. The therapist is attempting to stop dysfunction in one phase from automatically leading to dysfunction in other phases. The primary care physician should be able to identify the primary sexual disorders just mentioned and should have an established professional contact with a qualified sex counselor.

> *A principle of sexual counseling is to separate out the four different phases of the sexual response in order to avoid the otherwise inevitability of dysfunction in one phase automatically leading to dysfunction in the other phases.*

Despite good combined therapy with physician and therapist, persistent impotence, particularly when it is thought to be neurogenic, may require the use of tumescence devices. Available literature about them is increasing.[16,17] Intracavernous injection of prostaglandin E_1, (alprostadil, Caverject) has recently been approved by the FDA.[21] These can improve erectile function. Other prosthetic devices, including penile implants and prostheses,[17,22] have also been successful in men with persistent problems.

The management of sexual problems in institutional settings requires considerable tact and a balance between sensitivity to staff needs and recognition of residents' needs; at least for some, the institution is their continuing home. Nursing home staff frequently have problems with elderly men acting out.[10] Such incidents give the opportunity for staff education concerning patients' continuing sexual needs and about appropriate staff initiatives to ensure privacy for sexual expression.[23,24]

SUMMARY

Primary care physicians must be able to identify situations in which they should be presenting sexual information to their older patients. It is increasingly important for personal physicians to be able to discuss sexual problems, sexual positioning, and appropriate interventions for primary sexual disorders with their older patients.

POSTTEST

1. Sexual changes found in average aging men and women include all except which one of the following?
   a. Increased time before ejaculation can be re-achieved
   b. Reduced vaginal size
   c. Orgasm without ejaculation
   d. Increased variability of vaginal size during intercourse

2. Which one of the following statements concerning sexuality in old age is false?
   a. Counseling about sexuality has been shown to improve psychological factors following myocardial infarction.
   b. Caffeine is generally inhibitory to sexual performance.
   c. Osteoarthritis of the hips renders the dorsal sexual position uncomfortable.
   d. Impotent diabetic men rarely respond to behavioral interventions.

REFERENCES

1. Butler RN, Lewis MI: *Sex after 60: a guide for men and women in their later years,* New York, 1976, Harper & Row.
2. Masters WH, Johnson VE: Sex and the aging process, *J Am Geriatr Soc* 29:385-390, 1981.
3. Ham RJ: Sexual dysfunction in the elderly. In Ham RJ, ed: *Geriatric medicine annual: 1986,* Oradell, NJ, 1986, Medical Economics Books.
4. Masters WH, Johnson VE: *Human sexual response,* Boston, 1966, Little Brown.
5. Masters WH, Johnson VE, Kolodny RC: *Human sexuality,* Boston, 1982, Little Brown.
6. Kaiser FE et al: Impotence and aging: clinical and hormonal factors, *J Am Geriatr Soc* 36:511-519, 1988.
7. McCartney JR et al: Sexuality and the institutionalized elderly, *J Am Geriatr Soc* 35:331-338, 1987.
8. Szasz G: Sexual incidents in an extended care unit for aged men, *J Am Geriatr Soc* 31:407-411, 1983.
9. Comfort A: Sexuality in the old. In *Practice of geriatric psychiatry,* New York, 1980, Elsevier North Holland.
10. Goldstein MK, Teng NNH: Gynecologic factors in sexual dysfunction of the older woman, *Clin Geriatr Med* 7:41-61, 1991.
11. Jackson G: Sexual intercourse and angina pectoris, *Rehabil Med* 3:35-37, 1981.
12. Morley JE et al: UCLA geriatric grand rounds: sexual dysfunction in the elderly male, *J Am Geriatr Soc* 35:1014-1022, 1987.
13. Felstein I: Sexual function in the elderly, *Clin Obstet Gynecol* 7:401-420, 1980.
14. Mulligan T et al: The role of aging and chronic disease in sexual dysfunction, *J Am Geriatr Soc* 35:520-524, 1988.
15. Renshaw D: Sex, age and values, *J Am Geriatr Soc* 33:635-643, 1985.
16. Korenman SG et al: Use of a vacuum tumescence device in the management of impotence, *J Am Geriatr Soc* 38:217-220, 1990.
17. Morely JE, Kaiser FE, Johnson LE: Male sexual function. In Cassel CK et al, eds: *Geriatric medicine,* ed 2, New York, 1990, Springer-Verlag.
18. Clark A, Romm J: Effect of urinary incontinence on sexual activity in women, *J Reprod Med* 38:679-683, 1993.
19. Drugs causing sexual dysfunction, *Med Lett* 34(876):73-78, 1992.
20. Rowland KD, Haynes SM: Sexual enhancement program for elderly couples, *J Sex Marital Ther* 4:91-113, 1978.
21. Intracavernous injection of alprostadil for erectile dysfunction, *Med Lett* 37(958):83-84, 1995.
22. Johnson LE, Morley JE: Impotence in the elderly, *Am Fam Physician* 38:225-240, 1988.
23. Waasow M, Loeb MB: Sexuality in nursing homes, *J Am Geriatr Soc* 27:73-79, 1979.
24. Kass MJ: Sexual expression of the elderly in nursing homes, *Gerontologist* 18:372-378, 1978.

PRETEST ANSWER

1. d

POSTTEST ANSWERS

1. d
2. d

CHAPTER 30

Sleep

JEFFREY L. SUSMAN

OBJECTIVES

Upon completion of this chapter, the reader will be able to:

1. Recognize the normal changes in sleep that occur with aging.

2. Recognize common sleep disorders and be able to initiate appropriate treatment.

3. Understand appropriate use of pharmacological agents in the treatment of sleep disorders.

4. Recognize when a referral for sleep study is indicated.

PRETEST

1. Physiological changes in sleep with aging include:
   a. Decreased sleep latency
   b. Decreased rapid eye movement (REM) sleep
   c. Increased (deep) delta or stage IV sleep
   d. Decreased nocturnal awakenings
   e. All of the above
2. Which of the following may be associated with excessive somnolence?
   a. Amitriptyline (Elavil)
   b. Clonidine (Catapres)
   c. Alpha-methyldopa (Aldomet)
   d. Carbidopa/levodopa (Sinemet)
   e. All of the above
3. Symptoms and signs suggestive of sleep apnea include all the following except:
   a. Loud or unusual snoring
   b. Cor pulmonale
   c. Personality changes
   d. Hepatomegaly
   e. Morning headaches

Sleep, one of the body's most natural processes, is essential to health. It is usually more interrupted and less efficient as we age. Disrupted sleep is a sign of several significant illnesses of old age, including depression and a number of physical problems. A number of primary sleep disorders for which increasingly specific investigation and therapy are appropriate are described; these disorders must be differentiated and diagnosed. In dementia, the extreme disruption of day-night reversal sometimes occurs and can be difficult to correct. Sleep problems are stressful for all caregivers: interrupted sleep is the most common "last straw." Early recognition and intervention are optimal; sometimes a preventive approach can be used. Careful, comprehensive diagnosis and management are essential.

Complaints of insomnia rise in linear relationship to age; up to 45% of elders suffer from at least transient difficulty sleeping. Up to 14% habitually use sleeping pills. While regulations have restricted psychotropic use in nursing homes, sedative-hypnotics remain widely used.[1-3] Use of such medications has been linked to such complications as hip fractures and falls. Sleep disorders are associated with decreased well-being, with accidents, and with an increased risk of sudden cardiac death. Minor or physiological sleep disturbances must be differentiated from more serious difficulties, such as sleep apnea syndrome.

▼ ALICE GOLDMAN (Part I)

Mrs. Goldman, an 80-year-old woman, seeks your treatment, saying, "I just don't sleep as well as I used to." On close questioning, Mrs. Goldman says she spends more time in bed and sleeps less soundly than she did in her youth. She does not drink alcohol or caffeine, and for medication she uses only an occasional acetaminophen (Tylenol) for "rheumatism." She goes to bed at 11 o'clock, right after the evening news, and is asleep within 15 minutes. She wakes up several times nightly but falls back to sleep promptly. She does not snore, have abnormal movements, or experience other nocturnal problems. This information is corroborated by her husband. She feels refreshed in the morning and puts in a full day volunteering at a local hospital and participating in several civic organizations. Her physical examination shows only mild degenerative changes in the hands and right knee. Her mental and functional status is normal.

STUDY QUESTION

▪ How should you investigate and treat?

PHYSIOLOGICAL CHANGES WITH AGING

Insomnia is a symptom, not a diagnosis, and is defined as a subjective problem with the quality or quantity of sleep. Complaints about sleeping increase with age. These complaints mirror normal physiological changes in sleep.

Normal sleep is divided into two types on the basis of the electroencephalogram: non–rapid eye movement (non-REM, or NREM) and rapid eye movement (REM) sleep. NREM sleep is divided into four stages. Stages one and two are termed light sleep, and stages three and four compose deep sleep. Each night, sleep is initiated with NREM sleep. REM sleep begins approximately 2 hours from the onset of sleep and recurs in three to four regularly spaced, 10- to 15-minute cycles during each night. REM sleep is associated with skeletal muscle atonia, rapid eye movements, and dreaming.[3-5] The characteristic changes in sleep with age are summarized in Box 30-1.

▼ ALICE GOLDMAN (Part II)

You describe to Mrs. Goldman the ways in which sleep normally changes with aging. She remarks that this sounds just like her. You advise her to use acetaminophen (Tylenol), ibuprofen (Advil), or another nonsteroidal agent at night for her

---

BOX 30-1
Sleep Changes With Normal Aging

Increased nocturnal awakening
More time in bed with decreased time spent sleeping
Earlier awakening and falling asleep
Sleep generally less efficient
Increased sleep latency
Decreased deep sleep
Decreased REM sleep

BOX 30-2
Components of a Sleep Diary

Date and day of the week
Habits before sleep including food, drink (especially alcohol and caffeine), medication, etc.
Activities before bedtime (reading, television, telephone, sex, work, exercise, socializing, etc.)
Bedtime
How long it takes to fall asleep
Quality of sleep including awakenings and nightmares
Dreams, snoring, or unusual movements
Time awake
How you felt on awakening
Daytime sleepiness and naps
Other unusual or important factors

BOX 30-3
Some Medications Associated With Sleep Disturbance

Excessive Wakefulness

Theophylline
Amphetamines
Caffeine
Anticonvulsants
Alcohol
Nicotine
Triazolam (rebound phenomena)
Thyroid hormone
Methylphenidate
Sympathomimetics

Nightmares

β-Blockers (especially lipophilic agents such as propranolol)
Tricyclics
Antiparkinsonian agents
Quinidine

Excessive Somnolence

Benzodiazepine
Antihistamines
Tricyclics (especially amitriptyline, doxepin, trazodone)
Monoamine oxidase inhibitors
Antihypertensives (especially clonidine)

Other Symptoms

Diuretics can cause nocturia

---

osteoarthritis. At 1-month follow-up, she states that she feels much better when taking one ibuprofen nightly. While her sleep pattern remains much the same, she is relieved to know that she is normal.

▼ PAUL CUMMINGS (Part I)

Mr. Cummings is a 73-year-old man whose problem is that while he can promptly fall asleep, he wakes up about five times during the night. In the morning he feels tired and finds himself sleeping during the day. He takes digoxin (Lanoxin) 0.125 mg daily and furosemide (Lasix) 40 mg daily for congestive heart failure, and theophylline (Theo-Dur) 300 mg twice a day for chronic obstructive pulmonary disease.

STUDY QUESTIONS

▪ *Which factors already mentioned may be significant causes of insomnia?*
▪ *List the differential diagnosis of the sleeping problem.*

ASSESSMENT OF POTENTIAL SLEEP DISORDER

Insomnia is a symptom, not a diagnosis. It should prompt an appropriate history and physical examination.

The history should include the elements outlined in Box 30-2. Try to obtain corroborating evidence from the partner or a tape recording (especially if snoring or unusual noises are present, or if sleep apnea is a possible problem). Environmental conditions contributing to insomnia, including adverse temperature, noise levels, and light, should be explored. A careful psychosocial history, focusing on anxiety and depression as possibilities, is imperative. A mental status examination to rule out significant dementia may be helpful. Acute sleeping problems can be a symptom of delirium (i.e., there may be an underlying acute medical illness to be considered). Changes in social and environmental circumstances, including relocation and bereavement, can all prompt sleep disturbance. Many commonly used drugs can disturb sleep (Box 30-3), so a full medication history including over-the-counter and borrowed medication is vital.

Insomnia is a symptom, not a diagnosis: ask "what is the cause?"

Finally, treatable medical conditions should be sought. Symptoms such as pain, paresthesia, shortness of breath or cough may point to serious underlying conditions. Common problems leading to sleep disturbance include depression, neuropathy, gastrointestinal reflux, congestive heart failure, prostatism, urinary tract infection, and renal failure.[2-4]

> *Too often, sleeping pills are given to patients who are uncomfortable or simply not tired.*

▼ PAUL CUMMINGS (Part II)

On further evaluation, Mr. Cummings says he goes to sleep each night at 9 PM and promptly falls asleep. Tape recordings during two successive nights reveal no unusual noises or snoring. He does not drink alcohol and rarely drinks coffee, always decaffeinated. No major life events have occurred. However, his breathing has been "a little shorter" recently. He says he takes his medicine faithfully as directed: digoxin, furosemide, and theophylline each morning, and furosemide and theophylline before bedtime. A physical examination shows an intermittent S_3, rales one third of the way up both lungs, 3+ pitting edema of the ankles, a large soft prostate, and a 400 ml postvoid residual volume. Over the next several months you elect to consolidate Mr. Cummings' furosemide dosage to 80 mg in the morning, discontinue his theophylline and add captopril (Capoten) 0.625 mg, three times daily. After stabilization, a transurethral resection of the prostate is undertaken uneventfully. In follow-up, Mr. Cummings has forgotten that he originally had a sleep problem, saying, "I sleep like a baby." Now he wonders when he will be able to visit his granddaughter in Florida.

▼ BENJAMIN THOMAS (Part I)

Mr. Thomas is a 65-year-old patient of yours who says "I'm here because my wife made me come in." At this point, Mrs. Thomas interjects, "Something has to be done. I've moved down the hall and his snoring still keeps me awake."

STUDY QUESTION

- *What further evaluation should you undertake?*

SOME COMMON SLEEP DISORDERS

While environmental factors, predisposing symptoms, and other medical problems cause the majority of sleep disturbances in old age, several *primary sleep disorders* have an increased prevalence in the elderly. These should be suspected on the basis of characteristic historical and physical findings and a lack of response to usual therapy (Table 30-1). Sleep studies are often needed to evaluate

these disorders. Supervised studies in a qualified laboratory are still the standard of care; these should involve a history, physical examination, and measurements of muscle tone, oxygen saturation, respiratory effort, and polysomnography. Home sleep studies may be useful for follow-up but are inadequate for initial diagnosis.

Sleep cycle disturbances involve a disruption of the natural wake-sleep cycle. Although 95% of the population sleep between 5 to 9 hours, the rest have natural cycles of less than 5 or longer than 9 hours. These short and long sleepers are otherwise normal. Jet lag is an increasingly common disorder as the elderly remain in the work force longer and travel more frequently. A small delay in the sleep cycle (as with westbound travel) is easier to accommodate than a sleep advance (as with eastbound travel). This is in part because the natural sleep cycle is actually longer than 24 hours. Sleep cycle disturbances also include sleep phase problems where the natural circadian tendency to sleep is advanced, delayed, or irregular. The advanced sleep phase disturbance is commonly found in normal elders. People fall asleep earlier in the evening, sleep normally, and awaken earlier. In the hospital the delayed sleep phase problem is common. In this condition the patient has difficulty falling asleep, sleeps normally, and awakens later. The irregular sleep phase difficulty is often seen in nursing home patients. These individuals have disrupted sleep patterns with excessive time spent in bed and naps. The disorder is often associated with nocturnal wakefulness and poor sleep hygiene. The physician can play an important preventive role by recognizing such sleep disturbances early and providing appropriate advice and treatment. A particular opportunity to act preventively often occurs in patients with dementia, whose sleep cycles are often excessively disturbed, greatly increasing the stress on their caregivers.

Periodic movements are movement disorders during sleep. *Nocturnal myoclonus* is characterized by repetitive, stereotypical leg movements occurring during NREM sleep. These leg movements often interfere with both falling and staying asleep. *Restless legs syndrome* consists of an uncontrollable urge to move the legs. One third of these patients have a family history of this, which is associated with renal, circulatory, and neurological problems. The diagnosis of periodic movement disorders in sleep may be suggested by the history and can be confirmed by a sleep study.

The prevalence of *snoring* increases with age and is particularly associated with male patients. More than 60% of men and 45% of women over the age of 60 years snore. While snoring in itself may be disruptive, especially for the partner, the more serious problem of *sleep apnea syndrome* must be considered. This syndrome is characterized by loud or unusual snoring, daytime somnolence, morning headaches, and personality change and may be associated with obesity, cor pulmonale, hypertension,

Table 30-1   Selected Common Sleep Problems in Elders

Problem	Symptoms and Signs	Diagnosis
Advanced sleep phase disorder	Go to sleep early, sleep normally, and arise early	Careful history and rule out other disorders
Delayed sleep phase disorder	Go to bed late, sleep normally, and arise later	Careful history and rule out other disorders
Irregular sleep phase disorder	Irregular sleep patterns	Careful history and rule out other disorders
Nocturnal myoclonus (periodic leg movements of sleep)	Repetitive, jerky leg movements during sleep onset	History, physical, sleep study
Restless legs syndrome	Uncontrollable urge to move legs	Family history and association with renal, circulatory or neurological problems, sleep study
Obstructive sleep apnea syndrome	Loud snoring, daytime somnolence, morning headaches, cor pulmonale, hypertension, personality changes	History, ear, nose, and throat examination, cardiopulmonary evaluation, sleep study

dysrhythmias, and upper airway abnormalities. Obstructive sleep apnea is caused by obstruction to the nasal and oral airflow, while the central drive to breathe remains intact. An ear, nose, and throat examination, a cardiopulmonary evaluation, and a sleep study are indicated in any patient with signs or symptoms suggestive of sleep apnea. Sleep study interpretation in this condition is somewhat controversial: using the same criteria for apnea as in younger patients, as many as 70% of elders with daytime somnolence would be classified as having sleep apnea syndrome. Even among well elders the incidence of asymptomatic apneas increases with age.[6]

▼ BENJAMIN THOMAS (Part II)

Mrs. Thomas says her husband has been snoring for at least 10 years, but the snoring is becoming progressively louder. Recently it has been combined with awful grunting sounds. At times, Mr. Thomas even appears to stop breathing and thrashes around. Mr. Thomas wakes in the morning with a headache, which he ascribes to his sinuses. On physical examination, he has a blood pressure of 190/95 and weighs 275 lb. An ear-nose-throat (ENT) examination discloses macrognathia, confirmed by an ENT specialist. There are no signs of cor pulmonale, congestive heart failure, or arrhythmia. Laboratory evaluation including thyroid function is remarkable only for a hemoglobin level of 17.1 g/dl. A polysomnogram demonstrates periods of desaturation to 68% on multiple occasions, associated with periods of apnea up to 45 seconds long; the study is terminated after one such prolonged apneic episode. A vigorous weight loss program is suggested, and the patient is counseled concerning conservative vs. operative approaches to the sleep apnea syndrome. You institute a trial of nasal continuous positive airway pressure (CPAP). After a period of adjustment, Mr. Thomas tolerates this well. The follow-up polysomnogram and home trend oximetry confirm improvement in his apnea and his nocturnal oxygen desaturation.

▼ ADULT HOME PATIENTS (Part I)

During a bridge game at the local adult home, the partners are discussing their sleep problems. **Steven Lawrence** *says he's been despondent since the death of his spouse 2 weeks ago. "I just can't fall asleep," he says.* **Daniel Goldstein** *denies any problems himself but allows that the staff physician is concerned because of increasing nocturnal wandering and restlessness: "They say I get confused at night."* **Katharine McDowell** *says she too has been despondent since the death of her husband 2 years ago. Even now she cries and appears sad at the mention of his name. She wishes there could be an end to it all.* **Anne Kravitz** *says sleep is difficult for her. Her roommate stays up late at night listening to the midnight talk show. During the day, Mrs. Kravitz often naps after lunch and after dinner. She enjoys life and says she would be very happy if only she could sleep better.*

STUDY QUESTIONS

- *What would be the appropriate history, physical examination, and evaluation of each of these four individuals?*
- *Based on the history thus far, what is the differential diagnosis of each?*
- *Given the most likely diagnosis, what would be appropriate treatment in each case?*

TREATMENT

An accurate diagnosis is essential.[1-5] Some complaints of sleep disorder are within the normal range of sleeping patterns for older adults. Correction of environmental factors and treatment of underlying medical problems are needed. All drugs that have the potential to cause sleep disturbance should be evaluated. Psychophysiological problems should be considered. After underlying problems have been addressed, a trial of good sleep hygiene (a program of practices and habits to improve sleep) should be instituted (Box 30-4). Most sleep problems respond to these conservative measures.

> *Before resorting to medications for sleep, reorganize the day: exercise early, do not nap, and wind down to a warm familiar place, sleeping wherever you sleep best.*

Medication should be instituted only in selected cases. Over-the-counter preparations generally contain antihistamines, either diphenhydramine or doxylamine. Although they may be helpful transiently, antihistamines may cause serious anticholinergic side effects, carry-over sedation, and paradoxical wakefulness. Aspirin, acetaminophen, and other similar analgesics may relieve minor aches and pains. Patients often self-medicate with alcohol, but this should be avoided because of alcohol's disruption of the natural sleep cycle and its potential for disruption of REM sleep.

Prescription drugs should be used cautiously and only for appropriate indications (i.e., the target symptoms), and desired effects should be specified and shared clearly with the patient and family members. Antidepressants should be considered when any symptoms suggestive of depression are present. Sedating antidepressant drugs, such as trazodone (Desyrel) or doxepin (Sinequan), may be useful when sleep disturbance is prominent. Major tranquilizers may help in delirium or in dementia-associated disorders.

Three drug classes are useful for elderly patients with transient sleep disturbance: chloral hydrate, benzodiazepines, and zolpidem. Each of these classes of medication are for short-term use during a period of sleep disruption associated with external factors (e.g., recent bereavement, recent relocation, hospitalization, recent surgery). In all cases the possibility of using an analgesic instead of or in addition to the hypnotic should be considered. Chloral hydrate (Noctec) has few adverse effects on sleep and is well tolerated. Significant side effects include gastrointestinal upset and the possibility of potentiating the action of warfarin (Coumadin). The initial dose should be 250 to 500 mg.

Benzodiazepines, especially short- or intermediate-acting agents, are the other drugs of choice for sleep disturbance in the elderly. The basic metabolism of the benzodiazepines should be considered when choosing from available agents (Table 30-2). To act as an ideal sedative-hypnotic, a benzodiazepine should be absorbed and metabolized quickly. Since long-acting agents can lead to carry-over effects and significant accumulation, they should be avoided. Although the short-acting agent triazolam (Halcion) has been associated with rebound insomnia, it remains a potential choice because of its short half-life. Intermediate-acting agents are also useful. Drugs such as lorazepam (Ativan), temazepam (Restoril), or oxazepam (Serax) often must be given 1 to 2 hours before bedtime because of their slow onset of action. It is important to educate the patient about potential side effects and the possibility of withdrawal symptoms when initiating benzodiazepine therapy.

Zolpidem (Ambien) is a nonbenzodiazepine hypnotic whose selective binding to the benzodiazepine receptor is thought to be responsible for its sedative effects. Zolpidem appears to lack the anticonvulsant and muscle relaxant properties of the benzodiazepines. It may be started at 5 mg before bed.

BOX 30-4
Good Sleep Hygiene

Regular rising time
Daily exercise (not close to bedtime)
Correct environment (proper temperature, decreased noise and light)
Light snack (if not contraindicated)
Limiting or eliminating alcohol, caffeine, and nicotine
Short-term hypnotics (only)
Winding down before bedtime
Worry time early in evening
Going to bed when sleepy
Avoiding excessive sleep on weekends
Using relaxation techniques
Using bed for sleeping only
Eliminating naps (unless established as part of schedule)
Getting up if sleep does not occur in 15 to 30 minutes
Sleeping where the person sleeps best
Recognizing relocation phenomenon

▼ *ADULT HOME PATIENTS (Part II)*

*After a careful discussion with **Mr. Lawrence**, you propose a 2-week trial of triazolam (Halcion) 0.125 mg at bedtime. You educate him concerning possible rebound withdrawal and the time limits on such therapy. His condition is reviewed weekly. At the end of 2 weeks he has stopped the triazolam and declares, "I had a better night's rest than I've had in decades." You continue to counsel him informally for several months regarding the bereavement. You complete a mental status evaluation, and it is consistent with mild dementia. Instead of allowing Mr. Lawrence to remain in his room throughout the early evening, you have him brought out to sit with the other residents and encourage him to interact with family members and volunteer staff. He watches television and chats with other residents. With such modifications, no medication is needed to control his sleep disturbance.*

Direct questions asked of **Mrs. McDowell** *uncover evidence of major depression. A trial of a moderately sedating tricyclic, doxepin, is instituted at night. After 1 week, Ms. McDowell reports sleeping more soundly. By 3 weeks her crying jags are infrequent and she finds herself more interested in her crocheting and needlework than she has been in years.*

After a conference with **Mrs. Kravitz** *and her roommate, a change in room assignments is negotiated. Mrs. Kravitz is moved to a room with a morning person who turns in early and gets up early. Her nightly medications are given at dinnertime, and she is encouraged to have coffee with the nurses at 7 AM. At 3 months' follow-up, Mrs. Kravitz reports no further sleeping difficulties.*

REFERRAL FOR SLEEP STUDIES

Referral for a sleep study is sometimes needed to rule out a primary sleep disorder such as sleep apnea syndrome. Indications for referral include the following: (1) the problem persists despite conservative management; (2) there is a suspicion of sleep apnea, periodic leg movements, or a serious disturbance of the sleep-wake cycle; (3) there is periodic hypersomnia associated with functional impairment; or (4) the patient believes the problem is of such importance that referral is necessary.

SUMMARY

Careful history and physical examination narrow the differential diagnosis of sleep disorders in most cases. Correction of treatable problems and a trial of good sleep hygiene improve sleep for many patients. Specific illnesses (such as depression) and the factors that tend to wake the patient (nocturnal frequency, nocturnal dyspnea, musculoskeletal pain, etc.) should be defined and addressed with specific therapy when possible. When clearly indicated, chloral hydrate and shorter-acting benzodiazepines are the drugs of choice for short-term treatment of transient sleep disorders.

Table 30-2   Selected Sedative Hypnotics: Their Onset of Action, Rate of Metabolism, and Starting Dose

Generic Name	Trade Name	Onset of Action	Rate of Metabolism	Starting Dose (mg)
Alprazolam	Xanax	Intermediate	Intermediate	0.25
Chloral hydrate	Noctec	Intermediate	Intermediate	500
Lorazepam	Ativan	Intermediate	Intermediate	0.5
Oxazepam	Serax	Slow	Intermediate	10
Temazepam	Restoril	Slow	Intermediate	15
Triazolam	Halcion	Intermediate	Fast	0.125
Zolpidem	Ambien	Intermediate	Fast	5

POSTTEST

1. Which statement about benzodiazepine use in the elderly is true?
   a. They should be used no longer than 3 to 4 weeks.
   b. Chlordiazepoxide and diazepam are good agents to use because of their rapid metabolism.
   c. Rebound insomnia is a significant side effect of triazolam.
   d. Sedating tricyclics such as amitriptyline should be used instead of benzodiazepines in the nondepressed patient.
   e. a and c are correct.
2. Physiological changes of sleep with aging include:
   a. Increased time in bed
   b. Decreased deep sleep
   c. Decreased REM sleep
   d. Increased sleep latency
   e. All of the above
3. Nocturnal myoclonus is characterized by which one of the following:
   a. Stereotypical leg movements
   b. Occurrence in REM sleep
   c. An association with an uncontrollable urge to move one's legs
   d. An association with benzodiazepine use
   e. Treatment with nasal continuous positive airway pressure

REFERENCES

1. Swift CG: Sleep and sleep problems in elderly people, *Br Med J* 306:1468-1471, 1993.
2. Bachman DL: Sleep disorders with aging: evaluation and treatment, *Geriatrics* 47:53-61, 1992.
3. National Sleep Foundation: *Insomnia: its diagnosis and treatment,* Los Angeles, 1994, The Foundation.
4. Hauri PJ: *Sleep disorders,* Kalamazoo, Mich, 1992, Upjohn.
5. Feinsilver SH, Hertz G: Sleep in the elderly patient, *Clin Chest Med* 14:405-411, 1993.
6. Fleury B: Sleep apnea syndrome in the elderly, *Sleep* 15:S39-41, 1992.

PRETEST ANSWERS

1. b
2. e
3. d

POSTTEST ANSWERS

1. c
2. e
3. a

CHAPTER 31

The Mouth and Teeth

DOUGLAS B. BERKEY and INGRID H. VALDEZ

OBJECTIVES

Upon completion of this chapter, the reader will be able to:

1. List the major risk factors for oral cancer, its sites, and its public health significance.

2. Explain the increased susceptibility of older adults to dental caries and periodontal disease.

3. Discuss the clinical significance of xerostomia and its causes.

4. Report the reasons why denture wearers need follow-up care.

5. Review the factors preventing older people from seeking dental care and name the indications for immediate referral to a dentist.

6. Discuss the role of oral hygiene in controlling plaque and dental diseases.

7. Relate the benefits of good oral health to systemic health and the relationship of medical conditions to oral health.

8. Understand the American Heart Association guideline for antibiotic prophylaxis in cardiac patients at risk for infective endocarditis.

1. Which of the following is an outcome associated with poor oral health?
   a. Bacteremias of dental or periodontal origin
   b. Difficulty chewing solid food
   c. Changes in speech
   d. Declining self-esteem
   e. All of the above
2. Which of the following trends in oral health of Americans is false?
   a. More natural teeth are being retained in old age.
   b. Institutionalized patients generally have poor oral hygiene.
   c. Most patients over 65 are toothless.

d. The peak incidence of oropharyngeal cancer is in elderly persons.
3. Which of the following statements about infective endocarditis is false?
   a. Prophylactic antibiotic coverage can prevent most cases of infective endocarditis.
   b. Clindamycin is the drug of choice in the American Heart Association guidelines for antibiotic prophylaxis.
   c. Infective endocarditis is correlated with poor dental and periodontal health.
   d. Tooth brushing and chewing can cause transient bacteremias.

Oral disease can be detrimental to systemic health in numerous ways, particularly in the medically compromised elderly. Our society, however, generally regards dental care as elective; oral problems may inappropriately appear trivial.

Oral health is an essential part of primary care; oral health screening and appropriate referrals will optimize the health and well-being of patients.

▼ THELMA CAINE (Part I)

Thelma Caine, a 69-year-old black woman returns to your office for follow-up. You have been treating her depression, hypertension, and osteoporosis for several years. Current medications are imipramine, enalapril, estrogen, and calcium supplement. Today she says "my teeth keep breaking off" and "they've caused a sore on my tongue." She states that an ulcer has been present "for months it seems." She has smoked one pack of cigarettes daily for the last 50 years. You inspect the mouth and find a 0.5 × 0.5 cm ulcer on the left lateral border of the tongue. The lesion is posterior to the tooth-bearing area and does not appear to be associated with physical trauma.

STUDY QUESTIONS

- How is the smoking history relevant to oral health?
- What suspicions are raised by the oral ulcer?

OROPHARYNGEAL CANCER

Oropharyngeal cancer is a life-threatening condition most likely to occur in the aged. Cancers of the oral cavity and pharynx are diagnosed in about 40,000 Americans annually, making it more prevalent than leukemia, Hodgkin's lymphoma, thyroid cancer, or cervical cancer.

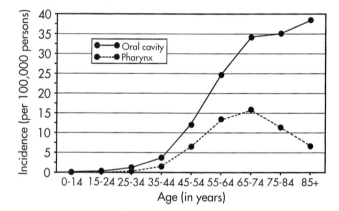

FIG. 31-1 Age-specific incidence per 100,000 population for cancer of the oral cavity and pharynx (1983-1987) in the United States. About 70% of tumors occur in the oral cavity. Advanced age is the number one risk factor for oral cancer. The peak incidence occurs after age 85, whereas pharyngeal tumors reach their peak between age 65 and 74. (Adapted from CDC monograph.)

Approximately 70% of oropharyngeal tumors occur in the oral cavity. Nearly all tumors are squamous cell carcinomas that spread via the lymphatic system. Mortality is high, approximately 50% at 5 years. Blacks have a lower survival rate than whites for both oral and pharyngeal sites. Morbidity is high among survivors and includes the complications of surgery (such as disfigurement and loss of oropharyngeal function) and radiation (loss of teeth, severe xerostomia, vascular damage).

Advanced age is the number one risk factor associated with development of oral cancer (Fig. 31-1); tobacco and alcohol use are the other important risk factors. About 75% of oropharyngeal cancers are associated with tobacco use (including both smoked and smokeless tobacco).[1] Heavy smokers who are also heavy drinkers have a risk 15 to 20 times that of nonsmokers and nondrinkers.[2]

CASE DISCUSSION

Both the frequency and duration of Ms. Caine's smoking make it more likely that she will develop oral cancer.[1] Any long-standing ulcer in the mouth raises suspicion of malignancy. Immediate referral to an oral surgeon is indicated.

▼ THELMA CAINE (Part II)

The soft tissues of the mouth appear dry, glossy, and friable; no other discrete lesions are noted. Scanty saliva is observed in the floor of the mouth. There are many chipped and broken teeth, as well as brown spots near the gum line on several teeth where the gums have receded.

STUDY QUESTIONS

- *What could be contributing to the fractures of her teeth?*
- *What is the most likely cause for her dry mouth?*
- *How does it relate to her dental condition?*

DENTAL CARIES AND PERIODONTAL DISEASE

The proportion of Americans with natural teeth has grown during the latter half of this century. The average number of teeth retained has also increased. These changes are attributed to preventive dentistry practices, such as water fluoridation, improved oral hygiene, and regular professional care with emphasis on maintaining the dentition. Unfortunately, the expanding elderly population has not enjoyed these benefits, so more older adults have dental problems such as dental caries and periodontal disease.

> *The quickest way to make many older patients feel better is to make their mouths more comfortable.*

Although late adulthood has not historically been thought of as "the cavity-prone years," dental caries (tooth decay) is a common problem in this age group. Dental caries is the progressive destruction of tooth structure caused by acid metabolites of plaque bacteria.[2] The longer a tooth has been in the mouth, the more likely it is to have had decay and to have been restored (filled). Two tooth areas are especially vulnerable to decay in mature patients, margins (border between filling and tooth surface) and tooth root surfaces (Fig. 31-2). Decay around margins is more likely to result from mi-

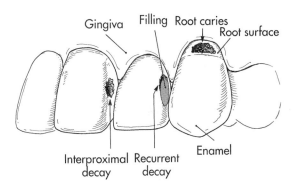

FIG. 31-2   The most common form of dental caries in older adults is root caries: decay that attacks the portion of tooth not protected by enamel, that is, the root. Root caries may appear as a tan, orange, brown, or black discoloration in this area or as frank cavitation. Untreated root caries commonly amputates the tooth at the gumline. Recurrent caries develops adjacent to a filling at its margin. Interproximal caries occurs between teeth and may not be observed clinically.

croscopic imperfections; this is known as recurrent caries. A recent study found that 30% of elderly patients had untreated decay on the coronal (enamel) surfaces of teeth, and that half the affected teeth had recurrent caries.[3]

Second, the gingiva commonly recedes over the years, exposing the tooth roots. These surfaces are not protected by enamel and are prone to root caries. This type of decay progresses rapidly and can amputate the tooth at the gum line if untreated. The prevalence of root caries is clearly age related, increasing throughout adulthood,[4] and it is currently the most common form of tooth decay in the elderly population. There are other risk factors for root caries: nonuse of dental services, poor oral hygiene, and inadequate preventive behaviors are significant. The influence of functional status of the patient is reflected in the observation that 25% of community-dwelling elders exhibit root caries, whereas 80% of institutionalized elderly have some root caries. This finding may also reflect the prevalence of xerostomia in institutionalized elders, another risk factor for caries development.

Periodontal disease or periodontitis is a progressive degenerative condition of the periodontium (gingiva and alveolar bone supporting the teeth). This chronic infection is caused by the microorganisms in dental plaque and calculus (mineralized plaque or tartar). The relationship between age and the prevalence and severity of periodontitis is a complex one. Since periodontitis is a progressive condition, its cumulative effects are often observed in older patients. Up to 70% of elderly individuals have some degree of periodontitis. The severity of periodontal involvement ranges from gingivitis (gingival inflammation) to severe periodontitis (advanced bone

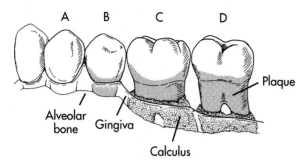

FIG. 31-3   The periodontium consists of alveolar bone and gingiva, the anatomical foundation for sound teeth *(tooth A)*. This condition is maintained by thorough oral hygiene practices. When plaque bacteria accumulate on the teeth, gingivitis develops *(tooth B)*. The accumulation of plaque and calculus on teeth results in destruction of the periodontium known as periodontitis *(tooth C)*. Periodontitis is considered severe when over 50% of supporting bone has been lost *(tooth D)*.

BOX 31-1
Medications That Can Cause Marked Decrease in Salivation

Antidepressants	Anticholinergics
Amitriptyline	Atropine
Nortriptyline	Scopolamine
Clomipramine	Propantheline
Imipramine	
Desipramine	**Antihistamines**
Maprotiline	Diphenhydramine
Chlorpromazine	
Triflupromazine	**Opiates**
Doxepin	Dipipanone
Antihypertensives	
Clonidine	

Modified from Atkinson JC, Fox PC: Salivary gland dysfunction, *Clin Geriatr Med* 8(3):499-511, 1992.

---

loss) (Fig. 31-3). Severe periodontitis is relatively uncommon in older adults because the most diseased teeth have already been extracted.[5]

XEROSTOMIA

Adequate saliva is essential for maintaining oral health and function, as well as the integrity of the upper gastrointestinal tract. Xerostomia (mouth dryness) is a common symptom among older adults. Prevalence ranges from 15% in community-dwelling seniors to 45% of institutionalized patients.[6] Early physiological studies suggested that salivary function declines with age. Today the high prevalence of xerostomia and salivary dysfunction in older adults is thought to represent the influence of medical conditions and their treatment rather than age.

> *A dry mouth makes a patient feel ill: this can be treated, and it can often be prevented.*

The most common cause of salivary dysfunction is probably medication. Patients taking multiple medications are more likely to have xerostomia than patients taking one or two drugs. Certain classes of medications are more likely to cause xerostomia: sedatives, antipsychotics, antidepressants, antihistamines, diuretics, and anticholinergics. However, only selected drugs have been studied and found to inhibit salivation (Box 31-1). Other forms of xerostomia include Sjögren's syndrome (an autoimmune condition characterized by dry mouth and dry eyes) and radiation-induced xerostomia (a permanent

complication of radiation therapy to the head and neck region).

Xerostomia and salivary dysfunction are clinically significant for a number of reasons. From the medical standpoint, constant mouth dryness may reduce compliance with prescription medications; patients may alter dosage or stop the drug altogether. Xerostomia restricts dietary choices and compromises nutrition by making chewing and swallowing uncomfortable, altering the taste sense, and disrupting food enjoyment. Lack of adequate salivation is associated with impaired esophageal acid clearance and chronic esophagitis, predisposing patients to gastroesophageal reflux disease.[7] From the dental perspective, the frequency and severity of dental caries are markedly increased. Patients with xerostomia often have rampant, rapidly progressive decay that is difficult to manage. Patients' ability to tolerate a full or partial denture is compromised as well because of the friable, sensitive mucosa caused by lack of lubrication.

EDENTULOUSNESS

As noted previously, the proportion of Americans with natural teeth has grown steadily in recent years. Yet edentulousness (toothlessness) remains a health concern for our older population. Edentulousness currently affects 32% of patients age 65 to 79 and nearly 50% of patients over 80.[4] Many adverse outcomes are associated with the loss of the natural teeth, including difficulty chewing solid food, undesirable dietary choices,[8] trouble enunciating clearly, poor esthetics, and lower self-esteem.

Complete dentures are the mainstay of treatment for restoring the edentulous mouth. Many people share a common misconception that one set of dentures will last a lifetime and that follow-up care is not needed. Older denture wearers typically report the chewing efficiency of their dentures is satisfactory. Only 13% of denture wearers seek annual dental care. Almost half of patients studied had not seen a dentist in 5 years.[4]

> *Dentures are not fitted "for life": they will get looser with time and need to be regularly serviced.*

In fact, the edentulous ridge (remaining alveolar bone) undergoes continuous resorption over the years, ultimately compromising the fit and stability of dentures. Most older patients tolerate these gradual changes, but their oral tissues do not. As many as 30% of denture wearers have oral lesions caused by the denture. Most lesions are inflammatory, infectious, or fibrous. As the fit and stability of dentures decrease, chewing efficiency is compromised. Thus follow-up care is essential for maintaining the functional benefits of dentures, as well as maintaining health of the edentulous mouth.

▼ EDWARD SPENCER (Part I)

Mr. Spencer, an 86-year-old white male patient of yours, has had multiple health problems and hospitalizations over the last 20 years. He has survived prostate cancer, lung cancer, and chronic obstructive pulmonary disease (COPD). He has been clinically stable the last few years despite some difficulty maintaining his weight. At a routine follow-up visit, his wife reports, "He's not eating good" and "He has bad teeth."

STUDY QUESTIONS

- *What prevents an older patient from seeking dental care?*
- *What should you do next?*

LOW UTILIZATION OF DENTAL SERVICES

The elderly have the lowest dental services utilization rate of any age group. It is extremely common for an older patient not to have sought dental care for years. The primary reasons are that older persons do not perceive a need for dental care, do not have dental insurance, and dismiss oral problems as an inevitable part of aging (Box 31-2).

> *Older patients go to see physicians but not dentists: the physicians need to send them to the dentists.*

> **BOX 31-2**
> *Factors Preventing Older People from Seeking Dental Care*
>
> No perceived need for dental care
> Tendency to dismiss oral problems
> Attention to other illnesses
> Financial concerns
> No dentist available
> Transportation problems
> Fear of dental procedures

Older adults tend to use medical services more frequently and repeatedly than dental services. This creates opportunities for primary care personnel to screen for oral disease. Primary care is the link between the older patient and adequate dental care. If these screenings are not performed in medical settings and patients are thus not referred for treatment, oral problems are less likely to be diagnosed and managed.

NEED FOR ORAL SCREENING

Oral cancer screening is advocated as a public health tool for reducing oral cancer mortality. The 50% survival rate among oral cancer patients has not improved significantly in the past 15 years. Early detection of these cancers greatly improves the prognosis: the 5-year survival rate for patients with distant metastasis at the time of diagnosis is 18%, whereas the survival is 75% when disease is localized at the time of diagnosis. It is clear that oral cancer screening has the potential to improve prognosis. A recent survey conducted by the Centers for Disease Control and Prevention showed that only 13% of community-dwelling elderly reported ever having had an oral cancer screening.[9] The American Cancer Society and American Dental Association recommend an oral examination annually for all elderly persons. In addition, a panel of health care experts recently advocated routine oral examination by physicians for all individuals over age 65.[10] An annual examination is mandated by federal regulations for the institutionalized elderly.

▼ EDWARD SPENCER (Part II)

Mr. Spencer has not seen a dentist since he first became ill. His wife states, "He's been in and out of the hospital so much, who has time to see the dentist?" Your screening examination reveals that all the upper teeth are decayed to the gum line, with some caries of the lower teeth as well. When questioned about this, Mr. Spencer denies any symptoms related to the mouth but admits that "some foods" are difficult to chew.

STUDY QUESTIONS

- Is the lack of symptoms consistent with the physical findings?
- What can be done to improve dietary intake?

Oral Health Screening

Screening for oral disease is accomplished by a few simple additions to routine history and physical examination technique. Questions on oral health are easily added to the review of systems. The patient may be questioned as to any sores in the mouth, painful or broken teeth, bleeding gums or loose teeth, the fit of dentures, and so forth. Age, smoking history, and drinking history are the chief risk factors for oral cancer. Several specific questions are predictive of salivary dysfunction (Box 31-3).[11]

It is important to note the tendency of older patients to have reduced symptoms. As in many organ systems, the presentation of oral disease may be altered, lessened, or delayed. Moreover, many oral conditions such as root caries and periodontitis are clinically inapparent. The clinician's level of suspicion should *not* be based on the report of symptoms.

> *Any examination of an elderly patient is incomplete until you have seen inside the mouth.*

The screening examination should include both extraoral and intraoral structures. The head and neck are inspected and palpated for asymmetry, masses, and lymphadenopathy. The soft tissues of the oral cavity proper are then inspected. *The highest risk locations in terms of malignancy are the lateral tongue, ventral tongue, and floor of mouth.* Any mass, red lesion, white lesion, mixed red and white lesion, ulcer, or erosion should be evaluated further for malignant potential. The periodontium and dentition are inspected last. Findings that indicate immediate referral to a dentist are summarized in Box 31-4.

The caveat to oral screening is that the possibility of false-negative findings is significant. Occult disease of the jaws, periodontium, and dentition includes chronic abscesses and other osseous pathologic conditions, periodontal disease, interproximal caries (decay between teeth) (see Fig. 31-2), and root tips (necrotic teeth submerged below the gum line). A thorough dental examination with appropriate radiographs is necessary to rule out these conditions.

A patient with acute oral infection may seek emergency treatment from a physician. Dental infection may be characterized by pain in one specific tooth, typically unprovoked, continuous, and unremitting. Swelling may occur in the gingiva or vestibule or may progress to involve the fascial spaces. Medical management should include antibiotic therapy, pain control, and immediate referral to a dentist. Penicillin-V is generally considered the drug of choice for odontogenic infection. Supportive care and hospitalization are needed in cases of advanced infection or debility.

We have emphasized referral to a dentist as the means to initiate individualized oral care for each patient, whether dentate or edentulous. A general dentist with interest and willingness to treat older patients is appropriate in most cases. The dental profession, like most health care fields, has become increasingly specialized. The primary care geriatrics team should be aware of these special interest areas. Geriatric dentists are an emerging group who have obtained additional training in geriatrics. Oral surgeons have extensive training in surgeries such as extractions, biopsies, and jaw reconstruction. Periodontists focus on the management of periodontitis, while endodontists restore the tooth with root canal therapy. Prosthodontists specialize in replacement of missing teeth. Hospital dentists and oral medicine specialists are often affiliated with medical centers and have training in the dental management of medically compromised patients.

PREVENTIVE AND LONG-TERM CARE

While the goal of dentistry remains to restore the mouth to health and function, dental practice has changed dramatically in recent decades. More emphasis has been placed on disease prevention and the maintenance of the

---

BOX 31-3
Evaluating Xerostomia

Does the amount of saliva in your mouth seem to be too little, too much, or not noticeable?
Do you have trouble swallowing your food?
Does your mouth feel dry while you are eating a meal?
Do you sip liquids to help you swallow dry foods?

Modified from Fox PC, Busch KA, Baum BJ: *J Am Dent Assoc* 115:581-584, 1987.

BOX 31-4
Immediate Referral to a Dentist

Tooth or gum pain
Facial swelling
Mobile teeth
Erythroplasia or leukoplakia
Ulceration or erosion

natural teeth. Primary prevention of dental diseases consists of daily oral hygiene (mechanical plaque removal by the patient or caregiver). Dental research in the 1960s clearly demonstrated that dental caries and periodontitis are infectious diseases. These diseases can be prevented or controlled by eliminating dental plaque, the complex of microorganisms that colonize the teeth and periodontium. Brushing and flossing are the chief methods of oral hygiene. Both procedures require an understanding of their purpose, as well as adequate eyesight and manual dexterity. Therefore these activities can be practiced by well-motivated, healthy elders. When cognition, vision, motivation, or dexterity is impaired, however, oral hygiene self-care declines and caregiver assistance is needed. The vast majority of nursing home residents, for example, have hard and soft deposits on their teeth, placing them at high risk for dental disease.

Chemotherapeutic adjuncts to mechanical plaque removal have an important role. Fluoride is effective in fortifying both enamel and root structure against decay. Prescription fluoride gels that are applied directly to the teeth are believed to be most effective. Antimicrobial agents such as chlorhexidine are also employed to reduce the oral microbial burden.

Long-term follow-up is recommended to maintain the oral health of both dentate and edentulous patients. The dentist typically establishes recall (reevaluation at intervals such as every 4 months, 6 months, or 1 year) for each patient based on the patient's condition. Thus success or failure of dental interventions can be monitored and treatment modified as needed.

DENTAL HEALTH AND GENERAL HEALTH

Good oral health has numerous benefits to systemic health. Acceptable facial esthetics are valuable to a healthy self-image, whereas poor dental health in the elderly has been correlated to low self-esteem. The ability to speak clearly, so important in human existence, depends largely on tooth support and position. Chewing ability is determined in large part by dental status. Persons with a full complement of teeth or with appropriate prostheses have higher chewing efficiency than persons without teeth; this allows the patient to select a more varied diet.

▼ EDWARD SPENCER (Part III)

Mr. Spencer is referred to a general dentist, who finds that root caries has devastated his upper teeth. They are extracted and a complete denture is fabricated. The lower teeth are preserved by routine fillings. Mr. Spencer is placed on daily prescription fluoride therapy and scheduled for a 4-month recall cycle. At follow-ups, Mrs. Spencer reports that her husband is eating a greater variety of solid foods than he has in years.

Medicine and Dentistry: The Interrelationship

More Americans are entering old age with their natural teeth than ever before, so more dental procedures will be indicated among medically compromised older adults in the future. Good communication between medical and dental personnel is paramount. The physician should be confident of understanding the nature of the dental procedure and potential risks before "approving" the patient for dental work. For example, what is the extent of invasiveness and mental stress expected? What is the typical postoperative condition of patients following this procedure? How will bleeding and postoperative discomfort be managed?

The well-being of patients with a variety of systemic conditions may be directly affected by poor oral health or by dental procedures. Patients with cardiovascular disease are potentially susceptible to the physical or emotional challenges of dental treatment. For example, stressful dental procedures could precipitate myocardial infarction or stroke in persons with angina pectoris or hypertension. Patients with diabetes mellitus must be encouraged to maintain good oral health; controlling dietary intake and avoiding infection are both necessary for diabetic control. Patients with prosthetic joints are considered at risk for infection of their prostheses because of bacteremia and are often premedicated with antibiotics before dental treatment. Cancer patients being prepared for chemotherapy or head and neck radiation therapy should be evaluated and treated by a dentist to avoid acute and chronic oral complications. Other conditions such as organic heart murmur, mitral valve prolapse, or rheumatic heart disease may predispose the patient to infective endocarditis.

PREVENTING INFECTIVE ENDOCARDITIS

Infective endocarditis (IE) is a serious complication of dental treatment that may occur in susceptible patients. It is important to note that IE has become more common in the elderly.[12] The proportion of IE cases in patients over age 65 has increased from 30% (from 1944 to 1964) to 55% (from 1965 to 1983). Even with appropriate medical therapy, mortality ranges from 10% to 65%. It appears that infective endocarditis can be prevented in most cases by using adequate prophylactic antibiotic coverage.

A number of cardiac conditions place the patient at risk for endocarditis.[13] These are listed in Box 31-5. About 30% of cases occur in patients with rheumatic heart disease, 10% to 33% in patients with mitral valve prolapse, and 10% to 20% in patients with congenital heart disease.

The oral cavity is a source of bacteremia during dental treatment and during routine use of the mouth. Invasive dental procedures and minor manipulation

BOX 31-5
Cardiac and Vascular Lesions Posing Infective Endocarditis Risk

Relatively High Risk*

Prosthetic heart valve
Aortic valve disease
Mitral insufficiency
Patent ductus arteriosus
Ventricular septal defect
Coarctation of aorta
Marfan's syndrome

Intermediate Risk*

Mitral valve prolapse with regurgitation
Pure mitral stenosis
Tricuspid valve disease
Pulmonary valve disease
Previous infective endocarditis
Calcific aortic sclerosis
Hyperalimentation or pressure-monitoring line that reaches right atrium
Nonvalvular intracardiac prosthetic implant
Hypertrophic cardiomyopathy

Low or Negligible Risk

Atrial septal defect
Arteriosclerotic plaques
Coronary artery disease
Syphilitic aortitis
Cardiac pacemaker
Surgically corrected cardiac lesion (without prosthetic implants, more than 6 months after surgery)

From Durack DT: Infective and non-infective endocarditis. In Hurst JE, ed: *The heart, arteries, and veins,* ed 7, New York, 1990, McGraw-Hill, pp 1230-1254.
*The American Heart Association recommends antibiotic prophylaxis.

BOX 31-6
American Heart Association–Recommended Prophylactic Regimen for Dental Procedures in Patients at Risk

Standard Regimen

Amoxicillin, 3 g PO 1 hr before procedure, then 1.5 g 6 hr after the initial dose

For Amoxicillin/Penicillin-Allergic Patients

Erythromycin ethylsuccinate, 800 mg, or erythromycin stearate, 1 g PO 2 hr before procedure, then half the dose 6 hr after initial dose

OR

Clindamycin, 300 mg PO 1 hr before procedure, then 150 mg 6 hr after initial dose

Modified from Dajani AS et al: *JAMA* 264:2919-2922, 1990.

such as cleaning can result in transient bacteremia. Normal daily activities such as chewing and tooth brushing are associated with bacteremia. The frequency of such bacteremias is correlated to poor dental and periodontal health. In susceptible patients, blood-borne bacteria may lodge on damaged or abnormal heart valves or endocardium, resulting in bacterial endocarditis. Streptococci and staphylococci are the causative agents in 80% of cases.

> *Be aware of who among your patients is at risk for infective endocarditis, a life-threatening illness of elders that can be prevented.*

The clinician's goal is to prevent endocarditis from occurring in susceptible patients. To accomplish this, the clinician must do the following:

1. Identify all at-risk patients. Dentists often consult primary care providers as to whether the cardiac status places a patient at risk. Questions most often arise when the patient relates a history of a heart murmur (is it functional or organic?) or a history of rheumatic fever (is there evidence of rheumatic heart disease?). Patients who are at risk for IE should be informed about antibiotic prophylaxis for dental procedures.

2. Use American Heart Association (AHA) guidelines for antibiotic prophylaxis. The most recent AHA guidelines were published in 1990 (Box 31-6).[14] This regimen involves oral amoxicillin, one dose before the procedure and a second dose afterward. Erythromycin or clindamycin is recommended for patients who are allergic to penicillins. If a patient is already taking penicillin for rheumatic fever, or is taking penicillin for other reasons, erythromycin or clindamycin should be used for IE prophylaxis.

3. Maintain the best possible oral health to reduce the further risk of bacteremia. Bacteremia of oral origin can occur secondary to daily activities, particularly in patients with poor oral health. Fewer than one in five cases of subacute bacterial endocarditis have in fact been associated with a dental or medical *procedure.* Therefore patients should be encouraged to keep the mouth as healthy as is achievable, by appropriate oral hygiene and follow-up with their dentist. All at-risk patients should be referred to a dentist for counseling about the medical reasons for complying with dental recommendations.

TREATMENT OF DRUG-INDUCED XEROSTOMIA

Xerostomia is deleterious to systemic well-being and oral health. Steps should be taken to reduce mouth dryness and to control its sequelae. If a patient's medication is known to inhibit salivation, an alternative drug in the same class should be considered. Some have recommended modifying medication schedules, so that the peak xerostomia effect occurs during mealtime when there is a natural stimulus for salivation. Oral stimulants can be used by patients to overcome the salivary-inhibiting effects of medication, such as sugarless gum or sugarless lemon drops. Systemic salivary stimulants such as pilocarpine may also be beneficial. Pilocarpine has been used successfully to treat patients with Sjögren's syndrome and radiation-induced xerostomia, but it has not been tested as a therapy for drug-induced xerostomia. Preventive oral care should be stepped up in patients with xerostomia to control their predilection for dental caries.

▼ THELMA CAINE (Part III)

Ms. Caine is referred to an oral surgeon for evaluation of the tongue lesion. Excisional biopsy reveals a stage I localized squamous cell carcinoma with margins free of tumor. She also sees a general dentist who extracts the nonrestorable teeth, builds up the remaining teeth, and constructs partial dentures to replace the missing teeth. It is thought that the imipramine may be contributing to the patient's mouth dryness, so this is discontinued and she is given a trial of fluoxetine. On 6-month follow-up, Ms. Caine's depression is adequately controlled. She has regularly scheduled follow-up with her general dentist and oral surgeon.

SUMMARY

Older adults present a wide range of oral diseases and conditions, many of which can have a significant impact on systemic health. Because they are among the most prevalent of chronic conditions experienced by older adults, the primary care physician must screen for dental problems and provide appropriate referral. Oral cancer, xerostomia, dental caries, periodontal disease, dentate status, oral screening, infective endocarditis, and a preventive approach are the major issues.

POSTTEST

1. Which one of the following is not true concerning oropharyngeal cancer?
   a. It is most likely to occur in the aged.
   b. More tumors develop in the pharynx than in the oral cavity.
   c. Tobacco and alcohol are notable risk factors.
   d. Mouth dryness may be a complication of radiation treatment.
2. Which one of the following statements is true?
   a. Periodontal disease is generally an acute infection.
   b. Active dental caries is most frequently found on the enamel surfaces of the teeth.
   c. Dental caries is a common problem of the aged.
   d. Gingivitis is a very severe form of periodontal disease.
3. Which one of the following statements about mouth dryness is false?
   a. The clinical signs of mouth dryness include friable and glossy tissue.
   b. The most likely cause for dry mouth in the elderly is the physiological aging process.
   c. Xerostomia may lead to restricted dietary intake.
   d. Mouth dryness can lead to rapid and progressive dental decay.
4. Which of the following statements is false?
   a. The vast majority of those over 65 years old are totally edentulous.
   b. Alveolar bone resorption is a typical result of tooth extractions.
   c. Dental utilization rates for edentulous elderly are lower than utilization rates for those with teeth.
   d. Medical utilization rates exceed dental utilization rates for the elderly.

REFERENCES

1. Centers for Disease Control and National Institutes of Health: Cancers of the oral cavity and pharynx: a statistics review monograph, Atlanta, 1973-1987, CDC.
2. Beck JD, Watkins C: Epidemiology of nondental oral disease in the elderly, *Clin Geriatr Med* 8(3):461-482, 1992.
3. Beck JD, Hunt RJ: Oral health status in the United States: problems of special patients, *J Dent Ed* 49(6):407-425, 1985.
4. National Institute for Dental Research: *Oral health of United States adults, the national survey of oral health in the US employed adults and seniors: 1985-1986,* US DHHS, NIH Pub No 87-2868, August 1987.
5. Burt BA: Epidemiology of dental diseases in the elderly, *Clin Geriatr Med* 8(3):447-459, 1992.
6. Atkinson JC, Fox PC: Salivary gland dysfunction, *Clin Geriatr Med* 8(3):499-511, 1992.
7. Valdez IH, Fox PC: Interactions of the salivary and gastrointestinal systems. II. Effects of salivary gland dysfunction on the gastrointestinal tract, *Dig Dis* 9:210-218, 1991.
8. Palmer CA: Nutrition and oral health of the elderly. In Papas AS, Niessen LC, Chauncey HH, eds: *Geriatric dentistry: aging and oral health,* St Louis, 1991, Mosby.
9. Centers for Disease Control Morbidity and Mortality Weekly Report: *Examinations for oral cancer—United States, 1992,* US DHHS 43:198-200, March 1994.
10. Sox HC: Preventive health services in adults, *N Engl J Med* 330:1589-1595, 1994.
11. Fox PC, Busch KA, Baum BJ: Subjective reports of xerostomia and objective measures of salivary gland performance, *J Am Dent Assoc* 115:581-584, 1987.
12. Little JW, Falace DA: *Dental management of the medically compromised patient,* ed 4, St Louis, 1993, Mosby.
13. Durack DT: Infective and non-infective endocarditis. In Hurst JE, ed: *The heart, arteries, and veins,* ed 7, New York, 1990, McGraw-Hill.
14. Dajani AS et al: Prevention of bacterial endocarditis: recommendations by the American Heart Association, *JAMA* 264:2919-2922, 1990.

PRETEST ANSWERS

1. e
2. c
3. b

POSTTEST ANSWERS

1. b
2. c
3. b
4. a

CHAPTER 32

The Feet

HAROLD RUBENSTEIN

OBJECTIVES

On completion of this chapter, the reader will be able to:

1. Describe the clinical features and management of hallux limitus/rigidus.

2. Describe the features and management of two common diabetic foot complications: neurotrophic infected ulceration and nail bed infection.

3. Understand the value of periodic and comprehensive foot examination in the diabetic.

4. Understand the scope of practice of podiatric medicine and surgery and the role of the podiatrist on the health team.

PRETEST

1. Which one of the following statements is false?
   a. Delays in referring diabetic foot problems have been shown to be associated with an increased amputation rate.
   b. Most diabetic foot ulcers, even if extensive, are painless.
   c. Hallux limitus implies absence of movement at the first metatarsophalangeal joint.
   d. Podiatrists can prescribe narcotics.

Many older persons lose their independence because painful or poorly functioning feet restrict ambulation. The problem may be as simple as a plantar corn with underlying capsulitis or as complex as ischemic neuritis. Accumulated microtrauma, trophic changes of the soft tissues, musculoskeletal pathologic conditions, manifestations of diseases such as diabetes, the arthritides, and vascular and neurological disorders often combine in an individual patient, profoundly affecting comfort and mobility.

Some problems can be prevented. Many more can be adequately managed. Evaluation and management of many foot complaints require knowledge of the biomechanics of foot function. Podiatrists are important allies in the care of such patients; they are trained in problems of the foot and ankle and those structures of the lower leg that affect the conditions and operations of the foot and ankle. The American Podiatric Medical Association defines podiatric medicine as that branch of the health sciences concerned with the prevention and diagnosis of problems affecting the human foot, ankle, and lower limb and the treatment of such problems by all appropriate means, including surgery and prescription drugs, including narcotics.

▼ ALAN CHASE (Part I)

Mr. Chase is a 75-year-old retired C.E.O. who comes to your office with a chief complaint of swelling and pain in his left forefoot of 2 weeks' duration. He denies any history of recent injury and states that his feet have never caused him any problems; he is an avid jogger, having run 5 miles a day, 7 days a week, for the past 25 years.

STUDY QUESTIONS

- What are the possible diagnoses?
- What will you specifically seek on examination?

▼ ALAN CHASE (Part II)

Mr. Chase is a trim, alert man who is concerned because his painful foot interferes with normal walking and jogging, which is a passion for him. Examination reveals edema and erythema of the left forefoot metatarsophalangeal joints (MTPJs). There is tenderness both to deep palpation and to motion of the third MTPJ. Palpable enlargement of the first MTPJ is present bilaterally without medial bunion or hallux abducto valgus deformity, but with almost complete restriction of motion. There is no crepitation or pain.

There has been no change in Mr. Chase's running shoes, his running surface, or anything else. However, when questioned about recent medical events, he reminds you that your partner recently sent him for a cardiologic opinion when a life insurance examination had shown an unexpected dysrhythmia. Although he had been told to refrain from jogging, he insisted on continuing. Exercise stress testing at the cardiologic office was carried out for 15 minutes on the treadmill, with him wearing his everyday dress shoes; the cardiologic examination was normal.

STUDY QUESTIONS

- How does this recent activity affect the possible diagnosis?
- What investigations are now indicated?

▼ ALAN CHASE (Part III)

Mr. Chase's radiographs (Fig. 32-1) show severe degenerative arthritis of both first MTPJs; the joint space is poorly visualized. On the left third toe a slightly displaced avulsion fracture is found, involving the lateral condyle at the base of the proximal phalanx.

CASE DISCUSSION

Although the initial diagnostic impression included degenerative joint disease of the first MTPJs and a number of musculoskeletal problems such as capsulitis, gout, and some other arthritis, it is evident that Mr. Chase has actually developed an avulsion fracture (i.e., a stress fracture), probably precipitated as a result of running in his dress shoes on an incline, which did not allow him his usual compensatory mechanism for his extremely stiff first MTPJs. This case demonstrates the relationship between the presence of just one pathological state (hallux limitus) and other biomechanical problems of the foot and lower extremities.

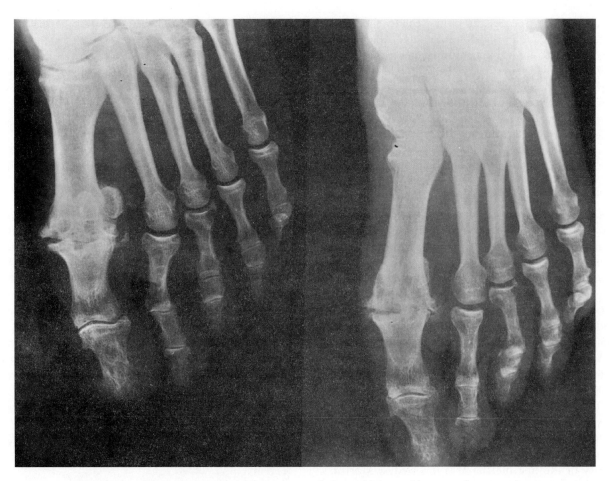

FIG. 32-1   Degenerative arthritis in metatarsophalangeal joints, with a stress fracture at base of left third proximal phalanx.

> *Always examine older people's feet, and watch them walking in their usual footwear.*

HALLUX LIMITUS/RIGIDUS

Limitation of motion at the first metatarsophalangeal joint is commonly referred to as hallux limitus (HL), whereas hallux rigidus (HR) indicates a total absence of motion. HL/HR ranks second in frequency to hallux valgus as a disorder of this important joint of the foot.[1] Both are characterized by degenerative joint disease at the first MTPJs. HL/HR most frequently affects middle-aged and elderly individuals and males more than females; it occurs more often in blacks.

Etiology

Primary causes of HL/HR include biomechanical abnormalities, which may be related to functional or structural aberrations of the foot and extremity. Secondary HL/HR has been attributed to trauma, including prior surgery, osteoarthritis, blunt trauma, and systemic arthritides.

Presentation

The patient frequently seeks attention for pain at the first metatarsophalangeal joint (MTPJ). Symptoms are usually gradual in onset, occurring with ambulation or prolonged weight bearing; with time the symptoms become more disabling.

Assessment

Palpation of the joint reveals enlargement, especially dorsal enlargement. The firm nonmoveable enlargement is bone or cartilage, and frequently a bursa or ganglion is present. Impingement of the dorsal hallucal nerves may be the source of symptoms. Passive dorsiflexion at the MTPJ is limited and may be associated with crepitation and pain.

During gait, 65 to 75 degrees of MTPJ dorsiflexion is required.[2] To compensate, individuals with HL alter their gait in one of several ways:

- A propulsive gait with vertical toe-off: This compensation, often seen in the old, is energy inefficient, causes fatigue, and significantly alters the ratio of one- or two-limb support during the gait cycle.

- Forefoot inversion: This compensation allows the individual to roll off the lesser MTPJs, exerting less stress on the compromised first MTPJ. This gait alteration may cause reactive skin lesions under the lesser metatarsal heads, especially the fifth, or pain involving the lateral column of the foot or the lateral side of the lower extremity joints.

Nonsurgical Treatment

The objectives of treatment are the alleviation of symptoms and the restoration or improvement of function. The risks of nontreatment require discussion, since HL is a progressive disease.

Nonsurgical management includes advice regarding foot gear and activities. Shoes with stiff soles and a high toe box without stitching over the joint are helpful. Avoidance of excessive stair or hill climbing may reduce symptoms. To reduce the need for first MTPJ dorsiflexion, *rocker bars* can be strategically placed on leather-soled shoes; this may reduce symptoms. Design of such bars is important: when they are tapered distally to the sole, there is less chance of tripping and injury. Alternatively, the available range of dorsiflexion can be increased by "dropping" the first metatarsal and stabilizing the medial column of the foot. *Orthoses* may help when hypermobility of the first metatarsal is involved; a Morton's extension to an orthosis has been suggested. If there is considerable pain on even slight motion at the first MTPJ, placing a *rigid material within the sole* of the shoe from under the metatarsal shaft to the tip of the toe will likely eliminate that pain, but symptoms may appear elsewhere, especially on the lateral column of the foot and side of the leg.

Physical therapy, NSAIDs, and injection therapy have limited roles in the management of the inflammatory process.

Surgical Management

Surgery is indicated when the symptoms and disability are significant and conservative therapy fails or is not practical. Because of compensatory stresses on the rest of the extremity, surgery to an otherwise asymptomatic HL is occasionally recommended, although this would be rare in the elderly.

Older patients must be evaluated to determine if they are surgical candidates. Surgical procedures range from soft tissue release to joint destructive procedures. The simplest osseous procedure, cheilectomy, involves removal of the osteophytic processes and remodeling of the joint contours and is limited to the early stages of the disease process. Joint destructive procedures include resectional arthroplasty with or without joint replacement or fusion of the joint. Osteotomy procedures to decom-

press or change sagittal plane position of the joint are other options.

Consider to what extent surgical intervention will affect the patient's life-style. A vibrant, energetic individual who cannot even do necessary grocery shopping without considerable pain will probably be gratified, whereas a patient with advanced Parkinson's disease would do as well with a rigid sole shoe.

CASE DISCUSSION

Mr. Chase used to run 5 miles every day with no symptoms despite the severe degenerative joint disease of the first MTPJs (for which he unconsciously compensated). It was the cardiac stress testing that was disastrous for his foot health because he wore inappropriate footgear. It is difficult to run up hill without flexing the hallux, which he couldn't do. This altered the stresses on his feet, and the result was his stress fracture.

Mr. Chase's case illustrates that patients with diagnosed disorders may not have to give up favorite physical activities. Teaching them how to walk to compensate for their problem may be sufficient. Specific footgear, orthoses, shoe modifications, choice of walking terrain, warming up, and stretching all may play a role in helping the patient adapt.

> *Many foot problems in the old are insidiously symptomatic, so patients learn to adapt to them, frequently in ways that produce musculoskeletal problems elsewhere.*

THE DIABETIC FOOT

Foot problems in diabetic patients often develop insidiously, from something as simple as a callus, fissure, incurvated or thickened toenail, or blister. If treated promptly, the majority of these problems resolve and do not produce serious sequelae. However, the complications of diabetic foot problems consume a high proportion of health care expenditures. This is in part due to inadequate patient recognition of early warning signs and, even worse, health care providers' failure to provide appropriate care or to refer the patient on a timely basis to those who can provide care. Delays in referring patients with foot lesions have been shown to make therapy more difficult and to contribute to greater morbidity and an increase in (and more extensive) amputations.[3]

▼ *MARY LONG (Part I)*

Mary Long is a 67-year-old widow who has been an insulin-dependent diabetic for 14 years. She has just moved to town to live nearer her daughter. She is seen in your office with two concerns: a thickened discolored right great toenail and a hemorrhagic, discolored, thick callus under the first MTPJ of her left foot. Neither is painful, but when she was hospitalized 2 weeks earlier for an unexplained fever, a nurse observed them and suggested she have them seen by a doctor; you are seeing her for the first time.

STUDY QUESTIONS

- What should you routinely look for on examination of a diabetic foot?
- What is the likely etiology for these two lesions?

Studies demonstrate that diabetic foot complications can be better controlled or eliminated.[4-6] The Centers for Disease Control and Prevention, the American Diabetes Association, and state and local health departments have set goals for reducing the number of amputations in the diabetic population by 50% by 2000.[7]

In the United Kingdom, patients with diabetic foot complications take up more hospital beds than the total number of beds occupied by patients with all other diabetic complications[8]; one out of five U.K. hospital admissions is for the treatment of foot problems in the diabetic.[9] In the United States, the estimated cost per hospitalization for treating diabetic foot infections, without resultant amputation, is $6,600.[10] The direct costs per amputation, including hospitalization, surgery, and anesthesia are approximately $20,000 to $25,000.[11] Forty-five percent to seventy percent of all amputations performed are on the extremities of diabetic patients.[12,13]

Most amputations or hospitalizations for infections are extensions of simpler foot problems, so the focus of health professionals must be on preventive strategies. The physician's task is to identify those patients most susceptible and then to intervene early enough to prevent a cascade of events. Recent data confirm that foot examinations in diabetics are not performed frequently enough.[14-16] A number of clinic-based studies (although not definitive nor controlled) demonstrate that intensive attention to foot care may dramatically alter morbidity statistics and result in positive outcomes.

▼ MARY LONG (Part II)

Ms. Long has no symptoms of foot discomfort. She reports that this is the first time her feet have been fully examined. She has poor understanding of the relationship between her diabetes and potential foot complications, although she vaguely remembers receiving a pamphlet on foot care years ago. During her recent hospitalization, she received IV antibiotics. Since then her blood sugar was in the 250s when she once tested it. She smokes a pack of cigarettes a day. There is no history of intermittent claudication.

On examination, Ms. Long is wearing a loafer-style shoe with excessive wear under the left first MTPJ. There is a bulge at the toe box of the right shoe, where the great toe is push-ing distally. Pedal pulses are reduced, but there are no significant trophic changes of the skin or nails. The feet are warmer than the lower leg. Plantar reflexes are absent; the patellar reflexes are present. Vibratory sense is absent at the toes and malleoli. Position sense is disturbed. The ability to distinguish between hot and cold and sharp and dull is significantly disturbed. The toe extensors are weak. The first ray is flexible but is plantar-flexed more than the rest of the forefoot. Weight bearing causes external rotation of the left foot, with excessive pronation. A slight slapping of the left forefoot during gait is observed.

A large hemorrhagic plantar callus is present under the first MTPJ and is surrounded by a zone of erythema; there is mild localized edema. The right great toenail is thickened and the central portion has a bluish coloration; it is slightly mobile on the nail bed.

STUDY QUESTIONS

- What diabetic problems have been identified in Ms. Long's feet?
- What other aspects of diabetic education should be undertaken here?
- What management would you suggest?

▼ MARY LONG (Part III)

You refer Ms. Long to a podiatrist with whom you have worked for many years. You recommend debridement of the right great toe nail, which is carried out without anesthesia because of the neuropathy. The nail bed culture grows Candida albicans.

The callused area on the left foot is also debrided, and blood-tinged exudate is drained. After the removal of the necrotic and hyperkeratotic tissue, there is a grade 1 ulcer; probing confirms nonextension to underlying bone. Cultures are obtained, and a broad-spectrum antibiotic is prescribed by the podiatrist. X-ray examinations are ordered and the results are unremarkable. The patient is instructed in the use of povidone-iodine compresses (diluted 1:3) three times daily and the use of sterile dressings. Bed rest, except for use of the bathroom, is prescribed.

CASE DISCUSSION

It is possible that Ms. Long's "unexplained fever" arose from this neurotrophic ulcer. Multiple bacteria are often present in diabetic wounds, and it is important to obtain both superficial and deep cultures. It is likely that prior antibiotic therapy caused a flare-up in the monilial infection and the poorly fitting footwear played a role. Given this patient's prior disinterest in diabetic foot care, active follow-up will be required. A topical antifungal should be used as the new nail regrows, and further debridement may be necessary. This patient also requires increased surveillance in all aspects of her diabetic care and should be counseled to reduce smoking if at all possible; she needs to be educated in many aspects of diabetic self-care.

Managing Diabetic and Neurotrophic Ulcers

The care of diabetic and neurotrophic ulcers requires an intensive and persistent approach.[17] Attempts must be made to eliminate infection, although this may be difficult if the circulation is inadequate. Attempts to improve the vascularization should be made if possible. Since most diabetic, infected wounds have multiple bacteria, with as many as four or five organisms, both deep and superficial cultures should be obtained with sensitivities, and antibiotic treatment should be adjusted accordingly.[10] As with other ulcers, the important principle is to debride necrotic or hyperkeratotic tissue and then to carry out conventional, sterile wound care. Concurrently, diabetic control must be optimized. While there is active infection in such an ulcer, it is generally advised to have complete non–weight bearing. Once the infection is controlled, weight bearing on the ulcer site must be reduced if possible, using padding or in some cases even total contact casting. If structural deformity or abnormal positioning of the foot is a factor in the production of the ulcer, modifications to the patient's footwear, an orthotic device, or even a short leg brace would all be considerations to be discussed between the podiatrist and the physician. In some cases, surgical correction of structural deformities should be considered.

> *Diabetic foot ulcers are painless, so the patient won't know about them; you must look for them.*

Especially since diabetic neuropathy frequently deprives the diabetic foot of sensation, patients are sometimes amazingly unaware of extensive necrotic areas in their feet. The only way to find these is by regular examination, preferably by a health professional, but the surveillance can be increased by training family members to do the examination and telling them what to look for if the patient is unable to examine himself or herself. Many elderly people find it difficult to examine their feet because of reduced range of movement.

SUMMARY

The management of the frequent structural deformities, which older individuals often tolerate, requires an attentive primary health care team, with the physician and nurse always considering the underlying cause of abnormal gait or foot pain. In collaboration with a podiatrist, and sometimes an orthopedic surgeon, many chronically uncomfortable and potentially disabling foot problems in elderly individuals can be considerably ameliorated, with reduction in pain and improvement in mobility. Diabetics are predisposed to considerable, sometimes life-threatening or limb-threatening, complications that can occur insidiously without pain and that therefore require organized surveillance of the lower extremities in order to prevent problems and to treat them promptly and aggressively whenever they should occur. A collaborative approach between the primary care physician, his or her immediate team, and the podiatrist, who is specialized in the medical and surgical care of the foot and ankle, is advised in all such instances.

POSTTEST

1. Which one of the following statements is false?
   a. With an infected diabetic foot ulcer, weight bearing must be continued to maintain circulation.
   b. Most diabetic infected ulcers have multiple bacteria present.
   c. Forefoot inversion is a common compensatory mechanism for hallux limitus/hallux rigidus.
   d. Podiatrists are expert in the management of the lower limb as it relates to foot and ankle function.

REFERENCES

1. Cohn I, Kanat IO: Functional limitation of the motion of the first metatarsophalangeal joint, *J Foot Surg* 23:477-488, 1984.
2. Root M, Orien W, Weed J: Normal and abnormal function of the foot, *Clin Biomechanics* 3:358, 1977.
3. Mills JL, Beckett WC, Taylor SM: The diabetic foot: consequences of delayed treatment and referral, *South Med J* 84:970-974, 1991.
4. Davidson JK et al: Assessment of program effectiveness at Grady Memorial Hospital. In Steiner G, Lawrence PA, eds: *Educating Diabetic Patients,* New York, 1981, Springer.
5. Edmonds ME et al: Improved survival of the diabetic foot: the role of a specialized foot clinic, *QJ Med* 60:763-771, 1986.
6. Runyan JW: The Memphis chronic disease program, *JAMA* 231:264-267, 1975.
7. National Diabetes Advisory Board: *1994 Annual Report: Diabetes,* NIH Publication, No 94-1587, Washington, DC, 1994, US Department of Health and Human Services.
8. Dyck PJ et al, eds: *Diabetic neuropathy,* Philadelphia, WB Saunders.
9. Masson EA, Angle S, Roseman IP: Foot ulcers: do diabetic patients know how to protect themselves? *Pract Diabetes* 78:371-378, 1988.
10. Wheat LJ, Allen SD, Henry M: Diabetic foot infections: bacteriologic analysis, *Arch Intern Med* 146:1935-1940, 1986.

11. Reiber GE: Diabetic foot care: guidelines and financial implications, *Diabetic Care* 15(suppl 1):29-31, 1992.

12. Levin ME, O'Neal FW: *The diabetic foot,* St Louis, 1993, Mosby.

13. Most RS, Sinnock P: The epidemiology of lower extremity amputations in diabetic individuals, *Diabetic Care 6* 1:87-91, 1983.

14. Cohen SJ: Potential barriers to diabetes care, *Diabetes Care* 6:499-500, 1983.

15. Bailey TS, Yu HM, Rayfield E: Patterns of foot examinations in a diabetic clinic, *Am J Med* 78:371-374, 1985.

16. Payne TH et al: Preventive care in diabetes mellitus: current practice in urban health care system, *Diabetes Care* 12:745-747, 1989.

17. Kozak GP et al: *Management of diabetic foot problems,* Philadelphia, 1995, WB Saunders.

PRETEST ANSWER

1. c

POSTTEST ANSWER

1. a

CHAPTER 33

The Skin

MARLENE J. MASH and MARIA FEDOR

OBJECTIVES

Upon completion of this chapter, the reader will be able to:

1. Differentiate between chronologically aged and photo-aged skin.

2. Describe and recognize common benign dermatoses: solar lentigines, sebaceous hyperplasia, milia, acrochordons, seborrheic keratoses, Favre-Racouchot, xerosis and pruritus, erythema ab igne, seborrheic dermatitis, purpura, cherry hemangiomas, and venous lakes.

3. Contrast the appearance of: bullous pemphigoid, erythema multiforme bullosum, allergic contact dermatitis, herpes zoster, and vesicular tinea pedis.

4. Describe the appearance and management of the common malignant skin neoplasms: actinic keratoses, basal cell carcinoma, squamous cell carcinoma, Kaposi's sarcoma, and malignant melanoma.

5. Arrange skin diseases by their color (flesh, white, brown, red, and yellow) to help classify the condition.

PRETEST

1. All of the following statements concerning skin changes in old age are true except:
   a. Seborrheic keratoses have a "stuck-on" appearance.
   b. Leathery, deep furrowed skin is caused by sun exposure, not aging.
   c. Sweat gland activity increases with age.
   d. Sebaceous glands increase in size but decrease in output with increasing age.

2. Multiple flat, scaly lesions, 2 mm to 1.5 cm in diameter, on sun-exposed areas of individuals with fair skin are most likely:
   a. Benign
   b. Actinic keratoses
   c. Caused by xerosis
   d. Only cosmetically significant

Prevention remains the best treatment for every disease, including disorders of the skin. Both benign and malignant skin conditions can often be prevented by avoiding sun exposure or by using appropriate sunscreens. Understanding the difference between normally aged and photo-damaged skin not only will help clinicians convey the importance of these preventive measures, but also will help the early detection of benign and malignant skin conditions. Early detection and appropriate management of these disorders reduces morbidity and is very rewarding. The most common skin problems in the elderly, their recognition, and their treatment are described in this chapter. Since a picture is worth a thousand words, color plates of pathological skin changes clinicians may observe in the elderly patient are included (Plates 1-12, following pg. 426). Primary care physicians are encouraged to refine their diagnostic and treatment skills of the skin problems commonly seen in the aged by using clues such as appearance and color (Box 33-1).

▼ RUTH HINES

Mrs. Hines is an 85-year-old singer who is a semiprofessional entertainer. She complains of deep facial wrinkling and blackheads on the outer aspect of her eyes. In addition, she is concerned about unsightly brown spots (which she calls liver spots) around her neck, on her chest, and on the dorsal surfaces of her hands and forearms. She admits to lifelong sun-worshipping summers at the beach.

On physical examination, Mrs. Hines has generalized dry skin. The skin on the lateral periocular and temporal areas is thickened, yellowish brown, and atrophic with wrinkling, deep furrows, comedones, and numerous small nodular cysts. The skin of her neck shows multiple pedunculated growths, some irritated by her gold necklace. Her cheeks, forehead, chest, back, and the dorsal aspect of her hands and forearms contain multiple 2 to 3 mm, slightly scaly, erythematous lesions. Interspersed with these areas are multiple blanchable telangi-

ectasias. *On the right nasal ala is a 1 cm raised pearly lesion with central ulceration. Over all sun-exposed areas are oval, 1 to 2 cm brown lesions, with a stuck-on appearance. A loss of subcutaneous tissue is noted around her face, hands, shins, and feet.*

BOX 33-1
Clinical Features of Elderly Skin

Non–Sun-Damaged Aging Skin	Sun-Damaged Skin
Shallow, fine wrinkles	Deep, coarse wrinkles (rhytides)
Animation lines of the face (e.g., frown lines, "crow's feet")	
Loss of skin resiliency and elasticity resulting in "sagging"	Thickened, leathery, inelastic skin, yellowish discoloration, irregular pigmentation, comedones, telangiectasias
Atrophy or thinning of skin (loss of collagen)	
Sebaceous gland hyperplasia	Clinically more apparent in photodamaged skin
Loss of hydration caused by reduced hyaluronic acid with moderate xerosis	Excessively dry skin, xerosis
Thinning of vascular walls with propensity to easy bruising	Telangiectasias, purpura (easy bruising more pronounced)
Smooth, unblemished surface	Cutaneous neoplasms (e.g., actinic keratoses, basal cell cancer, squamous cell cancer)

STUDY QUESTIONS

- *Your diagnosis of Mrs. Hines includes which of the following: skin changes secondary to chronological aging, photoaging, solar lentigines, sebaceous hyperplasia, seborrheic keratosis, Favre-Racouchot syndrome, or skin tumor?*
- *Which skin changes observed are due to the normal or intrinsic aging process, and which are secondary to chronic sun exposure?*
- *Which findings require intervention and which lesions should undergo biopsy?*

NORMAL AGING VS. PHOTO-AGING OF THE SKIN

At one time or another we have all observed how the sun-exposed skin of whites develops signs of premature aging. This prematurely aged look is really an acceleration of the normal aging process caused by cumulative exposure to sunlight. We usually see deep wrinkling, irregular pigmentation, telangiectasias, yellowing, and a dry, leathery appearance of the sun-exposed areas of the skin. In addition to causing a prematurely aged look, chronic sun exposure also increases an individual's risk of basal cell cancer, actinic keratoses, squamous cell cancer, and malignant melanoma. Many people in the United States still think that a tan "looks healthy." As a result, the incidence of all types of skin cancer has increased at an alarming rate. In contrast to the clinical features of the photo-aged skin, a leathery appearance, and deep wrinkles, chronologically aged skin has shallow, fine wrinkles. See Table 33-1.

CASE DISCUSSION

Mrs. Hines' skin changes are the result of both chronological aging and photo-aging. The deep facial wrinkling and blackheads on the outer aspects of her eyes, called Favre-Racouchot syndrome, are the result of cumulative sun exposure. Similarly, the so-called liver spots on her neck, chest, and the dorsal surface of her hands and forearms (solar lentigines), the multiple telangiectasias and scaly lesions (actinic keratoses), and the thick furrowed wrinkling and blotchy pigmentation in her sun-exposed skin areas are caused by UV radiation.

The pathology report from a biopsy of the pearly lesion on her nose confirms a basal cell carcinoma. On follow-up the lesion is removed by primary excision and closure. Later the importance of preventing further photo damage and cancers is discussed, and she is counseled to wear hats, avoid the midday sun, and use a sunscreen at all times.

Clinically, it is difficult to make a distinction between the basic biological effect of aging and the effect of photo-aging on the skin. Over the past decade a considerable amount of research to define these two separable effects on the skin at the cellular level has been conducted.[1-3] Without question the most damaging and cosmetically compromising effects on the skin have been found to be environmental and, more specifically, attributable to repeated sun exposure.

> *Sun exposure far outweighs aging itself as a cause of pathological and cosmetic changes in the skin in old age.*

BENIGN DERMATOSES
Solar Lentigines

"Brown spots," or solar lentigines, are circumscribed, pigmented, nonmalignant macules. They are approximately 0.5 cm in diameter and induced by natural or artificial sources of UV radiation. In rare cases, and over a period of many years, dark brown areas develop into a melanoma (lentigo-maligna melanoma). These malignant lesions are usually larger than lentigines (ranging from 3 to 6 cm); and they are irregularly pigmented and irregularly shaped, whereas lentigines are usually circumscribed. If adequate treatment of a lentigo-maligna melanoma (e.g., complete surgical excision with adequate margins) is not provided, there is a 50% chance that the lesion will become invasive malignant melanoma and a 10% chance that it will metastasize.[2]

Sebaceous Hyperplasia

Clinically, hyperplastic glands look like yellow nodules that may have a central pore (Plate 2—multiple sebaceous hyperplasia). The number of sebaceous glands remains constant as a person ages, but they increase in size and become more visible, particularly in chronically sun-exposed skin. Paradoxically, sebum production decreases over time, contributing to the dry skin seen in normally aged as well as photo-aged skin. It is important to distinguish sebaceous hyperplasia from nodular basal cell cancer (Plate 11—basal cell carcinoma). In contrast to basal cell cancer, the sebaceous gland is not translucent and does not have telangiectatic blood vessels. Nevertheless, if in doubt, it is always best to perform a biopsy.

Milia

Milia are the tiny, 1 mm, white, epidermal cysts frequently seen on sun-damaged skin. Patients sometimes need to be reassured that these cysts are not malignant and can be removed with a comedone or needle extractor for cosmetic reasons.

Acrochordons

Acrochordons are flesh-colored skin tags. They are most commonly seen on the neck and axillae of the elderly, especially the obese. Composed of normal skin, acrochordons are always benign. If their presence is irritat-

Table 33-1   Common Skin Lesions in Old Age, Their Color and Type

Lesion	Color	Type
Actinic keratoses	Yellow, skin colored, or brown	P
Basal cell carcinoma	Skin colored	M
Blue nevus	Blue	N
Cherry hemangiomas	Red	N
Compound nevus*	Brown	N
Cysts (inflamed or infected)	Red	N
Dermal nevi	Skin colored	N
Dermatofibroma	Brown	N
Dysplastic nevus	Brown	P
Epidermoid (sebaceous) cyst	Skin colored	N
Erythema nodosum	Red	N
Erythema ab igne	Red	N
Freckles	Brown	N
Hypersensitivity reactions	Red	N
Erythema	Red	N
Urticaria	Red	N
Erythema multiforme	Red	N
Toxic epidermal necrolysis	Red	N
Vasculitis	Red	N
Insect bites	Red	N
Junctional nevus	Brown	N
Kaposi's sarcoma	Blue, red, or brown	M
Keratoacanthoma	Skin colored	N
Lentigines	Brown	N
Lipomas	Skin colored	N
Melanoma	Brown or multicolored	M
Milia	White	N
Molluscum contagiosum	Skin colored	N
Nodular malignant melanoma	Blue	M
Pityriasis alba	White	N
Postinflammatory hypopigmentation	White	N
Sebaceous hyperplasia	Yellow	N
Seborrheic dermatitis	Red	N
Seborrheic keratoses	Brown or skin colored	N
Skin tags	Skin colored	N
Squamous cell carcinoma	Skin colored	M
Tinea versicolor	White	N
Venous lakes	Bluish-red	N
Vitiligo	White	N
Warts	Skin colored	N
Xanthomas	Yellow	N

N, Nonmalignant; M, malignant; P, premalignant.
*Biopsy if suspicious.

ing or if the patient wants them removed for cosmetic reasons, scissors excision or electrodesiccation can be performed.

Seborrheic Keratosis

Brown-black, stuck-on lesions resembling barnacles, sometimes called "postage stamp lesions," are common in the elderly and can appear anywhere on the body. They occur most frequently in the seborrheic areas (e.g., the back, chest, face, and inframary areas). Seborrheic keratosis has a hereditary predisposition and is not related to sun exposure. Most elderly have at least one, but many elderly have multiple seborrheic keratoses. Many feel that these lesions are cosmetically unacceptable. Superficial removal of the lesions can be accomplished by the use of a razor blade held parallel to the skin surface.[5] All specimens should be submitted for pathological diagnosis.

Favre-Racouchot Syndrome

Favre-Racouchot syndrome encompasses a variety of primarily sun-induced skin changes, including nodular elastosis with cysts and comedones (Plate 1) and alterations in the superficial vascular system and pigmentation. Changes in the vascular system, such as friable, thin blood vessels, cause persistent erythema and telangiectasias. Irregular melanocyte distribution, the alteration in pigmentation, can be seen as multiple areas of hyperpigmentation, hypopigmentation, and scattered lentigines. Sebaceous hyperplasia can also be observed.

Erythema ab igne

"Redness from the fire" (Plate 5) is the clinical manifestation of the presence of melanin and hemosiderin in the dermis. Hyperpigmentation, hypopigmentation, telangiectasias, and atrophy of the skin can be observed. Acute or prolonged heat exposure is the direct cause of erythema ab igne, and patients should be warned about the danger of a severe burn when using heating pads or portable heaters to keep warm.

Seborrheic Dermatitis

Although seborrheic dermatitis is common in adolescence and young adulthood, it is often seen in the nursing home population in general and in patients with Parkinson's disease in particular. Redness and scaling can be observed on the scalp, around the ears and the nose, in the eyebrows, and on the anterior chest. Medical treatment with topical ketoconazole (Nizoral) is usually effective in these patients. Use of prescription shampoos such as ketoconazole (Nizoral 2% shampoo) and chloroxine 2% (Capitrol shampoo) can also be helpful in the treatment of seborrheic dermatitis of the scalp.

Purpura

With aging, thinning of the dermis leads to increased fragility of the dermal capillaries, and blood vessels rupture. The resultant extravasation of blood into the surrounding tissue, commonly seen on the dorsal forearm and hands, is referred to as purpura or ecchymosis. Minimal trauma is the direct cause of ecchymosis and skin tears. Patients with senile purpura should be reassured that they do not have a "bleeding disorder" and should be advised to protect their skin against trauma and friction. Long-sleeved shirts reduce shear and friction, and nursing home personnel should be advised that gentle handling of the patient is crucial in preventing bruising and skin tears. If a skin tear does occur, nonadherent dressings secured with tubular retention bandages should be used to prevent trauma of the surrounding skin.

Cherry Hemangiomas

Cherry hemangiomas, bright red, 1 to 5 mm papules, often increase in number with advancing age. They are most commonly seen on the trunk and their pathogenesis is unknown. The occurrence of these capillary hemangiomas does not appear to be related to sun exposure and, except for cosmetic reasons, therapy is not needed. If removal is desired, cherry hemangiomas respond to light electrodesiccation.

Venous Lakes

Benign venous angiomas, called venous lakes, occur most often on the lower lips or on the ears of older persons. They are soft, compressible, flat, approximately 4 to 6 mm in size, and bluish red. Except for cosmetic reasons, treatment is usually unnecessary. However, if the lesion cannot be clinically differentiated from a melanoma, it should be removed for histological examination.

▼ LEO WASHINGTON

Mr. Washington is a 74-year-old nursing home resident. He has a history of Parkinson's disease, progressive Alzheimer's disease, and hypertension. His caregivers have asked if they can apply mittens to reduce the skin irritation caused by frequent scratching. His only medications are furosemide and carbidopa/levadopa (Sinemet).

On physical examination, Mr. Washington is mildly demented and complains that he is "itchy all over." He has dandruff of the scalp, as well as erythematous and slightly scaly areas behind his ears, over his eyebrows, around his nose, and on the anterior chest. His family complains that he cannot see because of the flakiness around his eyes. Multiple linear purpuric lesions of the arms and legs, specifically under his restraints, are observed as well, but the skin is intact.

STUDY QUESTIONS

- *How should you investigate Mr. Washington's itching?*
- *Are the linear purpuric lesions indicative of a bleeding disorder?*

Pruritus and Pruritus with Xerosis

The most common cause of pruritus, a symptom that evokes scratching, is dry skin or xerosis. [6] Also known as asteatosis, winter itch, or eczema craquele, xerosis is quite common in the elderly (see Box 33-1) and the unfortunate reference to "senile itch" implies that the condition is intrinsic to old age. Xerotic skin looks dry, rough, and scaly. Changes are most pronounced over the anterior legs, extensor aspects of the arms and forearms, and dorsum of the hands. Chronic rubbing and scratching cause thickening of the skin. Xerosis is usually more severe in the winter because low humidity, cold and windy weather, dry heat, and excessive bathing aggravate the condition. Severe cases (eczema craquele) can result in superinfection and cellulitis.

Before treatment of the dry skin is begun (or if xerosis treatment does not alleviate pruritus), it is important to rule out other potential causes of itching, such as contact allergy, medication or food allergies, scabies, meta-

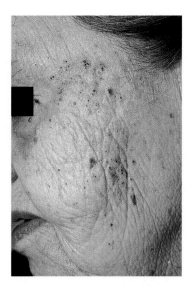

PLATE 1
Favre-Racouchot, or periorbital cysts, comedones, and solar elastoses caused by sun damage.

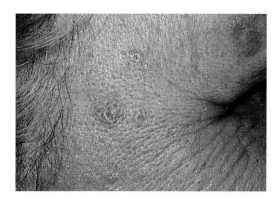

PLATE 2
Multiple sebaceous hyperplasias.

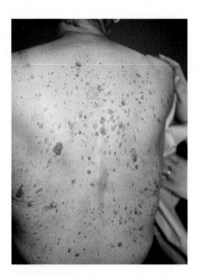

PLATE 3
Multiple seborrheic keratoses.

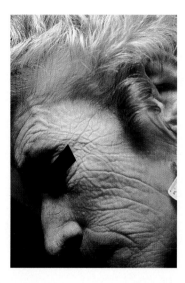

PLATE 4
Solar elastosis (note basal cell carcinoma near the left ear).

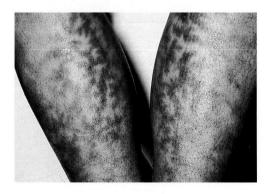

PLATE 5
Erythema ab igne of lower extremities caused by space heater.

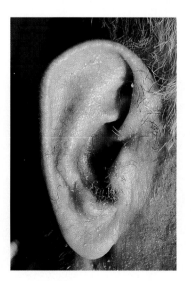

PLATE 6
Seborrheic dermatitis.

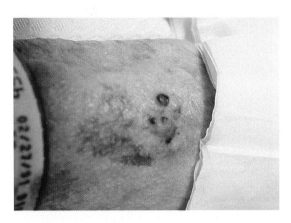

PLATE 7
Nodular malignant melanoma of forearm in 95 year old
(Level 4; 3.1 mm in depth).

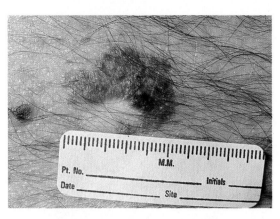

PLATE 8
Superficial spreading malignant melanoma of the back.

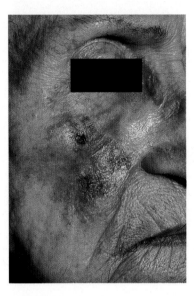

PLATE 9
Squamous cell carcinoma of the cheek.

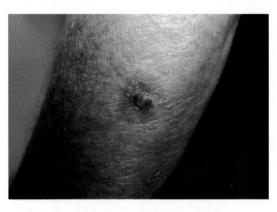

PLATE 10
Squamous cell carcinoma of the forearm arising from actinic
keratoses.

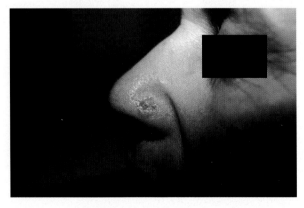

PLATE 11
Basal cell carcinoma (nasal ala).

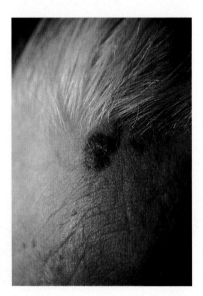

PLATE 12
Pigmented basal cell carcinoma of the temple.

bolic diseases, diseases of the liver or pillary ducts, neoplasia, and psychogenic causes.

Treatment of dry skin includes use of a humidifier and both patient and caregiver counseling. Patients should be advised to bathe less frequently, to use warm instead of hot water when bathing or taking a shower, and to use mild, moisturizing soaps (e.g., Aveeno moisturizing soap, Basis, or Dove) only. Following a bath or shower, the skin should be lightly patted dry and a moisturizer (e.g., hydrophilic ointment, Vaseline, Eucerin, or Moisturel) applied. Elderly patients should not use bath oil, since it makes the tub or shower slippery and hazardous.

If the above mentioned regimen does not reduce skin dryness and alleviate the pruritus, Lac-Hydrin 5% (over-the-counter) or prescription strength Lac-Hydrin 12% moisturizers have been found to be effective. If the skin is cracking or inflamed (eczema craquele) topical corticosteroids may be used.

CASE DISCUSSION

Mr. Washington's itchy skin cleared with elimination of detergent soaps, the use of moisturizers, and a humidifier in his room. Application of Nizoral shampoo for 10 minutes three times a week as an antifungal lotion on his eyebrows, perinasal areas, and chest, followed by washing his hair with the same shampoo, was effective.[7] The efficacy of these treatments confirmed the initial diagnosis of xerosis.

The purpuric lesions around Mr. Washington's wrists were not caused by a bleeding disorder, but by the restraints. Friction and trauma of his fragile skin had resulted in purpura. After Mr. Washington's dry skin and seborrhea had been treated successfully, his caregivers did not have to use restraints to stop him from scratching.

PREVENTION OF SUN-INDUCED SKIN CHANGES

Photo-damage, rather than the normal aging process, has been estimated to account for 90% of age-associated cosmetic problems.[8] Clinicians need to educate patients about the relationship between sun exposure or exposure to ultraviolet light from other sources (e.g., tanning booths) and cosmetic problems and cancer. Patients need to understand that there is no safe tan and that, even if sun-induced skin changes have occurred, further damage can be prevented.

Using a sunscreen with SPF 15 or higher will help protect the skin against further photo-damage. The relationship between SPF and degree of protection is not linear. An SPF 15 sunscreen will block 85% of UVB radiation, whereas UVB blockage is approximately 90% when using an SPF 20 sunscreen. Above this SPF level the degree of added protection is minimal.

Ideally, a sunscreen protects against UVA and UVB radiation; product labels usually specify this. The patient should be taught to apply a sunscreen ½ hour before going out into the sun, enabling it to bind to the skin, and to cover *all* exposed areas. The importance of reapplying the sunscreen every few hours as well as after swimming or perspiring should also be emphasized.

TREATMENT OF SUN-INDUCED SKIN CHANGES

Topical tretinoin (Retin-A) has received widespread attention for its role in treating sun-damaged skin, and controlled studies have shown that it is an effective treatment for many of the changes associated with photo-aged skin.[9] Retin-A can be used in long-term therapy to reverse photo-damage. The major side effects of topical tretinoin use are skin dryness and increased sensitivity to sun exposure. Patients should be started at the lowest available concentration (.025%) and instructed to apply the cream twice a week at first, gradually increasing the number of applications to twice a day. If the treatment is well tolerated, the tretinoin concentration can also be increased after several months. Patients who use tretinoin must be advised to avoid the sun and to use a sunscreen at all times.

Photo-damaged skin can also be treated surgically by means of dermabrasion, chemical peels using trichloroacetic acid or glycolic acid, or by augmenting soft tissue using collagen injections. For additional information on surgical treatments, the reader is referred to the bibliography.[10-12]

BULLOUS DISORDERS
Bullous Pemphigoid

Bullous pemphigoid is a blistering disease characterized by the presence of tense bullae with straw-colored fluid arising from normal or red skin. Usually, bullae first appear on the distal extremities, followed by the groin and axillae. Eventually, lesions are generalized and may include mucous membranes. Bullous pemphigoid is fairly common in the elderly and is the result of an autoimmune reaction to the epidermal basement membrane. If there is itching, it is usually severe. Diagnosis is made by biopsy with routine and direct immunofluorescence. The disease is self-limited, but if untreated, bullous pemphigoid may last from a few months to several years with periodic remissions and exacerbations. Mortality is low, but patients are uncomfortable. Treatment with oral corticosteroids (40 to 60 mg/day) is usually effective. For mild disease, dapsone or tetracycline may be prescribed.

Erythema Multiforme Bullosum

Red, nonscaling papules and plaques with central bullae and oral membrane erosion are the clinical signs of erythema multiforme bullosum, also known as Stevens-Johnson syndrome. The distribution is typically generalized, including the palms, soles, and mouth. Erythema multiforme bullosum is a hypersensitivity reaction to, among others, a medication, bacteria, virus, or food. The condition can be life threatening, especially if it results in toxic epidermal necrolysis. Prompt referral to a dermatologist and aggressive treatment (usually requiring hospitalization) are warranted.

Allergic Contact Dermatitis

Vesicles and bullae occurring in the area of exposure to an allergen (e.g., poison ivy on the forearm) are classified as allergic contact dermatitis. There is usually, but not always, a pattern suggestive of external causation such as lines from wearing a cap, ring, or necklace. If widespread, allergic contact dermatitis can be effectively treated with high-dose steroids (e.g., 40 to 60 mg) for 5 to 10 days. When symptoms are less severe, topical corticosteroids and lubrication are adequate. Determining the cause of the reaction is important to prevent recurrence.

Herpes Zoster

Herpes zoster, a self-limiting infection caused by the varicella virus, typically presents as a grouped band of inflammatory vesicles and bullae, often in a pattern following a dermatome. They can occur anywhere in the skin. Severe pain and a tingling sensation often precede the eruption. It is important to differentiate herpes zoster from herpes simplex. The latter does not occur in a dermatome pattern and is recurrent. Diagnosis is usually made following a careful history and inspection of the skin.

Treatment with acyclovir (Zovirax) 800 mg orally five times a day for 7 to 10 days has been found to reduce pain and facilitate healing. Acyclovir may reduce the incidence of postherpetic neuralgia. If the ophthalmic branch of the trigeminal nerve is involved (e.g., lesions on the tip of the nose), clinicians should be concerned about uveitis and corneal ulceration. In these instances an immediate ophthalmological consultation is warranted. The use of corticosteroids to prevent postherpetic neuralgia is controversial. If corticosteroids are prescribed for this purpose, they should be started early in the course of the disease. Prednisone 60 mg is usually initiated and tapered over a 3-week period.

The pain of herpes zoster can be severe and difficult to treat. Analgesics, carbamazepine, and amitriptyline have been used with varying success. Topical capsaicin (Zostrix) can be recommended for postherpetic neuralgia, providing the lesions have healed. Application of topical capsaicin on open, active lesions is extremely painful.

Vesicular Tinea Pedis

Vesicular tinea pedis is an intensely inflammatory infection characterized by vesicles with surrounding erythema in the instep, toe webs, and soles of the feet. The diagnosis is confirmed by KOH prep, but this can be falsely negative. Treatment with oral griseofulvin (500 mg bid) or ketoconazole (200 mg daily) is usually effective. Gram-negative infections, often present in chronically wet or macerated areas, must be treated with antifungals and appropriate antibiotics.

SKIN CANCER

Skin tumors can be classified as benign (see benign dermatoses) or malignant. Malignant tumors are further categorized as nonmelanoma (e.g., actinic keratoses, basal cell carcinoma, squamous cell carcinoma) or melanoma.

Actinic Keratoses

Actinic keratoses usually appear as multiple, flat or slightly elevated, rough, scaly macules or papules on a hyperemic base. They measure approximately 0.2 to 1.5 cm and occur on the sun-exposed areas of patients who are already genetically predisposed; hence they are most commonly seen in fair-skinned individuals.

Curettage or application of liquid nitrogen is an effective method of removing a limited number of lesions. If multiple lesions are present, the treatment of choice is fluorouracil cream. Fluorouracil 1% cream can be applied to the more delicate areas (e.g., the face), whereas 2% or 5% cream has been found to be effective for less delicate areas (e.g., forearms and dorsum of the hands). Approximately 5% to 10% of actinic keratoses progress to squamous cell carcinoma (SCC).

Basal Cell Carcinomas

Basal cell carcinomas (BCCs) are the most common skin cancers. For example, the ratio of basal cell to squamous cell carcinomas is 4:1. The most common BCCs are classified as nodular or ulcerative. BCC starts as a small papule. While the BCC slowly enlarges, a central depression, ringed by a pearly or waxy border with overlying telangietactic vessels, is formed. BCCs are most often found on sun-exposed areas of the body, especially the face and neck. They are slow growing and rarely metastasize.

Squamous Cell Carcinoma

The clinical appearance of squamous cell carcinomas (SCCs) varies, but most appear as solitary, keratotic nodules with nondistinct borders on an erythematous base (see Plates 9 and 10). SCCs can occur anywhere on the skin, including mucous membranes, but are most commonly found on sun-damaged skin and arise from actinic keratoses. They can also develop in burn scars, radiation-damaged skin, lesions of hidradenitis suppurativa, and chronic wounds (ulcers). SCCs are usually slow growing but can, although rarely, metastasize to the regional lymph nodes.

Treatment of Basal Cell and Squamous Cell Carcinomas. A variety of methods can be used to remove basal cell and squamous cell carcinomas, including curettage, electrodesiccation, excision, or radiation therapy. Primary care clinicians frequently remove smaller lesions (<0.5 cm) by curettage, which allows histological examination, or electrodesiccation. Patients with larger lesions are usually referred to a dermatologist for Mohs' surgery, skin grafting, or a primary advancement flap.

Keratoacanthoma

A keratoacanthoma resembles a carcinoma. However, this rapidly growing, bud-shaped, skin-colored to slightly reddish lesion that arises from a hair follicle is benign and occurs most often on exposed hairy skin in people over 60 years of age. Sometimes the lesion becomes ulcerated. Sun and exposure to chemical carcinogens (pitch, tar) have been found to be related to the development of keratoacanthoma. The lesion rapidly grows to approximately 10 to 25 mm followed by slow involution over 2 to 6 months. Occasionally, involution takes more than a year. For cosmetic and practical reasons, excision of the entire lesion is often recommended. Clinically as well as histologically, these lesions resemble a carcinoma, and complete excision helps confirm the diagnosis.

Malignant Melanoma

The importance of being able to evaluate any suspicious skin lesion has increased with the rising incidence of malignant melanoma in people of all ages. Early detection and prompt, aggressive treatment are essential for a cure. Widespread use of the A B C Ds of melanoma, adapted by the American Cancer Society, has helped to increase awareness.

Patients should be taught to look for: A—Asymmetry of the lesion; B—Border irregularity; C—Color variation; D—Diameter > 0.6 cm; and the recently added E—Elevation.

An originally flat lesion that becomes elevated should arouse suspicion. It is important however to tell patients that if their lesion meets only one of these criteria, they probably do not have a melanoma. If a patient is at risk for melanoma, concerned, or unsure about the ABCD's, we tell them to make an appointment every 6 months or so because it is better to: A-lways, B-e, C-hecked by their D-octor. Finally, health care professionals should be aware that only 20% of malignant melanomas arise on sun-exposed areas, so it is important to examine the *entire* body.[13,14]

SUMMARY

Skin problems in the elderly are common. Patients with chronologically aged as well as photo-aged skin may seek a physician's help to alleviate pain or itching, express their concerns related to a skin growth, or ask advice on improving the appearance of their skin. Fortunately, the vast majority of skin problems in the elderly can be treated, greatly improving their quality of life. After all, being older doesn't mean one has to be uncomfortable or itchy or live with unwanted skin lesions. In addition, physicians can play an important role in educating patients about the importance of sun protection to prevent (further) photo-damage. Since commonly encountered skin conditions in the elderly range from presenting a cosmetic concern or minor irritation to a stage IV melanoma with a 5-year survival rate of less than 50%, early recognition of the specific condition is crucial.[15] Understanding the appearance of chronologically aged and photo-aged skin (Box 33-1) and the potential diagnostic value of the color of a lesion (Table 33-1) will help clinicians guide their treatment plan.

POSTTEST

1. Which one of the following statements concerning skin disease in old age is false?
   a. The most common cause of pruritus in the elderly is xerosis (dry skin).
   b. Screening for malignancy should be considered in patients with herpes zoster.
   c. Actinic keratoses are not precancerous.
   d. Keratoacanthoma is not malignant.

2. Which one of the following statements concerning skin disease in old age is false?
   a. Malignant melanomas can occur in non–sun-exposed areas.
   b. Squamous cell carcinoma is generally preceded by actinic keratoses.
   c. Asymmetry of a lesion is a good indication that it is not malignant.
   d. Basal cell carcinomas are four times more common than squamous cell carcinomas.

REFERENCES

1. Fenske NA, Lober CW: Structural and functional changes of normal aging skin, *J Am Acad Dermatol* 15:571-587, 1986.
2. Beacham BE: Common skin problems in the elderly, *Am Family Phys* 46:163-168, 1992.
3. Selamnowitz VJ, Rizer RL, Orentreich N: Aging of the skin and its appendices. In Finch CE, Hayflock L, eds: *Handbook of the biology of aging,* New York, 1977, Van Nostrand Reinhold.
4. Kligman AM, Grove GL, Balin AK: Aging of human skin. In Finch CE, Hayflock L, eds: *Handbook of the biology of aging,* New York, 1985, Van Nostrand Reinhold.
5. Shelly WB: The razor blade in dermatologic practice, *Cutis* 16:843, 1975.
6. Denman ST: A review of pruritus, *J Am Acad Dermatol* 14:375, 1986.
7. Jacobs PH: Seborrheic dermatitis: causes and management, *Cutis* 41:182, 1988.
8. Gilchrest BA: Skin and aging process, Boca Raton, Fla, 1984, CRC Press.
9. Kligman AM: Guidelines for the use of topical tretinoin (Retin-A) for photoaged skin, *J Am Acad Dermatol* 21:650-654, 1989.
10. Alt TH: Technical aids for dermabrasion, *J Dermatol Surg Oncol* 13:638, 1987.
11. Ayres S III: Superficial chemosurgery, *Arch Dermatol* 395, 1964.
12. Elson ML: Soft tissue augmentation of periorbital fine lines and the orbital groove with Zyderm-I and fine gauge needles, *J Dermatol Surg Oncol* 18:779-782, 1992.
13. Wriggle DS et al: Importance of complete cutaneous examination for the detection of malignant melanoma, *J Am Acad Dermatol* 14:857-860, 1986.
14. Chiarello SE: The comprehensive skin examination: reasons for, facts, and methods, *J Geriatr Dermatol* 2:99-102, 1994.
15. Johnson TM et al: Current therapy for cutaneous melanoma, *J Am Acad Dermatol* 32:689-707, 1995.

ADDITIONAL SUGGESTED READINGS

Fitzpatrick TB et al: Dermatology in general medicine, New York, 1993, McGraw-Hill.
Young A, Newcomer VD, Kligman AM: Geriatric dermatology: color atlas and practitioner's guide, Philadelphia, 1993, Lea & Febiger.

PRETEST ANSWERS

1. c
2. b

POSTTEST ANSWERS

1. c
2. c

CHAPTER 34

Pressure Sores

HENRY M. WIEMAN

OBJECTIVES

On completion of this chapter, the reader will be able to:

1. Define pressure sores (pressure ulcers) and describe how they are distinguished from other skin ulcerations.

2. Identify the risk factors, contributing causes, and situations in which pressure sores develop.

3. Identify the stages of pressure sores.

4. Identify the complications of pressure sores, including cellulitis, sepsis, and osteomyelitis.

5. Describe variants of pressure ulceration (other than stage), including the presence of necrotic tissue, the process of undermining, and eschar formation.

6. Distinguish between contamination and infection of a pressure sore.

7. Select correct treatment options for the various stages and complications of pressure sores.

8. Determine when referral to a surgeon is appropriate.

9. Identify the role of the physician in the team of caregivers in the treatment of pressure sores.

10. Place the pressure sore in the context of the condition of the whole patient and recognize that the treatment goals of the pressure sore must sometimes take second place to the treatment goals of the whole patient.

PRETEST

1. A nursing home resident has a stage 4 pressure sore over the trochanter of the left hip. Which treatment option is not appropriate?
   a. Referral to surgical service for possible closure with flap of adjacent skin
   b. Dressing with saline-soaked gauze
   c. Placement of a thick hydrocolloid occlusive dressing
   d. Debridement of necrotic tissue if it is visibly present in the wound

2. A chronically debilitated woman is admitted to the hospital because of ischemic ulcers of her toes related to peripheral vascular disease and diabetes mellitus. She has no other skin problems. After surgical evaluation, a comfort care approach is decided on. She is transferred back to the nursing home where a stage 3 pressure sore over the coccyx is discovered. Steps that should have been taken to prevent this in the hospital include all except which one of the following:
   a. Placement of a gastrostomy tube
   b. Orders to turn the patient every 2 hours
   c. Nursing assessment of skin integrity on admission and frequently thereafter
   d. Use of a footboard and transferring with a draw sheet

BOX 34-1
Why Physicians Hate Pressure Sores

They remind us of our morbidity.
They represent failure.
They represent futility.
They are diagnostically and theoretically uninteresting.

PRESSURE SORES: WHY PHYSICIANS HATE THEM

It is important to recognize and acknowledge the repugnance physicians feel toward pressure sores (Box 34-1).[1] In many ways pressure sores are emblematic of the negative aspects of geriatrics in general. Pressure sores are graphic, ugly, smelly evidence of health care providers' failure to take good enough care of the elderly. Pressure sores often fail to respond to treatment and may recur even when they do respond, so health care providers may feel a sense of futility about dealing with them. The natural reaction is to avoid pressure sores altogether; there can be no doubt that hiding from them allows them to become worse, and hiding from the possibility is often what allows them to happen in the first place.

> *Pressure sores are repugnant; physicians tend to avoid them, so they happen and worsen.*

Clearly, geriatric medical care seeks to provide elders with an active healthy life and a comfortable and dignified death. Just as confrontation with the fact of mortality is the first step to becoming a caregiver to the dying, confrontation with feelings of repugnance toward pressure sores is the first step toward preventing and healing them.[2]

Pressure sores can be prevented and healed.[2] More than anything else, persistence and painstaking attention are required.

DEFINITION AND DIFFERENTIAL DIAGNOSIS

Pressure sores are usually obvious. The old term "decubitus ulcer" implies that lying down is the cause. Since *pressure* is the necessary causative factor, they are now called pressure sores or pressure ulcers.[3,4] Estimates of frequency vary widely. Somewhere between 2% and 11%[2] of hospitalized people have pressure sores and between 3% and 50%[2] (about 20% is the best estimate) of nursing home patients have them on admission.[5] Although it would be desirable to have an idea of the incidence of pressure sores in long-term care, the data are uninterpretable because of the variables involved. Incidence data reflect the population being studied: a chronic hospital[6] had 10% new sores in the first 3 weeks after admission; a large nursing home with multiple levels had 38.5% of stage 2 or worse sores in the first 12 weeks.[5] The first months after admission are the highest risk time.

Pressure sores are usually found over a bony prominence, but they must be in an area of prolonged pressure. They range from redness that does not blanch or fade to deep ulcers exposing muscle and bone. Pressure sores may resemble ischemic ulcers, venous stasis ulcers, radiation injury, pyoderma gangrenosum, or other ulcerations. If pressure is not involved, it is not a pressure sore, although other factors often coexist.

Table 34-1   The Four Stages of Pressure Sores

Stage	Description	Comments
1	Area of redness that does not blanch or fade	May resemble cellulitis but is not warm; represents tissue injury
2	Area where keratin layer is removed but underlying dermis is intact	Resembles an abrasion; usually clean, but exudate or dry crust can form
3	Ulcer through the skin, exposing subcutaneous tissue but not fascia, muscle, or bone	May be clean with pink granulation tissue, or draining, or with necrotic tissue at the base; may undermine adjacent skin
4	Ulcer that exposes fascia, muscle, or bone	Same as stage 3; if bone is exposed, osteomyelitis is to be presumed; surgical treatment often necessary if healing is sought

Usually the distinction between pressure sores and other ulcers is based on the history. Debilitated immobile persons with a sore over a pressure point have a pressure sore unless there is strong evidence for something else. The diagnosis is sometimes in doubt in foot ulcers in the presence of vascular disease or diabetes. Arteriograms may be necessary, since surgical treatment for arterial occlusion may be helpful.

▼ *LORETTA LOGAN (Part I)*

Loretta Logan is an 89-year-old woman admitted to the nursing home under your care following discharge from the hospital. She has had two strokes. She has difficulty turning in bed, and she can't get out of bed. She is incontinent of both urine and feces. She has a feeding tube in place but still has evidence of malnutrition: serum albumin is 2.2, total lymphocyte count is 600, and cholesterol is 112. She does not speak. The information from the hospital states that she has a stage 3 pressure sore over the coccyx, an eschar of unknown stage over the left heel, and a stage 2 sore over the left trochanter.

STUDY QUESTIONS

- *What are the risk factors to the presence of pressure sores?*
- *What other factors may have been involved in the development of Mrs. Logan's sores?*
- *What is meant by stage 3 and stage 2 pressure sores?*
- *Why is the heel ulcer said to be of unknown stage?*

STAGING PRESSURE SORES

Pressure sores are classified into four stages[7] (Table 34-1). Treatment depends not only on staging but also on the presence or absence of necrotic tissue, drainage, and the involvement of deep structures.

A hard, dry, black eschar cannot be assigned a stage. Eschars must be removed, usually surgically, so that the depth of the ulcer can be assessed and proper treatment instituted.

Stage 1 pressure sores are not really ulcers. Nonetheless, they represent subcutaneous tissue injury. Stage 1 sores are a harbinger of worse things to come; they offer a chance to prevent serious ulcers.

Stage 2 pressure sores resemble abrasions and can be caused by shearing forces (as well as pressure) combined with maceration resulting from moisture. They are usually moist and clean. The dermis is exposed but not the underlying tissue. They can develop dirty exudate and dry crust, but necrotic tissue is not seen.

Stage 3 pressure sores represent a wide range of wounds. They expose subcutaneous tissue but not fascia or muscle. They may have necrotic tissue or be clean, and they may be simple or may undermine tissue underlying adjacent intact skin. Undermining occurs because subcutaneous tissue is more vulnerable to pressure-related injury than the skin itself. Tracks and loculated spaces can extend for great distances under the skin and should be explored.

Stage 4 pressure sores involve fascia, muscle, or bone. They can occasionally be healed with hard work and high-technology beds, but surgery is often required if healing is the goal.

Stage 4 sores and some stage 3 sores are often found in very sick people. Although compassionate care must include care of the ulcer, a goal of healing is sometimes inappropriate, just as goals of curing the very ill patient are sometimes inappropriate.[1]

CAUSES AND RISK FACTORS

Pressure is the necessary condition for pressure sores. However, injury to the skin from pressure is related to two other physical conditions: *moisture* and *shearing* forces. Prolonged moisture macerates and greatly reduces the strength of the keratin layer and its resistance to injury. Shearing, the lateral force produced by sliding or rubbing of the skin on another surface, can produce injury on its own, in which case it is termed a skin tear. Shearing also acts in combination with pressure to produce injury, especially in such areas as the heel and coccyx (Box 34-2).

Population studies[5,6] have defined risk factors for the development of pressure sores (Box 34-3). Many of the

---

BOX 34-2
Physical Causes of Pressure Sores

Pressure
Immobility
Moisture
Shearing

BOX 34-3
Risk Factors for Pressure Sores

Strong Evidence

Immobility
Age
Malnutrition

Weak or Inconsistent Evidence

Zinc or vitamin C deficiency
Stroke
Low diastolic pressure
Incontinence (especially fecal)
Impaired mental status

BOX 34-4
Preventing Pressure Sores

Strong Evidence of Usefulness

Vigilance: use of risk assessment tools
Pressure relief: frequent turning, positioning
Use of footboards
Avoidance of shearing and moisture
Attention to nutrition

Weak or Inconsistent Evidence of Usefulness

Equipment: boots, mattresses
Massage and emollients

▼ **CAROLINE HANDY (Part I)**
Caroline Handy is a 79-year-old woman who is admitted to the nursing home after an open reduction and internal fixation of a left intertrochanteric fracture. She has no pressure sores.

STUDY QUESTIONS

■ *What information is needed to determine whether Ms Handy is likely to develop pressure sores?*
■ *What measures can be taken to avoid them?*

PREVENTING PRESSURE SORES

data are hard to interpret because they compare factors in different patients with and without pressure sores in settings where most of the people have some risk, so studies tend to reveal more about the nature of the institution than the risk of pressure sores.

Malnutrition, both general undernutrition and specific nutrient deficiencies, is clearly related to pressure sores,[7] although the precise nature of the relationship is not as clear as is commonly supposed. Protein deficiency both in terms of visceral storage and in the diet is related to pressure sores. There is some evidence that the actual intake of protein and calories is more important than the serum albumin in the development of pressure sores.[6] Protein and fluid requirements rise because of losses from the ulcer itself,[7] but such losses are difficult to quantitate.

Vitamins and minerals have been discussed in relation to pressure sores. Data are mixed, but it is reasonable to provide vitamin C and possibly zinc supplements for patients with pressure sores.[7]

Some studies have indicated that *low diastolic blood pressure* is a risk factor[5]; whether this relates to lack of perfusion of the skin or is simply a marker for general frailty is unclear.

In one study the *diagnosis of stroke* was an independent risk factor for pressure sores,[6] but the significance of this study is unclear. The setting of that study, a chronic hospital, meant that only a subset of stroke patients would be represented there.

It cannot be proven, but the most important preventive measure for pressure sores appears to be vigilance. Education of staff has been shown to be cost effective.[8] If a physician and his or her staff care about ulcers, they will be prevented. If a physician examines the skin thoroughly, examines and treats pressure sores frequently, and orders preventive measures, he or she is communicating a commitment to pressure sore prevention. If a nurse assesses and brings stage 1 sores to the attention of physicians and other nursing staff and advocates for aggressive pressure sore prevention, he or she will prevent pressure sores (Box 34-4).

 If the physician cares about pressure sores, they will be prevented.

Several risk assessment tools are available, including the Braden and Norton scales.[5,9] They focus attention on patients at risk. The Minimum Data Set (MDS) system in nursing homes incorporates markers for targeting skin breakdown; if used correctly, it could serve to target patients in need of preventive attention.

Inspecting the entire skin frequently and carefully for the presence of stage 1 (nonfading redness) sores and then treating them should be considered prevention.

Animal studies show that damage to muscle occurs after 1 to 2 hours of pressure at 60 mm Hg.[3] This has led to the regimen of turning every 2 hours when patients lack bed mobility. Whether this is adequate or excessive has not been proved in humans. Immobility is clearly the most powerful risk, and frequent repositioning of the immobile patient is the most important preventive measure available. When a patient is turned side to side, the preferred position is such that the pelvis is tilted about 30 degrees from the horizontal.[3] This position puts the weight over the thickest flesh of the buttock and avoids the trochanters and coccyx. The head of the bed should not be raised any more than necessary in immobile patients because of the shear forces on the coccyx in that position. If the head is raised, a footboard should be used.[3,10,11]

> *To prevent pressure sores, the patient is positioned with the pelvis 30 degrees from the horizontal.*

"Egg crate" and other padded mattresses are widely used. No evidence that they are effective exists. One study[2] showed that water mattresses were actually associated with the development of ulcers, but the results may be misleading; the study was not controlled. Soft foam does not necessarily decrease pressure.[12,13] After foam is compressed, it forms pressure points. High-technology beds with vertical pillows leaking air and air-fluidized styrofoam beads are clearly effective, but they are so expensive that their use for prevention is prohibitive except for patients immobilized by a respirator or other intensive equipment.[1,10] Except for the most expensive mattresses, they are adjunctive at best.

The role of nutrition is probably great, but interventions are not always effective or feasible. Evidence that the concurrent intake of protein is as important as long-term deficiency[6] affords some hope that a changed diet might modify risk even in the very debilitated. Zinc and vitamin C have received some attention as micronutrients important in wound healing.[14] The evidence is not compelling, but both are likely to be deficient in the diets of frail elders, so supplementation is reasonable.

> *Position, nutrition, and vigilance are more important than mattresses and applications.*

▼ LORETTA LOGAN (Part II)

Mrs. Logan, immobilized in bed and incontinent of urine and feces, with her undernutrition and aphasia, has a stage 3 ulcer on her coccyx, a stage 2 ulcer on the left trochanter, and an eschar on the left heel. She has just arrived under your care in the nursing home, following discharge from the hospital.

STUDY QUESTIONS

- *What further information is required before a treatment plan can be formulated?*
- *What treatment measures should be used or considered at this point?*
- *What is the prognosis for the treatment of Mrs. Logan's ulcers?*

PRESSURE SORE TREATMENT

Treatment of pressure sores is challenging and requires a team. The principles of treatment are well established (Box 34-5). Multiple products and diverse methods exist, which is evidence that no one method is clearly superior. Some members of the team may become enthusiastic about one or another technique. Unless well-founded objections exist, the favored technique should be attempted; any reasonable enthusiasm for this problem is to be encouraged.

This section necessarily reflects the methods that I favor; other emphases or approaches may be acceptable. The many treatments are critically summarized in Table 34-2.

In addition to determinating the stage of the pressure sore, the practitioner should note the presence of necrotic tissue, eschar, or purulent drainage. Exposure of bone raises the specter of osteomyelitis. Osteomyelitis can be difficult to diagnose: x-ray examinations, computed tomography, and bonescans may be unreliable, and bone biopsy may be necessary.[13]

The same preventive efforts must be used when pressure sores appear, if healing is to be allowed and other ulcers are to be prevented. Pressure relief, frequent movement, dryness, and cleanliness are all needed. Urinary catheters are generally not used, but they are occasionally justified when urinary incontinence is causing constant moisture. But even with pressure sores, urinary catheters should not be routine. Adequate nutrition must be provided.

BOX 34-5
Principles of Pressure Sore Treatment

Pressure and other causes must be removed.
Necrotic tissue must be removed.
Healing tissue should be kept moist and undisturbed mechanically or chemically.
Avoid closed space in the wound.
Purulent drainage should be removed.
Sterility is impossible; wounds should be clean but not sterile.

Table 34-2   The Many Treatments of Pressure Sores

Treatment	Comments
Pressure relief mattresses	Affordable ones are only marginally effective; very expensive ones are very good
Thin occlusive dressings	Usable for stage 2; transparent ones are better; do not change more often than every 3 days unless drainage collects
Hydrocolloid and other thick occlusive dressings	Good for stages 2 and 3; do not create a closed space; avoid using on wounds with lots of drainage or necrotic tissue
Topical antibiotics	Rarely useful
Systemic antibiotics	Only if cellulitis occurs in skin adjacent to the wound or if sepsis arises
Povidone-iodine, Dakin's solution, etc.	Avoid; they damage healing tissue
Wet-to-dry saline dressings	Best dressing for nonsurgical debridement; avoid on clean tissue and stop as soon as possible
Constantly moist saline dressings (wet-to-wet)	Best dressing for deep stage 4 and stage 3 with exuberant drainage; must be changed frequently; fill all the spaces in the wound but do not "pack"
Surgical debridement	Mandatory for fixed necrotic tissue
Surgical repair	Needed for stage 4 if patient's status and prognosis justify
Enzymatic debridement	Rarely useful; must be stopped as soon as possible

A pressure sore must heal from the bottom up (secondary intention). Even if it were possible to close the wound directly, creation of the dead space and necrotic tissue at the margin of the ulcer would preclude healing. In extensive stage 4 wounds, surgical repair consists of plastic techniques involving full-thickness flaps and skin pedicles.[15]

The wound will not heal if necrotic tissue or pus is present. Healing takes place in a protected, moist environment. Drying or chemical agents such as povidone-iodine, acetic acid, hydrogen peroxide, and Dakin's solution destroy growing fibroblasts and should be avoided.[3,12] The best environment is clean physiological saline. Bacterial contamination should be removed and controlled surgically or with dressing changes. Table

34-3 summarizes the recommended methods at the different stages.

 Necrotic tissue and pus must be removed if the wound is to heal.

▼ CAROLINE HANDY (Part II)

Ms. Handy fails to achieve the rehabilitation goals. She becomes more depressed and rarely leaves her bed. Her appetite is poor. A reddened area develops over her coccyx and both trochanters. A black, dry area 6 cm in diameter also develops over her left heel.

STUDY QUESTIONS
- What is the best way to address the black area of Ms. Handy's heel?
- What is the advisable treatment for the area over the trochanters?

Air-fluidized beds, if provided along with other treatments, are effective; even extensive wounds can be healed with them. They are very expensive. Some less expensive versions are becoming available, but whether they will have the impressive effects of the original models remains to be seen. Medicare will pay for these beds only when a stage 4 wound is established or when immobilizing equipment is being used for other medical conditions.[10]

Occlusive dressings provide the moist, protected environment necessary for healing. Their principal drawback is that they may be "slapped on," hiding the wound from view. They should be removed every 3 days, when they become loosened by mechanical disruption, or when there is drainage or liquid under the dressing. Thick hydrocolloid dressings liquify; thus leaking of fluid does not necessarily mean there is purulence. Hydrocolloid aids in removal of liquid drainage and small amounts of wet necrotic tissue, but it is no substitute for surgical debridement of extensive necrotic areas. When drainage or necrosis is more than minimal, occlusive dressings are inappropriate. If an occlusive dressing is placed on the coccyx, care must be taken to place it in firm contact with the skin between the buttocks; otherwise a closed and septic space can be formed. In general, occlusive dressings must be in contact with tissue, either skin or the base of the wound, at all points to avoid the creation of a dead space.

Any "dead space" encourages infection; occlusive dressings must be in firm, thorough contact. Surgical debridement must be done if necrotic tissue is present.

Table 34-3   Recommended Pressure Sore Treatments

Stage	Clean	Wet Necrosis	Dry Necrosis	Purulent Drainage
Eschar			Debride	
Stage 1	Remove cause			
Stage 2	Thin occlusive dressing	Brief wet-to-dry dressing		Wet or absorptive dressing
Stage 3	Hydrocolloid dressing	Wet-to-dry dressing or surgical debridement	Debride	Wet or absorptive dressing
Stage 4	Wet dressing, possibly plastic surgery	Wet to dry dressing	Surgical debridement	Wet or absorptive dressing

Antibiotics, both local and systemic, are rarely of great benefit; they can cause overgrowth of resistant bacteria, as well as allergic reactions. Pressure sores are all contaminated and cannot be made sterile, so attempts to do so are self-defeating. Occasionally treatment of draining wounds with local antibiotics is justifiable[3]; if methicillin-resistant *Staphylococcus aureus* is present, mupirocin may be warranted. Silver sulfadiazine seems to be a good choice if local antibiotics must be used; it has been effective for burns. If redness and induration occur in the skin around the wound, invasive infection is probably present and systemic antibiotic treatment should be given. Culturing pressure sores should generally be avoided, since the information obtained is not useful and may well press the physician into futile treatment.[3] If cellulitis occurs, the bacterium involved is probably not one that is found in the body of the wound. Cultures should be obtained from the extreme margin of the wound; some therefore advocate needle aspiration through the intact skin adjacent to the wound.[13]

Pressure sores can be the source of bacteria in an episode of sepsis. As in the urinary tract, attempting to sterilize the contaminated ulcer does not prevent sepsis but instead leads to a more formidable bacterial adversary.

Surgical debridement is the only effective treatment if necrotic tissue is present. It can usually be done at the bedside without anesthesia; primary care physicians should perform it in all but the most extensive cases. Sharp instruments are often required, but dry gauze mechanical debridement can be useful. When the process produces pain or bleeding, viable tissue has been reached and debridement in that area should cease. Hard eschar should be removed surgically; however, very early eschars can sometimes be removed after being softened with constant moisturizers on gauze. Debridement of pressure sores causes bacterial seeding into the systemic circulation,[2] so people with artificial heart valves and valvular disease should receive antibiotic prophylaxis as they do for dental or urological procedures.

 Necrotic tissue must be removed, avoiding damage to healthy tissue beneath.

Saline-soaked gauze is the dressing of choice for newly debrided necrotic wounds and for draining wounds. Saline gauze that is allowed to dry in the wound and is then removed ("wet-to-dry dressings") is an effective method of debridement, especially for wet necrotic tissue that is not firmly attached. Wet-to-dry dressings are in fact debridement; they remove tissue. They remove healthy healing tissue as well as necrotic tissue and must not be used on clean wounds. Constantly wet saline dressings ("wet to wet") are the best way to treat "dirty" draining wounds. They should be changed several times a day. Stage 4 and undermined stage 3 wounds should be dressed with moist saline even if they are clean because use of occlusive dressing produces dead space. Undermined and deep areas should be filled but not packed tightly; the pressure inside the wound can cause further injury.

Avoid aggressive treatment that damages healing tissue or induces pressure; such treatment inhibits healing.

There is a temptation to apply a "magic solution" to the wound instead of performing arduous and distasteful dressings and debridements. Therefore *enzyme preparations,* sometimes in conjunction with antibiotics, are used. Enzymes can be harmful if left on too long or applied to healing tissue. But if a member of the team is fervent and wishes to prove that they work, they may succeed; nonetheless, their use should be time limited and reviewed frequently.

It has been said that stage 4 pressure sores cannot be healed without *reconstructive surgery.*[1] This is not universally true, but reconstructive surgery is often required.

However, in a debilitated elderly patient with a stage 4 sore, the sore, bad as it is, may not be the worst problem.[1] The patient's nutritional, metabolic, neurological, and psychological state, social milieu, and overall prognosis must be considered; if the patient's overall status is clearly not conducive to healing, a surgical approach to the wound may be unkind and futile. However, if future ulcers are likely to be prevented, nutrition is improving and is expected to remain good, and cure of the ulcer will afford the patient functional and emotional improvement, reconstructive surgery should be sought.

THE FUTURE

Pressure sores are common, distressing, and expensive; extensive efforts to find better treatments are being made and will continue. Beds that achieve the very impressive results of high-technology air-fluidized models without the need for great expenditure would be a boon and will probably become available.

Tissue growth factors using recombinant DNA technology and tissue culturing techniques may find a place in the anti–pressure sore arsenal.[16] We can hope that these will be affordable, practical, and effective, and not another "magic solution" that gives physicians an excuse to avoid the difficult and distasteful, but supremely important and often gratifying, task of giving the personal, high-quality care that is required; such care remains the mainstay of pressure sore treatment.

POSTTEST

1. Which statement is true about surgical debridement of pressure sores?
   a. Antibiotic prophylaxis before debridement is advisable for patients with artificial heart valves.
   b. Sterilization of the operative field with povidone-iodine before the procedure is mandatory.
   c. After debridement the base of the wound should be closed with absorbable sutures.
   d. Although "wet" necrotic tissue must be removed, dry eschar acts as a protective barrier and may be left in place.

2. Which statement is true about the bacteriology of pressure sores?
   a. Wounds should all be cultured so that appropriate antimicrobial treatment can be prescribed.
   b. Cultures should be obtained from the furthest extent of undermined areas.
   c. Only sterile wounds can heal.
   d. Wounds that are draining a large amount of purulent material should be treated with topical antibiotics.

3. Which one of the following can lead to pressure sores?
   a. Presence of *Escherichia coli* on the skin
   b. Moisture on the skin
   c. Vitamin E deficiency
   d. Bacteremia

4. Which one of the following would correctly be classified as a stage 3 pressure sore?
   a. An area on the heel of dry, black eschar involving the whole skin thickness
   b. An area on the coccyx with gray moist necrotic tissue over the base of visible fatty tissue
   c. An area of the right trochanter that is clean but at the base of which can be seen a stainless steel hip prosthesis.
   d. An area on the ear of a man with a stroke in which the edge of the cartilage of the pinna has eroded away

REFERENCES

1. Moss RJ, LaPalma J: The ethics of pressure sore prevention and treatment in the elderly: a practical approach, *J Am Geriatr Soc* 39:905-908, 1991.
2. Berlowitz DR, Wilking SB: The short-term outcome of pressure sores, *J Am Geriatr Soc* 38:748-752, 1990.
3. Allman RM: Pressure ulcers among the elderly, *N Engl J Med* 320(13):850-853, 1989.
4. Woolsey RM, McGarry JD: The cause, prevention and treatment of pressure sores, *Neurol Clin North Am* 9:797-807, 1991.
5. Bergstrom N, Braden BA: Prospective study of pressure sore risk among institutionalized elderly, *J Amer Ger Soc* 40:747-758, 1992.
6. Berlowitz DR, Wilking SB: Risk factors for pressure sores: a comparison of cross-sectional and cohort-derived data, *J Am Geriatr Soc* 37:1043-1050, 1989.
7. Shea JD: Pressure sores classification and management, *Clin Orthop* 112:89-100, 1975.
8. Moody BL et al: Impact of staff education on pressure sore development in elderly hospitalized patients, *Arch Intern Med* 148:2241-2243, 1988.
9. Spoelhof GD, Ide K: Pressure ulcers in nursing home patients, *Am Fam Phys* 47(5):1207-1215, 1993.
10. Levine JM, Simpson M, McDonald RJ: Pressure sores: a plan for primary prevention, *Geriatrics* 44(4):75-76, 83-87, 90, 1989.

11. How to predict and prevent pressure ulcers, *Am J Nurs* 7:52-60, 1992.

12. Parish LC, Witkowski JA: Do's and dont's of wound healing, *Clin Dermatol* 12:129-131, 1994.

13. Kertesz D, Chow A: Infected pressure and diabetic ulcers, *Infect Dis Clin Geriatr Med* 8:835-852, 1992.

14. Breslow R: Nutritional status and dietary intake of patients with pressure ulcers: review of research literature 1943 to 1989, *Decubitus* 4(1):16-21, 1991.

15. Granick MS, Eisner AN, Solomon MP: Surgical management of decubitus ulcers, *Clin Dermatol* 12:71-79, 1994.

16. Leigh IH, Bennett G: Pressure ulcers: prevalence, etiology, and treatment modalities: a review, *Am J Surg* 167:25S-30S, 1994.

PRETEST ANSWERS
1. c
2. a

POSTTEST ANSWERS
1. a
2. b
3. b
4. b

CHAPTER 35

Diabetes Mellitus

RICHARD L. REED and ARSHAG D. MOORADIAN

OBJECTIVES

Upon completion of this chapter, the reader will be able to:

1. Identify both the typical and atypical symptoms of diabetes mellitus in the elderly.

2. Understand which specific components of the physical examination are particularly pertinent to older patients with diabetes mellitus.

3. Know the laboratory evaluations necessary to confirm the diagnosis of diabetes mellitus, as well as those helpful in screening for associated diabetic complications.

4. Decide when treatment is most appropriately indicated and choose from among the various management options, including exercise, diet, and drug therapy.

5. Describe a health maintenance protocol that would be appropriate for an elderly patient with diabetes mellitus.

Diabetes Mellitus   CHAPTER 35   **441**

PRETEST

1. Atypical symptoms of diabetes include all of the following except:
   a. Incontinence
   b. Confusion
   c. Visual difficulty
   d. Coughing
   e. Anorexia

Table 35-1   Presentation of Diabetes Mellitus in Older Patients Compared with Presentation in Younger Patients

Metabolic Abnormality	Presentation in Young Patients	Presentation in Older Patients
Increased serum osmolality	Polydipsia	Dehydration, confusion, delirium, obtundation, decreased visual acuity
Glycosuria	Polyuria	Incontinence
Catabolic state caused by insulin lack	Polyphagia	Weight loss, anorexia

One of the most common medical conditions in older persons, diabetes mellitus occurs in approximately 18% of individuals over 65 years of age,[1] and it is estimated that more than half of diabetic patients are over the age of 65.[2] In older patients diabetes mellitus often has an atypical presentation; as a result, it is frequently underdiagnosed and left untreated. Once diabetes is diagnosed, elderly patients are especially challenging to follow up; yet proactive, efficient, long-term follow-up can dramatically reduce or prevent the many complications and problems to which diabetics are prone. Since diabetics are at special risk of some of the most debilitating long-term illnesses of elders, such as coronary artery disease and stroke, efficiently recognizing and aggressively and actively managing diabetes in old age is thought to be vital for everyone in view of the consequences and costs of inadequate care.

▼ FRANK JONES (Part I)

Mr. Jones is a 68-year-old man who comes to your office for a routine follow-up visit for mild hypertension. There are no problems with his blood pressure, but he has gained 20 lb since his remarriage a year ago.

▼ BLANCHE WHITE (Part I)

Mrs. White is a 78-year-old patient of yours who is in a nursing home. She was placed there because of mild dementia following a fractured hip. She has become increasingly confused over the last week and now cannot be aroused.

▼ CARLOS MORENO (Part I)

Mr. Moreno is 82; he is brought to you because he fell while going to the bathroom. When questioned further, he notes frequent urination during the day and as many as 10 times each night. He has decreased vision and a 10-lb weight loss. These changes have occurred in the last 4 months.

Diabetes mellitus is characterized by a relative or absolute deficit in insulin production. One of the roles of insulin is to allow glucose to enter cells. Therefore a deficit in insulin produces elevated blood glucose. Aging alters the capacity to respond to physiological changes, so diabetes produces different symptoms in the elderly from those seen in younger patients. The metabolic complications and typical responses commonly noted in older patients are summarized in Table 35-1.

▼ FRANK JONES (Part II)

Mr. Jones is 20 lb overweight. The rest of the findings are within normal limits.

▼ BLANCHE WHITE (Part II)

Mrs. White has a blood pressure of 90/60 mm Hg sitting and a pulse of 120 beats per minute. She has dry mucous membranes. Her cardiologic findings are normal except for tachycardia, but rales are noted in the left lower base of her lungs. Her neurological examination shows that she is responsive only to deep pain.

▼ CARLOS MORENO (Part II)

Mr. Moreno weighs 120 lb and is 5 ft 10 in tall. He has symmetrical loss of sensation in his feet, to midankle. He ascribes a small ulcer on his great toe to poorly fitting shoes. Visual acuity is 20/100.

PHYSICAL EXAMINATION

The physical examination of the patient with suspected diabetes mellitus should be directed toward the associated acute and chronic complications. Dehydration is a common acute complication. Three types of chronic complications are frequently noted: large vessel complications, small vessel complications, and neuropathy. Diabetes mellitus is associated with accelerated atherosclerosis, producing large vessel complications such as myocardial infarction, stroke, and peripheral vascular disease. Damage to microvessels causes retinopathy and nephropathy. In the nervous system the peripheral autonomic and central systems can be involved. Important clinical complications include foot ulcers, impotence, recurrent mycotic infections, glaucoma, cataracts, and myopathy. Physical signs are summarized in Table 35-2.

▼ FRANK JONES (Part III)

On testing the urine there is glycosuria, and you order a fasting plasma glucose, which is 230 mg/dl. A second fasting level is ordered for confirmation, and is 210. A screening biochemi-

cal panel shows a total cholesterol of 270 mg/dl and a triglyceride level of 310 mg/dl. The glycosuria persists, but there is no proteinuria and the serum creatinine level is normal.

▼ BLANCHE WHITE (Part III)

You order a stat plasma glucose level as part of your evaluation to look for metabolic causes of Mrs. White's changed mental status. It is 821 mg/dl. Her serum is negative for ketones.

▼ CARLOS MORENO (Part III)

Suspecting diabetes mellitus, you order a glucose level as part of Mr. Moreno's evaluation. The glucose level is 380 mg/dl. The cholesterol is 310 mg/dl, and the triglyceride level is 1210 mg/dl. The serum creatinine level is 1.7 mg/dl, and his blood urea nitrogen (BUN) level is 32 mg/dl. He has 3+ glucose in his urine and 2+ protein.

LABORATORY TESTS AND DIAGNOSIS

The laboratory evaluation is directed at two different issues: first, the diagnosis; second, the detection of several metabolic complications that may not be apparent from the history and physical examination (Box 35-1).

There are three diagnostic criteria for diabetes mellitus; any one is sufficient to confirm the diagnosis[3]:

- Fasting plasma glucose level of 140 mg/dl or greater on at least two occasions
- Random glucose of 200 mg/dl or greater with the typical signs and symptoms of diabetes mellitus (e.g., polydipsia, polyuria, and polyphagia)
- Fasting glucose level of less than 140 mg/dl with two abnormal glucose tolerance tests; an abnormal test is defined as an elevated plasma glucose level (200 mg/dl or greater) at 2 hours and at least one other time between 0 and 2 hours after a 75 g oral glucose load

The third criterion (the oral glucose tolerance test) is rarely necessary in the elderly unless the diagnosis is strongly suspected but other criteria have not been met.

Table 35-2   Diabetic Complications and Associated Physical Examination Abnormalities in the Older Patient

Complication	Associated Physical Examination Abnormality
Large Vessel	
Myocardial infarction	Dysrhythmia, heart murmur
Cerebrovascular accident	Abnormal neurological examination
Peripheral vascular disease	Loss of peripheral pulses, skin changes
Small Vessel	
Diabetic retinopathy	Decreased visual acuity, abnormal funduscopic examination
Diabetic neuropathy	Symmetric loss of peripheral sensation, postural hypotension
Other Complications	
Foot ulcer	Decreased peripheral sensation, poor peripheral pulses
Cognitive deficit	Impaired mental status

BOX 35-1
Minimal Laboratory Evaluation of Patients With Diabetes Mellitus

BUN, creatinine, total cholesterol, high-density lipoprotein, and serum triglycerides
Urine for protein determination
Baseline glycosylated hemoglobin or fructosamine

METABOLIC COMPLICATIONS

Other metabolic complications are often present. Frequently, the serum levels of *cholesterol* and *triglycerides* are elevated. *Renal function* may be impaired; BUN and serum creatinine should be measured, although these tests will not detect mild impairment. Serum creatinine is often normal even with established renal impairment; this is because of reduced endogenous creatinine, secondary to the reduced muscle mass of many older patients.

Hyperosmolar nonketotic coma often occurs in persons whose diabetes was previously unknown; it typically affects older, female, nursing home patients. Older patients with diabetes frequently have some insulin production, so there is partial protection against ketone production. Measurement of serum ketones and blood pH helps differentiate hyperosmolar nonketotic coma from *diabetic ketoacidosis,* the other common cause of severely elevated blood glucose. Hyperosmolar coma often occurs rapidly without previous abnormalities being present, although a variety of events can initiate its development: infections; certain drugs, such as hydrochlorothiazide, propranolol, and glucocorticoids; and other acute medical illnesses, such as myocardial infarction, gastrointestinal bleeding, pulmonary embolism, and pancreatitis.[4]

CASE DISCUSSIONS

Diabetes mellitus can be totally asymptomatic, as with **Mr. Jones.** *The diagnosis is established with the second elevated fasting plasma glucose. The recent weight gain is probably precipitated by dietary changes with Mr. Jones' recent marriage. There are no diabetic complications. However, because of the difficulty of diagnosing retinopathy with routine funduscopy, a referral to an ophthalmologist should be made.*

Mrs. White is severely ill with a life-threatening condition—hyperosmolar nonketotic coma—which has a high mortality rate. Intravenous hydration should be initiated immediately, and she should be quickly transported to a hospital emergency room where she can receive intensive treatment and monitoring. Pneumonia is diagnosed at the hospital, the probable precipitant of the hyperosmolar state.

In the case of **Mr. Moreno,** *polydipsia, a symptom commonly associated with diabetes, is not prominent, probably because of age-associated loss of thirst. Instead, he falls when he gets up at night to urinate; this is the problem for which treatment is sought. Swelling of the lens, secondary to the high blood glucose level, along with peripheral neuropathy, increased the risk of falling. The catabolic state caused by the deficit of insulin accounted for the recent weight loss. The diagnosis is confirmed by the significantly elevated plasma glucose. Mr. Moreno also has a foot ulcer that will require careful podiatric treatment.*

TREATMENT

Treatment for diabetes mellitus in the elderly includes diet, exercise, and drugs.

Dietary modification as a treatment for diabetes has been used for over 2000 years. The optimal dietary modifications are still unknown. In the overweight a weight reduction program can cause rapid normalization of hyperglycemia.[5] Elaborate dietary exchange lists are not necessary in older patients; such lists often confuse them and interfere with compliance. Although many patients with diabetes are overweight, obesity is less common in the older diabetic population. In a recent study of patients with diabetes in a nursing home, being underweight was as common as being overweight.[6] If a patient is not overweight, weight reduction will only increase the risk of malnutrition. For underweight patients, weight gain should be suggested.

> *Do not be too strict about diet in elderly diabetics: undernutrition is a real danger.*

There are a number of micronutrient (vitamin and mineral) deficiencies in older persons and in diabetics,[7] but routine supplementation is not recommended unless there is specific evidence of a vitamin or mineral deficiency. Calcium supplementation (1000 mg/day) is, however, desirable for all elderly patients. For those who consume less than 1000 calories per day (19% of all those over the age of 65 in a recent national survey[8]) and for those who are on a weight-reducing diet, a multivitamin and mineral supplement is recommended (Box 35-2).

Exercise is an important component of management. Definitive data on its value in elders are lacking. Exercise programs have potential risks (foot ulcers, myocardial infarction, acceleration of proliferative retinopathy). Despite these concerns, exercise is likely to benefit healthy older patients with diabetes. A modest increase

---

BOX 35-2
Dietary Modifications for Patients With Diabetes Mellitus

Weight reduction for the obese
Reduction of simple carbohydrates (sugars); (moderate amounts of simple carbohydrates with mixed meals are acceptable)
Multivitamin supplement if caloric intake is less than 1000 calories or if the patient is on a weight-reducing diet
Calcium, 1000 mg daily, for both men and women

Modified from Reed RL, Mooradian AD: *Clin Geriatr Med* 6:883-901, 1990.

in low-impact activities, with preexercise evaluation by the primary care physician, is recommended. The general recommendation is to increase aerobic activity to 20 minutes at 60% to 70% maximal aerobic capacity at least three times per week[9]; however, this advice should be individualized.

> **Exercise is frequently neglected as a part of the management of the elderly diabetic.**

Drug therapy decisions can be difficult in the older patient,[10] especially when diabetes is asymptomatic or mild. However, the risk of complications in the asymptomatic elderly patient is as high as that in younger patients. Many older patients will have had diabetes for several years before diagnosis. Increasing life expectancy means that older individuals have many potential years of exposure, with increased risk of complications. A good general goal is to keep the 1- to 2-hour postprandial plasma glucose levels below 200 mg/dl.

Dietary modification has minimal risk. Therefore a minimum 1 to 2 months of weight reduction and modest exercise for asymptomatic or minimally symptomatic obese patients should be tried unless the patient is absolutely deficient in insulin (type I diabetes mellitus). Type I diabetes mellitus is uncommon in the elderly and is differentiated by the presence of ketones in the blood; treatment of type I requires insulin. However, if diet and exercise fail and the postprandial glucose is below 300 mg/dl, a trial of an *oral hypoglycemic agent* is recommended. Controversy continues to exist over safety, but most clinicians believe that the convenience of an oral drug makes it the best first-line agent for mild to moderate diabetes mellitus. Choices of sulfonylurea agents are summarized in Table 35-3. Second-generation agents are preferred to first-

generation because they are less likely to interfere with other medications (such as warfarin [Coumadin] or phenytoin), and they generally have less side effects. Glipizide (Glucotrol) has fewer pharmacologically active metabolites than glyburide (DiaBeta, Micronase) and is theoretically the better agent. It should be given 30 minutes before a meal for maximal effectiveness.[11] This may create compliance problems in some patients, but an extended release glipizide obviates this problem. The cost of second-generation agents is higher; first-generation agents can be used when cost is a major concern. However, chlorpropamide (Diabinese) is associated with prolonged hypoglycemia and drug-induced hyponatremia and is contraindicated in the older age group. Starting doses are usually at the low-dose range, with minimal frequency (Table 35-3). Dosages can be increased weekly to keep postprandial blood glucose levels between 140 and 200 mg/dl. Glucose levels below 140 mg/dl indicate a decrease in the drug dosage because of the risk of hypoglycemia.

The other available antidiabetic agents are metformin and acarbose. Both these agents are antihyperglycemic and therefore do not cause hypoglycemia when used as monotherapy. Both agents are associated with significant gastrointestinal discomfort and therefore should be initiated at very low doses. Clinical experience with combination therapy of either of these drugs with sulfonylurea medications or insulin in the elderly is limited.

Metformin should be initiated at 500 mg once a day, titrating to adequate glucose control. Dosage should be changed on a weekly basis to a maximum dose of 500 mg three times a day. Because of the potential of metformin-induced lactic acidosis in patients with impaired renal function, extreme caution should be used when this agent is prescribed in the elderly.

Acarbose should be started at 25 mg once a day and gradually increased as tolerated to adequate glucose con-

Table 35-3 Choice of Oral Sulfonylurea Agents in the Elderly

	Duration of Action (hr)	Daily Dose Range (mg)	Doses per Day	Comments
First Generation				
Tolbutamide	6-24	500-3000	2-3	Shortest acting of first-generation agents, probably oral hypoglycemic agent of choice in renal failure
Acetohexamide	12-24	250-1500	2	Somewhat less efficacious than other agents, mild uricosuric effect
Tolazamide	12-24	100-1000	1-2	Most similar to second generation agents
Chlorpropamide	24-72	100-500	1	Contraindicated in elderly patients
Second Generation				
Glyburide	12-24	1.25-20	1-2	More pharmacologically active metabolites than glipizide
Glipizide	16-24	2.5-40	1-2	Should be given 30 min before a meal for maximum effectiveness

Data from Reed RL, Mooradian AD: *Drugs of Today* 26:109-123, 1990; and Gerich JE: *N Engl J Med* 231:1231-1245, 1989.

trol. Most patients do not need more than 50 mg three times a day, and this is the maximum dosage for patients who weigh less than or equal to 60 kg. For patients above 60 kg, the maximum dose should not exceed 300 mg per day. Although definitive studies are pending, acarbose appears to be well suited for the management of diabetes in the elderly when fasting blood glucose is less than 200 mg/dl.[13]

> With oral agents, keep the postprandial blood glucose between 140 and 200 if possible.

Insulin is reserved for those in whom an oral agent and diet fail to produce plasma glucose levels below 200 mg/dl or those whose plasma glucose is consistently above 300 mg/dl. Insulin is usually initiated as an outpatient procedure, using an intermediate-acting preparation. If the plasma glucose is above 400 mg/dL, hospitalization may be required. It is infrequently necessary to give two doses a day, since significant insulin secretory capacity remains in most patients with type II diabetes mellitus. Human insulin should be used in situations in which therapy will be short term, such as during surgery or in a patient who is likely to lose significant weight, since starting and stopping nonhuman insulin is associated with sensitization. In most other cases in which insulin treatment is likely to be lifelong, animal-derived insulin is less expensive. Nonhuman insulin production is likely to be discontinued in the future. The starting dose needs to be individualized. Usually it can be started at a dose of 10 U of intermediate-acting insulin for normal- or low-weight individuals and 15 U for the obese.

MAINTAINING DIABETIC CONTROL

A mechanism for monitoring the individual's diabetic control is vital. Urine glucose measurement has little role given the greater accuracy of *glucometers* (home blood glucose monitoring); their use should be taught by a nurse. Color vision changes, such as the blue-green discrimination loss common to older individuals, can cause errors when visual readings are used. Glucometers that read the levels can be purchased. Some are much easier to use than others.[12]

Other monitoring methods include *glycosylated hemoglobin* (hemoglobin A_1C), which measures diabetic control over the previous 2 to 3 months. Recent bleeding, alcoholism, azotemia, and high-dose salicylates interfere with the levels. High-affinity chromatography allows a reliable measurement. An alternative is the serum *fructosamine*, which reflects plasma glucose over the previous 2 weeks; it costs approximately one third as much and is increasingly available.

▼ *FRANK JONES (Part IV)*

Mr. Jones loses 10 lb after discussion with a dietitian. He regains this weight gradually, despite a moderate exercise regimen. The fasting serum glucose level stays persistently above 180 mg/dl; you decide to initiate glyburide, 1.25 mg daily. Blood glucose levels, cholesterol, and triglyceride ultimately normalize on 2.5 mg a day.

▼ *BLANCHE WHITE (Part IV)*

Mrs. White survives her hospitalization and is discharged on intermediate-acting insulin, 25 U subcutaneously each morning. Her plasma glucose level varies between 150 and 250 mg/dl. Fluid intake is prescribed to prevent recurrent dehydration. She does well until she dies of other causes 2 years later in the nursing home.

▼ *CARLOS MORENO (Part IV)*

Since Mr. Moreno's plasma glucose level is substantially over 300 mg/dl, he is started on 10 U of human intermediate-acting insulin each morning. His vision improves significantly with normalization of the blood glucose levels, and his urinary frequency resolves. A podiatrist provides him with special shoes to decrease pressure on his toes; his foot ulcer heals. After initiation of insulin he begins to regain weight. Since his triglyceride level remains above 500 mg/dl, gemfibrozil (Lopid) is initiated, which brings these levels to an acceptable range.

LONG-TERM MANAGEMENT

Once the diagnosis and treatment are established, it is essential to develop a proactive, planned management strategy including recall of the patient, if necessary, and involving education not only of the patient but also of the family caregivers. Only by such an active approach can the many potential complications be prevented. Good diabetic control reduces the likelihood of several major complications. Routine care by other disciplines, especially podiatry, dentistry, and nutrition, is indicated in many cases. Each time the patient is seen, the next visit should be scheduled. At each visit, body weight and blood pressure are measured. Lipids generally revert to normal levels with improvement of diabetic control, but if the fasting triglyceride level is above 500 mg/dl, specific treatment with gemfibrozil (Lopid) is recommended. The fundi should be examined at every visit by the primary care physician and yearly by an ophthalmologist. Home glucose monitoring should be reviewed at every visit, and glycosylated hemoglobin (or fructosamine) should be measured every 3 months. Yearly renal function and urinary chemistry examinations are also recommended (Box 35-3).

BOX 35-3
Brief Preventive Maintenance Protocol for Diabetes Mellitus

Every visit
  Body weight
  Blood pressure
  Evaluation of feet
  Funduscopic examination
  Review of home blood glucose monitoring
Every 3 months
  Glycosylated hemoglobin
Every year
  Funduscopic examination by ophthalmologist
  Fasting blood lipid panel
  Renal function and urine chemistry

Aggressive, active follow-up is vital in diabetes: if the patient won't come to the team, the team must go to the patient.

SUMMARY

Diabetes mellitus is a common medical problem in the elderly. Careful surveillance for symptoms often suggests the diagnosis. Elevated plasma glucose levels alone are often diagnostic even in asymptomatic persons. A weight reduction diet and modest increase in exercise may control the disease. Judicious use of drug therapy with close monitoring of blood glucose levels is indicated in some situations. A preventive and monitoring management plan is vital for long-term follow-up and to prevent unnecessary morbidity and mortality.

POSTTEST

1. The recommended frequency of glycosylated hemoglobin determination in an established diabetic patient is:
  a. Weekly
  b. Every 2 weeks
  c. Every 3 months
  d. Yearly
2. Which one of the following examples does *not* meet the criteria for diabetes mellitus:
  a. Two fasting plasma glucose determinations of 175 and 182 mg/dl
  b. A random glucose of 240 mg/dl with typical signs of diabetes mellitus
  c. A random glucose of 150 mg/dl and an abnormal glucose tolerance test
  d. A random glucose of 210 mg/dl and typical signs of diabetes mellitus
3. Which one of the following is *not* an appropriate dietary recommendation for management of an older patient with diabetes mellitus:
  a. Reduction of simple carbohydrates
  b. Use of a multivitamin supplement if on a weight reduction diet
  c. Use of supplemental zinc in all older men
  d. Supplemental calcium in both men and women

REFERENCES

1. Harris MI et al: Prevalence of diabetes and impaired glucose tolerance and plasma glucose levels in US populations, ages 20-74 years, *Diabetes* 36:523-534, 1987.
2. Center for Economic Studies in Medicine: *Direct and indirect costs of diabetes in the United States in 1987,* Alexandria, Va, 1989, American Diabetes Association.
3. Lebovitz H, ed: *Physicians guide to non-insulin-dependent (type II) diabetes: diagnosis and treatment,* ed 2, Alexandria, Va, 1988, American Diabetes Association.
4. Wachtel TJ: The diabetic hyperosmolar state, *Clin Geriatr Med* 6:797-806, 1990.
5. Reaven GM: Beneficial effect of moderate weight loss in older patients with non-insulin-dependent diabetes mellitus poorly controlled with insulin, *J Am Geriatr Soc* 33:93-98, 1985.
6. Mooradian AD et al: Diabetes mellitus in elderly nursing home patients: a survey of clinical characteristics and management, *J Am Geriatr Soc* 36:391-396, 1988.
7. Reed RL, Mooradian AD: Nutritional status and dietary management of elderly diabetic patients, *Clin Geriatr Med* 6:883-901, 1990.
8. Carroll MD, Abraham S, Dresser CM: Dietary intake source data: United States 1976-80, *Vital Health Stat (2),* 11(231):124, 1983.
9. Rosenthal MJ et al: UCLA geriatric grand rounds: diabetes in the elderly, *J Am Geriatr Soc* 34:435-447, 1987.
10. Reed RL, Mooradian AD: Drug treatment of diabetes in the elderly, *Drugs of Today* 26:109-123, 1990.
11. Wahlin-Boll E et al: Influence of food intake on the absorption and effect of glipizide in diabetics and in healthy subjects, *Eur J Clin Pharmacol* 18:279-283, 1990.
12. Bernbaum M et al: The reliability of self-blood glucose monitoring in elderly diabetic patients, *J Am Geriatr Soc* 42:779-781, 1994.
13. Mooradian AD: Drug therapy of non–insulin-dependent diabetes in the elderly, *Drugs* 51:931-941, 1996.

PRETEST ANSWERS
1. d

POSTTEST ANSWERS
1. c
2. c
3. c

CHAPTER 36

Thyroid Disease

PETER J. RIZZOLO

OBJECTIVES

Upon completion of this chapter, the reader will be able to:

1. Describe the atypical presentations of hypothyroidism and hyperthyroidism associated with increasing age.

2. Describe the place of thyroid suppression in the management of thyroid cancer.

3. Describe the management of compensated hypothyroidism in old age.

4. Describe the recognition and management of toxic nodular goiter.

5. Describe the relationship between thyroxine treatment and coronary artery disease.

6. Describe the recognition and management of the euthyroid sick syndrome (ESS).

1. Of the following statements concerning thyroid disease and its treatment in old age, which one is not true?
   a. In the majority of older persons with hyperthyroidism, the clinical and laboratory findings are similar to those in younger persons.
   b. The clinical symptoms of hypothyroidism are common in euthyroid older persons.
   c. In persons with thyroid cancer, exogenous thyroxine can cause reactivation.
   d. Thyroxine has been known to precipitate acute myocardial infarction.

Thyroid disease is the second most common endocrinological problem of older persons (after diabetes). Detecting thyroid disease becomes increasingly difficult as patients age because the symptoms of aging and of hypothyroidism overlap, and the symptoms of hyperthyroidism are often blunted in the elderly. Fortunately, improvements in laboratory testing have sharpened diagnostic capabilities. Nonetheless many difficult and controversial areas remain in the management of thyroid disease in older persons. This chapter will focus on those areas.

HYPOTHYROIDISM

The classic signs and symptoms of hypothyroidism are for the most part the same in older individuals as in younger persons. Unlike younger persons, however, many of those symptoms and signs are seen in older persons without thyroid disease. Although the majority of hypothyroid persons have typical signs and symptoms, 25% to 40% have an atypical presentation.[1-4] Classic signs and symptoms of hypothyroidism include the following: fatigue, weakness, dry skin, menstrual disturbance, cold intolerance, depression, voice change (hoarseness), bradycardia, carotenemia, macroglossia, cardiomyopathy, anemia, and nonpitting edema. Many of these features are found in euthyroid individuals and could easily be misattributed to normal aging. Because of this tendency, the presence of hypothyroidism is frequently missed.

It is not uncommon for older persons with hypothyroidism to have vague, nonspecific, and atypical signs and symptoms, including confusional state, memory impairment, behavioral changes, myopathy, neuropathy, Raynaud's phenomenon, and macrocytic anemia.

A variety of symptoms usually associated with Alzheimer's disease and multiinfarct dementia may also be seen in persons with hypothyroidism. These symptoms include mental confusion, clouded state of consciousness, memory impairment, behavioral changes, depressed affect, and muscle weakness.

Symptoms related to peripheral neuropathy, such as paresthesia, mild to severe burning, and knifelike pain in the extremities, may be the only presenting complaints.

Muscle weakness, stiffness, and slowed responsiveness may also be seen.

There are few if any physical findings in early hypothyroidism, but as the disease progresses, many changes become apparent on general physical examination. These changes include thinning of hair with loss of the lateral one third of the eyebrows; coarse, dry, thickened skin; large tongue; typical moon facies with puffy eyelids and full cheeks; yellowish tint to the skin; nonpitting edema; slow return phase of the deep tendon reflex; and slow heart rate.

HYPERTHYROIDISM

Hyperthyroidism in the majority of older persons presents with clinical and laboratory findings similar to those in younger persons. However, in 25% to 40% of older individuals the presentation is atypical. Twenty-five percent demonstrate an apathetic picture with depressed affect, failure to thrive, and absence of eye signs and skin changes.[5,6] Often the serum thyroxine level is in the high normal range. T_3 toxicosis is seen in 10% of older patients with hyperthyroidism; goiter is absent in 40%; and atrial fibrillation is present in 40%. Because the T_4 level is often in the high normal range, a thyrotropin-releasing hormone (TRH) stimulation test may be necessary to establish the diagnosis.

> *Hyperthyroidism presents an atypical apathetic picture in 25% of elders, but in the majority the symptoms are the same as in younger adults.*

▼ HILDA LEVY

Hilda Levy is an 86-year-old woman with severe coronary artery disease; she is receiving several cardiac drugs, including a calcium channel blocker, a β-blocker, a nitroglycerin patch, and sublingual nitroglycerin as needed. She has been receiving thyroxine replacement for 15 years following surgery for a solitary cold thyroid nodule. Histological cell type was a well-

differentiated adenocarcinoma limited to the nodule. Reliable thyrotropin-stimulating hormone (TSH) receptor assay was not available at that time, so she was placed on thyroxine suppression therapy on an empirical basis. There was no evidence of spread to regional lymph nodes. She currently takes 150 μg of thyroxine daily.

STUDY QUESTIONS

- Could thyroxine dosage in the recommended range for an older person adversely affect cardiac status?
- Without evidence of recurrent thyroid cancer, how long should you continue suppression therapy with thyroxine?
- How can you gauge the minimum dose of thyroxine necessary for suppression to prevent possible recurrence of the cancer?

THYROXINE SUPPRESSION FOLLOWING THYROID CANCER

It is known that thyroxine increases myocardial oxygen demand and that elevated levels can aggravate congestive heart failure and make control of angina more difficult.[7,8] In a person with severe coronary artery disease with poorly controlled angina, thyroxine replacement in hyperphysiological doses is undesirable. On the other hand, thyroid suppression with exogenous thyroxine is part of the treatment to prevent recurrence of thyroid cancer.[9] There is no definitive answer as to how much thyroxine is enough. Some thyrologists believe that serum T_4 in the slightly elevated range would suffice to suppress thyroid cancer cells. Serum T_4 levels in the 12 to 15 μg/dl range would be a reasonable end point. A serum T_4 level can be ordered and the thyroxine dose adjusted accordingly. With the currently available ultrasensitive TSH, the physician could adjust the dose of thyroxine to keep the TSH just at or slightly below the low normal limit.

CASE DISCUSSION

Because of the more proximate risk related to the coronary artery disease and advanced age, physicians should be inclined toward maintaining a euthyroid state in the high normal range for serum thyroxine. If the thyroxine dose could be lowered by 25% to 50%, Mrs. Levy might benefit by improved anginal control and improved general functional status. Consultation with a surgeon or endocrinologist experienced in treating patients with thyroid cancer is indicated in helping to decide what course would optimize her cardiac function without significantly increasing her risk of recurrent thyroid cancer.

▼ JULIA FREEMAN (Part I)

Julia Freeman is a 78-year-old woman with a history of hypothyroidism who took thyroxine for approximately 20 years. One year ago she decided to stop taking the medicine and did not notice any ill effects. She is seen for a routine annual examination and is feeling well. A thyroid panel and TSH are ordered. The results are as follows: T_4, 4.8 μg/dl; T_3 radioactive uptake (T_3RU), 32%; free thyroxine index (FTI), 3.2; TSH, 8.0 mU/L.

STUDY QUESTIONS

- What is the significance of the slightly elevated serum TSH?
- Since the patient is asymptomatic, does anything need to be done?
- Are the abnormal laboratory values or the patient's clinical state to be treated?

COMPENSATED HYPOTHYROIDISM

As primary thyroid failure develops, the serum T_4 level falls but remains in the low normal range as the rising TSH stimulates the thyroid gland to hypertrophy and produce more thyroxine. The gland also produces relatively more T_3 so that the FTI tends to remain in the normal range until later in the disease process. This stage is referred to as compensated hypothyroidism.[10] Treatment of compensated hypothyroidism is probably unnecessary as long as the patient is asymptomatic and the FTI remains in the normal range.

> *In compensated hypothyroidism, treatment is probably not needed if the patient is asymptomatic and the free thyroxine index remains in the normal range.*

It is currently believed that most adults with hypothyroidism have had one or more bouts of thyroiditis resulting in eventual thyroid failure. The presence of thyroid antibodies in most patients with hypothyroidism supports that theory. Persons with compensated hypothyroidism may have suffered only slight thyroid damage and may remain compensated if no further thyroid damage occurs, or more likely, they may have recurrent thyroiditis with eventual decompensation of their thyroid status. It is reported that persons with compensated hypothyroidism become metabolically hypothyroid at the rate of 7% per year. Therefore many older persons with compensated hypothyroidism never become clinically hypothyroid.

▼ JULIA FREEMAN (Part II)

One year later, Ms. Freeman is experiencing easy fatigability and weight gain. The TSH level is 14.7 mU/L and her FTI is slightly below the normal range. She is restarted on thyroxine. Her symptoms clear on initiation of thyroxine therapy with return of the T_4 and TSH to the normal range.

▼ MARTHA LINCOLN

Mrs. Martha Lincoln is an 81-year-old mother of 11 children who lives with an invalid spouse and mentally retarded 48-year-old daughter. Her own health is tenuous. Her medical problems include insulin-dependent diabetes mellitus, near blindness secondary to macular degeneration, compensated congestive heart failure, hypertension, angina, and hypothyroidism. She takes several medications, including thyroxine, which she has been taking for 16 years following subtotal thyroidectomy for thyroid goiter. The family was told that the goiter was benign and that she would have to take thyroid medicine indefinitely.

STUDY QUESTIONS

- *Would a trial withdrawal of thyroxine be safe?*
- *Is it necessary to taper the T_4 before discontinuing?*
- *After withdrawal, how soon would one expect the pituitary gland to respond by production of TSH above the normal range?*

REEVALUATING AND DISCONTINUING THYROXINE THERAPY

Since thyroxine has a 7-day half-life, a natural taper occurs when the medication is abruptly stopped. After thyroxine is stopped, the pituitary gland responds within 2 to 3 weeks to the lower-than-normal thyroxine levels by producing increasing amounts of TSH. This appears to be true even after suppression of TSH production by exogenous thyroxine for many years.[11]

> ✂ *Patients who have been on thyroid replacement for decades should be considered for a trial without medication in case the diagnosis was inaccurate or thyroid function has recovered. Use the TSH-off treatment to judge if the patient is truly hypothyroid.*

Many elderly persons may have been started on thyroxine at a time when today's accurate thyroid function studies were not available; the diagnosis of hypothyroidism was often based on clinical findings and indirect, less accurate measures of thyroid function such as basal metabolic rate and Achilles' reflex measures.[12] Thyroxine is not an innocuous drug in the elderly, considering the prevalence of coronary artery disease with advancing age. Unless one is certain of the diagnostic criteria on which the diagnosis was originally established, it is not only reasonable but may be potentially beneficial to proceed with a trial withdrawal. There is good evidence that the thyroid remnant in the majority of persons undergoing sub-

total thyroidectomy is eventually able to produce sufficient thyroxine to maintain the euthyroid state.[13]

A trial withdrawal in a patient on thyroxine after subtotal thyroidectomy can be performed as follows:

1. Obtain a baseline TSH.
2. Stop the thyroxine medication and repeat the TSH in 3 to 4 weeks.
3. If the TSH has not risen above the normal range, continue to withhold the thyroxine, since the patient probably does not require it.
4. Repeat the TSH in 3 months and then annually for 1 to 2 years.

If the TSH is elevated above the normal range, the patient is hypothyroid and the medication should be restarted.

CASE DISCUSSION

In Mrs. Lincoln's case the initiation of thyroxine therapy was based on a commonly held belief that all persons having subtotal thyroidectomy need to be maintained on thyroxine after surgery. However, almost two thirds of individuals having subtotal thyroidectomy eventually revert to normal thyroid function, often within several months of surgery. In Mrs. Lincoln's case, after withdrawal of therapy the TSH after 3 weeks rose to 14.7 mU/L, indicating her continued need for exogenous thyroxine.

APATHETIC HYPERTHYROIDISM

▼ LOIS ALDIN (Part I)

Mrs. Lois Aldin is an 81-year-old, thin, woman who has lived alone since the death of her husband in an auto accident 8 years ago. She is brought to you, her primary care physician, by her son because of concern about weight loss, low energy, poor memory, poor concentration, and loss of interest in many of her usual social and physical activities. Other medical problems included mild chronic obstructive pulmonary disease, essential hypertension, and a history of depression following her husband's death. At the time of onset of her present symptoms, 6 to 8 months previously, she witnessed an automobile accident close to her home. Following that, her family reports occasional times when she reported seeing strangers (both adults and children) on her property. Her descriptions of the strangers were vague, and her family was concerned that she may have been imagining them. Findings included depressed affect, stigmata of weight loss, temporal muscle wasting, mild resting tremor, hyperreflexia, tachycardia (resting pulse 85 beats per minute), and a nontender, slightly enlarged thyroid gland. Mental status screening revealed a Folstein Mini–Mental State score of 24/30 (just within normal range). On the Geriatric Depression Scale she scored in the mild-to-moderate depression range. Initial laboratory tests of significance included T_4, 9.4 µg/dl; T_3RU, 41%; FTI, 3.85; normal vitamin B_{12} and complete blood count, sedimentation rate, SMA-6/60, FBS (fasting blood sugar), VDRL, and electrocardiogram.

STUDY QUESTIONS

- Does she have early dementia?
- Should she be treated for depression?
- With a normal thyroid screening profile is any other thyroid testing indicated?

CASE DISCUSSION

Mrs. Aldin does have many clinical features consistent with early dementia, including poor memory, behavioral changes, and personality change. Since the onset is recent, that is, over the past several months, a search for reversible causes is indicated. The initial screening battery reveals none of the more common causes of reversible dementia. However, the clinical examination reveals several findings consistent with the diagnosis of apathetic hyperthyroidism. T_3 toxicosis is seen in 10% of older patients with hyperthyroidism, goiter is absent in 40%, and atrial fibrillation is present in 40%. Because the T_4 is often in the normal range, a TRH stimulation test may be necessary to establish the diagnosis. Approximately 20% of older persons present a confusing picture of both typical and atypical findings. These include tremor, weight loss, temporal muscle wasting, tachycardia, confusion, apathy, depression, and, at times, psychotic symptoms.

▼ LOIS ALDIN (Part II)

Computed tomography of the brain reveals mild atrophy but no other changes. An ultrasensitive TSH is slightly below normal at 0.2 (normal, 0.3 to 4.5 mU/L). To confirm mild hyperthyroidism a TRH stimulation test is done. It is suggestive but not conclusive for hyperthyroidism. A consulting endocrinologist decides that treatment for hyperthyroidism is not indicated.

Mrs. Aldin is given a course of tricyclic antidepressant therapy but becomes more confused and refuses to continue to take it. She begins propylthiouracil (PTU) and after several weeks has gained 12 pounds; she is less apathetic and has a normal pulse and no tremor. However, she continues to be confused and to have poor short-term memory.

CASE DISCUSSION

Ms. Aldin may have mild apathetic hyperthyroidism as well as early dementia. Careful clinical follow-up is necessary to ascertain progression of her behavioral and cognitive impairments.

▼ ALICE CLARK (Part I)

Mrs. Alice Clark is a 72-year-old retired accountant whose complaints are sleep disturbance, night sweats, hand tremor, and anxiety. She reports that an older sister has been treated for Graves' disease. Her history includes hypertension and x-ray treatments for acne as a teenager. On examination, she has a diffusely enlarged thyroid gland and a 1.5 cm nodule in the left lobe. Initial thyroid function studies include the following: T_4, 14.2 μg/dl; T_3RU, 46%; FTI, 6.3; TSH < 0.3 mU/L (before ultrasensitive TSH was available). She is now being seen to evaluate her present thyroid status.

STUDY QUESTIONS

- In the presence of this history and laboratory values, would you order further testing before initiating therapy for hyperthyroidism?
- Would thyroid ultrasound or a thyroid scan be helpful?
- What is the most likely diagnosis?

TOXIC NODULAR GOITER

Recurrent hyperthyroidism secondary to toxic nodular goiter can be controlled at times by treatment with PTU or other suppressive therapy until the patient is euthyroid and then treated with thyroxine to suppress TSH production. This sometimes prevents recurrences of hyperthyroidism. When this is not effective, ablative therapy with radioactive ^{131}I is required. Some physicians advocate going directly to ablative therapy.

In the absence of multiple thyroid nodules, a similar clinical picture results from recurrent bouts of thyroiditis with transient hyperthyroidism followed by transient hypothyroidism. Hypothyroid periods usually continue for several months and eventually persist with repeated thyroidal injury secondary to recurrent thyroiditis. High levels of thyroid antibodies help to establish this diagnosis.

CASE DISCUSSION

The symptoms, physical findings, and laboratory results are consistent with a hyperthyroid state. Graves' disease and other autoimmune diseases of the thyroid gland are often familial; the family history of Graves' disease in this instance is suggestive. However, the absence of ocular signs such as proptosis and extraocular muscle paralysis makes this diagnosis less likely.

The diffuse thyroid enlargement is consistent with Graves' disease as well as other types of hyperthyroidism. The presence of a solitary nodule is worrisome considering the history of x-ray treatments for acne, since radiation increases the risk of subsequent thyroid cancer.

▼ ALICE CLARK (Part II)

Thyroid ultrasound shows the presence of other smaller nodules that were not clinically palpable. Thyroid scan subsequently reveals that the palpable nodule of the left lobe is hypofunctioning, or a "cold" nodule. Other nodules are judged to be hyperfunctioning. Aspiration biopsy of the cold nodule reveals normal thyroid tissue. A diagnosis of diffuse nodular *goiter is made, and Mrs. Clark is placed on suppressive therapy with PTU. She improves clinically, but after 3 months of treatment a follow-up TSH is 15.6 mU/L. The PTU is discontinued, and her thyroid function test results return to normal on 6-week follow-up. Approximately 1 year later she is again experiencing sweats, weight loss, and tachycardia. Ultrasensitive TSH is < 0.1, indicating a return of her hyperthyroid state.*

▼ JENNY HOLMES

Mrs. Jenny Holmes is a 65-year-old gradeschool teacher with a history of coronary artery disease, atypical angina, adult onset diabetes mellitus, and hyperlipidemia. She presents with low energy, poor concentration, sleep disturbance, yellowish skin, and nonpitting edema. On physical examination you note a nontender, diffusely enlarged thyroid gland that is approximately twice normal size. You obtain thyroid function studies with the following results: T₄, 2 μg/dL; T₃RU, 33%; FTI, 0.66; and TSH, 115 mU/L.

STUDY QUESTIONS

- *Hypothyroidism seems obvious from the clinical history, physical examination, and laboratory results. Is further testing necessary?*
- *Given her medical condition, what treatment should be initiated?*

TRANSIENT HYPOTHYROIDISM

Both subacute thyroiditis (viral) and silent thyroiditis (Hashimoto's) can cause a transient period of hypothyroidism lasting from weeks to several months.[13] Since the onset of subacute thyroiditis is most often associated with neck pain, tenderness, and a history of a viral-like illness, history and physical examination may suggest this potential cause of hypothyroidism. An elevated sedimentation rate would support this diagnosis.

Hashimoto's thyroiditis may be associated initially with transient hyperthyroidism and then with transient hypothyroidism. A slightly enlarged thyroid gland would be consistent with this diagnosis. It is believed that progressive and repeated bouts of Hashimoto's thyroiditis cause primary thyroid failure. A high titer of antithyroid antibodies would be highly suggestive; histological confirmation can be obtained with fine needle aspiration cytology.

Other causes of transient hypothyroidism include postpartum thyroiditis, post–subtotal thyroidectomy, and radioactive iodine therapy.

CASE DISCUSSION

Although several conditions can cause transient hypothyroidism, Mrs. Holmes probably has primary hypothyroidism and

will need to take thyroid medication indefinitely. Since she is clinically symptomatic, she should be treated anyway; it would not make sense to subject her to the expense and the risks associated with further diagnostic studies. Any of the other possible conditions need not be considered in this patient in the absence of history of thyroid surgery or treatment with radioactive iodine.

THYROXINE TREATMENT AND CORONARY ARTERY DISEASE

Thyroxine treatment must be initiated cautiously in the presence of known coronary artery disease. Thyroxine increases cardiac muscle oxygen demand and in the presence of coronary artery disease can precipitate angina or myocardial infarction. It is necessary, therefore, to start with very low doses and proceed slowly. Since thyroxine has a half-life of approximately 1 week, if angina were to develop, it would take days to reduce the thyroxine level. Liothyronine (T₃), on the other hand, has a half-life of approximately 36 hours, and its metabolic effect can be more quickly reversed.

In the presence of coronary artery disease, some thyrologists suggest initiating therapy with liothyronine and switching to thyroxine when it becomes apparent that the patient can tolerate the thyroid replacement therapy. The following approach is recommended: start with 5 μg of T₃ daily for 1 week. If no increase in angina occurs, increase by 5 μg increments at weekly intervals until reaching a dose of 25 μg daily. At that dose, switch to thyroxine (T₄), 25 μg daily for 1 week, and if tolerated, increase by 25 μg increments weekly to 75 μg daily. It is best to give the minimal dose that maintains the patient in the euthyroid range. The serum TSH can be repeated at monthly intervals, aiming for a dose of thyroxine that will maintain the TSH in the high normal range.

In hypothyroidism, especially when the patient also has coronary artery disease, use just enough thyroxine to keep the TSH in the high normal range.

▼ ADELE BRENNER

Mrs. Adele Brenner is 76 years old and has severe degenerative arthritis of both hips, which requires her to ambulate with a walker. She has long-standing hypertension that is well controlled with an angiotensin-converting enzyme inhibitor. She enjoys reading, knitting, and watching soap operas on television. At a recent routine physical examination you palpate a firm 1.5 cm nodule in the left lobe of the thyroid gland. There is no tenderness, skin change, or adenopathy. During the neck examination she asks you if something is wrong. On being told there is a small lump in her thyroid gland, she tells you that no other doctor had ever mentioned that she had a lump in the thyroid.

STUDY QUESTIONS

- What, if anything, will you do as a first step?
- What clinical features and laboratory results would indicate a need for aggressive management?

SOLITARY THYROID NODULE

The prevalence of palpable thyroid nodule is 4% in the general population. This represents 40,000 nodules per million people. Death from thyroid cancer is 7 per million population per year. This equals one death annually for every 5700 palpable nodules.[14]

The probability of malignancy decreases as the age of the patient increases. The following features suggest malignancy: male, younger than 30 years of age, history of head and neck irradiation, family history of thyroid cancer, hoarseness, dysphagia, dyspnea, recent increase in size, fixation to adjacent structures, lymph node enlargement, and absence of other nodules.

Since virtually all benign thyroid nodules are physiologically active, a thyroid scan that shows normal or above normal uptake (hot nodule) is strong evidence that the lesion is most likely benign and nothing further need be done. A nodule that is not physiologically active (cold nodule) has approximately a 10% chance of being malignant. Finding a cold nodule on thyroid scan indicates the need for further diagnostic evaluation.

A hot nodule on a thyroid scan is benign; a cold nodule has a 10% chance of malignancy. Fine needle aspiration of a solitary cold nodule is 50% to 97% accurate.

A thyroid ultrasound study often yields useful anatomical information, better defining the size and location of a nodule and possibly identifying other nodules that were not clinically apparent.

Fine needle aspiration cytology of solitary cold nodules is a relatively safe, inexpensive diagnostic procedure that can yield useful information. It has a diagnostic accuracy of 50% to 97% depending on the skill of the person performing the biopsy, as well as the experience of the cytopathologist. Whereas a positive biopsy specimen indicates the need for surgical excision, a negative biopsy cannot in itself be taken as absolute evidence of benignity. However, when coupled with other clinical information suggesting low probability of malignancy, a negative biopsy further supports that diagnosis.

CASE DISCUSSION

Except for having a single nodule, the patient had none of the features that would suggest thyroid malignancy. In this patient, if the solitary nodule were shown to be cystic, it would be less likely to be malignant, although sometimes mixed solid and cystic nodules are malignant.

▼ BRADLEY BISHOP

Mr. Bishop is a 77-year-old man with gait instability and mental confusion. He has a history of chronic hypertension controlled with hydrochlorothiazide and non–insulin dependent diabetes mellitus controlled with diet. He is alert but offers no spontaneous speech, answering questions with a nod or an occasional yes or no statement. His daughter states that he never was a "talker," but over the past 2 years he has virtually stopped speaking. Several years previously he had a stroke that affected his right arm and leg and his speech. On physical examination he has evidence of moderate residual right-sided weakness and an abnormal gait. He has a broad-based stooped posture with flexion at the hips and knees, short stride, and a tendency to fall to the right. Mental status testing indicates severe cognitive dysfunction, with a Mini–Mental State examination score of 8/30. Initial abnormal laboratory tests included a blood glucose of 258 mg/dl; a serum sodium of 148 mmol/L; a blood urea nitrogen (BUN) of 36 mg/dl; a serum creatinine of 1.5 mg/dl; a TSH of 22.5 mU/L; a T_4 of 2.2 μg/dl; a T_3RU of 48%; and an FTI in the normal range. Tentative diagnoses are uncontrolled diabetes mellitus, probable multiinfarct dementia, gait disorder secondary to dementia and previous stroke, and combined early thyroid failure with probable superimposed euthyroid sick syndrome.

EUTHYROID SICK SYNDROME

Euthyroid sick syndrome (ESS) is a condition in which severely or chronically ill patients manifest abnormal laboratory values for some of the tests commonly used to evaluate thyroid function. Most often, T_4, T_3, and FTI are low. This syndrome is thought to be caused by decreased peripheral production of T_3 and, at times, decreased availability of thyroid binding proteins. The TSH value can help distinguish these sick persons from patients who are truly hypothyroid. ESS may be divided in four major types: the low T_3 syndrome, the low T_3 and T_4 syndrome, the high T_4 syndrome, and mixed forms.[15] The low T_3 syndrome is the most common and is caused by decreased peripheral conversion of T_4 to T_3 or decreased serum thyroid binding globulins (TBG). Low T_4 is less common and is usually seen in severely ill or moribund patients. It is believed to be caused by decreased thyroid production of T_4 and decreased serum protein binding. The FTI, a measure calculated from the total T_4 and T_3RU, is usually normal but may be low in ESS.

When this is seen, evidence suggests that measurement of serum reverse T_3 may be useful. Serum reverse T_3 has been shown to be normal or high in ESS with low T_4 and low FTI. In hypothyroidism, however, reverse T_3 is virtually always below normal. Serum TSH is usually normal in ESS, and in the presence of low T_4, it may suggest coexisting secondary hypothyroidism. A normal reverse T_3, however, would tend to rule out hypothyroidism.[16]

Suspect the euthyroid sick syndrome if T_4, T_3, and FTI are all low: use a TSH to distinguish true hypothyroidism.

The cause of blunted TSH responsiveness in nonthyroidal illness is unknown. Similarly, the response to TRH may be blunted.

In screening ill patients for thyroid disease, the serum TSH is more useful than the usual thyroid panel (total T_4, T_3RU, FTI). If the serum TSH is borderline or only slightly elevated, a TRH stimulation test may be a useful next step.

CASE DISCUSSION

Mr. Bishop has low total T_4 and elevated T_3RU consistent with nonthyroidal disease, since one would expect both the T_4 and the T_3RU to be decreased in hypothyroidism. However, his TSH is clearly elevated in a range consistent with hypothyroidism. How then does one explain the elevated T_3RU? The most likely explanation is that Mr. Bishop is indeed hypothyroid and also has a superimposed ESS related to decreased peripheral conversion of T_4 to T_3 or decreased serum thyroxine binding proteins.

SUMMARY

Thyroid disorders present many challenges in the elderly patient. Not only can hyperthyroid patients be apathetic, they can appear demented; indeed, many have this as a concurrent problem. Yet thyroid disorders are remediable—although thyroxine must be given cautiously in patients with coronary artery disease. Thyroid treatment was sometimes initiated inappropriately in the past, so careful attempts to discontinue it must be made when necessary. Sick individuals can have abnormal thyroid tests that can be misleading. The sensitive TSH has facilitated screening and follow-up in the majority of cases.

POSTTEST

1. Which one of the following statements concerning thyroid disorders in old age is incorrect?
   a. Between 25% and 40% of older persons have an atypical presentation of hyperthyroidism.
   b. Atrial fibrillation is present in 40% of elderly people with hyperthyroidism.
   c. There is often a family history in patients with Graves' disease.
   d. The low T_4 syndrome is the most common form of ESS.

2. In initiating thyroxine treatment in a cardiac patient, which one of the following statements is false?
   a. T_3 is preferred initially because of its shorter half-life.
   b. Dosage should be increased at weekly intervals.
   c. Anginal symptoms would be the signal to slow the rate of increase of dose.
   d. TSH should be kept within the low normal range.

REFERENCES

1. Klein I, Levey S: Unusual manifestations of hypothyroidism, *Arch Intern Med* 144:123-128, 1984.
2. Kavonian GD, Wong NC, Mooradian AD: Unusual manifestations of hypothyroidism in an elderly patient, *Geriatr Med Today* 6(8): 31-37, 1987.
3. Mokshagundam S, Barzel US: Thyroid disease in the elderly, *JAGS* 41:1361-1369, 1993.
4. Levy EG: Thyroid disease in the elderly, *Med Clin North Am* 75:1 151-157, 1991.
5. De Groot LJ et al, eds: *The thyroid and its diseases,* ed 5, New York, 1984, Wiley Medical Publications.
6. Isley WL: Thyroid dysfunction in the severely ill and elderly, *Postgrad Med* 94(3):111-128, 1993.
7. Levine HD: Compromise therapy in the patient with angina pectoris and hypothyroidism, *Am J Med* 69:411-418, 1980.
8. Ellyin FM, Kumar Y, Somberg JC: Hypothyroidism complicated by angina pectoris: therapeutic approaches, *J Clin Pharmacol* 32:843-847, 1992.
9. Riccabona G: *Thyroid cancer, its epidemiology, clinical features, and treatment,* Berlin, 1987, Springer-Verlag.
10. Rosenthal MF et al: Thyroid failure in the elderly microsomal antibodies as discriminant for therapy, *JAMA* 258:209-213, 1987.
11. Krugman LG et al: Patterns of recovery of the hypothalamic-pituitary-thyroid axis in patients taken off of chronic thyroid therapy, *J Clin Endocrinol Metab* 41:70-80, 1975.
12. Rizzolo PJ, Porr D, Fisher PC: Reevaluation of patients on thyroxine therapy, *J Fam Pract* 22:241-244, 1986.

13. Evered D et al: Thyroid function after subtotal thyroidectomy for hyperthyroidism, *Br Med J* 25-27, 1975.

14. Hamburger JI: The various presentations of thyroiditis diagnostic considerations, *Ann Intern Med* 104:219-224, 1986.

15. Molitch ME et al: The cold thyroid nodule: an analysis of diagnostic and therapeutic options, *Endocr Rev* 5:185-199, 1984.

16. Zaloga GP, O'Brian JT: Euthyroid sick syndrome, *Am Fam Physician* 31:236-248, 1985.

17. Chopra IJ et al: Misleadingly low free thyroxine index and usefulness of reverse triiodothyronine measurement in non-thyroidal illnesses, *Ann Intern Med* 90:905-912, 1979.

PRETEST ANSWER

1. c

POSTTEST ANSWERS

1. d
2. d

CHAPTER 3 7

Osteoporosis

J. CHRISTOPHER HOUGH

OBJECTIVES

On completion of this chapter, the reader will be able to:

1. Identify risk factors and diagnostic criteria for osteoporosis in older persons.

2. Discuss screening interventions, laboratory tests, and the effects of aging on the clinical usefulness of these tests.

3. Describe the mechanism and types of treatment for osteoporosis and their indications for osteoporosis in the perimenopausal and postmenopausal patient in both ambulatory and institutional settings.

PRETEST

1. Which of the following is false about osteoporosis?
   a. By age 90, nearly half of women sustain a hip fracture.
   b. The direct and indirect cost of osteoporosis in the United States is over $6 billion annually.
   c. In type I osteoporosis, bone loss is mostly trabecular.
   d. Excessive calcium carbonate may cause iron deficiency anemia.

2. The following is true about type II osteoporosis:
   a. It is caused by loss of estrogen at menopause.
   b. Vitamin D at 1200 international units/day is the preferred treatment.
   c. The most frequent fracture sites are the hip and vertebrae.
   d. There is secondary hypoparathyroidism.

Osteoporosis is a loss of bone density, which leads to increased vulnerability to fractures that may result from apparently insignificant movements or accidents. The most common fractures occur in the vertebral bodies, the distal radius, and the proximal femur. Osteoporosis is a major public health problem and affects more than 20 million Americans; by age 90 about 30% of women have sustained a hip fracture.[1] The direct and indirect costs of osteoporosis in the United States are upward of $6.1 billion annually.

▼ FLORENCE SMITH (Part I)

Mrs. Smith is a 78-year-old retired schoolteacher. She returns to you for a "complete checkup." She was last seen by you 3 years ago. She underwent a cholecystectomy in 1982 and a hysterectomy in 1964 for dysfunctional uterine bleeding. She has hypertension treated with hydrochlorothiazide, 25 mg/day, and tries to follow a low-salt diet. On physical examination, she is a thin white woman, her blood pressure is 155/90, and she has a slight kyphosis.

Her only symptom is intractable back pain. She denies both back injury and falls. Her back primarily aches in the upper portion; she occasionally takes some ibuprofen for it. She has one or two drinks a day, usually wine with her meal.

STUDY QUESTIONS

- *Is she at risk for osteoporosis?*
- *How should her back pain be assessed?*
- *Does anything here reduce her risk?*

DEFINITION AND CLASSIFICATION

Osteoporosis is the clinical manifestation of osteopenia, in which an imbalance occurs between bone formation and bone resorption. It is associated with an increased risk of skeletal fractures and may be accompanied by clinical signs and symptoms. There are two distinct syndromes of idiopathic osteoporosis (Box 37-1).[2] Type I,

> **BOX 37-1**
> **Epidemiological Classification of Osteoporosis**
>
> **Type I**
>
> Affects women predominantly, related to menopause
> Mainly trabecular bone loss
> Fracture sites usually involve vertebrae and distal radius
>
> **Type II**
>
> Affects men and women, related to aging
> Cortical and trabecular bone loss
> Fracture sites usually hip and vertebrae; humerus, tibia, and pelvic bones may be involved
>
> **Type III**
>
> Affects men and women
> Trabecular and cortical bone loss
> Fracture sites usually vertebrae
> Therapy-induced, mainly corticosteroid agents

postmenopausal, occurs predominantly in women within 15 to 20 years after menopause; type II, senile, occurs in men and women 70 years of age or older.

In type I osteoporosis, bone loss is mostly trabecular. The cause is mainly a loss of estrogen at the time of menopause, with subsequent rapid bone turnover. Vertebral fractures are most common, although fracture of the distal radius may also occur.

In type II osteoporosis, both cortical and trabecular loss occur. This type is caused predominantly by loss of vitamin D activity and decreased osteoblastic function; this leads to decreased calcium absorption and secondary hyperparathyroidism. The most frequent fracture sites are the hip and vertebrae, but pelvic, humeral, and tibial fractures may also occur.

An important type of secondary osteoporosis categorized as "drug induced" has recently been labeled "type III" osteoporosis.[3] Box 37-2 lists many of the therapeu-

BOX 37-2
Therapy-Induced Osteoporosis (Type III)

Precipitating Agents

Aluminum-containing antacids
Anticonvulsants
  Phenytoin (Dilantin)
  Phenobarbital
  Primidone
Cholestyramine
Cyclosporine
Furosemide
Glucocorticoids
Heparin
Methotrexate
Phenothiazines
Thyroid hormones
Tetracycline
Isoniazid

tic drugs that have been associated with type III osteoporosis. Secondary osteoporosis has also been found in association with the diseases listed in Box 37-3.[3]

DIAGNOSIS

The diagnostic evaluation for osteoporosis in high-risk patients includes not only history, physical examination, and laboratory tests, but also bone mass quantification.

Among the risk factors that predispose to the development of type I osteoporosis are female gender, postmenopausal state, Caucasian or Oriental ancestry, low lean body mass, and calcium deficiency (see Box 37-3).

The physical and laboratory evaluation should exclude the presence of primary hyperparathyroidism, multiple myeloma, osteomalacia, and other disorders that may represent secondary causes of osteopenia. Laboratory evaluation should include measurement of serum calcium, phosphatase, alkaline phosphatase, thyroxine, and 24-hour urinary calcium and creatinine. If secondary dis-

BOX 37-3
Risk Factors for Osteoporosis

I. Endocrine abnormalities
  A. Hypogonadism
    1. Congenital (e.g., Turner's or Klinefelter's)
    2. Hypopituitarism
    3. Ovarian failure
    4. Hyperprolactinemia
  B. Hyperparathyroidism
  C. Hyperthyroidism
  D. Cushing's syndrome
  E. Calcium deficiency
II. Caucasian and Asian race
III. Female gender
IV. Nutritional factors
  A. Deficiency states
    1. Calcium
    2. Trace metals
      a. Manganese?
      b. Boron?
      c. Zinc?
    3. Vitamin D
    4. Vitamin C
    5. Malnutrition and malabsorption
  B. Excess intake
    1. Insoluble fiber (phytase)
    2. Animal protein
    3. Phosphate
    4. Caffeine
    5. Salt
    6. Sugar
    7. Alcohol
    8. Vitamin D
    9. Vitamin A

V. Smoking
VI. Drugs (See Box 37-2)
VII. Physiological and other stress
  A. Pregnancy and lactation
  B. Lack of exercise
  C. Immobility
VIII. Congenital
  A. Osteogenesis imperfecta
  B. Ehlers-Danlos syndrome
  C. Gaucher's disease
  D. Homocystinuria
IX. Miscellaneous conditions
  A. Renal failure
  B. Postgastrectomy and malabsorption
  C. Bone marrow malignancy (especially myeloma)
  D. Metabolic acidosis (e.g., renal tubular acidosis)
  E. Rheumatoid arthritis
  F. Liver disease (especially primary biliary cirrhosis)
  G. Juvenile osteoporosis
  H. Mast cell disease
  I. Chronic pulmonary disease
  J. Hemochromatosis
  K. Ankylosing spondylitis
  L. Inflammatory bowel disease
  M. Scurvy
  N. Sarcoidosis
  O. Diabetes mellitus

orders are suspected, appropriate diagnostic studies should be performed. When osteomalacia is suspected, measurement of 1,25-dihydroxyvitamin D_3 and bone biopsy should be considered. Serum and urinary osteocalcin and urinary hydroxyproline are markers of bone turnover but are not applicable in the clinical setting at present.

> *In England, frail elderly patients were at one time (fondly) called "crumbles"—partly on the assumption that osteoporosis was part of "normal aging." Now it is more accurately seen as a preventable, treatable, debilitating disease.*

A number of techniques such as single and dual photon absorptiometry, computed tomography, and x-ray densitometry are available for bone mass quantification. In addition to their use in determining baseline bone mass, these techniques can be used to detect the rate of bone loss to identify the need for aggressive therapy and to assess therapeutic response. Bone mass quantification at the time of menopause is helpful in determining which patients are at risk and have conditions that may lead to secondary osteoporosis.

THERAPY

In the *asymptomatic* patient, bone marrow content should be measured and monitored, and therapy should be targeted at minimizing bone loss and stabilizing bone mass. In the *symptomatic* patient, bone mass measurement should be used to monitor therapeutic response. Therapy in these patients should be directed toward analgesia, restoration of functional capability, prevention of future fractures, minimization of bone loss, and possible increase in bone mass. In patients on long-term *steroid therapy,* baseline and periodic follow-up bone mass measurements should be obtained to prevent steroid-induced osteopenia.

The total clinical situation must be considered when selecting therapy for decreased bone mass. Prevention of falls and fractures in patients with established osteoporosis is vital.[4,5]

▼ FLORENCE SMITH (Part II)

Bone densitometry of the dorsal and lumbar spine reveals significant decrease in bone density. X-ray examinations confirm several wedge compression fractures of the thoracic vertebrae. Laboratory tests for secondary causes are normal.

STUDY QUESTION

■ *What specific therapy do you recommend, and why?*

Calcium

Because older patients frequently have low calcium intake and calcium absorption declines with age, calcium supplementation is suggested when patients are not obtaining sufficient calcium in their diet. The suggested total calcium intake is 1000 mg per day for premenopausal patients and 1500 mg per day for postmenopausal. The recommended dietary changes include increased low-fat dairy products, fish, and fresh leafy green vegetables.

As a calcium supplement, calcium carbonate is 40% elemental calcium by weight. It is inexpensive and available in preparations providing elemental calcium in amounts from 250 to 600 mg per tablet. Bioavailability varies among brands. Oral preparations of those tablets that dissolve in vinegar within 30 minutes may be considered to be bioavailable. Calcium citrate, 21% of which is elemental calcium, is an excellent choice for supplemental therapy; absorption of calcium from the citrate moiety is greater than from carbonate, and citrate is a natural inhibitor of renal stone formation.

Since indigestion or constipation may occur with calcium carbonate, it should be given before meals to minimize gastrointestinal side effects and to help increase absorption. With excessive doses of calcium carbonate there is a risk of kidney stones, iron deficiency, and hypercalcemia, although these are rare. Calcium citrate is not associated with gastrointestinal symptoms. Although calcium supplements are beneficial, the patient's diet is still regarded as the best source of calcium, and advising patients to eat low-fat dairy foods, fish, and green leafy vegetables as part of the total calcium intake is valuable.

Vitamin D

As a person ages, vitamin D levels decrease. Type II (senile) osteoporosis is associated with a relative deficiency of vitamin D. It is advisable to give approximately 400 to 800 units of vitamin D per day. Doses greater than 1000 international units (IU) per day, however, encourage resorption of bone; larger doses should therefore be avoided.[3]

> *When treating osteoporosis, estrogen, calcitriol, calcitonin, and alendronate are to be considered; calcium, vitamin D, and exercise are mandatory.*

Estrogen and Progesterone

Estrogen. As a potent antiresorption agent, estrogen is useful for the prevention of postmenopausal osteoporosis. Although estrogen has proven safe and effective for relatively short-term use in relieving menopausal symptoms and may reduce cardiovascular morbidity and mortality,[6] recent medical literature has raised serious questions about the safety of its prolonged use (15 to 20 years) for skeletal preservation. The relationship between long-term estrogen use and breast cancer is not yet resolved. Long-term estrogen use is associated with a higher incidence of endometrial carcinoma, but that risk is markedly diminished by the addition of progesterone.[7]

There is also an age-related concern about the usefulness of estrogen as an antiresorption agent. It is generally believed that women who are postmenopausal by more than 15 to 20 years may not benefit from estrogen therapy because of the low rate of bone turnover. Side effects (bloating, breast tenderness, and bleeding) are problematic in some patients too.

However, estrogen has been shown to prevent both cortical and trabecular bone loss and to decrease the incidence of hip fracture. It may be started in the perimenopausal period or later. It is thus extremely useful, provided there is constant vigilance by routine Pap smears, mammography, and endometrial biopsy if there is dysfunctional bleeding.

Progesterone. There are good reasons to be cautious about progesterone or progestational agents in long-term therapy. Although its long-term effects are uncertain, progesterone is a known mitogen. It may also adversely affect serum lipids, especially by decreasing the high-density lipoprotein (HDL).[7] A recent study suggests that the combination of estrogen and progesterone may lead to a greater incidence of breast carcinoma than estrogen alone, although this is a tentative conclusion.[7] Progesterone does protect against the development of endometrial carcinoma, and progesterone may have a positive clinical effect on bone formation.

The regimen for the woman with an intact uterus is cyclic therapy with conjugated estrogens (0.625 mg per day), days 1 through 25, plus medroxyprogesterone acetate (10 mg per day), days 14 through 25, allowing a break from day 26 through the first of the following month. It is also acceptable to administer estrogen on a continuous daily basis, with medroxyprogesterone acetate on days 1 through 12 of each calendar month. The transdermal patch may be substituted for oral estrogen, especially for patients with a history of hypertension[3]: begin with a low-dose patch (Estroderm 0.05 system) and apply a new patch on days 1, 4, 8, 11, 15, 18, and 22 of each calendar month. Medroxyprogesterone acetate, 10 mg per day on days 14 through 25 of each month, should also be administered.

The relatively new continuous estrogen regimens with daily low-dose progesterone have been developed for patient convenience, including lack of withdrawal bleeding. It is at this time only advisable to use cyclic therapy. It is not known whether daily estrogen and progesterone will prevent endometrial carcinoma with long-term use, and erratic menses occur for 6 months after initiating therapy, before menstruation ceases completely.

Before estrogen therapy is instituted, a baseline Pap smear and mammogram are suggested, with yearly Pap smears and mammogram thereafter. Should any abnormal bleeding occur, an aspiration curettage with cytology evaluation is indicated. Appropriate calcium intake should be assured as well.

Currently, conjugated estrogen used alone is the recommended therapy for a woman without a uterus.

Calcitriol Therapy

A significant reduction in the rate of new vertebral fractures over a 3-year period has been observed in women receiving continuous administration of calcitriol 1,25-dihydroxyvitamin D_3 as compared with women receiving calcium.[8] Calcitriol should certainly be considered in the treatment of osteoporosis. The therapeutic toxicity window is narrow with this agent; therefore it should be used cautiously, in a compliant patient, and with frequent monitoring of serum calcium, BUN, and creatinine levels, as well as 24-hour urinary calcium and creatinine clearance determinations.

Calcitonin-Salmon Therapy

Several studies have proven the effectiveness of calcitonin-salmon (Calcimar, Miacalcin) in postmenopausal osteoporosis patients. Controlled studies with Calcimar clearly demonstrate inhibition of bone resorption, increased bone mineral content in several cases, analgesic effectiveness, increased mobility, and a low toxicity profile. Pharmacologically, calcitonin-salmon appears to have actions essentially identical to calcitonin of mammalian origin, but its potency is greater, and it has a longer duration of action. Calcitonin-salmon decreases the number of osteoclast receptors, resulting in a decreasing number of osteoclasts and therefore a decrease in bone resorption. There is early in vitro evidence that bone formation may be augmented by calcitonin through increased osteoblastic activity.[9] The action of calcitonin-salmon appears to be dose related. In one study there was an 8.5% increase in bone mineral content of the lumbar spine in osteoporotic patients treated with 100 international units (IU) of calcitonin-salmon daily for 1 year, compared with an increase of 4% in a group treated at half that dose.[10] Calcitonin-salmon has also been shown to have a beneficial effect on glucocorticoid-induced osteopenia. It is now marketed only as an injectable, but it has been shown to be effective as a prophylactic agent, retarding bone loss in the perimenopausal patient when administered by the intranasal route. This route will extend its potential use as a prophylactic agent. Table 37-1 compares it with estrogens.

Analgesia. Calcitonin-salmon has a potent analgesic affect, with increased mobility noted in many patients. It not only stabilizes bone mass, but also improves quality of life for patients with postmenopausal osteoporosis.

Table 37-1   Estrogens and Calcitonin-Salmon Compared

Therapeutic Attribute	Estrogen Replacement Therapy	Calcitonin-Salmon
Rapid therapeutic action	−	+
Analgesia	−	+
Increased mobility	−	+
Long-term toxicity	±	−
Expense	Low	Moderate
Effect in high-turnover osteoporosis	Moderate	Great
Effect in elderly	Controversial	Moderate (with analgesic and mobility-enhancing effects)

Analgesia and subsequent increased mobility may occur after as little as 2 weeks of therapy. The analgesic affects are greatest for patients who have spontaneous pain, pain on mobility, provoked pain, or functional impairment that may be improved by increasing mobility and muscle strength.[12]

Regimen. The recommended dosage of calcitonin-salmon is 100 IU per day. When financial or other considerations necessitate decreasing the dosage, it is important to remember that, for a duration of therapy of up to 18 months, the response of bone mineral content to calcitonin-salmon is dose related. So, if possible, 100 IU per day should be continued for at least 18 months. If that is not possible, 50 IU every other day or even 50 IU four times per week has proved helpful in regard to both bone resorption and analgesic effect. Because of its analgesic effect, treatment with calcitonin-salmon may allow the discontinuation of nonsteroidal antiinflammatory drugs (NSAIDS) or narcotics, thus lowering the total economic burden. Because calcitonin-salmon has a dose-related response in bone mass for up to 18 months, the following intermittent regimen is suggested: subcutaneous calcitonin-salmon 100 IU/day for the first 12 to 18 months followed by 50 to 100 IU, 5 to 7 days per week, 3 months on, 3 months off in a cyclic fashion for at least an additional 3 years. The symptomatic patient may require less "off" time on clinical grounds. When this therapy is used, a supplement of 1 g of elemental calcium and 400 IU of vitamin D should be administered daily. Regular weight-bearing exercise is also an important part of the therapeutic program.[13]

Side Effects. Transient nausea and anorexia usually abate within the first 5 to 7 days of therapy; these side effects are seen in 10% to 30% of patients. An agent such as metoclopramide (Reglan) (10 mg) may be used a half hour before the injection to mitigate these symptoms. Facial flushing has been seen in 10% of patients, and dermatological hypersensitivity and systemic allergic reactions occur rarely.

Biphosphonates

Biphosphonates inhibit osteoclastic resorption. In 1990, two clinical trials confirmed the usefulness of the compound etidronate disodium in the treatment of postmenopausal osteoporosis.[14,15] These studies document a beneficial effect on vertebral bone mass (5% increase after 2 years of therapy) with a reduction of new vertebral fractures by one half. More recently, third-year follow-up data from one of these studies showed an increase in vertebral fractures, leading an FDA advisory committee in March 1991 to recommend disapproval of etidronate.[15]

The biphosphonate alendronate sodium (Fosamax) is now available by prescription, and there is increasing clinical experience with its use. Its exact place in long-term management of osteoporosis remains to be established, since long-term data beyond 4 years of use are not yet available. The recommended dose is conveniently once daily, but since absorption is greatly reduced by any concomitant oral intake, the patient must be able to comply with taking it in the morning at least 30 minutes before anything else is taken by mouth. Since its utility in men is not established, it is only indicated for the treatment of osteoporosis in postmenopausal women. (It is also recommended, in a different dose, for the treatment of Paget's disease of bone.) It cannot be used when the patient has severe renal insufficiency (creatinine clearance less than 25 ml/minute), but it can be used if there is only mild or moderate renal insufficiency (creatinine clearance 25 to 60 ml/minute). Pooled data support a practical outcome of significant reduction in the proportion of patients experiencing new vertebral fractures and less loss of height in those under treatment even in the absence of such fractures. It appears that treatment needs to be continued to maintain the effect. Adequate calcium and vitamin D intakes must be ensured, although calcium supplements and antacids as well as other medications will interfere with the absorption if taken less than half an hour after the alendronate. Currently, caution is urged with patients who have upper gastrointestinal problems, since such problems (although mild and not particularly common) are the main side effects.

Sodium Fluoride

It is well known that sodium fluoride stimulates osteoblastic bone formation and increases bone density. However, there is an increased incidence of hip fractures in

BOX 37-4
Pharmacological Management of Osteoporosis

Premenopausal

Prophylaxis: calcium, vitamin D, exercise
Treatment: calcitonin-salmon (in osteoporosis with high bone turnover), calcium, vitamin D, exercise

Perimenopausal

Prophylaxis: calcium, vitamin D, exercise, estrogen
Treatment: estrogen, calcitonin-salmon (in symptomatic osteoporosis with high bone turnover), calcium, vitamin D, exercise

Postmenopausal

Prophylaxis: estrogen replacement therapy (up to 20 years after cessation of menses), calcium, vitamin D, exercise
Treatment:
Asymptomatic: estrogen replacement therapy (up to 20 years after cessation of menses), calcitonin-salmon, calcium, vitamin D; calcitriol therapy for patients who cannot take estrogen
Symptomatic: calcitonin-salmon, calcium, vitamin D

Postmenopausal patients with osteoporosis:
1. Supplement the diet with elemental calcium: 1500 mg per day total intake.
2. Add vitamin D: 400 to 800 IU per day.
3. Prescribe weight-bearing exercise.
4. Use estrogen-progesterone therapy, especially in perimenopausal patients (careful screening required). Consider calcitriol therapy in the patient who cannot take estrogen.
5. For symptomatic patients, do not restrict treatment with calcitonin-salmon (Calcimar or Miacalcin) on the basis of age alone.
6. Use calcitonin-salmon therapy in patients beyond the age of estrogen therapy, patients who are poor candidates for estrogen therapy, and patients requiring long-term glucocorticoid therapy.

Treatment of the postmenopausal patient with an intact uterus is as follows:
1. Use conjugated estrogen 0.625 mg per day, days 1 through 25 of each month, *plus* medroxyprogesterone acetate, 10 mg per day, days 14 through 25 of each month.
2. Alternatively, use the transdermal estrogen patch: 0.05 mg on days 1, 4, 8, 11, 15, 18 and 22, with medroxyprogesterone acetate 10 mg on days 14 through 25 of each month.
3. Use calcitonin-salmon in the symptomatic osteoporotic patient with a high bone turnover.
4. Prescribe calcium, vitamin D, and exercise.

osteoporotic women treated with sodium fluoride.[16] Sodium fluoride increases the density of the axial skeleton at the expense of appendicular skeleton. A recent study concluded that a continuous dose of 75 mg per day does not appear more effective than calcium carbonate in reducing the vertebral fracture rate or height loss in women with postmenopausal osteoporosis.[17] Thus sodium fluoride should not be used outside clinical research protocols.[18]

Tamoxifen

Early studies have shown that tamoxifen may protect against bone loss. It may be useful in patients receiving tamoxifen for breast carcinoma, since estrogen is absolutely contraindicated in such cases.[19]

Hydrochlorothiazide may be protective against osteoporosis, but it is not recommended specifically as a treatment.[20]

SUMMARY OF TREATMENT

Prophylaxis and treatment of osteoporosis are summarized in Box 37-4.

▼ *FLORENCE SMITH (Part III)*

Mrs. Smith starts daily estrogen therapy and calcium and vitamin D supplementation and is advised regarding a walking program. In a follow-up visit 2 weeks later, she still complains of back pain and therapy with calciton-salmon is initiated at home with visiting nurse assistance. Further follow-up a month later reveals good relief of her back pain.

SUMMARY

Whereas osteoporosis was once regarded as an inevitable consequence of increasing age, it is now seen as a serious chronic illness, with major problems as its consequence. It is an illness that can be prevented to a large degree by oral nutritional supplementation and weight-bearing exercise long before "old age" and by estrogen and other therapies.

POSTTEST

1. Routine evaluation of postmenopausal osteoporosis includes all except which one of the following:
   a. History and physical examination
   b. Serum calcium
   c. Thyroxine
   d. 24-Hour urine and creatinine levels
   e. 1,25-Dihydroxyvitamin D_3

2. Which one of the following has been proved to prevent osteoporosis:
   a. Vitamin D (1200 IU per day)
   b. Progesterone (10 mg per day)
   c. Calcitonin-salmon (100 IU per day)
   d. Etidronate (5 g per day)

REFERENCES

1. Campion EW et al: Hip fracture: a prospective study of hospital course, complications, and costs, *J Gen Intern Med* 2:78-82, 1987.
2. Riggs BL, Melton LJ: Involutional osteoporosis, *N Engl J Med* 314:1676-1686, 1986.
3. Wisneski LA: Clinical management of post menopausal osteoporosis, *S Med J* 85:832-839, 1992.
4. Tinetti M, Speechley M, Gonter S: Risk factors for falls among elderly persons living in the community, *N Engl J Med* 319:1701-1707, 1988.
5. Ray W et al: Psychotropic drug use and the risk of hip fracture, *N Engl J Med* 316:369-386, 1987.
6. Stampfer MD et al: Post menopausal estrogen therapy and cardiovascular disease, *N Engl J Med* 325:256-262, 1991.
7. Bergkvist, L et al: The risk of breast cancer after estrogen and estrogen-progestin replacement, *N Engl J Med* 321:293-297, 1989.
8. Tilyard MW et al: Treatment of postmenopausal osteoporosis with calcitriol or calcium, *N Engl J Med* 326:357-362, 1992.
9. Farley JR, Wergedal JE, Hall SL: Calcitonin has direct effects on the proliferation and differentiation of human osteoblast-line cells in vitro, *J Bone Miner Res* 4 (suppl 1):S278, 1989.
10. Gennari C et al: Comparative effects on bone mineral content of calcium and calcium plus salmon calcitonin given in two different regimens in postmenopausal osteoporosis, *Curr Ther Res* 38:455-464, 1985.
11. Puu KK, Chan MB: Analgesic effect of intranasal salmon calcitonin in the treatment of osteoporotic vertebral fractures, *Clin Ther* 11:205-209, 1989.
12. Lyritis EP et al: Analgesic effect of salmon calcinonin in osteoporotic vertebral fractures a double blind placebo-controlled clinical study, *Calcif Tissue Int* 49:369-372, 1991.
13. Sinaki M: Exercise and osteoporosis, *Arch Phys Med Rehabil* 70:220-227, 1989.
14. Storm T et al: Effect of intermittent cyclical etidronate therapy on bone mass and fracture rate in women with postmenopausal osteoporosis, *N Engl J Med* 322:1265-1271, 1990.
15. Watts NB et al: Intermittent cyclical etidronate treatment of postmenopausal osteoporosis, *N Engl J Med* 323:73-79, 1990.
16. Hedlund LR, Gallagher JC: Increased incidence of hip fracture in osteoporotic women treated with sodium fluoride, *J Miner Res* 4:223-225, 1989.
17. Riggs, B et al: Effect of fluoride treatment on the fracture rate in postmenopausal women with osteoporosis, *N Engl J Med* 322:802-809, 1990.
18. Kleerekoper M et al: *Continuous sodium fluoride therapy does not reduce vertebral fracture rate in postmenopausal osteoporosis,* Abstract 1035, September, 1989, American Society For Bone and Mineral Research.
19. Love, RR et al: Effects of tamoxifen on bone mineral density in post menopausal women with breast cancer, *N Engl J Med* 326:852-856, 1992.
20. LaCroix, AZ et al: Thiazide diuretic agents and the incidence of hip fracture, *N Engl J Med* 322:286-288, 1990.

PRETEST ANSWERS

1. a
2. c

POSTTEST ANSWERS

1. e
2. c

CHAPTER 38

Estrogen Therapy

BONNY NEYHART

OBJECTIVES

Upon completion of this chapter, the reader will be able to:

1. Describe the hormonal changes that occur in the immediate postmenopausal period.

2. Describe the symptoms of estrogen deprivation.

3. Describe the relationship between osteoporosis and estrogen, and describe estrogen's place in therapy.

4. Describe the relationship of estrogen to cardiovascular disease.

5. Describe the relative risks of estrogen replacement therapy.

6. Describe the rationale for progestin cotherapy.

7. Describe different hormone replacement regimens and their indications.

PRETEST

1. Which is the single best completion of the following statement? After menopause, estrogen is:
   a. Normally absent
   b. Secreted principally by the adrenal glands
   c. Synthesized mainly in the ovarian tissue
   d. Derived from the conversion of endogenous androgens
2. An increased risk of all of the following diseases may be seen in women on unopposed estrogen replacement therapy except which one?
   a. Gallbladder disease
   b. Endometrial hyperplasia
   c. Hypertension
   d. Endometrial cancer
3. Progestin cotherapy is frequently prescribed with estrogen to prevent which one of the following?
   a. Breast cancer
   b. Gallstones
   c. Endometrial cancer
   d. Fibrocystic breasts

As women age, there is an inevitable and progressive loss of ovarian follicular units. This ongoing loss is unnoticeable until the onset of the climacteric, a time in the fifth decade of life when the ovary and remaining follicles are no longer capable of sufficient hormone synthesis to maintain cyclic reproductive function. Clinically, this manifests as erratic menstrual bleeding that ultimately progresses to the amenorrhea that characterizes the menopause.

Significantly lower levels of circulating estrogens are seen in postmenopausal women. The ovary ceases direct production of estrogen within a few years of menopause, and this is reflected by a gradual rise in serum gonadotropins. Consequently, an elevated level of follicle-stimulating hormone (FSH) is seen in postmenopausal women who are not receiving supplemental estrogen. Unsupplemented postmenopausal women continue to maintain low levels of estrogen by the conversion of endogenous androgens to estrone. This conversion process occurs mainly in the skin, liver, and fatty tissues. It follows therefore that obese postmenopausal women enjoy higher circulating levels of estrogen than their slender contemporaries. Unfortunately, higher levels of estrogen, whether produced by the individual or prescribed by the physician, are correlated with an increased risk of endometrial hyperplasia and cancer.

▼ CYNTHIA WELLS (Part I)

Mrs. Wells is a white 72-year-old who has come to you for a checkup following her husband's recent heart attack. She last saw you 6 years ago. At that time you told her that she had osteoporosis and prescribed estrogen. She soon developed breast tenderness, and a screening mammogram showed benign-appearing calcifications. Troubled by her symptoms and insufficiently reassured by the normal mammogram, she discontinued the estrogen. She takes supplemental calcium and an occasional ibuprofen for chronic back pain. Review of systems and medical history confirm urinary urgency and vaginal dryness. She experienced hot flashes around the time of her last menstrual period 20 years ago. A smoker, she has no symptoms suggestive of cardiovascular disease and her family history is unremarkable.

SYMPTOMS OF ESTROGEN DEPRIVATION

Symptoms of estrogen deprivation first appear during the climacteric, a term that encompasses the years of ovarian dysfunction that immediately precede and follow the menopause. Initial symptoms include vasomotor episodes (hot flashes), manifestations of urogenital atrophy (dysuria, dryness, and dyspareunia), and various psychological and somatic complaints. Although vasomotor episodes and associated symptoms usually subside within several years of the menopause, symptoms of urogenital atrophy continue to manifest well into the seventh decade and beyond. Findings on physical examination consistent with urogenital atrophy include thin, pale genital mucosa. On pelvic examination the cervix does not protrude into the vagina and the upper third of the vagina is often narrowed. Symptoms such as dyspareunia, incontinence, and vaginal irritation often associated with atrophic changes are exquisitely responsive to estrogen therapy. Although estrogen vaginal creams enjoy unique popularity for this condition, they are no more effective than estrogens administered by other routes. Also, the systemic absorption of vaginal estrogen results in endometrial stimulation and cancer risk comparable to that of orally administered estrogen.

▼ *CYNTHIA WELLS (Part II)*

Cynthia is a slender woman with a blood pressure of 140/80. She has slight tenderness of the midthoracic spine and an exaggerated thoracic kyphosis. Pelvic examination reveals atrophic changes; no breast abnormalities are noted. Mrs. Wells is advised that her pelvic symptoms can be attributed to estrogen deficiency and that osteoporosis probably accounts for the symptoms and changes in her thoracic spine. Treatment with estrogen is anticipated, pending the results of laboratory tests and imaging studies. In the interim, she is advised to continue supplemental calcium.

ESTROGEN AND OSTEOPOROSIS

An ever-growing body of evidence over the past two decades has established the role of estrogen deprivation in the genesis of osteoporosis in women. Symptomatic osteoporosis currently affects one of three postmenopausal women. It is estimated that over 220,000 hip fractures and 500,000 vertebral fractures occur annually as a direct consequence of osteoporosis.[1] The risk of dying within 1 year of a hip fracture is at least 12% to 20%.[2] Of those who survive hip fractures, up to 50% require long-term nursing home placement.[3] Add this to the pain and disability endured by those with vertebral and wrist fractures, and osteoporosis is revealed to be a health problem of grave magnitude.

Osteoporosis is an age-related disorder that is characterized by decreased bone mass and an increased susceptibility to fractures. An individual's risk of developing osteoporosis is a function of many variables including his or her peak bone mass at skeletal maturity. Peak bone mass is, in turn, affected by heredity, gender, and racial differences. In general, black men enjoy a high peak bone mass and are relatively immune to osteoporosis. Conversely, fair-skinned women often have a low bone mass, which increases their risk of developing osteoporosis. The risk of osteoporosis is further increased when a positive family history is present and among those who drink alcohol or smoke cigarettes.

Researchers have proposed two types of osteoporosis.[4] Type II osteoporosis is characterized by slow bone loss beginning around age 30 and continuing throughout life. Coincident with the menopause there is a dramatic increase in the rate of bone loss. This accelerated bone loss is related to menopausal estrogen deficiency and leads to the development of type I osteoporosis. Estrogen replacement therapy significantly slows the bone loss associated with type I osteoporosis. To have a maximal benefit, estrogen therapy should be initiated at the time of menopause. Persistent skeletal responsiveness to estrogen therapy has, however, been demonstrated in women up to 35 years following the menopause.

The minimum dose of estrogen required to prevent type I osteoporosis is 0.625 mg of conjugated estrogen daily. Transdermal estrogen preparations in doses of 0.05 mg seem to be equally effective. Smoking reduces the bioavailability of estrogen. Thus higher doses of estrogen may be required to prevent osteoporosis in postmenopausal women who smoke, although this hypothesis has not been clinically proved.

The optimal length of estrogen therapy for the purpose of skeletal protection has not been determined. Available data suggest that treatment should be continued for a minimum of 5 to 6 years. Investigators suggest that type I osteoporosis is merely postponed by estrogen therapy and that the withdrawal of estrogen will result in accelerated bone loss at any age. In view of this, many clinicians recommend long-term and in some instances lifelong estrogen replacement therapy.

Other therapeutic agents and methods used in the treatment and prevention of osteoporosis are detailed in Chapter 37. Calcium therapy, while ineffective as an isolated means of preventing type I osteoporosis, is an appropriate adjunct to estrogen replacement. Vitamin D (400 to 800 mg) and calcium supplements are especially appropriate in elderly women, many of whom are calcium deficient owing to malabsorption and nutritional inadequacy.

▼ *CYNTHIA WELLS (Part III)*

Two weeks later, Mrs. Wells returns to review her laboratory work. Plain radiographs of her thoracic spine reveal osteopenia and anterior wedging of several vertebrae. Her mammogram and Pap smear are normal. An extensive serum chemistry profile is normal, including albumin, Ca, and PO$_4$. Thyroid-stimulating hormone (TSH) level is normal, as is the serum protein electrophoresis. Cholesterol is slightly elevated at 220 mg/dl. This latter result is especially alarming to her, since her husband recently suffered a myocardial infarction.

ESTROGEN AND CARDIOVASCULAR DISEASE

Cardiovascular disease is the leading cause of death in U.S. women. As women age, there is a trend toward elevated low-density lipoprotein (LDL) cholesterol and reduced levels of high-density lipoprotein (HDL) cholesterol. Analyses of women going through menopause reveal that estrogen deficiency contributes to these adverse lipoprotein changes. Oral estrogen therapy alters lipoprotein levels and leads to a lower LDL cholesterol level and an increase in HDL after 1 year of therapy. The transdermal estrogen patch has a less favorable effect on lipids because of the direct absorption of estrogen into the bloodstream and lack of first-pass metabolism.

Owing to estrogen's beneficial effect on lipids, there

is overwhelming consensus that it is cardioprotective. Many studies show that estrogen users have as much as a 50% lower risk of cardiovascular events, including angina, myocardial infarction, and sudden death. Based on reductions in the risk of fracture and cardiovascular disease, it has been suggested that timely estrogen replacement (i.e., at the time of menopause) in selected patients could add 2 or more good-quality years to a woman's life. Most of this added longevity follows directly from the decrease in cardiovascular disease.[5]

> *Many things formerly characterized as "normal aging" are due to the lack of estrogen. It clearly helps osteoporosis and helps combat the leading cause of death in U.S. women: cardiovascular disease.*

RISKS OF ESTROGEN REPLACEMENT

The risks of estrogen are far outweighed by the benefits of replacement in most women. Much of the concern about the safety of hormone replacement dates back several decades to when estrogen was first linked with endometrial carcinoma. Subsequent information regarding the risks of oral contraceptives added to the popular bias against estrogen therapy. Many patients remain apprehensive about hormonal replacement, and the clinician is obligated to discuss the advantages and disadvantages of therapy[6] (Table 38-1).

Unopposed estrogen therapy is associated with a significantly increased risk of endometrial cancer, which is a valid concern in women in whom the uterus remains intact. However, when the proliferative effects of estrogen are countered by appropriate progestin cotherapy, this increased risk of endometrial cancer is eliminated. Progestin therapy should be taken for a minimum of 12 to 14 consecutive days per month.[7] When taken cyclically, progestin therapy is followed by regular withdrawal bleeding. Although noticeable withdrawal bleeding frequently ceases in women over age 65, some women are quite averse to resuming or perpetuating their menstrual flow. For these women, continuous combined therapy—daily estrogen and progestin—is proposed to achieve a stable, inactive endometrium with no withdrawal bleeding. Most women achieve endometrial atrophy on this regimen, although up to 80% may have erratic bleeding during the first year of therapy. It should be noted that the long-term efficacy of continuous combined therapy has not been established. The addition of a progestin is generally not warranted in women who have had a hysterectomy.

Medroxyprogesterone acetate is the most commonly used and generally preferred progestin. When used cyclically, the dose is 5 to 10 mg for the first 12 to 14 days of a month. Research to date suggests that the 10-mg dose is more effective in preventing endometrial hyperplasia. However, progestins have been noted to lower HDL-cholesterol and confound the beneficial effects of estrogen on cardiovascular risk. For this reason the minimum effective progestin dose for achieving endometrial stability should be used. One group of researchers notes that endometrial histology correlates with the timing of menstruation in women who take daily estrogen and a progestin for 12 days each month.[8] Favorable endometrial cytology results are seen in women whose menstrual bleeding begins after day 10 of progestin therapy. Thus a reasonable clinical approach in women taking estrogen is to prescribe 12 consecutive days of medroxyprogesterone acetate 5 mg and follow their menstrual calendar. Women who menstruate on or before day 10 benefit from an increased progestin dose and closer clinical monitoring, whereas women who menstruate after day 10 can be maintained on the 5 mg progestin dose.

The relationship between estrogen therapy and breast cancer has been studied extensively, but the data remain inconclusive. There appears to be no increased breast cancer risk among women who take estrogen for less than 5 years. However, an analysis of studies to date suggests that women treated with long-term estrogen therapy have a relative risk of 1.25 of developing breast cancer.[9] While worrisome, this risk is probably outweighed by the skeletal and cardiovascular benefits.

Estrogen therapy is contraindicated in women with active liver or gallbladder disease and in women with estrogen-dependent cancer. Hypertension is not a contraindication to estrogen replacement, since blood pressure is usually unaffected by therapy. Oral estrogen therapy is associated with an increase in plasma triglycerides and should be used cautiously in women with hypertriglyceridemia. In addition, estrogen therapy is associated with a twofold increase in the risk of gallbladder disease.

Current recommendations for hormone replacement

Table 38-1 Risks and Benefits of Hormone Replacement Therapy

Disease	Relative Risk	
	Estrogen (Unopposed)	Estrogen and Progestin
Breast cancer	1.01-1.25	0.6-4.4*
Endometrial cancer	2.31-8.22	1.0
Gallbladder disease	2.0	
Stroke	0.96	0.96
Osteoporotic hip fracture	0.75	Probably 0.75
Coronary heart disease	0.55-0.65	Probably <1.0

Data from Grady D et al: *Ann Intern Med* 117:1016-1033, 1993.
*Relative risk range of few studies, some of which have design flaws.

in women, both with and without a uterus, are summarized in Tables 38-2 and 38-3, respectively.[10]

▼ CYNTHIA WELLS (Part IV)

Following a discussion of the risks and benefits of therapy, Mrs. Wells consents to estrogen replacement, prescribed as conjugated estrogen 0.625 mg daily and medroxyprogesterone acetate 5 mg on days 1 to 12 of every month. You advise her to quit smoking, both to decrease her risk of cardiovascular and other diseases and to improve the efficacy of estrogen therapy. A lipid profile is ordered, and she is counseled to reduce dietary fat intake. A follow-up appointment is scheduled for 3 months, and she is urged to call sooner if problems develop.

A pretreatment endometrial biopsy is generally unnecessary in women who have experienced a normal menopause and in whom there is no history of abnormal uterine bleeding. With continuous estrogen and cyclic progestin therapy, regular withdrawal bleeding generally occurs after day 10. Patients should be advised to record

Table 38-2   Recommended Hormone Replacement in Women with Intact Uterus

	Estrogen	Progestin
Standard regimen	Daily conjugated estrogen 0.625 mg	Cyclic medroxyprogesterone acetate 5-10 mg on days 1-12
Alternative regimens	1. Continuous transdermal estradiol patch 0.05 mg* 2. Daily conjugated estrogen 0.625 mg	1. Cyclic medroxyprogesterone acetate 5-10 mg on days 1-12 2. Daily medroxyprogesterone acetate 2.5 mg†

*Consider in women intolerant of oral estrogen, or women with stable liver or gallbladder disease or a history of venous thromboembolism.
†Consider for women who reject resuming or continuing their menses. Note that this regimen has not been proved to protect against coronary heart disease.

Table 38-3   Recommended Hormone Replacement in Women after a Hysterectomy

	Estrogen	Progestin
Standard regimen	Daily conjugated estrogen 0.625 mg	None
Alternative regimen	Continuous estradiol patch* 0.05 mg	None

*Consider in women intolerant of oral estrogen or women with stable liver or gallbladder disease or a history of venous thromboembolism.

their bleeding patterns so that abnormal bleeding requiring an endometrial biopsy can be identified.

Every perimenopausal woman must seriously consider estrogen therapy.

For women to enjoy the maximum benefit from estrogen replacement, therapy should be initiated at or before the time of menopause. Timely replacement is especially critical in women who experience premature menopause, whether spontaneously or following oophorectomy. Optimally, all women seen during the climacteric should be evaluated and independently apprised of the risks and benefits of hormone replacement.

CASE DISCUSSION

In retrospect, initiation of estrogen replacement therapy at the time of menopause would have been a more desirable therapeutic course for Mrs. Wells. Now that she is 72 years old, estrogen therapy is appropriate treatment for her urogenital symptoms, although the impact of estrogen on her bone and cardiovascular system cannot be predicted with certainty. In view of the uncertain benefits of long-term estrogen therapy in this patient, the goals of hormone therapy should be reviewed periodically. In addition, the role of exercise and specific pharmaceutical treatment of osteoporosis should be addressed.

▼ POLLY WELLS-KANBE (Part I)

Several weeks later the daughter of Mrs. Wells comes in for a checkup. Ms. Polly Wells-Kanbe is a 50-year-old white woman whose health care has been episodic since her hysterectomy for uterine fibroids. She is a self-described "health nut" who exercises regularly, watches her diet, does not smoke, and drinks just an occasional glass of wine. Concerns about her family history of osteoporosis and heart disease have prompted this visit. When asked, she acknowledges symptoms that are suggestive of hot flashes.

MENOPAUSE

For many middle-aged women, menstrual irregularity and ultimate amenorrhea signal the onset of menopause. Women who have had a hysterectomy lack menstrual clues, although most experience vasomotor instability (hot flashes) at some point during the climacteric. The hot flash is commonly described as a warm, wavelike sensation beginning in the upper body and spreading to the neck and face. Often occurring at night and sometimes accompanied by palpitations, the duration of a hot flash varies from a few seconds to several minutes. The precise mechanism of hot flashes is not known with certainty. However, hot flashes can be entirely eliminated by appropriate doses of supplemental estrogen.

▼ POLLY WELLS-KANBE (Part II)

Except for physical findings that relate to her hysterectomy, a thorough examination of Ms. Wells-Kanbe reveals no abnormalities. Screening laboratory work and a mammogram are normal, although serum FSH is elevated.

Although troublesome and disruptive, hot flashes are a less compelling reason for hormone replacement than are the long-term consequences of estrogen deprivation. We know that estrogen replacement stabilizes bone mass and reverses the adverse lipid changes that follow the menopause. From this follows the long-term goal of estrogen replacement therapy: to reduce the risk of osteoporosis and cardiovascular disease in otherwise healthy perimenopausal women. Women must be advised of these benefits, or they are unlikely to adhere to a program of long-term therapy. Similarly, the risks of hormone therapy must be reviewed with all patients. When the objective is an enduring therapeutic alliance, patients must be encouraged to participate fully in decisions that affect their future health.

▼ POLLY WELLS-KANBE (Part III)

You inform Ms. Wells-Kanbe that the symptoms and laboratory studies are consistent with menopause. The risks and benefits of estrogen therapy are carefully reviewed. Since the patient has had a hysterectomy, endometrial cancer is not a concern and progestin cotherapy is unnecessary. She concludes that the benefits of therapy outweigh the risks. Conjugated estrogen 0.625 mg daily is prescribed, a mammogram is scheduled, and a follow-up appointment is made.

Although 0.625 mg of conjugated estrogen is the minimal dose known to maintain bone mass, younger women with hot flashes often require higher doses to control their symptoms. In such patients the dose of estrogen should be adjusted according to symptoms. Periodically, an effort should be made to taper down to bone maintenance therapy (conjugated estrogen, 0.625 mg; estradiol transdermal, 0.05 mg; estropipate, 1.25 mg). Since hot flashes may persist up to 10 years after the final menstrual period, initial tapering efforts are not always successful and may need to be reattempted after an interval.

An annual screening mammogram is desirable in all women over the age of 50 and may be especially warranted in women taking supplemental estrogen. In addition, a focused history and physical examination should be done annually, always with attention directed at health promotion strategies likely to result in successful aging.

POSTTEST

1. Which of the following benefits of timely estrogen therapy is the single most significant in reducing mortality?
   a. Alleviation of vasomotor instability
   b. Decreased postmenopausal bone loss
   c. Attenuation of genitourinary atrophy
   d. Improvement in lipid profiles and decreased cardiovascular risk
2. The following statements regarding cyclic progestin therapy are all true except:
   a. Progestins should be prescribed for 12 to 14 consecutive days each month.
   b. Progestins decrease the beneficial lipid effects of postmenopausal estrogen therapy.
   c. Appropriate progestin therapy eliminates the risk of endometrial cancer associated with estrogen therapy.
   d. Progestins are an appropriate addition to the therapeutic regimen of all women using estrogen.
3. True statements regarding estrogen therapy include all of the following except:
   a. The estradiol patch is an appropriate estrogen formulation for women with a history of thromboembolic disease.
   b. Estrogen replacement is contraindicated in women with known coronary artery disease.
   c. A pretreatment endometrial biopsy is generally unnecessary in women who have experienced a normal menopause.
   d. Ideally, estrogen therapy should be initiated at the onset of menopause.

REFERENCES

1. Riggs BL, Melton LJ: Involutional osteoporosis, *N Engl J Med* 314:1676-1685, 1986.
2. Bonnick SL: AMWA position statement on osteoporosis, JAMWA 45:75-79, 1990.
3. Weinerman SA, Bockman RS: Medical therapy of osteoporosis, *Orthop Clin North Am* 21:109-124, 1990.
4. Riggs BL: Pathogenesis of osteoporosis, *Am J Obstet Gynecol* 156:1342-1346, 1987.
5. Lobo RL: Cardiovascular implications of estrogen replacement therapy, *Obstet Gynecol* 75:18s-25s, 1990.
6. American College of Physicians: Guidelines for counseling postmenopausal women about preventive hormone therapy, *Ann Intern Med* 117:1038-1041, 1993.
7. Whitehead M, Fraser D: Controversies concerning the safety of estrogen replacement therapy, *Am J Obstet Gynecol* 156:1313-1322, 1987.
8. Padwick ML et al: A simple method for determining the optimal dosage of progestin in postmenopausal women receiving estrogens, *N Engl J Med* 315:930-934, 1994.
9. Grady D et al: Hormone therapy to prevent disease and prolong life in postmenopausal women, *Ann Intern Med* 117:1016-1033, 1993.
10. Belchetz PE: Hormonal treatment of postmenopausal women, *N Engl J Med* 330:1062-1071, 1994.

ADDITIONAL SUGGESTED READING

Greendale GA, Judd HL: The menopause: health implications and clinical management, *J Am Geriatr Soc* 41:426-436, 1993.

PRETEST ANSWERS

1. d
2. c
3. c

POSTTEST ANSWERS

1. d
2. d
3. b

CHAPTER 39

The Prostate

RICHARD G. ROBERTS

OBJECTIVES

Upon completion of this chapter, the reader will be able to:

1. Describe the clinical anatomy, principal functions, and aging of the prostate.

2. List the four diagnostic steps for the man with uncomplicated benign prostatic hyperplasia (BPH).

3. Describe the four treatment approaches recommended for BPH.

4. Describe the pharmacology, uses, and side effects and give one example (with dosages) for each of the two categories of medications approved for treatment of BPH.

5. Discuss two arguments both for and against routine screening for prostate cancer using the serum prostate-specific antigen (PSA) test.

6. Describe the staging of prostate cancer.

7. List and describe the treatments recommended for prostate cancer.

PRETEST

1. Which one of the following is the best criterion for determining when to initiate treatment for BPH?
   a. Tests indicate significant reduction in urinary flow rate.
   b. Prostate enlargement is noted on rectal examination.
   c. The patient desires relief of symptoms.
   d. Hematuria or pyuria is present.

2. Which one of the following statements is correct?
   a. Treatment of organ-confined (stage A or B) prostate cancer with radical prostatectomy or radiation therapy improves 5-year survival.
   b. Screening with prostate-specific antigen (PSA) can detect prostate cancer earlier than rectal examination.
   c. Prostate cancer is the second leading cause of mortality in American men.
   d. Screening for prostate cancer improves outcomes for men over 50 years of age.

Prostate symptoms are a prominent feature of the aging process for most men. Loss of urinary stream, nocturia, and hesitancy occur nearly as predictably as the passage of time and constitute a frequent source of derision and discomfort. Prostate cancer, which can lead to pain and death, is an important concern of older men and the physicians who treat them. Often, primary care physicians are uncomfortable trying to sort through an aged man's urinary complaints and can be quick to refer the patient to a urologist. The comprehensiveness and continuity of care provided to aging men are enhanced, however, when the primary care physician is knowledgeable about and confident in managing prostate conditions.

This chapter focuses on the two most common prostate ailments: benign prostatic hyperplasia and prostate cancer. Brief mention is made of infection, stones, and infarct.

AGING OF THE PROSTATE

The prostate grows from 1 g at birth to a usual adult weight of about 20 g in the human male. Acinar glands with their ducts and fibromuscular stroma are the two structures that make up the bulk of the prostate gland. Shaped like a walnut and wrapped around the urethral outlet of the bladder, the prostate enlarges during adolescence under the influence of the intraprostatic androgen dihydrotestosterone (DHT). DHT results from the conversion of testosterone by the enzyme 5-α-reductase. The principal functions of the prostate are to nourish, alkalinize, and liquefy semen; prostatic fluid also appears to have some antimicrobial properties.

▼ PETER BAHR (Part I)

Mr. Bahr is a 72-year-old self-employed attorney who has noticed increasing nocturia. He arises two or three times at night to void, urinates every hour or two during the day, and complains of postvoid urgency almost every time he urinates. His symptoms have left him feeling deprived of sleep and un-able to sit through prolonged negotiations during the day. He has no other health problems.

BENIGN PROSTATIC HYPERPLASIA

Benign prostatic hyperplasia (BPH) is a common cause of obstructive (weak stream, incomplete emptying, dribbling, straining) and irritative (nocturia, urgency, frequency) urinary symptoms in older men. Autopsy data indicate that microscopic BPH is prevalent in 50% of men by age 60 and in 90% of men aged 85. Nearly half of men over 60 have symptoms consistent with clinical BPH.[1] Time and testosterone are required for BPH to develop; BPH is rare in young men and in men with prepubertal testosterone deficiencies. No risk factors other than age and sufficient serum testosterone levels have been associated with BPH.

Diagnosis

This chapter follows the recommendations of the clinical practice guideline on BPH, which was developed by an expert panel convened by the federal Agency for Health Care Policy and Research (AHCPR).[2] The panel reviewed several thousand articles, conducted a meta-analysis of the literature to ascertain the outcomes resulting from available BPH treatments, and surveyed patients as to their preferences about those outcomes.

The panel recommended four steps in the diagnosis of BPH: history, focused physical examination, urinalysis, and serum creatinine measurement. The history should include a general health assessment but should focus on prior genitourinary problems, such as previous infections or urological procedures. Particular attention should be given to fluid intake and voiding patterns; abnormal voiding in the face of normal intake is most typical of BPH. A careful medication review should be conducted, looking particularly for drugs that have anticholinergic side effects; these include many over-the-counter allergy

American Urological Association Symptom Checklist
for Benign Prostatic Hyperplasia

Over the past month, how often have you...	Never	Less Than 1 Time in 5	Less Than Half the Time	About Half the Time	More Than Half the Time	Almost Always
		Circle One Response for Each Question				
1. Felt that your bladder did not empty completely when you urinated?	0	1	2	3	4	5
2. Had to urinate again less than 2 hours after you finished urinating?	0	1	2	3	4	5
3. Had your urine flow stop and then start again several times when urinating?	0	1	2	3	4	5
4. Found it difficult to postpone urination?	0	1	2	3	4	5
5. Had a weak urinary stream?	0	1	2	3	4	5
6. Had to push or strain to begin urination?	0	1	2	3	4	5
Over the past month, how many times . . .						
7. Did you typically get up to urinate from the time you went to bed at night until the time you got up in the morning?	0	1	2	3	4	5

KEY	0-7 = Absent or mild symptoms 8-19 = Moderate symptoms 20+ = Severe symptoms	Total score (sum of 7 circled numbers): _____

FIG. 39-1   American Urological Association symptom checklist for benign prostatic hyperplasia. This checklist can be used to quantitate the severity of BPH symptoms and to follow patients longitudinally. According to an AHCPR study panel, persons with mild symptoms should be treated with watchful waiting, and those with moderate or severe symptoms should choose among four treatment options. (Modified from Barry MJ, et al: The American Urological Association Symptom Index for benign prostatic hyperplasia, *J Urol* 148:1549-1557, 1992.)

and cold preparations, as well as many prescription drugs.

There are two general types of symptoms indicative of BPH: obstructive and irritative. Obstructive symptoms include weakening of the urine stream, dribbling at the end of urination, difficulty initiating urination, and involuntary stopping and starting of urine flow. Irritative symptoms include urinary frequency, urgency, and nocturia. The history should include a quantitative assessment of symptom severity. The American Urological Association Symptom Index (Fig. 39-1), a reliable and valid measure of BPH severity, is recommended by the AHCPR panel.[3] Based on his score, a man is said to have mild (score less than 8), moderate (8 to 19), or severe (greater than 19) BPH symptoms.

On physical examination, palpation and percussion of the lower abdomen can help determine whether the urinary bladder is enlarged. Rectal examination is performed to determine whether prostate cancer may be present (e.g., a nodule or area of firmness is palpated) or whether some another condition is the cause of the symptoms (e.g., a tender and enlarged prostate suggests prostatitis; a flaccid anal sphincter can indicate a prior stroke and neurogenic bladder).

On rectal examination a prostate with BPH feels rubbery and large. Prostate size should not be relied on, however, to determine the severity of BPH. Some men with huge glands have minimal symptoms, whereas others with small glands have significant distress from BPH. This apparent paradox reflects the fact that there are two major determinants of BPH symptoms: (1) a *static* component, representing a large, hyperplastic gland that mechanically obstructs the prostatic urethra, and (2) a *dynamic* component, in which a decrease in urinary flow is caused by increased adrenergic tone of the prostatic fibromuscular stroma or the decreased expulsive power of a hypotonic bladder.

BPH symptoms are caused by both static and dynamic components; hence the size on rectal examination is inconsistent with the symptoms.

The AHCPR guidelines recommend only two routine laboratory tests for the man with suspected BPH: urinalysis and serum creatinine. Urinalysis may point to other causes of urinary symptoms (e.g., hematuria may indicate bladder cancer; pyuria may suggest cystitis or prostatitis). Serum creatinine is used to screen for renal insufficiency caused by obstructive uropathy.

The panel's recommendation to use only the creatinine to screen for renal damage is somewhat controversial. Many urologists have routinely obtained an intravenous pyelogram or a renal ultrasound, in order not to miss significant ureteral dilation or other pathologic conditions (e.g., renal cancer). Studies indicate, however, that only 2% of such imaging studies change the management of the patient. Therefore it is recommended that primary care physicians restrict imaging studies to the one third of men with an atypical history, an abnormal examination, or an abnormal urinalysis or creatinine level.

▼ *PETER BAHR (Part II)*

You determine that Mr. Bahr has an AUA symptom score of 16 (moderate severity). His history, physical examination, urine, and creatinine are otherwise normal. You discuss treatment options with him and he decides to try α-blocker therapy.

Treatment

The treatment of BPH is directed primarily toward symptom relief. There are four general treatment approaches advocated by the AHCPR panel: watchful waiting, surgery, medication, and balloon dilation. The AHCPR panel recommended that men with mild symptoms be treated with watchful waiting. For men with moderate or severe symptoms the panel concluded that all four treatment options should be discussed with the patient (Fig. 39-2). The primary care physician should help the patient choose among these available therapies, taking into account the course of symptoms over time, the patient's health status, and relevant psychosocial issues. Reflective decision making over time is usually the best approach; many men with BPH have no change in symp-

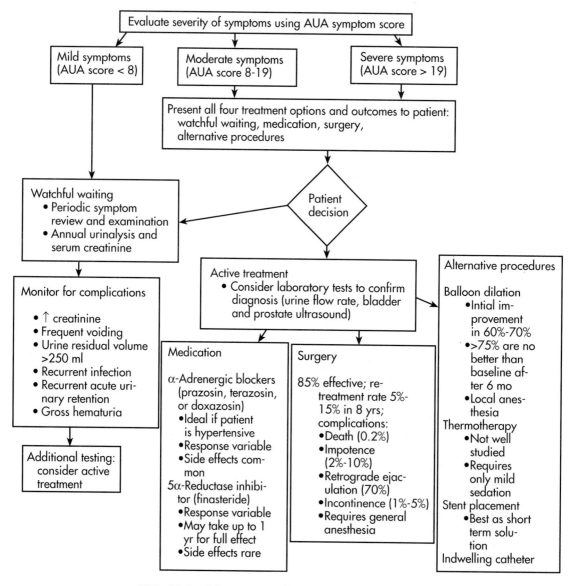

FIG. 39-2   Management of benign prostatic hyperplasia.

toms over many years, and in some cases disease symptoms improve with time.

> The four treatment approaches to BPH are watchful waiting, surgery, medication, and balloon dilation.

Watchful waiting includes active monitoring of the man's symptoms and further investigation if his symptoms change. If watchful waiting is chosen, another four-step assessment (history, examination, urinalysis, creatinine) should be repeated in 1 year. If the symptoms progress to the point at which further intervention is being considered, measurement of the peak urine flow rate (>15 ml per second is normal; 10 to 15 is borderline; <10 suggests significant obstruction) and bladder ultrasonography for residual urine may help quantify the degree of obstruction. The severity of symptoms, size of the gland, and urinary flow rate do not, however, predict reliably the natural history of BPH for any man.

Two classes of medication are most widely used to treat BPH: 5-α-reductase inhibitors and α₁-adrenergic blocking agents (Table 39-1). Finasteride (Proscar),[4,5] a 5-α-reductase inhibitor, prevents the conversion of testosterone to dihydrotestosterone, thereby gradually shrinking the prostate gland volume by an average of 20% to 30%. Symptoms improve in approximately 50% of patients. Side effects are infrequent (less than 5%) and include impotence and decreased libido. Dosing is usually at 5 mg daily; the drug may need to be continued for 6 months before its effect is fully realized. Finasteride reduces the PSA value by about half but does not obscure a rise that might reflect clinically important prostate cancer.

α-Blockers relax smooth muscle of the bladder outlet, the prostate gland, and the urethra, thereby reducing obstructive and irritative symptoms of BPH.[5] Only selective α₁-blocking agents should be used, since they have fewer side effects than nonselective agents. Of these, terazosin (Hytrin) and doxazosin (Cardura) have the advantage of once-a-day administration; prazosin (Minipress) is shorter acting but is available in generic form. Because these agents are approved for use as antihypertensive agents, they are particularly appropriate for patients who have both BPH and hypertension. Common side effects are weakness and dizziness (10%), postural hypotension (6%), a flulike syndrome (4%), and headache (3%). Side effects are best avoided by starting with low doses at bedtime and slowly titrating upward, while monitoring for symptom relief and adverse effects.

For men with moderate or severe symptoms, surgery provides the greatest amount and duration of symptom improvement. Transurethral resection (TURP) is the operation of choice for most men. More than 300,000 TURPs are performed annually in the United States, accounting for more than 90% of the surgeries for BPH. Open prostatectomy is preferred when the gland is large (greater than 50 g). A newer technique, transurethral incision (TUIP), may provide similar symptom relief with fewer complications. TUIP involves scoring one or both lobes of the prostate with a capsule-splitting incision. Laser prostatectomy is also under investigation. Surgical complications include anesthesia risk, bleeding, infection, pain, and a hospital stay of 2 (TUIP) to 5 (TURP) to 7 to 10 (open) days. Operative mortality risk is low (about 1%). Long-term effects include impotence, retrograde ejaculation, and (rarely) incontinence.

For patients who are poor surgical risks and fail to respond to medication, several alternative procedures are available that require only local anesthesia or mild sedation. Dilation of the prostatic urethra with an inflatable balloon was popular in the 1980s but appears to be losing favor because of high retreatment rates. Endoscopic placement of stainless steel or titanium stents can be performed on patients with urinary retention who need short-term relief. Thermotherapy involves using microwaves to heat the prostate gland, leading to localized tissue necrosis and, in successful cases, symptom relief. None of these alternative techniques is as successful as surgery, however, and all of them are still considered experimental.[6]

While managing patients with BPH, the physician

Table 39-1 Medications Commonly Used to Treat Benign Prostatic Hyperplasia

Medication	Class	Typical Dosage Range			Common Adverse Effects
		Starting	Maintenance	Maximum	
Finasteride	5-α-Reductase inhibitor	5 mg/day	5 mg/day	10 mg/day	Impotence, decreased libido
Prazosin	α₁-Adrenergic blocking agent	1 mg hs	1-2 mg tid	5 mg tid	Dizziness, headache, weakness, drowsiness, palpitations
Terazosin	α₁-Adrenergic blocking agent	1 mg hs	2-5 mg hs	10 mg hs	Dizziness, headaches, weakness, orthostatic hypotension
Doxazosin	α₁-Adrenergic blocking agent	1 mg hs	4 mg/day	16 mg/day	Dizziness, headaches, weakness, orthostatic hypotension

should monitor for complications such as urinary tract infection, hematuria, acute urinary retention, and renal failure. Urinary tract infections are more common in men with BPH because residual urine in a partially emptied bladder is a hospitable environment for bacteria. For this reason it may be useful to measure bladder residual urine (after treatment) by ultrasound; a residual urine above 250 ml may indicate the need for more active treatment.[6] Hematuria in older men is frequently caused by BPH. However, hematuria is not a common complication of BPH. It arises because the blood vessels lining the mucosa of an enlarged prostate are often more numerous and friable than in the normal prostate. When gross hematuria occurs, more serious bleeding sources should be ruled out by urinary tract imaging and cystoscopy. Acute urinary retention is another common complication of BPH; often it is triggered by a new anticholinergic medication or hospitalization. Finally, renal failure can result from chronic or acute obstruction resulting from BPH; monitoring patient symptoms and the serum creatinine level allows the physician to screen for this complication of BPH. Fortunately, severe complications from untreated BPH are rare and can usually be prevented with adequate monitoring.[7]

▼ PETER BAHR (Part III)

Mr. Bahr begins a 1 mg a day dose of terazosin. In spite of the low initial dose, bothersome orthostatic lightheadedness develops. You again review treatment options, and he elects to try finasteride. After 3 months of finasteride, his symptom score is 15; he considers himself only minimally improved, and he requests surgery. Four months after surgery he remains improved and is pleased with his results.

PROSTATE CANCER

Prostate cancer is primarily a disease of older men. It is becoming increasingly prevalent as a diagnosis and cause of death, to the point that its public health importance for men is approaching that of breast cancer for women.[8] It is now the most commonly diagnosed cancer and the second leading cause of cancer death among U.S. males. In 1994 prostate cancer was diagnosed in nearly 180,000 men and 40,000 died of it. Worldwide, between 10% and 30% of men aged 50 and older have the disease. Its prevalence doubles every 5 years beyond age 60, so that by age 80 nearly two thirds of men have histological evidence of prostate cancer.

> *Prostate cancer is the second leading cause of cancer death among U.S. males; however, far more individuals die* with *prostate cancer than die* of *it.*

The course of prostate cancer is often benign. Most cancers occur in older men and remain asymptomatic for years. Thus the average life expectancy for persons with the disease differs little from that of persons without the disease, and far more persons die *with* prostate cancer than *of* it.

Management of prostate cancer is embroiled in controversy. Often, different medical specialists have conflicting views about how to approach a specific patient. This is especially true in the management of asymptomatic disease. For example, specialists who treat advanced disease tend to be far more aggressive in recommending screening than are primary care physicians, whose experience is largely with nonprogressive disease and with the complications of treatment. Similarly, when localized disease is diagnosed, referral to a urologist usually results in a radical prostatectomy being recommended, whereas referral to a radiation oncologist leads to a recommendation that radiation therapy be administered. There is little evidence that either method is superior to doing nothing. Thus physicians who care for older men must make individualized decisions, balancing their understanding of the patient's unique circumstances with existing knowledge and opinion in this rapidly changing area.

> *With localized prostate cancer, there is little evidence that treatment is superior to doing nothing.*

▼ RICHARD GRAND (Part I)

Mr. Grand is a 74-year-old widowed retiree whose daughter has advised him to have a free prostate-specific antigen (PSA) blood test performed at your community hospital during Prostate Cancer Awareness Week. He asks your advice on whether he should have the test.

Prevention and Early Detection

No specific cause has been found for prostate cancer, but a number of risk factors have been identified (Table 39-2). As noted earlier, increasing age is the most powerful risk. Family history is important; a few families have very high prevalences of early onset disease, but overall the contribution of family history is moderate. High-fat, low-fiber diets have been implicated as an explanation for geographic variation in the disease, such as the threefold increase in disease prevalence in Japanese-Americans compared with persons living in Japan. Race contributes moderately to risk, with the disease being most prevalent among blacks. Vasectomy is associated with increased risk, although this conclusion remains debated. The role of heavy metal exposure is even more disputed;

cadmium exposure has been suggested to increase risk and zinc exposure to decrease risk, but neither appears to have a major role in disease pathogenesis. Smoking, socioeconomic status, sexually transmitted diseases, and benign prostatic hyperplasia have not been demonstrated to be independent risk factors.[9]

Since all known risk factors for prostate cancer convey only modest increases in risk, disease pathogenesis remains poorly explained. As a result, no effective primary prevention strategy has been identified. Therefore there is considerable interest in screening for early disease.

The time-honored screening method is the digital rectal examination (DRE). Both the National Cancer Institute and the American Cancer Society recommend an annual DRE for all men beginning at age 40; however, the Canadian Task Force on the Periodic Health Examination was unable to find adequate evidence for its use, and the U.S. Preventive Services Task Force recommended against its use in December 1995. When used for screening, the DRE has a sensitivity of approximately 43% and a positive predictive value of approximately 19%.[10]

Controversy around prostate cancer screening has been heightened by recent FDA approval and American Cancer Society endorsement of the serum prostate-specific antigen (PSA) test for mass screening. PSA is a nonspecific marker, produced by both benign and malignant prostate tissue. For this reason persons with prostatic enlargement caused by BPH often have elevated PSA levels, and persons with small tumors can have a normal PSA. Thus the sensitivity and specificity of the test are modest and the cost of following up borderline and abnormal PSA tests, if performed on all older men, would be staggering. Box 39-1 provides recommendations for use of the PSA in primary care.

Table 39-2 Identifying Men at High Risk for Prostate Cancer

Risk Factor	Approximate Magnitude
Age	Rare before age 55; approximately doubles in prevalence for every 5 years thereafter; microscopic disease present in over half of persons age 80+
Family history	Variable; family history in first-degree relatives approximately doubles risk of early onset disease
Black race	Increases relative risk by approximately 1.3
Vasectomy	Increases relative risk by 1.5-1.9
Diet high in saturated fat	Relative risk appears to be 1.6-1.9

From Pienta KJ, Esper PS: *Ann Intern Med* 118:793-803, 1993.

BOX 39-1
Use of the Prostate-Specific Antigen (PSA) Screening Test

1. It is not known whether aggressive treatment of prostate cancer detected by PSA screening actually extends life or reduces morbidity. Future longitudinal trials should help clarify this. Discuss the theoretical benefits and real risks (see Table 39-3) with each patient before PSA testing is undertaken, and be sure that patients with borderline or elevated PSA results understand the risks of treatment before referral.

2. The PSA is a better screening test than digital rectal examination, but its sensitivity and specificity remain modest. When screening studies were summarized, average test characteristics were as follows[10]:

Cutoff (ng/dl)	Sensitivity	Specificity	Predictive value of:	
			Positive Result	Negative Result
4.0	71	75	37%	91%
10.0	56	77	47%	88%

3. Do not screen men whose life expectancy is less than 10 years (i.e., those over age 75 or with chronic, progressive illnesses such as Alzheimer's disease, congestive heart failure, and chronic renal disease).

4. Invasive urological procedures definitely elevate PSA; therefore testing should be postponed for 2 to 3 weeks after such procedures. Putting a patient at bed rest reduces the PSA by 18% to 50%; therefore measurements should be obtained on ambulatory patients.

5. When interpreting test results, consider using age-specific reference ranges[11]:

Age	Normal value (ng/ml)
40-49	≤2.5
50-59	≤3.5
60-69	≤4.5
70-79	≤6.5

6. In patients taking finasteride (Proscar), expect the PSA (and the upper limit of normal for the PSA) to be reduced by about 50%.

7. Patients whose PSA is borderline can be followed with serial PSA. A rate of change above 0.75 ng/year, when observed in three serial measurements, increases the specificity of the PSA to around 90%.[10]

Do not do a PSA screen for men with a life expectancy of 10 years or less.

Transrectal ultrasonography (TRUS) has also received attention as a prostate cancer screening test, but its current role is confined largely to guiding biopsy needles. According to some physicians it is useful as a method of following up PSA elevations in persons without a palpable prostate nodule. This is because prostate cancer produces more PSA (averaging 3.5 ng/dl) than benign prostate tissue (0.3 ng/dl), so combining the PSA value with a measure of prostate size using TRUS yields the PSA density, which may be more specific and sensitive than either the PSA or the TRUS alone. Whether PSA density is superior to age-specific PSA norms (Box 39-1) is unproved, however.[11]

The test for any diagnostic procedure is whether its application actually improves patient outcomes. This is especially true for screening procedures applied to asymptomatic populations. The difficulty with prostate cancer screening is that early detection or treatment has not yet been proved to improve outcomes. Consequently, a man who contemplates being screened with a serum PSA must be willing to trade off the theoretical possibility of being helped by treatment against the real probabilities of complications from treatment. Table 39-3 illustrates such a balance sheet.[9] The challenge for the primary care clinician is to help men sort through the risks and benefits of the various strategies to help them arrive at a decision that best reflects personal risk and individual values.[10-16]

▼ RICHARD GRAND (Part II)

Mr. Grand decides to have a PSA done; the result is 3.7 ng/ml (normal <4). He is thought to have BPH, which he prefers to manage with watchful waiting.

One year later low back pain and increased urinary urgency and frequency develop. Infection is ruled out. On examination he is noted to have an area of firmness over the

right lobe of the prostate. PSA is now 34.6 ng/ml, and a bone scan indicates increased uptake over the fourth lumbar vertebra. Needle biopsy of the prostate shows a poorly differentiated cancer with a Gleason score of 8.[15] He decides to be treated with hormone therapy to control his bone pain.

CASE DISCUSSION

Mr. Grand's case illustrates some of the problems inherent in prostate cancer diagnosis. Even when combined with rectal examination and transrectal ultrasound (TRUS), the accuracy of PSA in predicting the presence of prostate cancer is still only about 65%. One third of men with PSA values greater than 4 have some cause other than prostate cancer to explain the elevation (e.g., BPH, prostatitis), and one fourth of men with prostate cancer have PSA levels less than 4. At the time his cancer is diagnosed, Mr. Grand has Whitmore-Jewett stage D_2 disease (Table 39-4).

Treatment

Once prostate cancer has been diagnosed, regardless of whether diagnosis was the result of screening or the evaluation of symptoms, treatment decisions should be directed toward the relief of any symptoms and the man's preferences regarding the trade-off between potential benefits of treatment and possible complications of therapy. There are four basic approaches to prostate cancer: watchful waiting, surgery (usually radical prostatectomy, although TURP may be done on occasion to relieve obstruction in metastatic disease), radiation therapy (external beam or interstitial implants), and hormonal therapy.

The four basic approaches to prostate cancer are watchful waiting, surgery, radiation, and hormones.

Prostate cancers are staged according to histology and extent. The Gleason system[15] provides a measure of tumor aggressiveness. Pathological slides are assigned a

Table 39-3   Prostate Cancer: A Balance Sheet for Decision Making

	Radical Surgery	Radiation Therapy	Watchful Waiting
Median annual mortality rate			
All causes	0.032	0.045	0.060
Cancer-specific causes	0.009	0.023	0.009
Persistent adverse outcomes after treatment			
Any urinary incontinence	26.6%	6.1%	—
Complete incontinence	6.8%	1.2-5.4%	—
Any bowel injury	2.7%	11.4-14.4%	—
Stricture requiring long term treatment	12.4%	4.5-9.8%	—
Impotence	84.6%	12.4-41.4%	—

Adapted from Wasson JH et al: *Arch Fam Med* 2:487-493, 1993.

score from 1 to 5, with 5 indicating chaotic histological architecture. The predominant area, called the primary grade, is added to a less representative area, the secondary grade, to develop a total Gleason grade of 2 to 10. Gleason grades of 2 to 4 are considered well differentiated; 5 to 7 moderately differentiated; and 8 to 10 poorly differentiated.[14] Two systems are available to stage tumor extension (see Table 39-4).

In general, for the man with organ-confined prostate cancer who prefers active treatment, radical prostatectomy is recommended if he has a life expectancy greater than 10 years; radiation therapy is recommended if he has a life expectancy less than 10 years. Surgery results commonly in impotence, and bladder incontinence is a frequent complication (see Table 39-3). Immediate risks of surgery include perioperative mortality, bleeding, pain, and infection. Risks associated with radiation therapy are lower than those associated with surgery (see Table 39-3).

For the man with metastatic disease, recommended treatments include radiation therapy and hormone therapy. Radiation therapy is particularly useful if local metastases are present or if symptomatic metastatic disease is confined to one area (e.g., the lumbar spine). Hormonal therapy aims at reducing the androgenic milieu that promotes prostate cancer growth. Hormonal treatments include castration, diethylstilbestrol 1 to 3 mg by mouth daily, leuprolide 7.5 mg intramuscularly (IM) monthly, goserelin implant 3.5 mg subcutaneously monthly, flutamide 250 mg 3 times a day, megestrol 40 mg by mouth 2 to 4 times a day, or ketoconazole 400 mg by mouth every 8 hours. Side effects of these treatments include decreased libido and sexual potency, hot flashes, gynecomastia, hepatotoxicity, and risk of thromboembolism.[16]

Some oncologists are using cytotoxic chemotherapy for hormone-refractory disease, even though response rates are below 50%. The two agents used most frequently are estramustine and vinblastine. Supportive care may require steroids (for cord compression), analgesics (bone pain), antiemetics, stool softeners, antidepressants, and psychological support.

OTHER PROSTATE DISEASES

Prostatitis, or prostate infection, usually represents an acute flare-up in a man with chronic prostatitis. Classic symptoms of acute bacterial prostatitis are fever, rigors, back or groin ache, and dysuria. In older persons, however, the symptoms are frequently milder: low-grade fever, muscle aches, malaise, and mild dysuria or increased frequency. Rectal examination should be undertaken carefully in men with suspected prostatitis because vigorous prostatic massage can cause gram-negative bacteremia and lead to sepsis. Men with mild or chronic prostatitis can be managed on an outpatient basis; those with acute and severe prostatitis usually require hospitalization and intravenous antibiotics. Successful treatment of prostatitis requires use of antibiotics with good penetrance into prostatic fluid (quinolones, sulfa drugs, tetracyclines) for at least 3 weeks.

Prostate stones are small calcifications that arise typically in men with a history of chronic prostatitis. They are usually asymptomatic and of little clinical consequence. Occasionally a palpable stone on physical examination is mistaken for a prostate cancer. Ultrasound usually resolves the issue.

Infarction of the prostate is another condition that can mislead the clinician into diagnosing prostate cancer; it typically presents acutely and causes temporary, localized prostate swelling and elevation the serum prostate-specific antigen (PSA) level.

SUMMARY

Medical treatment for symptoms of BPH is a serious consideration in patients with moderate symptoms, although surgery (TURP) remains the procedure of choice for those with moderate or severe symptoms. Prostate cancer management is controversial: the patient must consider the alternatives carefully. Watchful waiting is the appropriate management for many. The PSA test should not be used indiscriminately, since there may be little point in doing it if the patient is likely to live less than 10 years. Thus all prostatic management decisions must be carefully assisted by a well-informed primary care physician who can help the patient (and family if necessary) choose between different specialized treatments.

Table 39-4   Staging the Extensiveness of Prostate Cancer

Extent of Cancer	Whitmore-Jewett System	WHO System
Confined to the gland, nonpalpable	A	T_0
Confined to the gland, palpable	B	$T_{1,2}$
Local extra-capsular spread	C	$T_{3,4}$
Distant spread to		
Regional lymph nodes	D_1	T_4N
Skeleton (pelvis, spine)	D_2	T_4M

POSTTEST

1. Which one of the following tests is not recommended in the routine management of men with BPH?
   a. Urinary flow rate
   b. Symptom score
   c. Rectal examination
   d. Serum creatinine
2. For a man with moderate symptoms of BPH, which of the following is not a reasonable treatment option?
   a. Watchful waiting
   b. TURP
   c. Finasteride
   d. α-Blockers
   e. Hormonal treatment
3. Which of the following statements is true for prostate cancer?
   a. Screening with prostate specific antigen has been shown to save lives.
   b. African-American men have higher death rates from prostate cancer than other U.S. males.
   c. Organ-confined prostate cancer should be treated by surgery alone.
   d. Surgical or medical castration is not an acceptable therapy for stage D (T_4M) disease.

REFERENCES

1. Garraway M, Collins G, Lee R: High prevalence of benign prostatic hypertrophy in the community, *Lancet* 338:469-471, 1991.
2. McConnell JD et al: *Benign prostatic hyperplasia: diagnosis and treatment. Clinical practice guideline,* Number 8, AHCPR Publication No 94-0582, Rockville, Md, February 1994, Agency for Health Care Policy and Research, Public Health Service, US Department of Health and Human Services.
3. Barry MJ et al: The American Urological Association Symptom Index for benign prostatic hyperplasia, *J Urol* 148:1549-1557, 1992.
4. Gormley GJ et al: The effect of finasteride in men with benign prostatic hyperplasia, *N Engl J Med* 327:1185-1191, 1992.
5. Monda JM, Oesterling JE: Medical treatment of benign prostatic hyperplasia: 5α-reductase inhibitors and α-adrenergic antagonists, *Mayo Clin Proc* 68:670-679, 1993.
6. Bruskewitz RC: Benign prostatic hyperplasia: intervene or wait? *Hosp Prac Off Ed* 27(6):99-102, 105-106, 109-110, 1992.
7. Barry MJ: Epidemiology and natural history of benign prostatic hyperplasia, *Urol Clin North Am* 17:495-507, 1990.
8. Coffey DS: Prostate cancer: an overview of an increasing dilemma, *Cancer* 71(suppl):880-886, 1993.
9. Pienta KJ, Esper PS: Risk factors for prostate cancer, *Ann Intern Med* 118:793-803, 1993.
10. Canadian Task Force on the Periodic Health Examination: Periodic health examination, 1991 update. 3. Secondary prevention of prostate cancer, *Can Med Assoc J* 145:413-418, 1991.
11. Ruckle HC, Klee GG, Oesterling JE: Prostate-specific antigen: critical issues for the practicing physician, *Mayo Clin Proc* 69:59-68, 1994.
12. Wasson JH et al: A structured literature review of treatment for localized prostate cancer, *Arch Fam Med* 2:487-493, 1993.
13. Hahn D, Roberts RG: PSA screening for asymptomatic prostate cancer: truth in advertising, *J Fam Pract* 37:432-435, 1993.
14. Catalona WJ: Management of cancer of the prostate, *N Engl J Med* 331:996-1004, 1994.
15. Garnick MB: Prostate cancer: screening, diagnosis, and management, *Ann Intern Med* 118:904-918, 1993.
16. Dorr VJ, Williamson SK, Stephens RL: An evaluation of prostate-specific antigen as a screening test for prostate cancer, *Arch Intern Med* 153:2529-2537, 1993.

PRETEST ANSWERS

1. c
2. b

POSTTEST ANSWERS

1. a
2. e
3. b

CHAPTER 40

Constipation

HENRY M. WIEMAN

OBJECTIVES

On completion of this chapter, the reader will be able to:

1. Discuss the nature of constipation, and discuss alternative definitions and understandings of the problem.

2. Identify risk factors and causes of constipation.

3. Identify advantages and disadvantages of the various treatment modalities that are available for constipation.

4. Devise a treatment program for individuals with constipation and impaction.

5. Recognize the complications of constipation.

PRETEST

1. Which one of the following should never be used in elderly people?
   a. Oral mineral oil
   b. Stimulant laxatives
   c. Phospho-soda enemas
   d. Surgical treatment for constipation
   e. Advice to increase fluid intake
2. Which of the following is associated with parkinsonian-like side effects?
   a. Misoprostol
   b. Bisacodyl
   c. Milk of magnesia
   d. Metoclopramide
   e. Senna
3. Which one of the following statements concerning constipation in frail elders is false?
   a. Eleven percent of frail elders consider constipation a major problem.
   b. Fecal leakage in frail elderly is generally due to extreme constipation.
   c. Pelvic dyssynergia is a common condition of the elderly and causes constipation.
   d. Oral mineral oil is a safe adjunct to assist the smooth passage of hard stool.

CONSTIPATION: WHAT IS IT?

Constipation may be America's most common health complaint[1]; a recent survey[2] indicates that 45% of frail elderly home-dwelling people complain of constipation. Eleven percent consider it a major problem, and only 5% are satisfied with the treatment they take or are given for it.

Nonetheless, constipation eludes clear definition. Various clinicians, authors, and patients use various definitions.[3] Some consider fewer than three movements a week constipation. Others consider the defining characteristic of constipation as the need to strain or hard, painful bowel movements. Normal bowel function is an elusive concept. If the three bowel movement a week standard is used, constipation is probably not so common.[4] A number of problems may be misinterpreted as constipation (Box 40-1). As with "dizziness," it is worthwhile for the clinician to ascertain the meaning the patient attaches to the term "constipation" before proceeding to treatment.[3,5] People who are now elderly may have been exposed to the medical teaching in the early years of the century that regular purging bowel movements are necessary to cleanse the colon of the toxins of bacterial growth that accumulate there and cause many of the ills to which people are susceptible. Before deriding this view, it is well to remember that the medical profession promulgated it.

> *Constipation is present if there is a need to strain to pass firm, hard, or generally painful bowel movements.*

Constipation can appear as its apparent opposite: fecal leaking or scant watery "diarrhea" can be the presentation of *fecal impaction*. Symptoms produced by fecal impaction vary widely: some patients may be hardly aware of the problem, whereas others are clearly rendered ill and even confused, their cerebral clarity returning when the impaction is relieved. Fecal impaction is the most common cause of apparent fecal incontinence, which is perhaps one of the most distressing symptoms in somebody who is aware and a burden to caregivers. The leakage of feculent brown liquid from around rocklike impacted stool in a dilated rectum has been termed "spurious diarrhea." This phenomenon is one reason that it is not advisable to have standing orders for antidiarrheal medication in dependent elderly patients in nursing homes. Apparent "diarrhea" requires a rectal examination, not a reflex prescription.

BOX 40-1
Problems That May Be Termed "Constipation"

Straining at stool
Painful bowel movements (dyschezia)
Perceived infrequent bowel movements
Sensation of incomplete elimination
Abdominal discomfort relieved by bowel movements

▼ JANE BUTTON

Mrs. Button, 76, has never been constipated before. She is a healthy and vigorous person. She has been admitted to the hospital to have a knee replacement because her degenerative joint disease has been interfering with her tennis game. On the second postoperative day she becomes profoundly and painfully constipated.

BOX 40-2
Causes of Constipation

Chronic slow transit time
Pelvic dyssynergia
Irritable bowel syndrome
Environmental factors
   Immobility
   Poor hydration
   Dietary deficiency of bulk and fiber
Psychological factors
   Depression
   Neurosis
   Bowel obsession
Iatrogenesis
Laxative habituation
Colonic mass
   Cancer
   Diverticulitis
Bowel obstruction
Anal stricture or fissure

STUDY QUESTIONS

- *What is the most likely course of events leading to this new event in her life?*
- *How might it be addressed?*

CAUSES OF CONSTIPATION

Not all constipation is the same. Chronic slow transit time causes lifelong constipation that simply worsens in old age as further constipating factors ensue. This type of constipation may be severe and may even justify surgical intervention.

Pelvic dyssynergia occurs when the muscles controlling elimination fail to coordinate. When the rectum contracts the puborectalis sling, the internal and external sphincters fail to relax. Pain, incomplete evacuation, and failure to defecate in spite of the urge and effort may occur.[1] Pelvic dyssynergia is thought to be a common condition in elderly people.[6]

Irritable bowel syndrome is also usually a lifelong condition. The most common symptom is alternating periods of diarrhea and constipation. Abdominal discomfort relieved by bowel movements is another common symptom of irritable bowel syndrome.

Environmental causes include inactivity, poor hydration, and poor dietary intake. Although fiber deficiency is blamed for constipation, total caloric deficiency may be important.[7]

Drugs commonly contribute to constipation (Box 40-2).[4,8] Unfortunately, drugs that constipate are also popular and commonly indicated among elderly people. Constipation is a possible side effect of almost any drug. Medications with anticholinergic side effects are particu-

BOX 40-3
Basic Bowel Hygiene

Regular, unhurried, quiet, private toilet time
Extra dietary fiber
No less than 1500 ml of water intake per day
Regular exercise

larly prone to cause this problem and include many over-the-counter preparations such as antihistamines sold as allergy pills, cold remedies, and sleep aids.

Laxative habituation often arises from obsession for a clean bowel. Data are not complete, but it is likely that old age in itself does not cause constipation. The environmental and iatrogenic factors mentioned above are all much more common among the elderly and probably account for the increased prevalence of constipation in frail elders.[6]

Psychological factors affect and are affected by constipation. There is considerable evidence that depression and general irritability accompany constipation.[7,9] The relationships between psychological factors and bowel function are probably diverse.

Specific tissue pathologies can cause constipation; if usual treatments fail, investigation for bowel mass, either intrinsic or extrinsic, and for anal stricture should be undertaken.[10-12]

COMPLICATIONS OF CONSTIPATION

Straining to have a bowel movement can cause syncope, TIAs, and even myocardial infarction.[3] Hemorrhoids, rectocele, and rectal prolapse are also complications of constipation. Hernias of various kinds may result as well, but the major complication of constipation is fecal impaction.

BASIC BOWEL HYGIENE

Basic bowel hygiene should be achieved before using a prescription (Box 40-3). Constipation in the nursing home may originate from lack of regular private time on the toilet. Fluid intake is often low in elderly people; alcoholic or caffeine-containing beverages should not be included in the calculation of fluid intake.

Treatment and prevention of constipation involves three factors: fluid, fiber, and exercise; many older people's lives are deficient in all three.

Dietary fiber is low in most people's diets and even lower in the diets of the elderly, so increasing or supplementing it is reasonable. There are a number of methods and formulations for achieving higher fiber intake, and there are creative ways of making it more appetizing. It unfortunately causes colonic gas. This is distressing, particularly to fastidious people. If feasible, after dinner outdoor strolls are healthy for many reasons, not the least of which is gas relief. Gassiness and bloating can improve with continued use of fiber. Dosage is also a neglected issue: some people are sensitive to bowel stimulation, and others are more tolerant.

Exercise can help, although there is little data to support this. An immobilized patient is known to be predisposed to constipation, even if the fluid and fiber intake is adequate. Massage over the descending colon can help produce a bowel movement in the immobilized, as can any movement that compresses the abdominal contents. Abdominal "crunches" are likely to help if the patient can do them.

Another sometimes helpful technique is to take advantage of the "gastrocolic reflex." This is the tendency to evacuate when the stomach is filled. Many people have a sensation of abdominal fullness following meals, and, particularly if movement or exercise intervene, the period within 15 or 20 minutes of completing a meal (e.g., breakfast or lunch, but any meal will do) may be the optimal time to attempt to have a bowel movement. Thus toileting after meals may be helpful in "catching" bowel movements in the fecally incontinent, unaware patient.

> *The optimal time to attempt bowel movement is probably within a half hour of completing a meal, especially if some exercise intervenes.*

After basic bowel hygiene is established, more specific approaches can be undertaken. However, laxatives are drugs and have adverse effects like any others.

▼ THELMA MYERS (Part I)

Mrs. Myers is a widow who lives at home alone. Her family is distant both physically and emotionally. She has frequently been sick since her childhood. That she is chronically constipated is one of her many complaints. She takes many over-the-counter and prescription medicines. Among them are many laxatives, but she is still constipated and the problem seems to be getting worse. You examine her, and indeed there is firm to hard stool in the rectum, and the descending colon can be palpated, with small feculent masses present.

STUDY QUESTIONS

- *What situations or sequence of events underlie Mrs. Myers constipation?*
- *What approaches should you take?*

A PRACTICAL APPROACH TO CONSTIPATION

I. Basic bowel hygiene (Box 40-3)
  A. Diet
  B. Exercise
  C. Determine exact symptoms (and reassure if appropriate)
  D. Fiber supplements
    1. Mixed fruit or psyllium, whichever is acceptable
    2. Titrate dose: some will become too flatulent
    3. Use fiber tablets or mixtures if preferred
  E. Encourage serene, unhurried toilet time
  F. Consider underlying causes (Box 40-2)
    1. Laboratory chemistries
    2. Colonoscope or barium enema (mandatory to consider if bowel habit has changed, but pointless if the patient is too frail to be a surgical candidate)

II. If this fails, use drugs (Table 40-1)
  A. Remove constipating drugs if possible (Box 40-4)
  B. Milk of Magnesia at night
  C. Senna at night if above is ineffective
  D. Other drugs are available, but questionably cost effective

III. If this fails, approach from below
  A. Digitally disimpact (if rectal examination reveals need)
  B. Suppositories
    1. Glycerine; cheap, easy, safe
    2. Bisacodyl (if above is ineffective)
  C. Enemas
    1. Mineral oil retention first (retain as long as possible)
    2. Follow with saline lavage (especially for high impaction)
    3. Phospho-soda or hypertonic (only if others fail)
    4. Regular two- or three-time weekly water enemas for chronic recurrent impaction and incontinence

IV. Desperation measures
  A. Surgical evaluation[10] (rarely indicated in the elderly)
  B. Colectomy (sometimes needed in severe slow transit time constipation)[11]
  C. Surgery (rectal and anal dysfunctions such as rectocele and hemorrhoids may indicate this)

Physicians shy away from stimulant laxatives because they have seen stimulant-addicted colons. Nonetheless, judicious (not daily) use of mild stimulants such as senna is useful and fairly benign.[12, 13] Many more expensive (but no more effective) drugs are available. Docusate, one of the most widely sold preparations on the market, has very little evidence of effectiveness; it is probably a mucosal irritant instead of the pure softener it is said to

Table 40-1   Nondietary Constipation Remedies

Treatment	Comment
Softeners	
Docusate	Questionable effectiveness
Stimulants	Whole class is habituating
Senna	Probably best in group
Bisacodyl	Good alternative
Avoid others	
Saline and electrolytes	
Milk of magnesia	Old standby; contraindicated in renal failure
Magnesium salts: citrate and sulfate	Too harsh: enemas are better if the problem is this severe
Other electrolytes	Used only in preparation for bowel procedures
Sugars	
Lactulose	No better than much less expensive alternatives such as senna
Sorbitol	
Miscellaneous drugs	
Metoclopramide (Reglan)	Expensive and doubtfully better, plus has parkinsonian side effects
Suppositories	Advantage of local treatment for local problem, but undignified and may miss high impactions
Glycerine	Good, benign first step
Bisacodyl	Very useful and fairly safe
Enemas	Can cause life-threatening complications
Phospho-soda	Very popular; can cause electrolyte disturbance
Mineral oil	Very useful for impaction; hard to retain, but worth it
Tap water	Can cause water overload, but high volume is required for high impaction
Saline	Useful for lavage of high impactions
Hypertonic milk and molasses	Possible last resort but can be dehydrating
To be Avoided	
Oral mineral oil	Causes severe chemical pneumonitis if even small amounts are aspirated
Soapsuds enemas	Too irritating; saline lavage indicated for severe situations

be.[4,14] Powerful stimulants like magnesium salts can be distressing and dangerous if impaction or other obstruction prevents evacuation.

Enemas are by no means benign.[15] Nonetheless, in intractable cases of constipation they are indispensable. Mineral oil from an enema is safe and effective. It must be remembered that water-based enema solutions cause a dialysis across the colonic mucosa and affect salt and water balance. A dialysis solution would probably be the best solution to use, but failing that, saline or alternating saline and water is preferable.[10]

▼ *THELMA MYERS (Part II)*

On physical examination you find that Mrs. Myers is indeed constipated. You use the "plastic bag" technique to get all of her laxatives together, and you introduce a regimen of fiber, fluid, and exercise, but to no avail. A lifetime of laxative abuse has made it impossible to defecate without stimulation, and you resort to suppositories; glycerine does not work, but the regular use of bisacodyl every third day finally secures regular bowel movement for her. However, when she is hospitalized for repair of a hip fracture, on the fourth postoperative day she is found to be fecally incontinent, confused, uncomfortable, and distended and has signs of intestinal obstruction: the abdomen is extended and hyperresonant and a radiograph shows dilated loops of gas-distended bowel and huge amounts of feces filling her colon. Intensive laxative treatment from above and manual disimpaction, enemas, and eventually high colonic washouts from below are necessary to clear her long-standing constipation. Following hospitalization, colonoscopy is carried out, but no other problems are found. Rehabilitated after surgery, she eventually has to settle back to the bisacodyl suppository every second or third day and an occasional enema to keep things clear.

FECAL INCONTINENCE

Fecal incontinence may be one of the most depressing symptoms of the old. As with urinary incontinence, it is important to distinguish whether the patient is aware of the incontinence or not. If the patient is unaware (and this is generally because of dementia of some kind), management includes a regular toileting regimen and may even include inducing a degree of constipation so that the bowel movement can be controlled with regular suppository treatment or enemas to secure regular evacuation.

Another cause of fecal incontinence may be an extremely lax anal sphincter, so it is essential to assess the anal tone on examination. If it is lax, a simple surgical procedure (generally carried out as a 1-day procedure) can be effective. This is basically the same procedure that is used for rectal prolapse. Sometimes fecal incontinence is due to looseness of the stool, and the huge differential diagnosis of diarrhea then becomes applicable. Discussion of this is beyond the scope of this book, but it should be stated that new onset intractable diarrhea in old people often turns out to be due to underlying carcinoma, so colonoscopic investigation is the first priority, after stool analysis and culture, in such instances.

As a last resort the new diaper technology will contain stool, and even those with intractable fecal incontinence can thus be spared some of the indignity otherwise associated with their illness.[16]

THE FUTURE

If history is any guide, constipation will always be with us. Of all the common complaints, there seems to be less progress or change in the treatment of constipation than any other. It seems that this problem bothers patients more than it bothers the physicians who treat it. Recent developments have included diagnostic tests and procedures such as fecoflowometry, videodefecography, and radiodefecography. The clinical correlation of various findings of these tests and the usefulness of addressing those findings have yet to be defined.

POSTTEST

1. In cases of intractable constipation, which one of the following tests should generally not be considered if surgical treatment is an option?
   a. Colonoscopy
   b. X-ray examination of abdomen
   c. Serum calcium determination
   d. MRI of the colon
2. Recommended treatments for constipation include all the following except:
   a. Bisacodyl suppositories
   b. Senna
   c. Soapsuds enemas
   d. Mineral oil enemas
   e. Milk of Magnesia
3. Which one of the following statements concerning constipation in old age is false?
   a. In pelvic dyssynergia, rectal contraction coincides with the relaxation of the anal sphincter.
   b. The flatulence of dietary fiber becomes less with continuing use.
   c. Oral mineral oil is contraindicated in frail elders.
   d. Magnesium salts can produce extreme discomfort if fecal impaction is present.

REFERENCES

1. Donatelle EP: Constipation: pathophysiology and treatment, *Am Fam Phys* 42:1335-1342, 1990.
2. Wolfsen CR, Barker JC, Mitteness LS: Constipation in the daily lives of frail elderly people, *Arch Fam Med* 2:853-858, 1993.
3. Wald A: Constipation and fecal incontinence in the elderly, *Gastroenterol Clin North Am* 19:405-418, 1990.
4. Harari M, Gurwitz JH, Minaker KL: Constipation in the elderly, *J Am Geriatr Soc* 41:1130-1140, 1993.
5. Van Der Horst ML, Sykula J, Lingley K: The constipation quandary, *Can Nurse* 90(1):25-30, 1994.
6. Wald, A: Constipation in elderly patients: pathogenesis and management, *Drugs and Aging* 3(3):220-231, 1993.
7. Towers AL et al: Constipation in the elderly: influence of dietary, psychological and physiological factors, *JAGS* 42:701-706, 1994.
8. Monane M et al: Anticholinergic drug use and bowel function in nursing home patients, *Arch Intern Med* 153(5):633-638, 1993.
9. Heymen S, Wexner SD, Gulledge AD: MMPI assessment of patients with functional bowel disorders, *Dis Colon Rectum* 36:593-596, 1993.
10. Marshall JB: Chronic constipation in adults: how far should evaluation and treatment go? *Postgrad Med* 88:49-60, 1990.
11. Heine JA, Wong WD, Goldberg SM: Surgical treatment for constipation, *Surg Gynecol Obstet* 176:403-409, 1993.
12. Pemberton JH: Evaluation and surgical treatment of severe chronic constipation, *Ann Surg* 214(4):403-413, 1991.

13. Passmore AP et al: Chronic constipation in long stay elderly patients: a comparison of lactulose and a senna-fibre combination, *Brit Med J* 307:769-771, 1991.

14. Castle SC et al: Constipation prevention: empiric use of stool softeners questioned, *Geriatrics* 46(11):84-86, 1991.

15. Korzets A et al: Life-threatening hyperphosphatemia and hypocalcemic tetany following the use of Fleet enemas, *JAGS* 40:620-621, 1992.

16. Goldstein MK et al: Fecal incontinence in an elderly man: Stanford University Geriatrics Case Conference, *J Am Geriatr Soc* 37:991-1002, 1989.

PRETEST ANSWERS
1. a
2. d
3. d

POSTTEST ANSWERS
1. d
2. c
3. a

CHAPTER 41

Hypertension

DARLYNE MENSCER

OBJECTIVES

Upon completion of this chapter, the reader will be able to:

1. Define hypertension and outline its prevalence and role as a risk factor in cardiovascular disease.

2. Discuss the pathophysiology of hypertension.

3. Describe the appropriate evaluation of the elderly patient with hypertension.

4. Discuss the evidence that treating hypertension, both systolic and diastolic, is beneficial in the elderly.

5. Discuss pharmacological and nonpharmacological therapies for hypertension, including the tailoring of drugs to concomitant disease, where present.

PRETEST

1. The prevalence of hypertension in the elderly is approximately:
   a. 5% to 10%
   b. 20% to 25%
   c. 50% to 60%
   d. 70% to 80%
2. The most common change in the blood vessels of elderly patients with hypertension is:
   a. Increased peripheral vascular resistance
   b. Decreased peripheral vascular resistance
   c. Increased response to β-adrenergic stimulation
   d. Increased response to the renin-angiotensin system
3. What change in the structure of the heart, caused by hypertension, can be reversed by some drug therapies?
   a. Aortic valve diameter
   b. Mitral valve diameter
   c. Right ventricular hypertrophy
   d. Left ventricular hypertrophy

Hypertension is one of the most common medical diagnoses in persons over the age of 60. Even though the disease is common, it is important to apply the label "hypertension" carefully because not every elevated blood pressure reading deserves this name. The implications for the patient are considerable, including the fear of heart disease and stroke and the need to consider life-style changes, such as restricting dietary sodium and taking medication regularly. Choosing appropriate medication and deciding how aggressively to treat the patient require considerable clinical judgment from the primary care provider. Older individuals are frequently undertreated *and* overtreated for this condition.

▼ FRANCES LONG (Part I)

Mrs. Frances Long is a 70-year-old white woman who visits you regularly for treatment of type II diabetes mellitus for which she takes insulin. She is 5 ft 9 in tall, and weight and blood pressure readings for her last three office visits were:

6 months ago: 190 lb, 170/70 mm Hg
3 months ago: 192 lb, 175/74 mm Hg
Today: 194 lb, 180/78 mm Hg

Her blood pressure is 175/80 mm Hg after she has been standing for 2 minutes. She denies chest pain, shortness of breath, or claudication. She does not smoke or drink alcohol.

▼ PHILIP GARVIN (Part I)

Mr. Philip Garvin is a 78-year-old black man with a long history of hypertension. He had a heart attack 3 months ago. Since discharge from the hospital, he has been taking these medications: furosemide (Lasix), 40 mg/day; metoprolol (Lopressor), 25 mg twice daily; and nifedipine (Procardia XL), 30 mg/day. He is 6 ft tall, and weight and blood pressure readings for his last three office visits were:

2 months ago: 190 lb, 140/90 mm Hg

1 month ago: 195 lb, 145/95 mm Hg
Today: 198 lb, 150/100 mm Hg

His blood pressure is essentially the same when measured after 2 minutes of standing. He reports that he is a little tired and somewhat short of breath. He has not had any chest pain. Although he quit smoking after his heart attack, he had been a pack-a-day smoker for 60 years.

STUDY QUESTION

■ *What should be specifically sought on physical examination of these two individuals?*

PREVALENCE

Estimations of the prevalence of hypertension differ somewhat because the definition of hypertension is not the same in every study. The Third National Health and Nutrition Examination Survey in the USA, completed in 1991, showed that hypertension was present in 54% of all persons aged 65 to 74.[1] The prevalence is even higher in black populations.

DEFINITION

With the publication of the fifth Joint National Commission report in 1993, the definition of hypertension became: diastolic blood pressure readings of at least 90 and systolic readings of greater than 140, for all ages.[2] Since blood pressure readings are quite variable in the elderly, multiple readings at more than one visit should be taken. Each reading should be taken with the patient seated and after at least 5 minutes of rest. Systolic blood pressures normally rise with age, whereas diastolic blood pressures usually peak between the ages of 55 and 60. In the Systolic Hypertension in the Elderly Program (SHEP) study,[3] systolic hypertension was defined as greater than 160 mm Hg, and this number is now often considered the highest "normal" blood pressure of elderly persons.

Systolic values between 140 and 160 are at least borderline, however, and probably warrant treatment in patients under age 85. Data on extremely old patients are inconclusive.

MEASUREMENT

Measurement of blood pressure should always be performed with a cuff that is large enough to cover at least one third of the patient's upper arm. In the elderly, rigid blood vessels that remain palpable after the cuff has been inflated above the true systolic pressure can cause overestimation of the blood pressure. It is reasonable to check to ensure that in persons with very high blood pressure readings and no signs of target organ damage the brachial and radial arteries are not still palpable when the cuff pressure exceeds systolic pressure (Osler's maneuver). Recent reports indicate that this maneuver may not be reliable and suggest that electronic oscillometric devices may be used to provide readings closer to intraarterial levels without requiring an invasive procedure.[4] It may also be important to check blood pressure readings measured in the patient's home or in a setting other than the physician's office, since these readings may be lower and correlate better with the actual blood pressure.

> *First get a reliable set of blood pressure readings, preferably away from the physician's office*

Hypertension is not feared for itself, but for its consequences, especially its role in the development of heart disease, stroke, and kidney failure. Although the relative risk of cardiovascular disease conferred by a particular level of elevated blood pressure is greater in younger and middle-aged persons than in the elderly, the absolute risk of cardiovascular disease is actually greater in older persons. Not only is an increasing blood pressure level related to an increasing risk of cardiovascular disease of all types in the elderly, but there is some evidence that increased systolic blood pressure is related to mortality from all causes.[3,5] Although this observation may be an association rather than a direct cause-and-effect relationship, it does confirm that although elevated blood pressure may be common in the elderly, it should not be considered benign. The evidence that treating hypertension improves the morbidity and mortality of older persons is discussed later.

ETIOLOGY

Separating normal aging phenomena from changes associated with hypertension is difficult. The elasticity of blood vessels normally decreases with increasing age, and atherosclerosis hastens this process. Less compliant arter-ies result in increased peripheral vascular resistance. With age, blood vessels also become less responsive to β-adrenergic stimulation, which ordinarily would lead to vasodilation, so aging blood vessels have increased peripheral resistance. Higher blood pressures accelerate these normal phenomena.

The renin-angiotensin system is unlikely to play a central role in the etiology of hypertension in the elderly. Plasma renin levels decline with age even though plasma volume decreases. Renin response to sodium depletion, diuretic administration, and upright posture declines with age as well. Physiological changes in the elderly that influence development of hypertension are summarized in Box 41-1.

PHYSICAL EXAMINATION

Once the diagnosis of hypertension has been made, the patient should be carefully examined for a significant difference in the pressure measured in each arm and for any evidence of target organ damage. The optic fundi should be examined for hypertensive retinopathy. Bruits should be assessed in the carotid, abdominal, and femoral areas. The heart should be auscultated for murmurs, gallops, and extrasystoles. The lungs should be examined for evidence of congestive heart failure. The abdomen should be palpated for evidence of passive congestion of the liver and aneurysmic dilation of the abdominal aorta. The extremities should be examined for evidence of edema and the quality of the peripheral pulses. In addition to noting these specific positive and negative findings, it is important to obtain a complete history and physical examination, since the treatment of hypertension requires an understanding of the total patient and the consideration of any concomitant disease.

BOX 41-1
Physiological Changes Influencing the Development of Hypertension in the Elderly

Reduced cardiac output and myocardial reserve
Left ventricular hypertrophy
Reduced aortic elasticity and baroreceptor sensitivity
Increased susceptibility to orthostatic hypotension
Increased peripheral vascular resistance and atherosclerosis
Reduced intravascular volume and plasma renin activity
Reduced regional blood flow
Reduced renal and hepatic reserve
Increased salt sensitivity
Increased plasma catecholamine levels with decreased β-adrenergic responsiveness

Burris, James F: *Am Fam Physician* 44(1):139, 1991.

▼ FRANCES LONG (Part II)

On physical examination Mrs. Long has a cataract obscuring the view of one eye, but normal vessels can be seen in the other. She has a somewhat diminished carotid upstroke on the left with a soft bruit. The lung fields are clear, and the heart examination is only significant for an S_4. The abdominal examination is benign. She has 2+ dorsalis pedis pulses and no peripheral edema.

▼ PHILIP GARVIN (Part II)

On physical examination Mr. Garvin has moderate arteriovenous nicking in the fundi. The carotid arteries have normal upstrokes. He has bibasilar rales, and the heart examination is significant for an occasional irregular beat and a soft systolic murmur heard best in the aortic area. The liver is slightly enlarged, and he has 2+ peripheral edema. His peripheral pulses are only barely palpable.

STUDY QUESTION

■ What laboratory and other investigations are appropriate in these cases?

INVESTIGATION

The laboratory workup of the elderly patient with hypertension is controversial. Many physicians think that a complete blood count, a battery of blood chemistries, an ECG, and a chest x-ray examination are essential, although not all have been shown to be cost effective. As a minimum, electrolytes, creatinine, and hematocrit are needed. It would be useful to have an inexpensive method of determining left ventricular hypertrophy (LVH), since therapies that can reverse this process may be helpful to the patient.[6] An echocardiogram is a more accurate method of making this diagnosis than an ECG and chest x-ray, but it is more expensive. In the future it may become a standard part of the initial workup of an elderly patient with hypertension.

In addition to evaluating hypertension thoroughly, it is appropriate to evaluate the patient for other cardiovascular risk factors. The presence of hyperlipidemia in the elderly in the absence of coronary artery, peripheral vascular, or cerebrovascular disease has uncertain significance. It is not clear that treating hyperlipidemia is helpful at all in persons over the age of 70, even if target organ damage exists. The presence of hyperlipidemia, however, may result in the decision to treat a borderline blood pressure that might otherwise be only observed.

▼ FRANCES LONG (Part III)

Mrs. Long has a hematocrit of 45%, sodium of 138 mmol/L, potassium of 4.0 mEq/L, creatinine of 1.2 mg/dl, and glucose of 257 mg/dl. The electrocardiogram shows some nonspecific ST and T wave changes in the lateral leads. Her chest x-ray shows clear lung fields, some calcium in the aortic arch, and a normal-sized heart.

▼ PHILIP GARVIN (Part III)

Mr. Garvin has a hematocrit of 35%, sodium of 140 mmol/L, potassium of 3.2 mEq/L, creatinine of 2.5 mg/dl, and glucose of 90 mg/dl. His ECG shows an anteroseptal myocardial infarction, unifocal premature ventricular contractions, and diffuse nonspecific ST and T wave changes. His chest x-ray shows moderate cardiomegaly, fluid in the fissures, and small bilateral pleural effusions.

STUDY QUESTION

■ How do these findings influence your management of these cases?

SMOKING AND ALCOHOL

Smoking cessation is helpful to reduce the risk of cardiovascular risk factors at any age and is certainly worth encouraging in the elderly patient with hypertension. Excessive alcohol consumption elevates the blood pressure of all patients, and the elderly should certainly receive advice regarding the need for moderation.

SECONDARY HYPERTENSION

Secondary causes of hypertension, other than renal artery stenosis, are rare in the elderly. The indications for a workup for secondary hypertension include the following:

■ Sudden onset of diastolic blood pressure (BP) >105 in a person known to be normotensive before
■ Diastolic BP >100 on rational three-drug therapy
■ Accelerated hypertension (rapid worsening) in a previously known hypertensive
■ Presence of spontaneous hypokalemia (without drug therapy)
■ Symptoms suggestive of pheochromocytoma[7]

Even when renal artery stenosis is present, angioplasty or surgical therapy is not indicated unless the blood pressure cannot be controlled by a rational three-drug regimen or there is rapid deterioration in renal function. Even successful treatment of renal artery stenosis is likely to require the continuation of antihypertensive drugs, so neither the patient nor the physician should view this condition as a cause of reversible hypertension.

▼ FRANCES LONG (Part IV)

Mrs. Long asks if it is recommended that she begin to take medication for her blood pressure.

▼ *PHILIP GARVIN (Part IV)*
Mr. Garvin asks why his blood pressure is going up when he is taking all of his medicines.

STUDY QUESTION

■ *What will your prescription for each of these patients be?*

TREATMENT

The evidence that treating hypertension in the elderly is effective in lowering morbidity and mortality is relatively new. Table 41-1 presents the features of six trials involving treating hypertension in the elderly that were published from the mid-1980s to early 1990s.[3,5,8-11] Most studies included patients who had both diastolic and systolic hypertension, but the SHEP study patients had systolic hypertension only.[3] All studies except the Australian one [8] showed a significant decrease in stroke events for treated patients. Only the SHEP study showed a significant decrease in coronary disease and all cardiovascular mortality in treated patients. However, because the SHEP study screened 450,000 persons to obtain fewer than 5000 participants, it is not certain that these data are representative of most patients over 70. Nevertheless, it is reassuring to see that even these very functional, otherwise healthy patients did benefit from medication to lower their blood pressure when only their systolic blood pressure was elevated.

There is reason to be especially cautious in treating very elderly hypertensive patients, however. In the European Working Party Study,[5] those over the age of 80 experienced a mild negative effect with drug treatment. Most experienced health care providers have seen elderly patients who did not function as well when their blood pressure was lowered. Separating the effects of particular medications from the effect of blood pressure lowering itself is difficult, of course, but Table 41-2 shows factors that may contribute to increased risk in treating elderly patients with medications.[12]

One of the most controversial issues in treating hypertension in the elderly is whether there is a diastolic blood pressure—usually said to be about 85 mm HG—below which coronary perfusion is compromised and therefore patients have increased rather than decreased cardiovascular complications. Most studies fail to demonstrate this "J curve" phenomenon, but careful monitoring of patients known to have coronary artery disease seems prudent.

▼ *FRANCES LONG (Part V)*
You counsel Mrs. Long that she is at least 20 lb over her ideal body weight and that losing these extra pounds will probably make her diabetes easier to control. You note that weight loss will be easier if she also exercises and suggest that she begins walking for at least half an hour three times a week at a pace that does not leave her winded. You warn her that if decreasing her calories and exercising give her symptoms of hypoglycemia, she should monitor her blood sugar level and call your office for an adjustment in her insulin dose. You also suggest that she restrict the sodium in her diet to no more than 4 g daily. In addition to giving Mrs. Long handouts on a 1500 calorie diet and low-sodium foods, you schedule an appointment for her with the dietitian next week.

▼ *PHILIP GARVIN (Part V)*
You advise Mr. Garvin that his blood pressure may be rising because his weight is increasing, and you tell him that some of his weight gain is caused by congestive heart failure. Therefore, although medication changes may be needed, he will need to restrict the sodium in his diet. In addition to giving him handouts on a 4 g sodium diet, you schedule an appointment with the dietitian for him as soon as his wife (who cooks for him) can be present.

Although the usefulness of treating hypertension in the elderly is still being studied, most people with hypertension will want some form of treatment if there are possible benefits and if the treatment is not too expensive or the side effects too bothersome. As with many other chronic medical conditions, hypertension is best initially treated with dietary and life-style changes that should continue even if drug therapy is also needed.

Weight

Elderly patients with hypertension who are overweight should be encouraged to lose to within 15% of their ideal body weight.[13] However, some studies have shown benefit in reducing blood pressure if overweight patients lose only 15 to 20 lb, even if this does not lower their total weight to anywhere close to ideal body weight.[14] Counseling elderly patients to make dietary modifications often requires more understanding of their social situation than similar recommendations in other age groups. Elderly patients are more likely to be eating in group living situations where they do not prepare their own meals; they are also likely to have limited financial resources to purchase fresh foods, which usually have fewer calories and less sodium than packaged or processed foods. When counseling elderly patients to lose weight, it is also important to remember that older persons' ideas of the size they should be may be pounds heavier than what the ideal body weight charts suggest is best. In many cultures, particularly Afro-American and Hispanic, thinness is not considered healthy. Indeed, patients and their families or friends may associate weight loss with diseases such as cancer. Therefore it is important that the amount of weight loss that is "prescribed" be negotiated with the patient.

Table 41-1   Features of Six Trials of Hypertension in the Elderly

	Australian	EWPHE	Coope and Warrender	STOP-Hypertension	MRC	SHEP
No. of patients	582	840	884	1627	4396	4736
Age range (years)	60-69	60-97	60-79	70-84	65-74	70-≥80
BP entry criteria						
Systolic	<200	160-239	190-230	180-230 or <180	160-209	160-219
Diastolic	95-109	90-119	105-120	90-120 or 105-120	<115	<90
Mean blood pressure at entry	165/100	182/101	197/100	195/102	185/91 (43% ISH)	170/77 (100% ISH)
BP goal						
Systolic	—	—	<170	<160	<160/<150*	<160/↓20*
Diastolic	<90/<80†	<90	<105	95	—	—
Treatment						
Initial	Chlorthalidone	Hydrochlorothiazide/triamterene	Atenolol	Hydrochlorothiazide/amiloride, or atenolol, or metoprolol, or pindolol	Hydrochlorothiazide/amiloride, or atenolol	Chlorthalidone
Add on	Various	Methyldopa	Bendrofluazide Methyldopa	Atenolol or metoprolol or pindolol Hydrochlorothiazide	Atenolol, or hydrochlorothiazide/amiloride	Atenolol
BP obtained						
Treatment group	143/87	149/85	162/77	167/87	152/79	—
Placebo group	155/94	172/94	180/88	186/96	167/85	—
Events per 1000 patient years (treated versus placebo)/relative risk						
Stroke	0.67	0.64‡	0.58‡	0.53‡	0.75‡	0.67‡
Coronary disease	0.82	0.80	1.03	0.87§	0.81§	0.73‡
Congestive failure	—	0.78	0.68	0.49‡	—	0.45‡
All cardiovascular	0.69	0.71‡	0.76‡	0.60‡	0.83‡	0.68‡

From Kaplan NM: *Am J Med Sci* 305(3):190, 1993.
ISH, Isolated systolic hypertension.
*Depending on entry systolic pressure.
†Initial goal <90 mm Hg, reduced to <80 mm Hg after 2 years.
‡Statistically significant.
§Myocardial infarction only.

Table 41-2 Factors That Might Contribute to Increased Risk from Pharmacological Treatment of Hypertension in the Elderly

Factors	Potential Complications
Diminished baroreceptor activity	Orthostatic hypotension
Impaired cerebral autoregulation	Cerebral ischemia with small falls in systemic pressure
Decreased intravascular volume	Orthostatic hypotension Volume deficiency Hyponatremia
Sensitivity to hypokalemia	Arrhythmia, muscular weakness
Decreased renal and hepatic function	Drug accumulation
Polypharmacy	Drug interaction
Central nervous system changes	Depression, confusion

From Kaplan M: *Am J Med Sci* 305(3):189, 1993.

Exercise

Most patients will find it easier to lose weight if they also engage in some form of exercise. Consider the patient's total medical condition, including any musculoskeletal and visual limitations, as well as cardiovascular risk factors, before an exercise prescription is given. Walking is usually a safe activity for elderly patients, but in those with significant arthritis or other orthopedic limitations in the lower extremities, swimming or an indoor skiing machine may be better choices.

> *Weight loss is good for the overweight, and exercise is good for everyone, but sodium restriction is to be used with care. Not all patients need it, and it may compromise some patients' nutrition.*

Sodium Restriction

In addition to losing weight, sodium restriction is often recommended to lower blood pressure in hypertensive patients of all ages. Studies have shown that limiting sodium in the diet is at least as effective in the elderly as in younger patients.[13] The amount of sodium that has been permitted in the diets of the study groups has usually been about 1.5 to 2.5 g per day. Diets containing less than 4 to 6 g of sodium can be unpalatable and may result in a decline in the patient's overall nutritional status. The use of salt substitutes containing potassium in patients with normal renal function can improve the taste of food. Several studies have even shown a hypotensive effect of potassium supplementation in hypertensive (but not in normotensive) patients.

BOX 41-2
Nonpharmacological Treatment of Hypertension in Elderly Patients

> Sodium restriction to 4 g/day
> Weight reduction (even 15-20 lb)
> Moderate exercise program
> Reduction in alcohol consumption to less than two drinks a day
> Cessation of smoking

In many patients both weight loss and sodium restriction are appropriate recommendations and can be expected to have additive benefits. It may be helpful to enlist the help of the spouse and a dietitian in an individual or group setting to give assistance with these often difficult life-style adjustments. Scheduling follow-up office visits to assess the effectiveness of these nonpharmacological interventions is important. If the provider gives less attention to weight loss and sodium restriction than to compliance with medications, the patient will do the same.

Summary recommendations regarding the nonpharmacological treatment of hypertension are given in Box 41-2.

▼ FRANCES LONG (Part VI)

You advise Mrs. Long that you do not want to suggest any medication to control her blood pressure until the effects of weight reduction and salt restriction can be assessed. You schedule visits every 2 months for the next 6 months so that her progress can be monitored.

▼ PHILIP GARVIN (Part VI)

You advise Mr. Garvin that two of his medications, metoprolol and nifedipine, could be making his heart pump less efficiently, allowing fluid to build up in his lungs, liver, and feet. Because he has had a heart attack, you suggest that metoprolol be continued for now. However, you do discontinue nifedipine, because it can cause peripheral edema and can reduce cardiac function. Because he is in congestive heart failure, you suggest beginning captopril (Capoten) in low doses. You advise him that there is a chance that his kidney function may decrease on this medication and that you will want to recheck his creatinine and electrolytes within 1 week. Because the first dose of an angiotensin-converting enzyme (ACE) inhibitor can lower blood pressure in a person who is sodium depleted from a diuretic, you tell Mr. Garvin to discontinue his diuretic for 24 hours before starting the lowest dose of captopril—6.25 mg—at bedtime.

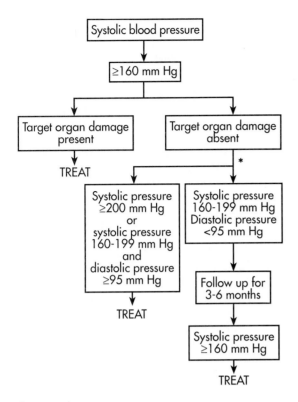

*Repeated measurements.

FIG. 41-1   Thresholds and factors in drug treatment of hypertension. (From Sever P et al: *Br Med J* 306:985, 1993.)

Drug Therapy

Even when diet and life-style changes have been incorporated into the regimen, some patients will still have blood pressures in a range that warrants drug therapy. Fig. 41-1 shows an algorithm, based on repeated blood pressure measurements, that suggests how to decide whether to start drug therapy.[15]

Orthostatic Blood Pressures

Before any antihypertensive agent is chosen for an elderly patient, it is important to measure blood pressure not only sitting but also after 1 to 2 minutes in the standing position (orthostatic blood pressures). If systolic blood pressure drops as much as 20 mm Hg, the patient may already have a dizzy feeling on initially changing position. Even if the patient has no symptoms, medications that tend to increase the orthostatic drop will increase the patient's instability and tendency to fall. Some patients notice similar symptoms within 30 to 45 minutes after eating a meal (postprandial hypotension), although the drop in blood pressure is usually only 10 to 15 mm Hg systolic. Those who experience postprandial hypotension tend to be older. Eating smaller meals at more frequent intervals may improve this symptom.

Always take an elderly patient's blood pressure sitting or lying and standing: even without medications, orthostasis must be sought.

Diuretics

Most clinical trials of drug therapy for hypertension in the elderly have included thiazide diuretics or their equivalents. These drugs have been shown to be effective in lowering both systolic and diastolic blood pressures. Diuretics can be taken only once daily and generally are quite inexpensive. However, their role as first-line therapy has been questioned because of concerns over whether their metabolic side effects may compromise their clearly demonstrated efficacy in lowering overall cardiovascular morbidity and mortality.

Thiazide diuretics may cause hypokalemia, especially in persons who do not limit their sodium intake. Hypokalemia is associated with a higher incidence of cardiac dysrhythmias, especially in men who have an abnormal electrocardiogram before treatment. For at least the first few months of therapy, thiazide diuretics may have an adverse effect on lipid metabolism. With continued treatment, however, this effect may not continue, so the overall effect on blood lipids may not be truly significant. Because of these concerns, however, thiazide diuretics may not be the best for persons with significant lipid abnormalities or an abnormal ECG unless they are expected to be compliant with monitoring potassium. Even if a diuretic is not chosen initially, many patients who require two or more drugs to control their blood pressure will need a diuretic because of the fluid retentive effects of the other medications. This is especially true in Afro-American patients. Thiazide diuretics are effective only when the patient's creatinine clearance is above 30 mL/min. Loop diuretics are needed at lower levels of creatinine clearance. A formula for computing creatinine clearance is as follows[16]:

$$\text{Creatinine clearance (ml/min)} = \frac{140 - \text{age (yr)} \times \text{weight (kg)}}{72 \times \text{serum creatinine (mg/dl)}} \times \begin{pmatrix} 0.85 \\ \text{for women} \end{pmatrix}$$

β-Blockers

β-Blockers have been available for the treatment of hypertension for over 20 years. Although there are theoretical physiological reasons why these drugs may not be ideal antihypertensive agents for the elderly, two large randomized trials comparing a β-blocker with a diuretic as initial therapy of hypertension in the elderly have shown that the β-blocker and the diuretic were equivalent in efficacy and in rates of side effects.[17,18]

β-Blockers do increase peripheral vascular resistance, a phenomenon that already occurs with normal aging,

Table 41-3   Characteristics of Antihypertensive Drugs

Drug Class	Effect on Potassium	Effect on Lipids	Effect on Peripheral Resistance	Effect on LVH	Expense of Cheapest Agent	Especially Useful in These Disorders	Consider Avoiding in the Following Disorders
Diuretics	↓	Negative	↓	0/↓	$	CHF	Potassium-sensitive dysrhythmia, sexual dysfunction, gout, hypercholesterolemia, diabetes mellitus
β-Blockers	0	Negative	↑	0/↓	$$	Angina, post-MI, migraine, anxiety	Sexual dysfunction, diabetes mellitus, depression, asthma/COPD, peripheral vascular disease, CHF/conduction abnormality, hypercholesterolemia
Calcium channel blockers	0	0	↓	↓	$$$	Angina	CHF, AV conduction defects (some agents)
ACE inhibitors	↑	0	↓	↓	$$$	Diabetes mellitus, CHF, post-MI	Renal artery stenosis
Peripheral α-blockers	0	Positive	↓	↓	$$	Prostatic outlet obstruction, hyperlipidemia	Postural hypotension
Vasodilators	0	0	↓	—	$$		Angina, postural hypotension
Central agents	0	Positive	↓	↓	$		Sexual dysfunction, depression

so these drugs may precipitate or worsen the symptoms of claudication in patients with peripheral vascular disease. They have a negative inotropic effect and tend to suppress atrioventricular node function; therefore they should be used carefully in elderly patients with poor cardiac output or conduction abnormalities. For persons who have survived a myocardial infarction, β-blockers have been shown to improve life expectancy. Thus they are probably the best agent to choose to treat hypertension after myocardial infarction, even though their long-term effect on blood lipids, especially high-density lipoproteins, may not be favorable.

β-Blockers may cause central nervous system side effects, including depression, forgetfulness, and nightmares. These side effects may be misinterpreted by an elderly patient as effects of old age, and the patient may not report them unless the provider specifically inquires. Fatigue may also be a side effect that is similarly misunderstood. These side effects may adversely affect the quality of the patient's life and may necessitate another choice of drug or a trial without medication.

Calcium Channel Blockers

Calcium channel blockers decrease peripheral vascular resistance and therefore are theoretically ideal antihypertensive agents in the elderly. Recent data comparing the use of verapamil and the β-blocker atenolol in a small number of persons over the age of 60 demonstrated that verapamil reduced left ventricular mass and lowered blood pressure, whereas atenolol did not.[19] β-Blockers with intrinsic sympathomimetic effects may decrease left ventricular hypertrophy, however. Because calcium channel blockers have no adverse effects on serum lipids and are less likely than β-blockers to cause fatigue, they are generally well tolerated. Some preparations of calcium channel blockers are available in sustained release formulations, which can be taken once a day.

Calcium channel blockers do have side effects that are important for some patients. Verapamil can cause cardiac conduction defects and may impair myocardial contractility. Nifedipine may cause peripheral edema. Headache may occur somewhat more frequently than with β-blockers, possibly because these drugs are vasodilators. All calcium channel blockers are at least moderately expensive in comparison with other antihypertensive agents.

ACE Inhibitors

Since older individuals generally have low renin activity, angiotensin-converting enzyme (ACE) inhibitors are theoretically not the most appropriate drugs. However, possibly because of effects on kinins and prostaglandins,

ACE inhibitors are known to lower blood pressure in some patients who do not have elevated renin values. In one large descriptive study[20] of the use of captopril in elderly patients with hypertension, the drug did reduce blood pressure, but only 15% of the cases were controlled long-term with captopril alone. There are not yet any large studies available comparing captopril or any other ACE inhibitor with other classes of antihypertensive drugs in the elderly. However, in younger age groups, ACE inhibitors have been shown to reduce left ventricular hypertrophy.[21]

ACE inhibitors can increase the serum creatinine level, particularly in patients who are also receiving diuretics. In patients with renal artery stenosis, ACE inhibitors can even cause renal failure. However, ACE inhibitors improve intrarenal blood flow and decrease proteinuria in patients with diabetes mellitus. ACE inhibitors have been shown to prolong life in patients with congestive heart failure (CHF) by improving overall cardiac function. ACE inhibitors have recently been approved for use in post–myocardial infarction (MI) patients, even if CHF is not clinically present. Especially in elderly patients who would also benefit from one of these indications, ACE inhibitors could be an excellent choice for antihypertensive therapy. All the agents in this category are relatively expensive. Some ACE inhibitors have a long enough duration of action to be used once a day.

> *ACE inhibitors improve overall cardiac function and extend life in those with CHF.*

Vasodilators and Peripheral α-Blockers

Vasodilators such as hydralazine directly lower peripheral vascular resistance and are therefore theoretically excellent agents to treat hypertension in the elderly. Reflex tachycardia may occur and precipitate angina, although this happens less often in the elderly than in younger patients. Agents that have α-adrenergic blocking activity, such as terazosin and labetalol, also lower peripheral vascular resistance and are effective in lowering both systolic and diastolic blood pressure in the elderly according to several small studies.[22,23] α-Blocking agents decrease symptoms of prostatic outlet obstruction and may be useful for men with hypertension who also have this problem. Peripheral α-blocking agents reduce left ventricular hypertrophy, but there are very little data on vasodilators.

Both vasodilators and peripheral α-adrenergic blocking agents can cause postural hypotension and are there-

---

BOX 41-3
Guidelines in Treating Hypertension in the Elderly

1. Check for postural and postprandial hypotension before starting.
2. Choose drugs that will help concomitant conditions.
3. Start with small doses, titrating gradually.
4. Use longer acting, once daily formulations.
5. Avoid drug interactions, particularly from over-the-counter medications, e.g., nonsteroidal antiinflammatory drugs.
6. Look for subtle drug-induced adverse effects, e.g., weakness, dizziness, depression, confusion.
7. Monitor home blood pressures to avoid over and under treatment.
8. Aim for the goal of systolic BP = 140-145, diastolic = 80-85.

From Kaplan M: *Am J Med Sci* 305(3):194, 1993.

---

fore unlikely to be appropriate choices for patients who have a pretreatment drop of 15 mm Hg or more in their systolic pressure on standing. Hydralazine is relatively inexpensive, however, and may be a good choice if it can be tolerated.

Central Adrenergic Inhibitors

Central adrenergic inhibitors lower peripheral vascular resistance and are effective in treating hypertension in the elderly. This class of agents does reduce left ventricular hypertrophy. However, in many elderly patients, sedation is a limiting side effect. Reserpine may also cause depression if given in high doses or nasal stuffiness in lower therapeutic doses. If it can be tolerated, reserpine can be helpful because it is the least expensive antihypertensive drug available in any class and is taken only once a day. A summary of pharmacological agents useful in the treatment of hypertension in elderly persons is given in Table 41-3. Summary recommendations regarding treatment of hypertension in the elderly are given in Box 41-3.[12]

It is important to discuss thoroughly the potential benefits and side effects of any therapy with the patient before any course is recommended. It is the responsibility of the primary care provider to be sure that the patient does not reject potentially helpful therapies out of fear or misunderstanding. As with all chronic conditions that affect the elderly, the appropriate treatment of hypertension requires considering the patient as a whole.

POSTTEST

1. Mr. S is a 72-year-old white man who has a long history of chronic obstructive pulmonary disease and now requires pharmacological therapy for hypertension. The class of drugs that should be avoided when choosing an agent for him is:
   a. Central adrenergic inhibitors
   b. β-Blockers
   c. Calcium channel blockers
   d. ACE inhibitors
   e. Diuretics

2. Mrs. M is an 82-year-old black woman who has had hypertension for many years. Recently she has developed congestive heart failure. The class of drugs that would be best for her antihypertensive therapy now is:
   a. Central adrenergic inhibitors
   b. β-Blocker

   c. ACE inhibitors
   d. Calcium channel blockers

3. Mr. M is a 70-year-old white man who has had hypertension for years and now has left ventricular hypertrophy noted on an echocardiogram. He is a retired physician and is worried about this finding. He wants to be treated with a drug that may reverse this condition. An agent from which of the following classes is most likely to be beneficial?
   a. β-Blockers
   b. Diuretics
   c. Calcium channel blockers
   d. Vasodilators

REFERENCES

1. National Health and Nutrition Examination Survey (NHANES III), 1988-1991. In The fifth report of the Joint National Committee on Detection, Evaluation, and Treatment of High Blood Pressure, *Arch Intern Med* 153:154-183, 1993.

2. Joint National Committee on Detection, Evaluation, and Treatment of High Blood Pressure. In The fifth report of the Joint National Committee on Detection, Evaluation and Treatment of High Blood Pressure, *Arch Intern Med* 153:154-183, 1993.

3. SHEP Cooperative Research Group: Prevention of stroke by antihypertensive drug treatment in older persons with isolated systolic hypertension: final results of the Systolic Hypertension in the Elderly Program (SHEP), *JAMA* 265:3255-3264, 1991.

4. Kaplan NM: Southwestern Internal Medicine Conference: the promises and perils of treating the elderly hypertensive, *Am J Med Sci* 305(3):183-197, 1993.

5. Amery A et al: Mortality and morbidity results from the European Working Party on high blood pressure in the elderly trial, *Lancet* 2:1349-1354, 1985.

6. Pfeffer MA, Pfeffer JM: Reversing cardiac hypertrophy in hypertension, *N Engl J Med* 322:1388-1389, 1990.

7. Applegate WB: Hypertension in elderly patients, *Ann Intern Med* 110:908, 1989.

8. Management Committee of the Australian Therapeutic Trials in Mild Hypertension: the Australian Therapeutic Trial, *Lancet* 2:1261-1267, 1980.

9. Coope J, Warrender TS: Randomized trial of treatment of hypertension in elderly patients in primary care, *Br Med J* 293:1145-1151, 1986.

10. Dahlof B et al: Morbidity and mortality in the Swedish Trial in old patients with hypertension (STOP-Hypertension), *Lancet* 338:1281-1285, 1991.

11. MRC Working Party: Medical Research Council trial of treatment of hypertension in older adults: principal results, *Br Med J* 304:405-412, 1992.

12. Kaplan N: Southwest Internal Medical Conference: the promises and perils of treating the elderly hypertensive, *Am J Med Sci* 305(3):194, 1993.

13. Kumanyika K: Weight reduction and sodium restriction in the management of hypertension, *Clin Geriatr Med* 5:770, 1989.

14. Kaplan N: Non-drug treatment of hypertension, *Ann Intern Med* 102:361, 1985.

15. Sever P et al: Management guidelines in essential hypertension: report of the second working party of the British Hypertension Society, *Br Med J* 306:983-987, 1993.

16. Weder, Alan B: The renally compromised older hypertensive: therapeutic considerations, *Geriatrics* 46(2):43, 1991.

17. Andersen GS: Atenolol vs bendroflumethiazide in middle aged and elderly hypertensives, *Acta Med Scand* 218:165-172, 1985.

18. Wikstrand J et al: Antihypertensive treatment with metoprolol or hydrochlorothiazide in patients aged 60-75 years, *JAMA* 255:1304-1310, 1986.

19. Schulman P et al: The effects of antihypertensive therapy on left ventricular mass in elderly patients, *N Engl J Med* 322:1350-1356, 1990.

20. Jenkins AC, Knill JR, Presilinski GR: Captopril in the treatment of elderly hypertensive patients, *Arch Intern Med* 145:2020-2031, 1995.

21. Graettinger WF, Weber MA: Left ventricular hypertrophy and antihypertensive therapy, *Am Fam Physician* 46(2):483-491, August 1992.

22. Buell JC et al: Hemodynamic effects of labetolol in young and older hypertensives, *J Clin Pharmacol* 28:327-331, 1988.

23. Abernathy DR, Bartos P, Plachetka JR: Labetolol in the treatment of hypertension in elderly and younger patients, *J Clin Pharmacol* 27:902-906, 1987.

PRETEST ANSWERS
1. c
2. a
3. d

POSTTEST ANSWERS
1. b
2. c
3. c

CHAPTER 42

Congestive Heart Failure and Dysrhythmias

ROBERT J. LUCHI and GEORGE E. TAFFET

OBJECTIVES

On completion of this chapter, the reader will be able to:

1. Understand how the basic elements of congestive heart failure (CHF) diagnosis, history, physical examination, and chest x-ray examination are altered in the older patient.

2. Appreciate that CHF may be caused by systolic dysfunction or diastolic dysfunction of the heart.

3. Understand the important role of ACE inhibitors in the prevention and treatment of CHF associated with left ventricular systolic dysfunction.

4. Learn the basic approaches to treatment of CHF associated with left ventricular diastolic dysfunction.

5. Understand the importance of controlling ischemia and atrial fibrillation complicating the course of CHF.

PRETEST

1. Atypical manifestations of congestive heart failure in the elderly are most frequently related to reduced perfusion of which of the following?
   a. Brain
   b. Heart
   c. Extremities
   d. Kidneys
   e. Lungs
2. In patients with congestive heart failure, the best indicator of left ventricular systolic function is
   a. Left ventricular ejection fraction
   b. ECG
   c. Chest x-ray examination (CXR)
   d. Distended jugular veins
   e. Atrial fibrillation
3. In patients with congestive heart failure, the angiotensin-converting enzyme inhibitor enalapril is contraindicated when which one of the following is present?
   a. Creatinine clearance 45 ml/min
   b. BUN 32 mg/dl
   c. Blood pressure 105/60
   d. Serum K 5 mEq/L
   e. History of captopril-induced angioedema

Congestive heart failure (CHF) is one of the most common disorders in geriatric practice. Approximately 400,000 new cases occur annually in the United States among all age groups, but the incidence and prevalence of CHF increase dramatically with age—for those over 75 years of age the prevalence approaches 10%. The frequency of CHF has not decreased to any great extent despite improved treatment for hypertension and ischemic heart disease. Survival continues to be poor despite advances in treatment. CHF poses challenges for those taking care of older people because of the difficulty in recognizing atypical symptoms and because of the frequency of age- and disease-related changes that complicate therapeutic strategies.

▼ MARY BURKITT (Part I)

Mrs. Burkitt, an 82-year-old patient of yours, has a past history of myocardial infarction. She comes to your office with dyspnea, fatigue, nocturnal cough, and restless sleep. Vital signs include BP 150/80, P 92 and regular, RR 26/min, T 97°. Positive physical findings related to the cardiovascular system include peripheral edema, increased abdominal girth, jugular venous distention, positive hepatojugular reflux, bilateral basilar rales, S_4, and a 2/6 systolic ejection murmur heard best at the base of the heart. ECG shows a regular sinus rhythm with evidence of an old anterior myocardial infarction. Chest x-ray examination reveals cardiac enlargement, pulmonary venous vascular congestion exemplified by enlarged hila that appear indistinct because of perivascular edema, increased prominence of the pulmonary veins draining the upper lobes ("cephalization of flow"), and moderate right-sided pleural effusion. Hemoglobin and hematocrit are 13 g and 32%, WBC is normal, urinalysis shows 1+ protein. BUN/creatinine are 30 mg/dl and 1.6 mg/dl. Serum albumin is 3.6 g/dl.

STUDY QUESTIONS

- What is the significance of the S_4?
- What one type of drug should be used for initial treatment?
- What further test will guide optimal treatment and why?
- What other precipitating factors should be ruled out?

DEFINITIONS, ETIOLOGY, AND PATHOPHYSIOLOGY

Heart failure is strictly defined as impairment in heart function leading to symptoms such as fatigue and dyspnea because of reduced cardiac output. *Congestive heart failure* represents a more advanced stage of this condition with evidence of fluid retention, manifested clinically by edema and congestion of the veins of the pulmonary and systemic circuits. The focus of this chapter is on congestive heart failure (CHF).

CHF may result from either systolic or diastolic ventricular dysfunction. *Asymptomatic left ventricular systolic dysfunction* frequently progresses to either heart failure or congestive heart failure. This progression can be retarded by the use of angiotensin-converting enzyme (ACE) inhibitors.[1]

CHF in the elderly patient is due to left ventricular systolic dysfunction in 50% to 60% of cases. In the remainder, left ventricular systolic function is normal but evidence of restriction in filling of the ventricles is present.[2] This condition is called left ventricular diastolic dysfunction. Left ventricular systolic function is most conveniently measured by determining the left ventricular ejection fraction (LVEF) either by echo or by radionuclide techniques (MUGA scan). Normal LVEF is generally considered to be 50% or more. Significant left ventricular systolic dysfunction is defined as an LVEF of less than 40%. An equally simple measure of diastolic dysfunction

---

BOX 42-1
Classic and Atypical Manifestations of CHF in the Elderly

Classic	Atypical (nondementia)	Atypical (dementia)
Dyspnea	Chronic cough	No history
Orthopnea	Insomnia	Falls
Paroxysmal nocturnal dyspnea	Weight loss	Anorexia
Peripheral edema	Nausea	Behavioral disturbances
Unexplained weight gain	Nocturia	Decreased functional status
Weakness	Syncope	
Poor exercise tolerance		
Abdominal pain		
Fatigue		

---

is not available clinically. In the absence of significant valvular or pericardial disease, congestive heart failure with an LVEF of 50% or more is primarily due to diastolic dysfunction.

DIAGNOSIS

Diagnosis of heart failure is based on history, physical examination, and chest x-ray.[3] Diagnosis of heart failure in the elderly may be difficult because the history is often atypical (Box 42-1), or unobtainable, or symptoms are minimized or attributable to age. One of the most common atypical presentations is that of delirium. Delirium may or may not be superimposed on a preexisting dementia.

> *JVD, hepatojugular reflex, S₃ gallop, and a good chest x-ray are the best ways to look for and diagnose CHF (lung rales and ankle edema are too nonspecific).*

Physical signs of CHF are often overlooked in the elderly. Jugular venous distention and hepatojugular reflux are excellent signs of "right-sided failure"; S_3 gallop is an excellent sign of heart failure but is often difficult to hear. In contrast, the S_4 is a normal finding in an older patient. Pedal edema is less reliable, especially in immobilized patients who spend all day in their chairs. A good quality chest x-ray may be difficult to obtain, especially in the frail, older patient. Persistence until an adequate film is obtained pays rich diagnostic dividends. Often, performing the x-ray examination with the patient sitting upright in the wheelchair provides a reasonable image. Key findings are an enlarged heart, enlarged hila with indistinct margins (perivascular edema), and prominence of veins draining the upper lobes ("cephalization of flow").

BOX 42-2
Factors that Precipitate CHF

Anemia
Arrhythmias
Exacerbation of chronic obstructive pulmonary disease
Digoxin withdrawal
Drugs: cardiac depressants (e.g., antiarrhythmics, antineoplastics)
Hypoxia
Hyperthyroidism
IV fluid overload*
Infection
Myocardial infarction/ischemics
Dietary or medication noncompliance†
Pulmonary embolism
Renal insufficiency
Sepsis

*Most common precipitating cause in hospitalized patients.
†Most common precipitating cause outside of hospital.

PRECIPITATING FACTORS

Any condition placing extra strain on the cardiovascular system can precipitate heart failure in a patient with heart disease who otherwise would be in a compensated state (Box 42-2). Precipitating factors of particular relevance to the elderly form the mnemonic DAM NIH: *D*rugs, including digitalis withdrawal and administration of NSAIDS; *A*rrhythmias—bradyarrhythmias including heart block and tachyarrhythmias, especially atrial fibrillation; *M*yocardial ischemia, which often presents atypically (consider some form of stress test if suspicion high); *N*oncompliance with diet, fluid restriction, or medications; *I*ntravenous fluid administration; and *H*yperthyroidism (TSH and free T_4 determination should be part of the workup of elderly patients with CHF). In patients for whom exercise testing is not obtainable, a pharmacological stress test such as dipyradimole-thallium (Persantine) can be used.

> Look for precipitants to CHF. Once these are treated, ongoing CHF treatment may not be necessary.

▼ MARY BURKITT (Part II)

Mrs. Burkitt is treated at home with furosemide 10 mg PO daily for 2 days. Furosemide is then increased to 40 mg PO every other day. A 4 g sodium diet is prescribed. She reports significant relief of symptoms with the diuresis. LVEF by echocardiography is 35%; hypokinesis of the apical and inferior wall of the heart is noted. TSH and free T$_4$ are normal. Captopril 12.5 mg PO bid and digoxin 0.125 mg PO daily are started. Blood pressure does not decrease either in the recumbent or upright position. At this point enalapril 10 mg bid is substituted for captopril. The patient eventually tolerates enalapril 10 mg bid without significant effect on renal function, serum K, or blood pressure. Serum digoxin level stabilizes at 1.6 ng/dl.

STUDY QUESTIONS

- Mr. Burkitt is shocked at the cost of the ACE inhibitor. Why is it justified?
- How would you assess renal function in order to guard against digoxin toxicity?

TREATMENT

There are two lines of treatment, one that addresses the underlying heart failure and one that addresses the precipitating factors. Both need to be addressed aggressively.

General Measures

General measures include sodium restriction, appropriate exercise after acute symptoms have been controlled, and control of precipitating factors. Patient education and support groups will help to promote compliance. Prognosis should be discussed openly and completion of advanced directives regarding health care preferences encouraged.

Restriction of dietary sodium intake to 3 or 4 g per day, and omission or reduction in alcohol intake are recommended. Smoking is discouraged. Instruction of the person preparing the patient's food by a dietitian promotes compliance. Mild aerobic exercise, mainly walking or cycling, increases functional capacity and quality of life.

Diuretics

The use of medications in the elderly is complicated by altered pharmacokinetics and by pharmacodynamics resulting from age- and disease-related changes in various organ systems.[3] The goals of treatment are increased quality of life and improved survival. Loop diuretics (furosemide, bumetanide, ethacrynic acid) are used most frequently because glomerular filtration rate (GFR) in the elderly is often less than 30 ml/min, rendering thiazides ineffective. The goal is gentle diuresis, thus avoiding hypotension and its consequences. Equivalent doses of loop diuretics are furosemide 40 mg, bumetanide 1 mg, and ethacrynic acid 50 mg. Whether given orally or intravenously, the first dose of furosemide should not exceed 20 mg because of the danger of an exaggerated "first dose diuresis"; sometimes an effective diuresis can be obtained with an initial furosemide dose of 10 mg. The usual maintenance dose is 40 mg furosemide daily, but doses of 160 mg per day are not unusual. Equivalent doses of bumetanide may be used if a diuretic with a shorter duration of action is desired. Ethacrynic acid is rarely used because of ototoxicity, but it may be of use in patients allergic to furosemide and bumetanide. Major toxic effects of loop diuretics include hypotension, hypokalemia, hyponatremia, and hypomagnesemia. Hypotension can be avoided by monitoring orthostatic blood pressures and BUN/creatinine and by reducing the dose of the loop diuretic at the first sign of volume depletion. Removing the last trace of peripheral edema or pleural effusion may decrease preload to the point at which the patient becomes symptomatic because of poor cardiac output. Serum magnesium and potassium should be measured routinely and replaced as indicated. Magnesium oxide supplements 400 mg 1 to 2 times daily for several days usually suffice to restore magnesium levels. Treatment of hyponatremia depends on the cause: sodium depletion consequent on excessive diuresis calls for reduction in diuretic dose and lessening or omission of sodium restriction; hyponatremia secondary to retention of free water is treated by fluid restriction. Diuretic-related incontinence can be avoided by appropriate timing of diuretic doses or by giving bumetanide, which has a relatively short duration of action. Major drug interactions include other drugs with hypotensive potential and NSAIDS, which by their action on GFR can completely inhibit a brisk loop diuretic–induced diuresis. Potassium-sparing diuretics are most useful in combination with loop diuretics to reduce potassium loss. Their major side effect is hyperkalemia, which can be additive to the hyperkalemia of ACE inhibitors (see below). Another useful combination is the addition of metolazone to a loop diuretic when the patient is resistant to the action of the loop diuretic alone. A 2.5 mg test dose of metolazone is recommended to avoid profound volume depletion.

Subsequently, one may give 5 mg PO 1 hour before administration of the loop diuretic.

> *Diuretics are the most widely used drugs and can be lifesaving, but ACE inhibitors are the drugs that definitely increase survival.*

ACE Inhibitors

In patients with left ventricular systolic dysfunction and heart failure, ACE inhibitors both improve quality of life and increase survival.[4] ACE inhibitors both reduce myocardial oxygen consumption and increase cardiac output by decreasing afterload and reduce pulmonary vascular congestion by decreasing preload. All patients with left ventricular systolic dysfunction characterized by LVEF less than 40% should be given a trial of an ACE inhibitor unless contraindicated. Contraindications to ACE inhibitors include significant renal insufficiency or hyperkalemia, severe hypotension, and previous allergic reaction (angioedema) to any one of the members of this class of drugs. Before beginning ACE inhibitor therapy, one should reduce the dose of commonly administered diuretics and either withhold or reduce the dose of other drugs with hypotensive effects. Hyponatremia (serum sodium level less than 135 mEq/L) and hyperkalemia should also be corrected. Because older people correct hypotension poorly, one should consider beginning ACE inhibitor therapy with a short-acting agent such as captopril (Capoten), using a test dose of either 6.25 mg or 12.5 mg. If no significant hypotension occurs, the dose can then be gradually increased. For older people the maximum doses generally are 25 mg of captopril three times a day, enalapril (Vasotec) 20 mg twice daily, and lisinopril (Prinivil, Zestril) 20 mg once daily. In addition to monitoring orthostatic blood pressures, one must monitor BUN, electrolytes, and creatinine. Small increments in BUN, creatinine, and potassium do not necessarily contraindicate the continuation of ACE inhibitor therapy. However, reduction in the dose or even stopping the ACE inhibitor is indicated if the serum potassium rises to 6 mEq/L, the creatinine increases by 0.75 mg to 1 mg/dl, or the patient develops symptomatic orthostatic hypotension. Cough is a common side affect of ACE inhibitor therapy, often caused by mild angioedema of the larynx and tracheobronchial tree. Patients often tolerate a mild cough if they understand the clear benefits of ACE inhibitor therapy. Severe cough, dyspnea, and wheezing are causes for discontinuing ACE inhibitor therapy. An alternative vasodilator program is the combination of nitrates and hydralazine.[5]

Digoxin

Digitalis glycosides (e.g., digoxin) remain extremely useful agents in the management of congestive heart failure with left ventricular systolic dysfunction. Digoxin is also useful in the management of patients whose heart failure is complicated by atrial fibrillation. Digoxin pharmacokinetics are altered in the elderly because of diminished volume of distribution, decreased renal clearance, and, less frequently, poor absorption of the drug. Digoxin is mainly excreted by the kidney, but one should be aware that a normal serum creatinine concentration is not always indicative of a normal GFR in the elderly patient. Calculate the GFR by the Cockcroft-Gault equation:

Calculated creatinine clearance* =
$$\frac{140 - age}{serum\ creatinine} \times \frac{lean\ body\ mass\ (kg)}{72}$$

> *Digoxin still has a place in treatment, especially when CHF involves atrial fibrillation.*

In nonemergency situations it is not necessary to give a loading dose of digoxin. Treatment is best initiated and maintained by the daily administration of an oral maintenance dose. For patients with creatinine clearance below 10 ml/min, give 0.125 mg every second or third day; for those with creatinine clearances between 10 and 30 ml/min, 0.125 mg daily; and for those with creatinine clearance above 30 ml/min, 0.25 mg daily. These dosage schedules usually result in a steady-state serum digoxin concentration between 1 and 2 ng/ml within 5 to 15 days. It is important to check a serum digoxin concentration to confirm that an appropriate steady-state serum digoxin concentration has been achieved. Subsequently, serum digoxin concentrations are not needed unless there is reason to suspect that the patient is not absorbing digoxin (lack of continued digoxin effect; coexistent administration of antacids, kaolin, pectin, and cholestyramine), the patient's renal function is changing, or drugs that raise the serum digoxin concentration are administered (quinidine, amiodarone, and calcium channel blocking drugs). Digitalis toxicity may present atypically in the elderly. In addition to the common symptoms of anorexia, nausea, vomiting, and visual disturbances, confusion, fatigue, and irritability may dominate. Any new disturbance in the cardiac rhythm should be considered as possible evidence of digitalis toxicity. It is well to remember that digitalis toxicity in older people may occur at serum concentrations usually considered to be in the therapeutic range.

---

*Multiply the result by 0.85 for women.

▼ MARY BURKITT (Part III)

The furosemide dose is decreased to 40 mg PO three times a week. On this therapeutic program Mrs. Burkitt does well for 4 months, but she returns to your office because of acute symptoms of intermittent rapid heart beat, increasing dyspnea, nocturnal cough, and typical anginal pain occurring both at rest and with limited exertion. Congestive heart failure and an irregular heart rhythm of 110 beats per minute are found on physical examination. ECG reveals a sinus tachycardia with multiple, multifocal ventricular premature beats, one 14-beat run of nonsustained ventricular tachycardia, and new, significant ST segment depression in the anterolateral chest leads. You admit her to the hospital for treatment of recurrent CHF, her cardiac dysrhythmia, and her chest pain and to rule out acute myocardial infarction. Pertinent laboratory studies included a CXR showing findings of recurrent CHF, normal thyroid function studies, and a serum digoxin level of 0.9 ng/ml. MB-CK enzymes exclude myocardial infarction. Treatment consists of O_2 by nasal cannula, daily doses of furosemide, and a nitroglycerin patch worn 20 hours each day. On this regimen her heart failure clears, her anginal symptoms disappear, and the ST segments no longer reflect ischemia. The frequency of ectopy also decreases markedly. Mrs. Burkitt elects against cardiac catheterization. She is discharged on furosemide 40 mg daily, enalapril 10 mg bid, digoxin 0.125 mg daily dose, and transdermal nitroglycerin 0.1 mg/hr worn 20 hours each day. Scheduled follow-up is arranged in your office, with routine electrolyte and digoxin level monitoring and reevaluation for subtle signs or symptoms of CHF or angina.

MYOCARDIAL ISCHEMIA AND CONGESTIVE HEART FAILURE

Angina may be a precipitating factor in, or the result of, CHF. Ischemia can worsen myocardial contractility and increase diastolic dysfunction, thus promoting CHF. Alternatively, CHF may cause angina pectoris because increasing left ventricular diameter and end diastolic pressure increases myocardial oxygen consumption and compromises perfusion of the subendocardium. Controlling angina and heart failure is the first step. If the patient is willing to consider revascularization, cardiac catheterization is advised. Angioplasty or coronary artery bypass graft (CABG) improve myocardial perfusion, relieve angina, and increase myocardial systolic and diastolic function. Life expectancy is increased by CABG in patients with unstable angina and compromised LVEF.[6]

▼ HARVEY HALL (Part I)

Harvey Hall, a 94-year-old white man, lives at home and has long-standing hypertension and mild vascular dementia. He comes to see you because of increased confusion. He has been taking hydrochlorothiazide (HCTZ) 50 mg/day. His family re-

lates subtle worsening of his functional status over the past few weeks and increasing pedal edema. They also comment that he seems to sleep in his chair a lot during the day and is eating poorly. He denies dyspnea on exertion, orthopnea, or paroxysmal nocturnal dyspnea. His vital signs reveal an apical heart rate of 105 with a pulse deficit of 21. His respirations are 20 breaths/min and BP is 120/76; he is afebrile. On examination he has evidence of pleural effusions with crackles above bilateral basal dullness, an irregularly irregular rhythm with an S_3 and a systolic ejection murmur, and 2+ pedal edema. He has no jugular venous distention nor a hepatojugular reflex. ECG shows atrial fibrillation with a ventricular rate of 110. Chest x-ray examination shows mild cardiac enlargement, bilateral pleural effusions, and cephalization of flow. Initial laboratory workup is essentially normal.

STUDY QUESTIONS

- How does the pathophysiology of this case of CHF differ from that of Mary Burkitt?
- How will this modify the management?
- What relatively recent group of medications may be specifically useful in long-term maintenance?

CASE DISCUSSION

This case is similar to the first, yet the pathophysiology of the CHF is entirely different. In this patient systolic function is preserved and diastolic dysfunction is present. Atrial fibrillation with a rapid ventricular response is the precipitating factor, and the patient worsens with the loss of atrial systole and the reduced duration of diastole (less time for filling the stiff ventricle) because of the increased heart rate.

CONGESTIVE HEART FAILURE WITH DIASTOLIC DYSFUNCTION

The ability to discriminate clinically between those with primarily systolic dysfunction and those with diastolic dysfunction is poor.[3] The prevalence of potential etiologies such as hypertension, coronary artery disease, prior myocardial infarction, and diabetes mellitus is high in both groups. In addition, there is no difference in the frequency of presenting signs, symptoms, precipitating factors, or historical factors between those with CHF caused by left ventricular systolic dysfunction and those with CHF caused by left ventricular diastolic dysfunction.

> *In the absence of significant valvular or pericardial disease, CHF with an LVEF of 50% or more is primarily due to diastolic dysfunction.*

The presenting symptoms of older patients with CHF exacerbations are frequently not classic (Box 42-1). Certain symptoms, such as paroxysmal nocturnal dyspnea and orthopnea, may not be evident, but evidence of stress, such as sleeping during the day in a chair, may be the equivalent. Confusion and decreasing functional status may be the primary clues that a new illness is present. Pedal edema is consistent with the diagnosis of CHF, but in a patient sitting all day with legs dependent it may merely be a marker of venous insufficiency. In contrast, an S_3 on examination, new atrial fibrillation, bilateral pleural effusions, and other chest x-ray findings are important signs of CHF.

ATRIAL FIBRILLATION WITH CONGESTIVE HEART FAILURE

CHF due primarily to diastolic dysfunction comprises 40% to 50% of those with CHF. One reason that CHF caused by primarily diastolic function is so common in the elderly is that impairment in diastolic function is part of normal aging. In contrast, left ventricular systolic function, as measured by LVEF, is unaltered by normal aging.[7,8] To compensate for lesser early filling (impaired ventricular relaxation), there is an age-associated increase in the dependence on atrial systole for filling of the left ventricle during diastole. Thus, as in this patient, atrial fibrillation often precipitates CHF. Atrial fibrillation may also precipitate CHF by increasing the oxygen demands of the heart because of the rapid heart rate. In addition, the loss of atrial contraction (atrial kick) decreases preload and thereby decreases myocardial contractility. Alternatively, CHF may predispose to atrial fibrillation; worsening heart failure distends the atria, leading to development of atrial fibrillation.

In CHF with diastolic dysfunction, use calcium channel blockers, digoxin, and other antiarrhythmics; but be careful with diuretics!

Digoxin and Calcium Channel Blockers

When both heart failure and atrial fibrillation coexist, the first priority is control of congestive heart failure by the usual measures and by control of heart rate. This can be accomplished by digitalis alone or in combination with calcium channel blocking drugs. Since calcium channel blocking drugs (verapamil, diltiazem) have negative inotropic effects, they should be used with caution in patients with impaired systolic function when digitalis alone fails to control the ventricular rate. Calcium channel blockers (verapamil and diltiazem) are often effective first-line therapy for rate control in patients with atrial fibrillation and normal LVEF. β-Receptor blocking drugs may also be useful, but contraindications to the use of β-receptor blocking drugs are common in the elderly. Digoxin is also

useful, but digoxin can (theoretically) exacerbate diastolic dysfunction by increasing myocardial diastolic calcium concentrations. Adequate control of the ventricular rate in patients with atrial fibrillation is defined as a postexercise (any level of mild exercise of which the patient is capable) apical rate of under 100 beats per minute.

Calcium channel blockers have been recommended for treatment of patients with normal LVEF CHF. Recently the use of high doses of verapamil has been shown to increase diastolic function in older persons without heart disease or CHF.[9] In older persons with CHF caused by diastolic dysfunction, this may be an important therapeutic approach. The ultimate role of high-dose verapamil in treatment of very elderly patients awaits confirmation.

Cardioversion and Anticoagulation

Once heart failure is controlled, attention can be given to restoring sinus rhythm. At times, sinus rhythm will result simply from control of CHF. If it does not, and if there is no contraindication to cardioversion (such as a greatly enlarged left atrium), direct current countershock or chemical cardioversion (quinidine, procainamide, amiodarone) may be tried. Anticoagulation must be given 3 weeks before and 2 weeks after cardioversion to reduce the possibility of systemic embolization. Given the increased frequency of systemic embolization (including stroke) in persistent atrial fibrillation, if cardioversion is not advisable, long-term anticoagulation with warfarin (Coumadin) or possibly acetylsalicylic acid (ASA) should be considered.

Diuretics

The judicious use of diuretics is necessary for symptom control in patients with diastolic dysfunction. Because filling of the stiff ventricle is already impaired, overly vigorous diuresis will lower ventricular filling to the point where cardiac output is compromised. The presence of a small amount of pedal edema may be necessary to maintain filling pressures and systemic perfusion.

▼ HARVEY HALL (Part II)

Mr. Hall has a good response to furosemide and rate control is initially obtained with oral digoxin. Thyroid function is normal, echocardiogram reveals an LVEF of 55% with left ventricular hypertrophy. Digoxin is tapered and ventricular rate and symptoms are well controlled with verapamil 240 mg/day and alternate-day furosemide. He improves and returns to baseline functional status. Follow-up is scheduled at your office with a "tickler" file in case of noncompliance in view of his known cognitive difficulties.

The prognosis of elderly patients with CHF caused by impaired diastolic function is not significantly different from those with impaired systolic function. In our experience with an elderly male population, mortality is very high (28%) the first year after diagnosis in both CHF groups, but in subsequent years the mortality is not different from age-matched controls.[10] This observation has two important implications. First, discussion of treatment preferences should not be delayed and needs to be addressed early. Second, a full and appropriately vigorous therapeutic program should be instituted at the time the diagnosis of CHF is made.

POSTTEST

1. The *best* way to differentiate between patients with normal LVEF and low LVEF is by:
   a. History
   b. Physical examination
   c. Echocardiography
   d. ECG
   e. Chest x-ray examination
2. Beneficial effects of converting atrial fibrillation with heart rate of 120 beats per minute to severe rhythm with heart rate 80 beats per minute include all of the following except:
   a. Increase time for ventricular filling
   b. Restoration of atrial contributors to ventricular filling
   c. Decreased myocardial oxygen consumption
   d. Increased myocardial contractility
   e. Reduction in ventricular hypertrophy
3. Which of these presenting symptoms would not be consistent with onset of CHF in an elderly patient?
   a. Dyspnea
   b. Worsening ability to self-care
   c. Anorexia
   d. Falls
   e. None of the above

REFERENCES

1. SOLVD investigators: Effect of enalapril on mortality and the development of heart failure in asymptomatic patients with reduced left ventricular ejection fractions, *N Engl J Med* 327:685-691, 1992.
2. Luchi RJ et al: Left ventricular function in hospitalized geriatric patients, *J Am Geriatric Soc* 30:700-705, 1982.
3. Luchi RJ, Taffet GE, Teasdale TA: Congestive heart failure in the elderly, *J Am Geriatr Soc* 39:810-825, 1991.
4. SOLVD investigators: Effect of enalapril on survival in patients with reduced left ventricular ejection fraction and congestive heart failure, *N Engl J Med* 325:293-302, 1991.
5. Cohn, JN et al: A comparison of enalapril with hydralazine-isosorbide dinitrate in the treatment of chronic congestive heart failure, *N Engl J Med* 325:303-310, 1991.
6. Luchi RJ et al: Coronary bypass surgery improves survival in high-risk unstable angina, Results of a Veterans Administration Cooperative study with an 8 year follow-up, Veterans Administration Unstable Angina Cooperative Study Group.
7. Lakatta EG: Cardiovascular regulatory mechanisms in advanced age, *Physiol Rev* 73:413-467, 1993.
8. Wei JY: Age and the cardiovascular system, *N Engl J Med* 327:1735-1739, 1992.
9. Setaro JF et al: Usefulness of verapamil for congestive heart failure associated with abnormal left ventricular diastolic filling and normal left ventricular systolic performance, *Am J Cardiol* 66:981-986, 1990.
10. Taffet GE et al: Survival of elderly men with congestive heart failure, *Age Ageing* 21:49-55, 1992.

PRETEST ANSWERS
1. a
2. a
3. e

POSTTEST ANSWERS
1. c
2. c
3. e

CHAPTER 43

Myocardial Infarction and Angina

PATRICK P. COLL

OBJECTIVES

Upon completion of this chapter, the reader will be able to:

1. Appreciate the potential for the altered presentation of myocardial infarction (MI) in an older patient.

2. Know the clinical management of an MI in an older patient.

3. Know and understand the important aspects of prevention and rehabilitation following an MI in an older patient.

4. Know and understand the management of angina in an older patient.

PRETEST

1. Which one of the following medications is *not* of benefit in the emergency management of acute myocardial infarction in a 80-year-old man with normal ventricular function:
   a. Streptokinase
   b. Aspirin
   c. Captopril
   d. Tissue plasminogen activator
   e. Metoprolol

Myocardial infarction (MI) is the most common cause of death and is an important cause of morbidity in patients over 65. Its clinical presentation may be altered by age. Management should be based on clinical trials that have included older patients and should take into consideration the patient's functional status and comorbidity. Prevention is the single most important aspect of this condition. It should be practiced in patients with and without identifiable cardiovascular disease and in all age groups.

▼ BARBARA MILS (Part I)

Ms. Mils is an 83-year-old white woman who began to live with her son following her husband's recent death. She is active and independent. Medical history includes diet-controlled non–insulin dependent diabetes mellitus and hypertension. She takes hydrochlorothiazide, 25 mg per day. You have seen her once in your office to check her blood pressure and to refill her antihypertensive medications. Today you receive a call from her son, who sounds anxious. He states that his mother has become increasingly short of breath over the preceding 24 hours and is mildly confused. You ask to speak to her, and although she has some difficulty being attentive to your questions, she denies any chest pain, fever, or sputum production. You ask her to have her son accompany her to meet you in the emergency room of the local hospital. There your examination reveals congestive cardiac failure. An electrocardiogram (ECG) shows a recent inferior myocardial infarction and frequent multifocal premature ventricular contractions (PVCs).

STUDY QUESTION

- *What management decisions should be made at this time?*

Myocardial infarction is the leading cause of death in the Western world today. The prevalence of coronary heart disease increases with age in both men and women. The increase in women occurs predominantly after menopause. The presentation of myocardial infarction in older patients may be atypical, although the majority still present with classic symptoms of crushing central chest pain or pressure, associated with diaphoresis and nausea.[1]

Atypical presentations cause diagnostic difficulty. The frequency of myocardial infarction without chest pain or pressure increases with age. Dyspnea associated with new-onset congestive cardiac failure may be the only presenting complaint. Other atypical presentations include syncope, stroke, acute confusion, weakness, and anorexia. True silent myocardial infarction does occur.[2] This is usually discovered on an ECG performed in the course of a preoperative assessment or other incidental reason. Data from the Framingham study indicate that approximately 15% of myocardial infarctions in persons over 65 are silent.[3] A significant number of myocardial infarctions resulting in death go unrecognized while the patient is alive. Failure to diagnose these ultimately fatal events occurs more often in older patients.[3]

> The "silent MI" really does occur; consider MI in the differential of many acute illnesses.

The high incidence of coronary heart disease and the greater likelihood of an atypical presentation warrant inclusion of myocardial infarction in the differential diagnosis of many acute illnesses in older patients. It should be considered a possible etiology for acute confusional states, acute onset of dyspnea, a fall, acute abdominal symptoms, a syncopal episode, or a stroke. The criteria by which a myocardial infarction is judged to occur are the same for older patients as for young: chest pain, characteristic ECG changes, and elevated cardiac enzymes. An older patient who has fallen, or who has spent time lying on a hard surface, may have an elevated creatinine phosphokinase (CPK) level because of skeletal muscle damage; hence the necessity of looking for a rise in the CPK-MB fraction in order to establish myocardial damage.

▼ BARBARA MILS (Part II)

You place Ms. Mils on 6 L of oxygen per minute by nasal cannula. She is given adult aspirin, 325 mg, to take by mouth and is placed on a cardiac monitor. A chest x-ray examination confirms congestive cardiac failure and shows an enlarged heart. She is given 20 mg of furosemide IV for initial treatment of the pulmonary edema. Because her myocardial infarction is suspected to be at least 24 hours old, thrombolytic therapy is not used. No therapy for the frequent PVCs is instituted. She is transferred to the coronary care unit, where she has an uneventful course.

STUDY QUESTIONS

- *What further investigations if any should be pursued after she leaves the coronary care unit?*
- *What does the rest of her management plan entail?*

Treatment of acute myocardial infarction in older patients is similar to that in younger patients. Because of the continued underrepresentation of those over 85 years in clinical studies, the benefits of certain interventions in this age group have to be deducted by extrapolating from data on younger patients. All patients, regardless of age, should have initial therapy directed toward controlling pain, supporting blood pressure if necessary, reducing myocardial oxygen demand, and ensuring an adequate supply of oxygen. Myocardial damage is caused by hypoxia, so oxygen should be started for anyone suspected of having myocardial infarction or experiencing angina. Assuming the patient is not allergic to it, chewable aspirin between 160 and 325 mg should be given as soon as possible. There is strong evidence to support the benefit of aspirin for acute MI, even in patients over 75 years of age.[4]

> *If an MI is suspected, start oxygen and aspirin immediately and control pain.*

There is increasing evidence that patients over 75 benefit from thrombolytic therapy as much as, if not more than, younger patients.[5] The debate rages as to whether IV tissue plasminogen activator (TPA) or IV streptokinase is the drug of choice for the treatment of acute MI in patients over 75.[6] There appears to be a marginal benefit for TPA when all MI sufferers are considered together. But, because of an increased hemorrhagic stroke rate, especially in older patients, streptokinase is a perfectly reasonable alternative in this age group. The excessive cost of TPA is a factor that must be considered in the decision analysis. There is no additional benefit to adding IV heparin when using IV streptokinase, except in the patient with anterior myocardial infarction. Streptokinase should be avoided if it has been given in the last 6 months. A number of patients, particularly those for whom thrombolysis is risky or contraindicated, will benefit from immediate coronary angioplasty.[7] A β-blocker should be given unless there are contraindications.

The appropriate use of antiarrhythmic agents in pa-

BOX 43-1
Key Components in Managing Acute Myocardial Infarction in the Elderly

Immediate transfer to emergency room
Adequate oxygenation
Relief of pain
Blood pressure support if necessary
Cardiac monitoring
Aspirin
Appropriate and timely use of thrombolytic agents (when indicated)
β-Blocker if not contraindicated

---

tients with MI is controversial. Prophylactic lidocaine is not recommended, it has not been shown to decrease mortality in this setting, and older patients in particular are susceptible to its central nervous system side effects, even when given in therapeutic doses. Antiarrhythmic agents such as lidocaine should be used only for patients with sustained ventricular tachycardia or ventricular fibrillation. The key components in the management of acute MI are shown in Box 43-1.

▼ BARBARA MILS (Part III)

Ms. Mils starts in-hospital cardiac rehabilitation, and a coronary angiogram is arranged. This shows extensive coronary disease, with an 80% occlusion of the left anterior descending artery. Based on these findings and the risk of further cardiac damage, coronary bypass surgery during the hospitalization is recommended by the cardiology team. She tolerates this well and returns home to her son 2 weeks later.

STUDY QUESTIONS

- *She asks you at the time of discharge what can be done to minimize the occurrence of another heart attack. What do you recommend?*

Coronary artery bypass grafting (CABG) for patients over 75 years of age is now common; CABG for patients over 85 is not unusual. No randomized controlled trials compare medical to surgical management of coronary heart disease in the elderly. Older CABG recipients tend to have higher complication rates, including mortality and longer lengths of hospital stay, when compared with younger patients. However, comorbidities such as heart failure, unstable angina, and valvular heart disease, all of which are more common in older patients, are stronger predictors of a poor outcome than age alone.[8] The clinician needs to perform a risk assessment comparing the risks and benefits before recommending CABG. Increased life expectancy is neither the only nor the most important benefit to be considered. Relief of pain, increased exercise tolerance, and overall improvement in functional capacity are important potential benefits of CABG.

> *Cardiac comorbidities may deter you from CABG, but age alone should not.*

Elective coronary angioplasty continues to play an increasing role in cardiac reperfusion. Lower morbidity, less discomfort, and lower cost make it an attractive procedure. However, the greater need for repeating the procedure and its unsuitability for extensively and diffusely diseased coronary arteries will most likely prevent it from supplanting CABG completely.

Risk factor reduction deserves attention in the elderly just as it does in younger patients: smoking cessation, reduction of hyperlipidemia, use of β-blockers, and exercise. Smoking cessation should always be pursued, especially in those who already have evidence of coronary artery disease. Smoking at any age increases cardiovascular mortality; limited evidence suggests that smoking cessation, even in the elderly, can reduce cardiovascular mortality.

Hypercholesterolemia is a risk factor for coronary artery disease across all age groups. Yet the efficacy and cost effectiveness of lowering cholesterol in older patients, especially by pharmacological means, are not clear.[9] In spite of this, many physicians prescribe expensive cholesterol-lowering agents for patients in their 70s and 80s. Once again the choice is between extrapolating from data on younger patients and prescribing cholesterol-lowering medication or waiting for the results of controlled trials that contain a larger number of older patients. If hypercholesterolemia is addressed, however, a low-fat, low-cholesterol diet should be emphasized. All other proven risk reduction interventions should be used before prescribing cholesterol-lowering medication.

> *β-Blockers, ACE inhibitors, and careful exercise are recommended post MI in elderly patients.*

β-Blockers have been shown to have a cardioprotective effect for older patients after MI; their use should be considered in all older patients who have had an MI.[4] Potential contraindications include chronic obstructive airway disease and peripheral vascular disease. Angiotensin-converting enzyme (ACE) inhibitors appeared to offer benefit to post-MI patients who have symptomatic CHF or a left ventricular ejection fraction of less than 40% in one study in which 15% of the subjects were over 70;

however, a subset analysis of these older patients was not reported.[10]

The efficacy of exercise for the older patient after MI is not proven. However, exercise within the guidance of a cardiac rehabilitation program should be encouraged for psychological as well as potential physical benefit.

▼ BARBARA MILS (Part IV)

Ms. Mils attends the outpatient cardiac rehabilitation program and is started on timolol before discharge. You arrange for a follow-up office visit at which you plan to discuss the use of a low-fat, low-cholesterol diet and a long-term exercise program.

▼ JAMES KELLY (Part I)

During a routine visit for preoperative evaluation for cataract removal, your patient Mr. Kelly, who is 91, reports that he is having chest pain and pressure while walking up stairs. He has previously been noted to have lower leg claudication while walking long distances. He previously smoked heavily but stopped 10 years ago. He has been hypertensive for many years and has mild benign prostatic hypertrophy. His only medications are prazosin (Minipress) and aspirin. On examination his pulse is 90 beats per minute and regular in rate, blood pressure is 150/85, his lungs are clear, and he has a soft ejection systolic murmur. After you discuss with him the possible causes of his pain and potential investigations and treatments, he is adamant that he does not want any kind of invasive or surgical procedure.

STUDY QUESTIONS
- *What further testing, if any, would you do?*
- *What treatment, if any, would you recommend?*

Coronary artery disease (CAD) and associated angina are common in old age. As with myocardial infarction the presentation of myocardial ischemia may be atypical. Silent ischemia can occur or ischemia may be manifested by dyspnea or decreased exercise tolerance.[11] Other conditions, in particular upper gastrointestinal disorders (hiatal hernia, peptic ulcer disease), may have symptoms similar to angina. A variety of conditions, including anemia, hyperthyroidism, and participation for the first time in an exercise program, may precipitate angina in the older patient.

Initial assessment should include a detailed history emphasizing potential risk factors for CAD (smoking, family history, hyperlipidemia, and hypertension); GI symptoms (regurgitation of food, dyspepsia, and heme-positive stool); and symptoms or diseases that will modify the choice of therapy (COPD, peripheral vascular disease, benign prostatic hypertrophy, orthostatic hypotension). The examination should search for anemia, hyper-

thyroidism, additional heart sounds, and signs of congestive heart failure (CHF).

Investigations should include hemoglobin and hematocrit (Hgb/Hct), thyroid function tests, and a resting
electrocardiogram (ECG). Further investigations should
be tailored to history and physical findings. There is no
point in proceeding with cardiac stress testing or angiography if the patient is not a candidate for, or is not willing to undergo, a revascularization.

The mainstays of pharmacological treatment for angina in older patients (as in younger) are β-blockers, nitrates, calcium channel blockers, and aspirin.[12] No one
of these three groups is clearly preferable to the others.
There are an increasing number of new medications
within each of the categories. Table 43-1 outlines the
pharmacotherapy for angina.

CASE DISCUSSION

*Mr. Kelly has blood drawn for Hgb, Hct, and thyroid func-
tion, which are within normal limits. An ECG is normal. He
is prescribed isosorbide mononitrate each morning and sublingual nitroglycerin to take for episodes of chest pain or pressure. You instruct him to contact you if the pain persists after*
*taking two sublingual nitroglycerin. You decide that if his
pain should continue in spite of the above treatments, he will
change his antihypertensive medication from his current
α-blocker to a calcium channel blocker. The cataract extraction goes ahead.*

SUMMARY

Myocardial infarction and angina, two of the major manifestations of coronary artery disease, frequently present
atypically or are clinically inapparent in older individuals. Most of the evidence is that treatment standards for
younger patients should be applied to elderly patients.
These conditions represent a major cause of morbidity
and mortality. Increasingly, procedures previously reserved for younger patients, such as coronary artery bypass grafts (CABGs) and coronary angioplasty, have
proved to be applicable to many elders, with resultant
improvement in morbidity as well as mortality. In these
often asymptomatic or atypical situations, laboratory and
particularly cardiographic investigations are of particular
importance in selecting patients at risk and ensuring their
access to therapy.

Table 43-1   Choosing Medication for Angina in the Elderly

Group	Relative Contraindication	Side Effects	Special Considerations
Nitrates	Hypotension; orthostatic hypo-tension	Hypotension; orthostatic hy-potension; reflex tachycar-dia; headache	Patients may develop toler-ance; nitropatch should be removed at night; long-acting mononitrate once a day may help avoid toler-ance
β-Blockers	Congestive heart failure (CHF); peripheral vascular disease; chronic obstructive airway dis-ease	Fatigue; anorexia; depression; bradyarrhythmia; CHF	Ideal for patient with prior MI or supraventricular tachycar-dia
Calcium channel blocker	CHF (verapamil, diltiazem)	Constipation (verapamil); hy-potension; reflex tachycardia (dihydropiridines); brady-arrhythmia (verapamil); ankle edema (dihydropiri-dines)	Good choice if concurrent hypertension; verapamil and diltiazem: avoid with β-blockers

POSTTEST

1. Which of the following cardiac medications in a
   therapeutic dose is most likely to cause a change in
   mental status in an 87-year-old with a recent myocardial infarction:
   a. Nitroglycerin
   b. Lidocaine

   c. Furosemide
   d. Verapamil
   e. Digoxin

REFERENCES

1. Bayer AJ et al: Changing presentation of myocardial infarction with increasing old age, *J Am Geriatr Soc* 34:263-266, 1986.
2. Bayliss RS: The silent coronary, *Br Med J* 290:1093-1094, 1985.
3. Kannel WB, Abbott RD: Incidence and prognosis of unrecognized myocardial infarction, *N Engl J Med* 318:1144-1147, 1984.
4. ISIS-2 Collaborative Group: Randomized trial of intravenous streptokinase, oral aspirin, both or neither among 17,187 cases of suspected acute myocardial infarction ISIS-2, *Lancet* 2:349-360, 1988.
5. Forman D, Gutierrez Bernal JL, Wei J: Management of acute myocardial infarction in the very elderly, *Am J Med* 93:315-326, 1992.
6. Gusto Investigators: An international randomized trial comparing four thrombolytic strategies for acute myocardial infarction, *N Engl J Med* 329:673-682, 1993.
7. Grines C et al: A comparison of immediate angioplasty with thrombolytic therapy for acute myocardial infarction, *N Engl J Med* 328:673-679, 1993.
8. Gold S et al: Invasive treatment for coronary artery disease in the elderly, *Arch Intern Med* 151:1085-1088, 1991.
9. Eisenberg JM: Should the elderly be screened for hypercholesterolemia, *Arch Intern Med* 151:1063-1065, 1991.
10. Pfeffer M et al: Effect of captopril on mortality and morbidity in patients with left ventricular dysfunction after myocardial infarction, *N Engl J Med* 327:669-677, 1992.
11. Lazar EJ, Lazar JM, Frishman W: Angina pectoris and silent ischemia in the elderly: a management update, *Geriatrics* 47:24-36, 1992.
12. Fleg J: Angina pectoris in the elderly, *Cardiol Clin* 9(1):177-187, 1991.

PRETEST ANSWER

1. c

POSTTEST ANSWER

1. b

CHAPTER 44

Peripheral Vascular Disease

DOUGLAS C. WOOLLEY

OBJECTIVES

Upon completion of this chapter, the reader will be able to:

1. Describe the major risk factors associated with the development of peripheral atherosclerotic occlusive disease.

2. Describe the common patterns of lower extremity atherosclerotic disease, its clinical presentations, and the characteristics of the patients who typically develop it.

3. Describe the appropriate steps in making a diagnosis when lower extremity arterial insufficiency is suspected.

4. Describe a sequential approach to the management of lower extremity arterial disease with mention of prevention, rehabilitation, and the uses and limitations of drug and surgical treatment.

PRETEST

1. Patients who have peripheral arterial occlusive disease are most likely to die of:
   a. Peripheral vascular disease
   b. Renal failure
   c. Cardiovascular or cerebrovascular disease
   d. Diabetes mellitus
2. Which one of the following statements is false?
   a. Middle-aged men are twice as likely as middle-aged women to suffer symptoms of lower extremity arterial disease.
   b. Peripheral vascular symptoms often occur in the absence of significant coronary artery or cerebrovascular disease.
   c. Degenerative joint disease of the lumbar spine produces claudication pain on straight leg raising.
   d. Dangling the legs generally worsens venous stasis pain.

Symptoms of lower extremity arterial insufficiency are common in old age. Associated ischemia often leads to suffering and disability and may lead to loss of limb or life. Assisting patients to reduce risk factors is the key; diagnosis and management must be skilled and proactive.

▼ ALBERT BERN (Part I)

Your patient, Mr. Bern, is a 67-year-old retired waiter. He complains of burning calf pain that forces him to stop climbing after two flights of stairs. The pain is predictable and moderate and disappears after a brief rest. He was a heavy smoker until 2 years ago when he suffered a stroke with minimal sequelae. He has hypertension and hyperlipidemia.

▼ ROBERT AYRENS (Part I)

Mr. Ayrens is a 76-year-old retired accountant. His type II diabetes mellitus has been poorly controlled for two decades. His ankles are edematous and sore, and he has venous stasis and congestive heart failure. To help reduce the edema, you have prescribed custom-fit compression stockings. When he walks in the stockings, he experiences a new pain in the anterior tibial muscles and in the arches of both feet.

STUDY QUESTIONS

- *What modifiable risk factors for peripheral vascular disease do these two patients show?*
- *What could be the mechanism for the new pain Mr. Ayrens is experiencing?*
- *What is the differential diagnosis?*
- *What should be emphasized in your history and clinical examination?*

Peripheral vascular disease refers to any occlusive process that limits blood flow to limbs or to vital organs other than the heart. Lower extremity arterial disease (LEAD), which will be the focus of this chapter, is most often due to enlarging atherosclerotic plaques in the distal aorta and its branches. Victims of LEAD often complain of pain in the lower limb muscles, particularly the calves, while walking; this exercise-induced pain is called intermittent claudication.

Framingham study data show that those aged 65 to 74 experience the highest rate of newly symptomatic LEAD.[1] It affects middle-aged men twice as often as middle-aged women, but the gender disparity begins to disappear after age 65.

Risk factors are the same as for coronary artery disease: smoking, hyperlipidemia, hypertension, diabetes mellitus, and family history.[2] The atherosclerosis is rarely confined to the lower extremities; by the time lower limb ischemia is symptomatic, cerebrovascular disease and coronary artery disease are usually present as well. Although LEAD can be disabling, its victims more often die from their coronary or cerebrovascular disease.[1]

ATHEROSCLEROSIS

Atherosclerosis is a slowly evolving process of damage to the artery walls. It is first seen peripherally at the origins of major branches of the aorta and at their more distal bifurcations. The vessels may be under more stress from torsion, turbulent flow, and high pressure at these points than elsewhere. When stresses disrupt the endothelium, deeper tissues are exposed. Platelets adhere to this denuded vessel wall, forming small thrombi. They then release factors that induce smooth muscle cells and macrophages to migrate to the area. These cells proliferate and lay down a lipid and connective tissue matrix. With further injury these plaques thicken, stiffen, and develop cholesterol and calcific deposits. These complex atheromatous plaques further enlarge by mechanically injuring adjacent endothelium. Their surface may become quite rough and ragged, shedding thrombi and plaque fragments into the distal circulation.

Atherogenic risk factors work by amplifying vessel injury or disturbing healing. For example, elevated blood pressure tends to injure the endothelium, hyperlipidemia speeds up cholesterol plaque formation, and smoking promotes vessel spasm and platelet aggregation (along with many other harmful effects).

CLINICAL PRESENTATIONS OF LEAD

Clinical presentation of LEAD has three general patterns. The first is typified by a rather young smoking man, between the ages of 40 and 60, with hyperlipidemia and a family history of vascular disease. He complains of weakness and exercise-induced aching of the proximal lower extremities, that is, of the pelvic girdle musculature and thighs. He also may complain of decreased penile erection and poor sexual function. Examination shows a decrease of lower extremity muscle mass and tone, bruits over the distal aorta and iliac arteries, and decreased femoral pulses. Atheromatous lesions are found in the distal aorta and its branches. Symptoms stem from inadequate blood supply to the pelvic girdle and thighs, worsened by the increased oxygen demands of exercise.

The second common clinical presentation is of a man or woman aged 65 to 75 years who complains of calf aching or burning. This pain emerges after predictable amounts of exercise. Such a patient generally has several atherosclerosis risk factors, usually including smoking, and typically has coronary or cerebral vascular disease. Examination shows adequate femoral pulses, but weak popliteal and distal pulses. Widespread atheromatous disease may be present, but the major occlusive lesions are in the femoral and popliteal arteries. When symptoms first appear, tissue perfusion is usually still adequate to supply resting needs. Smaller auxiliary vessels (collateral circulation) may channel blood flow around the occlusive lesions to distal tissues. Evidence of advanced peripheral ischemia, such as pain at rest, thinning of the skin, nonhealing ulcers, absent toe hair, and thickening and distortion of toenails, is not usually present.

The third clinical pattern is typified by a diabetic patient of either sex, with years of suboptimal control. The patient complains of aching pain in the anterior tibial muscles and the foot, particularly the metatarsal arch, while walking. Examination shows absence of peripheral pulses, but proximal pulses may be intact. The ankle and foot may show trophic changes, suggesting significant ischemia at rest: fragile skin with a mottled rubor, absence of toe hair, thickened nails, muscle wasting, and nonhealing ulcers. Rest pain may be present, particularly at night, and must be differentiated from the dysesthesias of peripheral neuropathy. The occlusive lesions are found in the distal tibial and peroneal arteries and in the dorsal arch of the foot.

CAD and cerebrovascular disease are usually present by the time lower limb ischemia is symptomatic.

Very old or infirm patients may not ambulate enough to experience exercise-related ischemia. Their progressive LEAD may be silent until perfusion is inadequate to meet even basal tissue needs. They then suffer pain at night or at times when the feet are elevated so that perfusion pressure is not augmented by gravity. Their feet and legs may show advanced ischemic changes, as previously described.

HISTORY

The patient's history should bring out the quality, intensity, and location of the limb discomfort, as well as the pattern of how it develops and subsides. This will serve to differentiate vascular disease from other causes of lower limb pain. *Degenerative joint disease of the lumbar spine* can lead to stenosis of the spinal canal and impingement on the cauda equina and exiting nerve roots; this produces aching and burning pain of the buttock, thigh, and calf muscles when nerve compression is accentuated, such as during straight leg raising or with prolonged standing. Because this condition is often misinterpreted as intermittent claudication, it has been referred to as pseudoclaudication.[3] *Venous stasis* can cause aching of the thighs and calves. Whereas patients with rest pain from LEAD may find relief by dangling their legs, patients with venous disease report that this amplifies their symptoms. Patients with *peripheral neuropathy* often complain of burning or throbbing distal lower extremity pains. As in severe arterial insufficiency, these pains may be more frequent at night. Dangling the feet typically does not help, but light foot exercise might.

Dangling the legs may relieve rest pain from LEAD, but it will not help neuropathic pain, and it will worsen venous stasis pain.

EXAMINATION

During the physical examination, signs of vascular disease should be carefully sought. Is there evidence of old cerebral infarct or myocardial damage? Is there evidence of retinal vascular changes, arcus senilis, carotid bruits, left ventricular hypertrophy, asymmetry of upper extremity pulses or blood pressure, aortic aneurysm, abdominal or flank bruits? The pelvic girdle and lower extremities should be examined for muscle bulk and strength. The presence, symmetry, and quality of the femoral, popliteal, dorsalis pedis, and posterior tibialis pulses are noted. The distal skin, hair, and nails are examined for the trophic changes of ischemia described earlier. The differential diagnosis of LEAD is summarized in Table 44-1.

Two easy office tests may demonstrate vascular insufficiency: (1) While the patient is supine, the lower extremity is passively raised to a 45- to 60-degree angle. The patient then flexes and extends the ankle a few times. A thigh blood pressure cuff is pumped to above 200 mm Hg. The leg is returned to the horizontal position at the same time that the cuff is released. The time it takes for toe color to return gives a qualitative assessment of perfusion: 10 to 15 seconds is normal, and greater than 30 seconds suggests significant vascular disease, in proportion to the delay in refill.[4] (2) The systolic blood pressure measured at the ankle is compared with that measured in the arm. This is termed the ankle/brachial index. Return of blood flow is measured with a hand-held Doppler device as the cuff is slowly deflated. The normal index should be 1 or greater. In the active older individual who gives a classic history of exercise-induced claudication, the ratio is usually between 0.5 and 1. In patients who have rest symptoms it may be much lower than 0.5.[5]

▼ ALBERT BERN (Part II)

Mr. Bern is slim and vigorous. His blood pressure is 170/90 and heart rate 80, with occasional ectopy. He has bilateral arcus senilis and early hypertensive retinal vascular changes. He has a right carotid bruit, a laterally displaced apical impulse, and an audible S_4. There are abdominal aortic and femoral bruits. His femoral pulses are equal and easily felt, but his popliteal pulse on the left and both dorsalis pedis pulses are diminished. Lower extremity skin and musculature appear normal. The blood pressure measured at his ankle is abnormally low.

▼ ROBERT AYRENS (Part II)

Mr. Ayrens becomes short of breath with minimal exertion. Bibasilar rales, an S_3, and symmetric ankle edema are present. The calves, ankles, and feet have thin, ruborous, shiny skin with no hair. The nails are thick and gnarled. The toes are gaunt and have a violaceous hue that darkens toward the tips. Peripheral pulses are not palpable. During the capillary refill test described above, return of color takes more than 30 seconds even when the feet dangle.

STUDY QUESTIONS

- What is your assessment of the severity of disease in these two patients?
- Why has Mr. Ayrens suffered little pain?
- What management would you recommend for both of these patients?

CASE DISCUSSION

Mr. Ayrens has severe bilateral occlusive disease of the tibioperoneal vessels. Painful ischemia had not been evident because he does not walk much. The quality of the distal pulses is difficult to assess through edematous tissue. However, wearing the compression stockings further reduces the already low arterial pressure, so that the need for increased muscle perfusion during walking cannot be met: claudication symptoms result. **Mr. Bern** has extensive vascular disease. If he continues to walk regularly, lowers changeable risk factors, and takes proper care of his feet, worse peripheral disease may not develop. However, his existing cardiovascular and cerebrovascular problems are likely to produce further illness in the future.

Table 44-1   Differential Diagnosis of Lower Extremity Arterial Disease (LEAD)

	LEAD	Venous Stasis	DJD of Lumbosacral Spine	Peripheral Neuropathy
Peripheral pulses	Generally reduced or absent	May be disguised by edema	Normal	Normal
Trophic skin, muscle, and nail changes	Only if advanced or in diabetics; possibly thin, wasted muscles	Skin fragile if edematous, can be "tight" and "shiny," even ulcerated, but no associated muscle loss	Not associated	Often present, generally associated with diabetes
What makes the pain worse, and is it present at rest?	Pain worse with specifiable quantity of exercise; rest pain only if advanced	Typically worse with prolonged standing; association with exercise unpredictable	Typically worse with prolonged standing or straight leg raising on examination; association with exercise unpredictable	Pain often worse at night; association with exercise unpredictable
Does dangling the feet affect the pain?	May relieve	Usually worsens	No help	No help (light exercise may relieve)

FURTHER INVESTIGATION

A well-equipped vascular laboratory can help define the presence and extent of LEAD. The sensitivity of the ankle/brachial index may be improved by measuring it before and after exercise. After exercise the ratio is somewhat increased in healthy subjects but in patients with significant occlusive disease it drops, sometimes dramatically. The resting perfusion pressure of the great toe can be determined as a measure of whether ischemia exists and whether existing lesions such as pressure sores will heal.[5] Vascular duplex scanning, which combines Doppler ultrasound (for the study of blood flow) with imaging ultrasound (for the study of vessel anatomy), can provide useful pictures of both the location and severity of lower limb occlusive disease in the larger arteries.[6] Arteriography, an invasive test with higher risks than the tests discussed so far, is typically not performed unless surgery is being considered. Magnetic resonance angiography is a noninvasive imaging technique that may soon supplant conventional angiography as the routine preoperative study, since it appears to be at least as useful in delineating diseased vessels and is significantly safer.[7]

MANAGEMENT

Management of LEAD begins with prevention by helping individuals reduce all modifiable risk factors early in life. Those who already have vascular disease must avoid tobacco. Maintaining normal lipids, blood pressure, and blood glucose probably slows disease progress. Regular exercise has been shown to increase the distance a patient can walk before claudication emerges. This may be due to improvements in muscle efficiency, increases in collateral circulation, or both.[2]

Once LEAD is recognized, the patient must be helped to prevent complications. Poorly perfused tissue heals poorly, so the patient must avoid trauma, including extremes of hot or cold. Sturdy, well-fitting shoes must be worn at all times when the patient is up. The care of thickened and distorted toenails requires podiatric expertise. Poorly perfused feet, particularly those of a diabetic, are susceptible to fungous infections, interdigital maceration, and hard, scaly calluses. These sites are susceptible to smoldering and slowly deepening bacterial infections, which can threaten limb or even life. The patient must learn to inspect the feet daily for signs of trauma or infection and to keep the skin clean, soft, and free of callus and scaling.

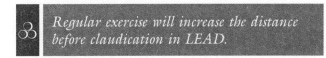

Regular exercise will increase the distance before claudication in LEAD.

MEDICATION

The role of medication in treating LEAD is limited. Though pentoxifylline (Trental) is the most respected drug for this indication, its clinical effectiveness is debated. By several mechanisms, including rendering the red blood cell more flexible in the microvasculature, it decreases blood viscosity and increases peripheral perfusion. Not all patients experience symptomatic improvement in claudication with pentoxifylline, and for those who do respond, the gains are usually modest. However, it appears to speed the healing of lower extremity diabetic ulcers.[8] Most elderly patients with lower limb vascular disease never need surgery. However, if the patient is quite disabled or limb survival is in question, several procedures may be considered. Dilating a localized proximal stenosis, as in the common and external iliac arteries, with a balloon catheter (balloon angioplasty) may be the procedure of choice. Longer or more distal stenotic lesions are best approached with bypass grafting. If disease is extensive in both proximal and distal vessels, surgery may not be possible. Laser angioplasty may yet have a role in LEAD treatment, but initial enthusiasm for this technology has waned.[9]

SUMMARY

Managing peripheral vascular disease begins by reducing risk factors in everyone at any age, whether or not they show evidence of disease. Functional rehabilitation and prevention of complications, including routine self and podiatric care, are indicated in those with established disease. Some will benefit from drug therapy and a few will eventually require angioplasty or surgery.

POSTTEST

1. Which one of the following statements is false?
   a. Magnetic resonance angiography will probably displace arteriography as the preoperative study of choice.
   b. Above age 65, the proportion of women suffering symptomatic LEAD increases significantly.
   c. Dangling the feet may relieve ischemic pain but not neuropathic pain.
   d. If the ankle/brachial index is over 1.0, the patient probably does have claudication.

2. Match the typical clinical presentation with the symptoms:
   a. 55-year-old male smoker
   b. 70-year-old diabetic with long history of noncontrol
   c. 72-year-old smoker

   1. Aching feet and anterior tibial muscles with exercise, fragile skin with nonhealing ulcers, and pain at night
   2. Aching or burning of the calves with exercise, with significant coronary artery or cerebrovascular disease
   3. Poor sexual function, with exercise-induced aching of the pelvic girdle and thighs

REFERENCES

1. Kannel WB et al: Intermittent claudication: incidence in the Framingham Study, *Circulation* 41:857, 1970.
2. Clyne CAC: Non-surgical management of peripheral vascular disease, *Br Med J* 281:794-797, 1980.
3. Stanton PE Jr et al: Differentiation of vascular and neurogenic claudication, *Am Surg* 53:71-76, 1987.
4. Halperin JL: Peripheral vascular disease: medical evaluation and treatment, *Geriatrics* 42:47-61, 1989.
5. Orchard TJ, Strandness DE: Assessment of peripheral vascular disease in diabetes, *Circulation* 88:819-828, 1993.
6. Kazmers A, Strandness DE Jr: Duplex scanning in vascular surgery, *Surg Ann* 19:23-40, 1987.
7. Carpenter JP et al: Magnetic resonance angiography of the aorta, iliac, and femoral arteries, *Surgery* 116:17-23, 1994.
8. Campbell RK: Clinical update on pentoxifylline therapy for diabetes-induced peripheral vascular disease, *Ann Pharmacother* 27(9):1099-1105, 1993.
9. Seeger JM, Kaelin LD: Limitations and pitfalls of laser angioplasty, *Surg Ann* 25(2):177-192, 1993.

PRETEST ANSWERS
1. c
2. b

POSTTEST ANSWERS
1. d
2. a–3
   b–1
   c–2

CHAPTER 45

Stroke

LAURA MOSQUEDA and KENNETH BRUMMEL-SMITH

OBJECTIVES

On completion of this chapter, the reader will be able to:

1. Describe the features of the most common causes of stroke: thrombosis, hemorrhage, and embolism.

2. Describe the initial treatment of the patient with stroke.

3. Describe the initial management of the common complications of stroke: pressure sores, malnutrition, pneumonia, venous thrombosis, contractures, nerve palsies, conjunctivitis, shoulder pain, depression, and confusion.

1. All of the following statements regarding stroke are true except which one?
   a. Forty percent of patients ultimately suffer severe disability following stroke.
   b. Thirty percent of patients have no ultimate disability following stroke.
   c. Eighty-five percent of completed strokes are due to infarction.
   d. The risk of stroke following a transient ischemic attack is 5% per year for 3 years.

2. All of the following statements regarding stroke are true except which one?
   a. The most common site of the lesion is the middle cerebral artery.
   b. Cerebrobasilar insufficiency characteristically involves cerebellar features.
   c. Left hemisphere lesions are often associated with aphasia.
   d. Right hemisphere lesions are associated with visuospatial deficits.
   e. Aphasia is rare in middle cerebral artery lesions.

The term "stroke" refers to a broad group of conditions that disrupt the blood supply to an area of the brain to the point of causing cellular death. Stroke is the third leading cause of death in older persons, and some 500,000 persons have strokes each year. More elderly individuals are disabled as a result of strokes than any other cause.[1] Among survivors some level of disability is usually present. About 10% have complete resolution of their impairments, 40% have mild-to-moderate disability, 40% are more severely impaired, and only 10% need institutional care.[2] Because most people who have a stroke survive, intensive rehabilitation should be considered in all patients.[3] Certain complications are sufficiently frequent and disabling that they should be anticipated and either prevented if possible or promptly recognized and treated if they occur.[4]

> *Most people survive stroke, so intensive rehabilitation should be considered in all patients.*

Age is the single most important risk factor for stroke. The incidence of stroke climbs from 30 per 100,000 before the age of 44 years to more than 1230 per 100,000 after the age of 75 years.[5] Other risk factors, both modifiable and nonmodifiable, are listed in Box 45-1. The response to stroke also changes with age. This is due to a combination of issues including normal changes of aging, polypharmacy, and common diseases that occur with aging. These issues influence both the acute and the long-term management of elderly people who have a stroke.

BOX 45-1
Risk Factors for Stroke

Modifiable

Hypertension
Diabetes
Cigarette smoking
Elevated LDL and triglycerides

Nonmodifiable

Advanced age
African-American race

LOCALIZATION OF THE LESION

Before the advent of computed tomography (CT) scanning, the patient's clinical picture was used to localize the site of the lesion (Table 45-1).

The most common lesion occurs as a result of occlusion of the *middle cerebral artery* (MCA). Contralateral hemiparesis, with the leg being less affected than the arm and face, is usually seen. Weakness may also be accompanied by sensory loss. Some may experience a homonymous hemianopsia. If the head and eyes are deviated, they are deviated toward the side of the lesion. When the *dominant* (usually the left) MCA is affected, aphasia may occur. The person's ability to speak (expressive aphasia) may be affected, as well as the person's ability to understand (receptive aphasia). Dominant hemisphere lesions are also associated with a high incidence of depression.

If the *nondominant* (usually the right) hemisphere is affected, visuospatial deficits occur. Often there is significant neglect, whereby the patient does not attend to ob-

Table 45-1   Sites of Lesions and Their Manifestations

Anatomical Location	Arterial Supply	Neurological Signs and Symptoms
Lateral Frontal and Parietal Lobes	Middle cerebral artery	
Dominant hemisphere		Contralateral hemiplegia (arm weaker than leg), contralateral sensory loss, emotional lability, aphasia
Nondominant hemisphere		Contralateral hemiplegia (arm weaker than leg), contralateral sensory loss, emotional lability, contralateral neglect, decreased awareness of deficit, visuospatial deficit
Medial Frontal and Parietal Lobes	Anterior cerebral artery	Contralateral hemiplegia (leg weaker than arm), urinary incontinence, apathy
Internal Capsule	Medial striate branches of anterior cerebral artery	Contralateral weakness
	Lenticulostriate branches of middle cerebral artery	Contralateral weakness
Thalamus	Thalamic branches of posterior cerebral artery	Altered sensation without weakness
Putamen	Lenticulostriate branches of middle cerebral artery	
Dominant hemisphere		Contralateral hemiparesis, conjugate gaze deviation (toward side of lesion), aphasia (nonfluent)
Nondominant hemisphere		Contralateral hemiparesis, conjugate gaze deviation (toward size of lesion), contralateral neglect, constructional apraxia
Occipital Lobe	Posterior cerebral artery	
Dominant hemisphere		Contralateral visual field defect, reading impairment
Nondominant hemisphere		Contralateral visual field defect
Pons	Penetrating branches of basilar artery	Tetraplegia, coma, horizontal eye movements lost
Cerebellum	Branches of vertebrobasilar artery (posterior inferior cerebellar, anterior inferior cerebellar, and superior cerebellar arteries)	Ipsilateral limb ataxia/ataxic gait, vertigo
Retina	Ophthalmic branch of internal carotid artery	Monocular blindness

jects in the left spatial area. Many lose their ability to modulate speech or become emotionally labile, presenting a picture that can be misinterpreted as depression.

> A dominant MCA stroke is associated with aphasia and depression; a nondominant MCA stroke is associated with visuospatial deficit, unilateral neglect, and emotional lability that can mimic depression.

Pure *anterior cerebral artery* occlusions are less common and have relatively greater leg weakness than face or arm weakness. Aphasia is uncommon. Frontal features predominate with emotionality, impairment of mood or personality, and intellectual deficits.

Vertebrobasilar insufficiency often presents with prominent cerebellar features. Vomiting, dizziness or vertigo, double vision, and dysarthria are commonly seen. Quadriparesis or bilateral numbness can occur. The person may exhibit ataxia. Crossed weakness with one side of the face and the other side of the body may also develop. Nystagmus may be present. Occasionally pseudobulbar palsy will develop with the triad of dysarthria, dysphagia, and emotional lability. If the brain stem is involved, the person may be stuporous.

Lacunar strokes are small occlusions of the penetrating arteries. Such strokes are subcortical and tend to occur in the basal ganglia, internal capsule, thalamus, or pons. Depending on the site, a wide variety of presentations may occur. Pure motor or pure sensory strokes are seen. A parkinsonian picture may develop with stiffness, increased tone, and a shuffling gait if the substantia nigra is affected. Pseudobulbar palsy may also occur.

▼ GEORGE PAUL (Part I)

Mr. Paul is an 80-year-old man brought into the emergency room by his wife, who says she heard him fall out of bed as he was trying to get up this morning. She noticed that his right side was weak and that he couldn't talk. He was fine when he went to bed the night before. On examination he is alert but cannot articulate clearly. His speech is hesitant and he appears frustrated. The right side of his face droops, and he drools from the right corner of his mouth. His right arm is flaccid, and the right leg moves only slightly. His reflexes are hyperactive on the right and normal on the left (except for an absent ankle jerk). He has an extensor response (positive Babinski's sign) on the right.

▼ MARIA HERNANDEZ (Part I)

Ms. Hernandez is a 65-year-old woman who was brought to the emergency room by the paramedics after she complained of a severe headache that began while she was gardening. She then fell to the ground and was unable to move her left arm or leg. Initially she seemed to be somewhat confused about her surroundings. On the way to the emergency room she had a generalized tonic-clonic seizure.

STUDY QUESTIONS

- What is the likely site and etiology in each case?
- What should the immediate management strategy be?

CAUSES OF STROKE

It is important to distinguish between the two major categories of strokes, ischemic and hemorrhagic, since the prognosis and approach to treatment differ significantly for each. Ischemic strokes account for approximately 80% of all strokes. They involve a blockage in an arterial vessel from either an embolic or a thrombotic event. Sometimes the blood supply is reestablished and the deficit resolves completely in less than 24 hours; this is said to be a transient ischemic attack (TIA). The less common hemorrhagic strokes are due to a bleeding event either in the subarachnoid space or in the parenchyma of the brain. A more detailed explanation of these categories follows.

Ischemic Strokes

When a mass, such as a blood clot, travels through the vascular system and causes significant blockage of a vessel that supplies the brain, it produces an *embolic stroke*. The most common source for an embolus is the heart. The prevalence of cardiogenic emboli increases with advancing age. Atrial fibrillation is the most common cause, although emboli from dyskinetic portions of the heart following a myocardial infarction or from vegetations from damaged or prosthetic valves may also occur.

The other category of ischemic stroke, called *thrombotic stroke*, involves clot formation at the site of the vessel. Atherosclerosis accounts for the majority of these strokes. The internal carotid arteries are most commonly affected, although the vertebrobasilar system can be affected as well. The atherosclerotic lesion in the artery gradually causes stenosis through plaque formation. Ulceration, which is thrombogenic, may occur in atherosclerotic plaques. Thrombi are also induced to form as a result of the turbulent blood flow within the stenotic area. Brain infarction occurs as a result of the thrombus itself or by microemboli from the ulcerated plaques. Because the process of occlusion is gradual, many patients experience TIAs before the completed stroke.

Transient Ischemic Attacks

A cerebral TIA refers to the temporary occlusion of a cerebral blood vessel such that the symptoms resolve spontaneously and completely within 24 hours. (The symptoms are typically gone within minutes to hours.) TIAs are an indication of significant underlying atherosclerotic disease and are therefore often a precursor to a stroke or myocardial infarction. A prospective study compared control subjects (matched for cardiovascular risk factors) with people who experienced one TIA and followed them for 3 years. Although all-cause mortality was similar for both groups, those with TIAs were approximately four times more likely to experience a stroke and more than twice as likely to experience a myocardial infarction during each year of the follow-up period.[6]

TIAs are usually caused by thromboembolism; for example, an ulcerated placque in a carotid artery leads to thrombus formation. Microemboli break off the thrombus and travel to intracranial vessels. As these small emboli lodge in a vessel, causing symptoms such as aphasia, they are quickly dissolved, leading to quick resolution of the symptoms.

The symptoms depend on the location of the microemboli. Those originating in the carotid artery system may travel into the ophthalmic branch of the internal carotid artery or may travel into the vasculature of the cerebral hemispheres. People who experience retinal ischemia often report a sensation of a shade being pulled down over one eye. Transient loss of vision in one eye is called amaurosis fugax. Transient ischemia in a cerebral hemisphere leads to contralateral symptoms such as hemiparesis or a sensation of numbness or may cause temporary aphasia.

Microemboli originating in the vertebrobasilar arterial system may travel to the brain stem, cerebellum, thalamus, or occipital lobes. Symptoms again vary with the location of the ischemia. Unlike the visual disturbance caused by an embolism to the retina, an embolism to the occipital lobes causes dim or blurry vision or may even cause temporary blindness bilaterally. Double vision, or diplopia, may occur if an embolism reaches the area in the brain stem responsible for conjugate gaze. Cerebellar symptoms include unsteady gait and difficulty with coordination of movement. TIAs in the vertebrobasilar system are often related to a sudden change in posture that causes a sudden drop in the blood pressure and thus cerebrovascular insufficiency. If an elder's blood pressure is being kept too low (overaggressive antihypertensive therapy) or if there is severe orthostatic hypotension (anticholinergic medication side effect), a TIA may occur. Many older adults have osteophytes in the cervical spine. These bony projections may impinge on the vertebrobasilar arterial system with certain movements of the head, such as hyperextension.

When a patient gives a credible history of having experienced a TIA, the clinician should view this as an opportunity to prevent a stroke. A targeted workup should begin immediately. Physical assessment may provide clues as to the pathological mechanism of the TIA. For example, cardiac arrhythmias or murmurs would make the clinician consider the possibility of an intracardiac thrombus or a vegetation on a valve. Echocardiography is the most useful tool for further assessment of these cardiac problems. Evaluation of the carotid arteries is often an important part of the workup. Cerebral contrast angiography is the gold standard for examination of the vasculature, although this may be replaced by the newer and safer method of magnetic resonance angiography (MRA). Carotid ultrasound is a useful noninvasive screening method for the detection of moderate to severe stenosis.

> ✂ *A credible history of TIA represents an opportunity to prevent stroke.*

Treatment, aimed at the prevention of further TIAs or strokes, includes medication and surgery. Unless the patient has atrial fibrillation, in which case warfarin (Coumadin) is generally the preferred agent, aspirin therapy is the first medication to use. The optimal dosage has not been established, but 325 mg is commonly recommended. If a person is unable to take aspirin or continues to experience symptoms while taking aspirin, ticlopidine (Ticlid) should be tried. This medication inhibits platelet aggregation. In patients who have 70% to 90% stenosis of the appropriately symptomatic carotid artery, surgical intervention in the form of carotid endarterectomy should be considered. Age itself is not a contraindication to surgery; however, the diseases that commonly accompany aging (e.g., congestive heart failure, diabetes) may increase the risks of surgery.

Hemorrhagic Strokes

Although cerebral hemorrhage is less common than infarction, it is much more lethal.[7] Symptoms of an intracerebral bleed usually evolve over several hours and are often associated with headache. Unlike infarctions, in which the level of consciousness is rarely affected, hemorrhages are often associated with obtundation. Other signs of raised intracranial pressure may develop, such as vomiting, seizures, or nuchal rigidity. Intracerebral bleeding, usually caused by hypertension, is more common in the elderly than is subarachnoid bleeding. Subarachnoid hemorrhages are usually caused by ruptured aneurysms or arteriovenous malformations. Elders who are taking anticoagulant therapy, such as warfarin, are also at increased risk of hemorrhage.

The most common site of a spontaneous intracerebral hemorrhage is the putamen. Other areas that are also affected include the subcortical white matter, thalamus, cerebellum, and pons.[8]

▼ GEORGE PAUL (Part II)

Mr. Paul is admitted to a monitored bed. An intravenous (IV) solution of 5% dextrose in 0.45% normal saline is begun. Laboratory tests are all normal except a blood glucose level of 315 mg/dl and occasional unifocal premature ventricular contractions. A CT scan of the brain, taken the day of admission, is normal except for mild atrophy. Nursing begins regular turning and range-of-motion exercises. Physical, occupational, and speech therapy consults are obtained on the third hospital day. However, by day 5 Mr. Paul is still having problems with choking and his oral intake is low.

▼ MARIA HERNANDEZ (Part II)

Ms. Hernandez' respiratory status deteriorates, necessitating intubation. An emergency CT scan of the head reveals an intracerebral hemorrhage in the internal capsule and thalamus. There is no evidence of increased intracranial pressure. Blood pressure on admission was 190/110 but decreased to 170/95 within an hour. By the second day Ms. Hernandez begins to open her eyes but still seems confused.

STUDY QUESTIONS

▪ Is Mr. Paul's essentially normal CT compatible with your original diagnosis?

▪ How should you address Ms. Hernandez' apparent hypertension?

ACUTE STROKE MANAGEMENT

At this time there is no treatment that will cure a stroke. Management is directed at (1) limiting the extent of the stroke; (2) preventing secondary complications (both immediate and delayed); and (3) alleviating risk factors for subsequent strokes.

The initial step is to obtain an adequate data base. While completing the history and physical examination, laboratory tests can be ordered (Box 45-2). A lumbar puncture is rarely needed and may be dangerous if there is evidence of increased intracranial pressure (pupillary inequality, third nerve palsy, or obtundation). If the patient is suspected to have had an embolic stroke, echocardiography is indicated. Blood cultures may also be helpful to look for evidence of bacterial endocarditis. Cardiac monitoring for 24 to 48 hours to detect the commonly seen arrhythmias is advised.

It is important to establish if the stroke was due to an ischemic or hemorrhagic event, since the treatment varies dramatically depending on this distinction. A CT scan is the most useful and efficient method for making the determination. Whereas a hemorrhagic stroke appears immediately as an area of increased density, an ischemic stroke may not cause a visible abnormality on CT scan

for 2 to 4 days after the onset of symptoms. If the lesion is suspected to be in the brain stem or cerebellum, magnetic resonance imaging (MRI) is more sensitive than CT. Lacunar infarcts that are not visible on CT scanning may be seen on MRI.

If the stroke was hemorrhagic, the scan will also reveal the degree of mass effect and brain stem compression. Neurosurgical consultation should be sought if there is significant mass effect or rapid deterioration of the patient's condition. Only some patients are considered reasonable surgical candidates, depending on the location of the bleed and the degree of mass effect. Those with large hemorrhages in the subcortical white matter or putamen, particularly if they are worsening, are more likely to benefit from a craniotomy than those with pontine or thalamic hemorrhages. Patients with cerebellar hemorrhage are prone to sudden decompensation because of the proximity of the cerebellum to the brain stem, leading to brain stem compression. Unless the patient has a small (less than 3 cm) bleed, neurosurgical consultation should be obtained.[9]

> *Craniotomy should be considered in a large subcortical white matter or putamen hemorrhage, especially if the condition is worsening.*

The most important measures to prevent acute complications are maintenance of blood pressure, hydration, oxygenation, and metabolic balance. Often the blood pressure rises dramatically in an attempt to maintain adequate cerebral perfusion. Therefore it is important not to overtreat hypertension. In ischemic stroke, aggressive treatment is probably not needed unless the systolic blood pressure is greater than 220 mm Hg or the mean blood pressure is greater than 130 mm Hg.[10] There is no clear evidence that gives the clinician an exact algorithm for lowering blood pressure following a stroke. It should probably be treated in such a way that a gradual reduction is achieved over a period of several days.[11] Approximately two thirds of patients with hypertension at the time of the stroke become normotensive *without* any targeted intervention in a few days following the acute event.[12] If the pressure remains high, treatment may begin with a low dose of a medication that has minimal side effects, such as a calcium channel blocker or an angiotensin-converting enzyme inhibitor. When the blood pressure is out of control (an uncommon but well-known possibility), an intravenous infusion of nitroprusside may be necessary to prevent further damage. Sublingual calcium channel blockers should not be given, since a sudden and rapid decline in blood pressure may increase the volume of brain damage.

BOX 45-2
Laboratory Evaluation of Stroke

Always

Complete blood count with differential
Platelet count
Electrolytes
Renal and liver function blood tests
Prothrombin time and partial thromboplastin time
Urinalysis
Chest x-ray examination
Electrocardiogram with rhythm strip
CT scan

Also consider

MRI scan
Arterial blood gas or pulse oximetry
Holter monitor

> *Hypertension immediately following stroke may be the body's attempt to maintain perfusion: treat with care.*

When hypotension is noted, hypovolemia is the most likely cause.[13] Restoration of volume is important for the maintenance of adequate cardiac output. However, the clinician must be mindful of maintaining euvolemia, particularly in patients with hemorrhagic strokes, because fluid overload encourages cerebral edema.

The benefit of using heparin during the acute phase of an ischemic stroke is controversial. It is logical to think that heparin would minimize the damage that occurs during an ischemic stroke, but heparin carries risks such as hemorrhagic transformation of the ischemic area. In fact, a group of experts who formulated guidelines for the management of patients with acute ischemic strokes wrote, "Because data about the safety and efficacy of heparin in patients with acute ischemic stroke are insufficient and conflicting, no recommendation can be offered."[13] Heparin treatment can be considered if the blood pressure is not out of control, the stroke seems to be progressing, and there is no apparent contraindication to heparin therapy.

Some patients have acute respiratory problems and require ventilatory support. It is not necessary to give supplemental oxygen unless there is evidence of hypoxemia. Clinical signs of hypoxemia are easily confirmed by an arterial blood gas measurement or pulse oximetry.

Some promising new agents, such as N-methyl-D-asparate (NMDA), may reduce the amount of cellular death that occurs in ischemic strokes. Similar in principle to the reperfusion technique commonly used in acute myocardial infarctions, "clot busters" such as tissue plasminogen activator (t-PA) are being studied for their use in restoring blood flow to the ischemic area. Nimodipine is an accepted treatment in people who experience a subarachnoid hemorrhage. It reduces delayed ischemic complications and disability.[14] As more data become available and patient selection criteria are established, new forms of treatment for an acute stroke are likely to become available in the near future.

PREVENTING SECONDARY COMPLICATIONS

Prevention of secondary complications must begin immediately. This requires excellent nursing and allied health care. Certain problems are common (Table 45-2). Immobile patients must be turned every 2 hours to prevent pressure sores. The skin must be checked at least once a day by rolling the patient over and inspecting the sacrum, ischial, and greater trochanter areas, and heels. A Foley catheter may be needed initially but should be discontinued as soon as possible. Adequate nutrition may help to prevent pressure sores.

Some elderly may be undernourished at the time of their stroke; others become malnourished following the stroke because of swallowing difficulties (often in combination with cognitive problems). Dysphagia is a common problem in the acute phase, affecting 25% to 45% of patients following a stroke. A swallowing evaluation by a speech therapist and, if necessary, videofluoroscopy are helpful in diagnosing feeding problems. An intact gag reflex does not mean that oral feeding is safe; tongue movement and swallowing response (the transit time of a food bolus from the base of the tongue to the esophagus) are important factors in determining aspiration risk.[15] If a patient is unable to receive adequate nutrition through an oral feeding program, early use of tube feedings is indicated. A tracheostomy, especially with brain stem strokes, may be necessary to protect the airway. Attention to a patient's swallowing function may prevent an aspiration pneumonia and thus is a critically important part of the evaluation.

> *In stroke, minidose heparin until the patient is ambulatory, or at least mobile, is recommended by most; full heparinization following ischemic strokes cannot yet be recommended because of a lack of data.*

Venous thrombosis (or deep vein thrombosis [DVT]) occurs in at least 30% of patients with strokes. This complication is more likely in those who are put at bed rest or who have significantly limited mobility secondary to the stroke. Most authorities recommend using minidose heparin (5000 U subcutaneously every 12 hours) until the patient is ambulatory (in ideal situations) or at least out of bed and more mobile. Support stockings and sequential compression devices are also of benefit in DVT

Table 45-2   Secondary Complications of Stroke

Complication	Treatment
Pressure sores	Turning, avoid moisture, nutrition
Malnutrition	Special foods, exercises, positioning, tube feeding
Venous thrombosis	Stockings, minidose heparin
Contractures	Range-of-motion exercises
Pneumonia	Food changes, positioning, intubation
Nerve palsies	Proper body positioning
Conjunctivitis	Eyedrops, taping
Depression	Counseling, medications
Confusion	Reduction of drugs, reality orientation, family presence

prophylaxis. Many ongoing trials are examining the use of low molecular weight heparin for DVT prophylaxis. Recent studies comparing it with heparin have produced mixed results in terms of its efficacy, and, particularly in view of its significantly higher cost, there is no clear choice of agent. Many trials are under way, and a more definitive answer may soon be available.[16,17]

Contractures begin within 24 hours and lead to permanent shortening of tendons if the joint is not stretched. Twice-daily range-of-motion exercises by a physical therapist, nurse, or even the family are imperative. Nerve palsies, such as a peroneal or brachial plexus injury, occur when the affected body parts are malpositioned. The arm must never be allowed to lie under the body, and the paralyzed leg should not be left across the unaffected leg.

 Positioning and range of movement must begin immediately following stroke.

Shoulder pain frequently develops but is usually preventable. Subluxation occurs when the shoulder capsule muscles are paralyzed. Prevention includes proper bed positioning, avoidance of pulling on the shoulder, and physical therapy. Reflex sympathetic dystrophy may develop in persistently subluxated shoulders. This condition is characterized by erythema, edema, and pain in the affected extremity. Treatment includes physical therapy, shoulder slings or other physical supports, and nonsteroidal antiinflammatory drugs. Prevention is the best treatment.

Depression is seen in the majority of patients with left hemisphere stroke and often occurs in other stroke patients. It frequently goes undetected by clinicians. Its presence can affect functional recovery. Early detection and treatment are strongly advised. Antidepressant medication often is beneficial. Appropriate choices for elderly patients include desipramine, nortriptyline, trazodone, sertraline, or paroxetine. Choice of antidepressant is based on factors such as cardiovascular status, types of vegetative symptoms, and side effect profile. Starting at very low doses and gradually working up is important (Table 45-3). In some patients, when a more rapid response is desired, methylphenidate is useful.

 Depression following stroke occurs in many patients (especially following left hemispheric stroke), but it is often undetected, to the detriment of the patient's prognosis and recovery.

Confusion commonly follows a stroke. It may be directly related to the brain injury or secondary to drug effects, hypovolemia or hypotension, sensory deprivation, or depression. Attempts should be made to decrease all unnecessary medications. Positioning the patient in the room so that any visual field deficit is minimized and providing a view out a window, familiar pictures or music, and contact with family help.

▼ *GEORGE PAUL (Part III)*

By the seventh day, Mr. Paul is beginning to recover some motion in his hand and leg. However, the speech therapist is concerned about Mr. Paul's swallowing. He also has lost 3 lb since admission. She recommends that a videofluoroscopic examination be performed. A significant amount of aspiration is noted. Because the special feeding program has not improved his intake, a decision regarding placement of a feeding tube is needed.

▼ *MARIA HERNANDEZ (Part III)*

Ms. Hernandez is much more alert on the fifth day. Her blood pressure is now 160-190/90-100 mm Hg. She has started occupational therapy. During feeding, she rarely eats food from the left side of her plate. When she calls the nurses to ask where her juice is, they point out that it is sitting in the left corner of her tray. She has been more irritable and prone to sudden crying spells.

STUDY QUESTION

■ *What special aspects of both cases need to be addressed as the rehabilitative phase is entered?*

CASE DISCUSSION

Both patients are heading toward rehabilitation; feeding and unilateral neglect problems, as well as emotionality, are issues

Table 45-3   Commonly Used Antidepressants for Poststroke Depression

Medication	Usual Therapeutic Dose (mg/day)	Side Effects
Trazodone (Desyrel)	100-200	Mild anticholinergic activity; moderately sedating
Nortriptyline	25-50	Moderate anticholinergic activity; moderately sedating
Desipramine	75-100	Mild anticholinergic activity; mildly sedating
Sertraline (Zoloft)	25-150	Insomnia; agitation; nausea
Methylphenidate (Ritalin)	2.5-10	(Should be used only for short-term treatment); tachycardia; hypertension; nervousness

that will need to be addressed. The further management and rehabilitation of these patients is detailed in Chapter 11.

PLANNING FOR REHABILITATION
Recovery

In general, the larger the area of brain damage, the poorer the prognosis for recovery. There is, however, a natural progression of neurological recovery after a stroke. Areflexia changes to hyperreflexia over the first 48 to 72 hours. An initially flaccid or hypotonic limb progresses to hypertonicity, then to patterned synergistic movements, and finally to isolated motor control for return of normal function. The person's motor recovery may cease at any of these stages. There is a correlation between the rate and the amount of motor recovery; patients who move through this progression early in the recovery phase tend to have the most functional neurological return.[3] Although most motor recovery occurs within the first 3 months, aphasia may improve for 2 years following a stroke. Predictors of poor recovery after a stroke include no motor return after 1 month, neglect, poor cognition, persistent bowel incontinence, and coma at outset.[19]

Preparation for rehabilitation must begin immediately in the acute phase. Such preparation involves prevention of secondary conditions and preservation of functional abilities. In anticipation of beginning a rehabilitation program, consultation with a physiatrist or rehabilitation team is recommended early. Decisions regarding whether the patient is an appropriate rehabilitation candidate should be made after the consultation. The criteria for admission to a rehabilitation program are discussed in Chapter 11. Even if the patient is to go home, a consultation is valuable to prepare for home modifications and ongoing therapy.

It is heartening to note that the incidence of stroke in elderly people is declining. This is probably due to improvement in the recognition and treatment of risk factors such as hypertension, diabetes, and heart disease.[18]

SUMMARY

The primary care physician has a vital role in the acute management of stroke. The alert physician may pick up the history of TIA and be given the remarkable opportunity of directly preventing stroke. Determining the site of stroke assists in management, especially in relation to the management of speech difficulties, potential depression, and visuospatial difficulties, including unilateral neglect. Careful blood pressure management must follow the acute episode. New treatments are being assessed for ischemic stroke. Minidose heparinization is recommended for virtually all patients. Since most patients recover from stroke, aggressive efforts, assuming that intense rehabilitation will be carried out, should be started immediately. Range of movement and careful positioning are essential immediately following the acute episode.

POSTTEST

1. In the differentiation of infarction vs. hemorrhagic stroke, which one of the following statements is false?
   a. TIAs are rarely precursors of hemorrhage.
   b. The onset of hemorrhage is characteristically sudden.
   c. Infarction often occurs in sleep.
   d. Vomiting is rare in infarction.

2. Which one of the following statements involving in stroke management is false?
   a. Raised blood pressure should be reduced only in the poststroke patient with symptoms of hypertension and encephalopathy.
   b. Most authorities recommend minidose heparin until the patient is ambulatory.
   c. Dysphonia is a better indicator of risk of aspiration than gag reflex.
   d. Depression occurs in the majority of cases of left hemisphere strokes.

REFERENCES

1. Wolf PA, Kannel WB, McGee D: Epidemiology of strokes in North America. In Barrett HJ et al, eds: *Stroke, pathophysiology, diagnosis, and management,* New York, 1986, Churchill Livingstone.
2. Brummel-Smith K: Rehabilitation. In Cassell CK et al, eds: *Geriatric medicine,* New York, 1990, Springer-Verlag.
3. Kelly JF: Stroke rehabilitation for elderly patients. In Kemp B, Brummel-Smith K, Ramsdell JW, eds: *Geriatric rehabilitation,* Boston, 1990, McGraw-Hill.
4. Kelly JF, Winograd C: A functional approach to stroke management in elderly patients, *J Am Geriatr Soc* 33:48-60, 1985.
5. American Heart Association: *1993 Heart and Stroke Facts Statistics,* Dallas, 1993, The Association.
6. Howard G et al: A prospective reevaluation of transient ischemic attacks as a risk factor for death and fatal or non-fatal cardiovascular events, *Stroke* 25:342-345, 1994.
7. Tuhrim S et al: Prediction of intracerebral hemorrhage survival, *Ann Neurol* 24:258-263, 1988.

8. Brott T, Thalinger K, Hertzberg V: Hypertension as a risk factor for spontaneous intracerebral hemorrhage, *Stroke* 17:1078-1083, 1986.

9. Kotapka MJ, Flamm ES: Surgical management of spontaneous intracerebral hemorrhage. In Adams HP, ed: *Handbook of cerebrovascular disease,* New York, 1993, Marcel Dekker.

10. Litin SC: *Mayo clinical update* 11(1)1-3, Winter 1995.

11. Shuaib A, Hachinski V: Mechanisms and management of stroke in the elderly, *Can Med Assoc J* 145(5):433-443, 1991.

12. Wallace JD, Levy LL: Blood pressure after stroke, *JAMA* 246:2177-2180, 1981.

13. Adams HP et al: Guidelines for the management of patients with acute ischemic stroke, *Stroke* 25(9):1901-1914, 1994.

14. Ohman J, Servo A, Heiskanen O: Long term effects of nimodipine on cerebral infarcts and outcome after aneurysmal subarachnoid hemorrhage and surgery, *J Neurosurg* 74:8-13, 1991.

15. Elliott JL: Swallowing disorders in elderly: a guide to diagnosis and treatment, *Geriatrics* 4(1):95-113, 1988.

16. Turpie AG et al: A low-molecular-weight heparinoid compared with unfractionated heparin in the prevention of deep venous thrombosis in patients with acute ischemic stroke, *Ann Intern Med* 117(5):353-357, 1992.

17. Sandset PM et al: A double-blind and randomized placebo-controlled trial of low molecular weight heparin once daily to prevent deep vein thrombosis in acute ischemic stroke, *Semin Thromb Hemost* 16(Suppl):25-33, 1990.

18. Albers GW, Cutler RP: Cerebrovascular disease. In Dale DC, Federman DD, eds: *Scientific American medicine,* New York, 1994, Scientific American.

19. Jongbleed L: Prediction of function after stroke: a critical review, *Stroke* 17:765, 1986.

PRETEST ANSWERS

1. b
2. e

POSTTEST ANSWERS

1. a
2. c

CHAPTER 46

Parkinson's Disease

JAMES Q. MILLER

OBJECTIVES

On completion of this chapter, the reader will be able to:

1. Describe the symptoms and signs to be sought when parkinsonism is clinically suspected.

2. Describe the alternative approaches to Parkinson's disease treatment when the symptoms are mild.

3. Describe the generally accepted treatment regimen for Parkinson's disease when function is impaired.

4. Describe the involuntary movements that are not parkinsonian and should be differentiated in elders.

5. Describe the Parkinson's-like side effects of antipsychotics and their management.

1. Which one of the following is not a feature of Parkinson's disease?
   a. Slow movements
   b. Poor balance
   c. Spasticity
   d. Resting tremor
   e. Soft voice

2. Which one of the following statements is false?
   a. Parkinson's patients generally have small handwriting.
   b. Posture in Parkinson's disease is forward-bent.
   c. Writhing, twisting movements can complicate dopamine therapy.
   d. Selegiline (Eldepryl) can be discontinued when carbidopa-levodopa (Sinemet) is initiated.

▼ RUTH JONES (Part I)

Mrs. Jones is the 66-year-old director of volunteer services at your local hospital. She notes that she has slowed down to an inconvenient degree, so that she requires 25 minutes to dress each morning and can no longer prepare her breakfast rapidly enough to get to work on time. Friends note the development of her impassive face, too quiet voice, and slow, small-stepped gait.

STUDY QUESTIONS

▪ *What should be specifically sought from the history and physical examination to confirm the likelihood of Parkinson's disease?*

▪ *What other illnesses need to be considered in the differential diagnosis?*

▪ *What is the initial choice of therapy if signs of Parkinson's disease are found?*

The incidence of involuntary uncontrollable movements increases with age. They are abnormalities of purposeful voluntary coordinative muscle activity that are recognized primarily on the basis of clinical examination. With rare exceptions there are no radiographic or clinical laboratory characteristics that aid diagnosis. Parkinson's disease is the most important of these movement disorders. It is a classic disease of the basal ganglia whose management has been revolutionized by the identification of neuron transmitter abnormalities and the development of pharmacotherapy.

Parkinson's disease, first described in 1817,[1] occurs in approximately 1% of Americans over 55 years of age. Its cause is unknown. Its increased incidence in the elderly suggests the possibility of environmental toxins as causal agents. Whatever the cause or causes may be, alteration in the basal ganglia is important: there is neuronal loss in the zona compacta of the substantia nigra and diminution of the neurotransmitter, dopamine, in the striate nuclei, putamen, and caudate nuclei. Since other neuron-depleting diseases (abiotrophies) may cause neuronal death in other areas of the basal ganglia and adjacent

BOX 46-1
Parkinsonism, Parkinson's, and Parkinson's Plus: Definitions

Parkinsonism

A clinical syndrome including bradykinesia, postural imbalance, cogwheel rigidity, and tremor at rest. Clinical manifestations also may include impassive face, poverty of associated movements, short-stepped forward-flexed gait, festination, soft voice, difficulty initiating walking, arising, or other girdle-moving actions, and resting tremor minimized during muscle activities.

Parkinson's Disease

One cause of parkinsonism; it is of unknown etiology and is associated with death of nerve cells in the zona compacta of the substantia nigra and other basal ganglia: an abiotrophy of nerve cells in the dopamine pathway.

Parkinson's Plus (Parkinson's-like diseases)

Other abiotrophies associated with neuronal loss, both in the dopamine pathways and also in other regional neuronal systems; there is a less favorable clinical response to dopamine replacement therapy:
   Supranuclear palsy
   Primary autonomic failure
   Olivopontocerebellar atrophy
   Corticobasal atrophy

brain, clinical manifestations of parkinsonism occur both in Parkinson's disease and in related disorders. Thus Parkinson's disease is one, but not the only, cause of the clinical syndrome of parkinsonism (Box 46-1).

PHYSICAL EXAMINATION

The clinical features of Parkinson's disease are summarized in Box 46-2. Effective diagnosis relies on maintaining an appropriate degree of clinical suspicion, recognizing that individuals with metabolic disorders and with depression may also appear bradykinetic and that poor

BOX 46-2
Features of Parkinsonism

Bradykinesia

All activities are performed more slowly than normal, including the acts of dressing, shaving, eating, etc.

Imbalance

The patient may be at risk of falling and may show a forward-bend posture, often with a tendency to fall backward.

Rigidity

There is poverty of movement associated with walking, such as decreased arm swing, and there is diminished facial animation. There may be a weak voice; examination reveals cogwheel resistance to passive extremity movement, especially when the patient is distracted.

Tremor at Rest

Tremor typically involves the distal extremities and diminishes or stops with voluntary actions; tremors may increase with excitement or agitation.

Other Features

Hesitancy initiating actions, such as when stepping out in walking

Decomposition of complex acts, such as requiring many steps to turn around

Gait arrest when encountering a doorway or reaching a corner

Micrographia

---

balance and muscular rigidity are nonspecific and frequent findings in many frail elders. The onset is often insidious, which easily delays diagnosis.

When parkinsonism is suspected, the examination must include an assessment of gait, with observation of the person walking freely if possible, so that diminished associated movements such as arm swing, for example, can be perceived. A sufficiently prolonged walk with the patient may show gait arrest when the patient encounters the need to turn a corner or reaches a doorway. The recommended tests of gait and balance to be conducted with any older person include asking the patient to turn around completely; this may demonstrate decomposition of this movement (the patient taking many steps to achieve it), which is also a parkinsonian sign.

The "push on sternum" test should be performed in patients with suspected Parkinson's disease.

Most clinicians favor, in suspected parkinsonism, a formal test of balance and its correction: the "push on sternum" test. The patient stands beside the examiner, and the examiner's hand is behind the patient's back. A clear explanation must be given to the patient as to what is to be done. A sharp push on the sternum would, in a normal individual, rapidly produce corrective action to maintain the upright posture. In patients with Parkinson's disease, and also in very deconditioned elders, a tendency to stagger backward without correction is revealed. It is usually clinically obvious if imbalance and a tendency to fall backward are part of generalized deconditioning; in an individual who is able to stand readily and yet exhibits these deficits, this is a parkinsonian sign. Examination of mental status is often indicated; but if no examination is conducted, an opportunity should be created to see the patient's handwriting and if possible compare it with previous efforts.

Mental status should generally be examined objectively in older patients with Parkinson's disease, and a very careful history regarding the onset should be obtained.

▼ RUTH JONES (Part II)

Physical examination reveals convincing signs of parkinsonism. Not only is Mrs. Jones bradykinetic, she has a forward-bent posture and tends to fall backward, walks with diminished arm swing, and has little facial animation. There is a hint of cogwheel-like resistance to passive movement of her arms, but little tremor. She is started on amantadine 100 mg bid and selegiline 5 mg bid with a 50% improvement in speed of gait and daily activities. She continues working. Eight months later her bradykinesia has increased and her effectiveness at work is impaired. She begins a leave of absence.

STUDY QUESTIONS

- *What caused the improvement in her symptoms?*
- *Was this the appropriate medication approach?*
- *What should you do next?*

DOPAMINE AND ACETYLCHOLINE

Proper function of the motor pathway in the brain depends on production of dopamine in the zona compacta of the substantia nigra and its conveyance via nigrostriatal axons to the striate basal ganglia. There should be a balance in the basal ganglia between the two neurotransmitters, acetylcholine and dopamine. The death of nerve cells in the substantia nigra causes depletion of dopamine in the striatum.

The treatment of parkinsonism relies primarily on strategies to *increase* dopamine or *decrease* acetylcholine and thereby restore the appropriate balance between these two neurotransmitters to the caudate nucleus. The major treatment of Parkinson's disease is dopamine replacement, although some benefit can be obtained from anticholinergic medication, amantadine, and dopaminomimetic drugs, such as bromocriptine, which activate postsynaptic dopamine receptors.

DOPAMINE REPLACEMENT THERAPY: TWO VIEWS

One school of thought holds that Parkinson's disease is a dopamine deficiency state and that carbidopa-levodopa is indicated from the onset, even in patients with little or no occupational or personal disability.[2-6]

The second perspective contends that dopamine metabolism itself may exert a toxic effect on Parkinson's disease neurons, termed "oxidative stress," and therefore that carbidopa-levodopa should be delayed in patients with minimal disease. In addition, there is evidence that selegiline (L-deprenyl, Eldepryl), a monoamine oxidase B inhibitor, has a neuroprotective function in Parkinson's disease, slowing the pace of neuronal damage otherwise associated with dopamine metabolism.[7,8] Supplementary to this perspective is the view that rapid blood dopamine fluctuations are hurtful to neuronal functional survival.

> *In early Parkinson's disease it is reasonable to delay levodopa-carbidopa until there is functional impairment; selegiline can be started immediately.*

TREATMENT STRATEGIES IN THE EARLY STAGES

For the primary care physician, early-stage treatment should seek these goals:

1. Delay institution of exogenous levodopa therapy while other parkinsonian medications, such as amantadine and anticholinergics, keep the patient functionally effective.
2. Use selegiline (Eldepryl) for its "neuroprotective" effects.
3. Institute levodopa-carbidopa (Sinemet) therapy whenever *functional impairment* commences.
4. Attend to the psychological, social, and rehabilitative aspects of each patient.

The mechanism of the antiparkinsonian drugs is summarized in Table 46-1, and the initial treatments while Parkinson's symptoms are mild are summarized in Box 46-3.

TREATMENT WHEN FUNCTION IS IMPAIRED

Undoubtedly, once there is functional impairment from the Parkinson's disease, carbidopa-levodopa (Sinemet) is the mainstay of treatment. (Boxes 46-4 and 46-5). It should replace drugs previously used in the patient, except for selegiline 5 mg bid, which should be continued. Adults should receive at least 75 mg of daily oral carbidopa for maximum benefit. A reasonable starting regimen would be 1 tablet of carbidopa-levodopa 25/100 bid taken half an hour before meals, with an increase to tid and at bedtime. The duration of therapeutic effect is 3 to 5 hours, with an onset 20 to 30 minutes after ingestion. Onset of benefit is delayed by food, particularly

Table 46-1 Mechanism of Antiparkinsonian Treatments

Treatment	Mechanism
Anticholinergics	Diminishes striatal acetylcholine
Amantadine	Enhances striatal dopamine release
L-Dopa (levodopa)	Restores striatal dopamine
Bromocriptine	Mimics dopamine
Pergolide	Mimics dopamine
Cryothalamotomy	Interrupts pathways from striatum to motor cortex and cord
Selegiline	Monoamine oxidase inhibition increases available dopamine

---

BOX 46-3
Treatment Strategy for Mild Parkinsonism

Anticholinergics (Artane, Cogentin, Akineton, etc.)
  Be attentive to urinary retention
  1-2 mg qd to tid (individualize)
Amantadine (Symmetrel) 100 mg qd to bid
  Mild symptomatic benefit in some patients
Selegiline (Deprenyl) 5 mg bid
  Its neuroprotective benefit is not agreed upon by all authorities

---

BOX 46-4
Treatment Strategy for Severe Parkinson's Disease

Carbidopa-levodopa (Sinemet)
  Start with 25/100 ½ tablet bid or tid, individualize stepwise increases to optimal response
  or
  Sustained release 50/200 1 tablet qd, and increase to optimal response
Discontinue anticholinergics and/or amantadine
Continue selegiline (Eldepryl) 5 mg bid

protein-rich meals. Sustained release carbidopa-levodopa may minimize the "wearing away" phenomenon (loss of dopamine benefit before the next dose takes effect). Some patients benefit from carbidopa-levodopa every 1½ to 2 hours during some parts of the day. Some patients change rapidly from parkinsonian akinesia to dopamine-induced hyperkinesia and back to akinesia. This complex "on-off" state is best addressed by careful attention to the scheduled dopamine administration. The patient should avoid any medication that blocks dopamine uptake, such as butyrophenone, haloperidol (Haldol), or the phenothiazines, since they interfere with the intended goal of levodopa replacement therapy. It is appropriate to teach the patient and family the principles of levodopa administration so that they can participate in the development of an optimal dosage sequence and titration; they also must be able to recognize and report levodopa side effects.

> *Levodopa-carbidopa (Sinemet) is the mainstay of Parkinson's treatment once function becomes impaired.*

▼ RUTH JONES (Part III)

You replace amantadine with carbidopa-levodopa 25/100 mg four times daily, with a return to 90% of her premorbid voice strength, vigor, and speed of activity. A mild distal pill-rolling tremor is observed in her hands when at rest. She returns to work. Over the next 2 years, with minimal increases in the carbidopa-levodopa to 25/100 mg six times daily, her parkinsonism is controlled sufficiently that she enjoys normal balance and gait. She continues work, despite a mild tremor of the hands at rest, but her face remains less animated than it had been before the onset of the Parkinson's disease. At the age of 69 she retires but is able to continue working as a volunteer hospital receptionist.

BOX 46-5
Principles of Carbidopa-Levodopa Therapy in Parkinson's Disease

Carbidopa-levodopa (Sinemet) should replace other
    parkinsonian drugs, except selegiline.
Onset of therapeutic action is delayed by protein foods.
Duration of effect is 3 to 5 hours in most patients.
Sustained release forms aid some patients to minimize
    response fluctuations.
Excessive dopamine levels may cause dopamine dyski-
    nesia: writhing and twisting movements, usually of
    neck, face, and torso, etc.

PRINCIPLES OF MEDICATION TREATMENT

There are different practical applications of therapy in the individual patient, but these principles are generally agreed upon:

1. Parkinson's disease is a dopamine-deficiency state secondary to progressive neuronal cell loss, and carbidopa-levodopa (Sinemet) by mouth is the most effective replacement therapy.
2. Amantadine (Symmetrel) maximizes available dopamine.
3. Anticholinergics benefit dopamine-deficiency Parkinson's disease, especially tremor.
4. Selegiline (Eldepryl) can provide minimal symptomatic improvement but may prolong the time before the need to start carbidopa-levodopa therapy.
5. The institution of dopamine agonists, such as bromocriptine (Parlodel) and pergolide (Permax), may benefit patients with Parkinson's disease who become unresponsive to medications or who do not respond well to levodopa replacement therapy; some authorities advocate coadministration of levodopa and dopamine agonists early in the treatment of Parkinson's disease.

Amantadine or anticholinergics might be a consideration *before* carbidopa-levodopa is initiated if the patient's symptoms are not disabling. Selegiline may be justifiable from the outset and for life. Bromocriptine or pergolide is generally a consideration later in the illness, when the patient is becoming less responsive to the levodopa.

▼ RUTH JONES (Part IV)

One year later, at her regular health maintenance checkup, Mrs. Jones mentions her readings about Parkinson's disease and her concern that levodopa is known to "wear off." She asks about other therapy that might be useful in the future. You describe the possibility of adjustment in dosage, but particularly mention the medications bromocriptine and pergolide, which can be used if the levodopa eventually stops working. You discuss the probable importance of continuing selegiline to maintain responsiveness to the levodopa. You encourage her to join the Parkinson's support group that meets regularly in your area.

> *Treatment should begin with amantadine or anticholinergics and selegiline and then progress to levodopa/carbidopa when functionally impaired; bromocriptine and/or pergolide should only be started when levodopa-carbidopa loses effect.*

PARKINSON'S AND COGNITION

Mental and psychological changes occur in patients with Parkinson's disease; the etiology is often unclear. Dementia occurs in about 30% of parkinsonian patients, some of whom show MRI evidence of diffuse cortical atrophy. In addition, levodopa therapy and anticholinergic therapy for Parkinson's disease are occasional causes of hallucinations, confusion, and psychotic thinking. The relationship between medication and mentation is unique to the patient; some develop disordered thought on medication, whereas others enjoy clear thought after appropriate antiparkinsonian medicines have been instituted, possibly by virtue of the increased mobility and social interaction made possible by the drugs. When mental changes are caused by levodopa therapy, it is usually relatively soon after institution of medication; it is also more common in patients who have a history of thought disorder before their Parkinson's disease.

SURGERY

The role of surgery in Parkinson's disease is extremely limited.[9] Thalamotomy does benefit refractory tremor in some parkinsonian patients. However, tremor is seldom disabling in parkinsonism, so surgery has limited applicability. Bilateral cryothalamotomy is particularly likely to result in pseudobulbar palsy. There is lively interest in the possible role of surgical transplantation of either fetal or cultured adrenal medullary tissue into the basal ganglia of parkinsonian patients. To date, results of such procedures are variable and generally disappointing. Transplantation remains an experimental strategy at present.

OTHER PARKINSON'S-LIKE CONDITIONS

Other neuron-depleting disorders may impede the dopamine pathway and produce parkinsonism. The clue for the primary care physician is the presence of neurological signs not found in classic Parkinson's disease *or* failure of clinical response to levodopa replacement therapy. These neurological conditions, although less frequent than Parkinson's disease, increase in prevalence in the older population. The most important of them and a clinical clue to the presence of each is summarized in Box 46-6.

NONPARKINSONIAN INVOLUNTARY MOVEMENTS

The many involuntary movements encountered in the elderly are summarized in Box 46-7.

BOX 46-6
Parkinsonian Syndromes Other Than Parkinson's Disease

Progressive supranuclear palsy (Steele-Richardson-Olszewski syndrome)
  Parkinsonism with impairment of vertical gaze
Primary autonomic failure (Shy-Drager syndrome)
  Parkinsonism with postural hypotension and urinary incontinence
Olivopontocerebellar degeneration
  Parkinsonism with cerebellar signs

BOX 46-7
Involuntary Movements in the Elderly

Tremors
Rhythmical alternating contractions of opposed muscle groups

Parkinsonian tremor: resting tremor; diminishes with action
Cerebellar tremor: absent at repose; intensifies with action; exaggerates at *end* of action
Essential, senile, or familial tremor: distal action tremor, especially in hands; may be familial; may have head nodding

Focal Dystonia
Slow sustained muscle contractions

Blepharospasm: forcible, repetitive eye closure
Torticollis, retrocollis: neck spasms
Spasmodic dysphonia: strangled speech

Generalized Dystonia
Slow sustained large muscle contractions

Often of trunk and girdle

Complications of Neuroleptic Drugs
Tardive dyskinesia
Dystonia
Akathisia
Rigidity

Tics
Can be mimicked; often are habits

Chorea
Arrhythmic, rapid jerks; patient may try to incorporate into voluntary movements

Athetosis
Slow, sinuous, writhing distortion of digits, face, and limbs

Cerebellar Tremor

Signs of cerebellar disease depend on the location of the lesions within the cerebellum: cerebellar hemisphere lesions produce ipsilateral incoordination and tremor; disease of the midline cerebellar vermis causes poor balance, titubation (shaking of the head and trunk), and a wide-based ataxic gait. There may or may not be nystagmus, and there is no sensory abnormality. The tremor of cerebellar hemisphere disease is in many ways the antithesis of parkinsonian tremor (Box 46-8). Minimal at rest, it intensifies with voluntary activity and may clearly disrupt handwriting, speech, feeding, etc. On finger-to-nose or heel-to-shin testing, it causes a dysrhythmic right-angle tremor toward the *end* of the action. In contrast, the patient with cerebellar vermis disease may have little tremor but, when erect, manifests titubation and has difficulty standing with approximated feet. Daily activities may be facilitated by providing support, such as eating in a chair with a high back or stabilizing the elbow on the tabletop. Drug therapy of cerebellar tremor is unsuccessful in most instances. Diazepam (Valium) or clonazepam (Klonopin) may minimize tremor, and occasional patients benefit from the anticonvulsant primidone (Mysoline).

Blepharospasm

Dystonia is sustained concurrent contraction of *opposing* muscle groups and leads to such movements as the repetitive head twisting of torticollis and retrocollis or the forcible eye closure of blepharospasm. When blepharospasm coexists with dystonic contraction of laryngeal muscles, it is called Meige's syndrome. Pharmacotherapy is variable in effect and usually disappointing. Careful injections of botulinum toxin provide temporary, but often long-lasting, paralysis of the offending muscles and may be used for spasmodic dysphonia, blepharospasm, and torticollis-retrocollis if pharmacotherapy fails. Appropriate drugs that are of occasional benefit include clonazepam (Klonopin), haloperidol (Haldol), amitriptyline, and anticholinergic antiparkinsonian medications. Occasionally, selective surgical destruction of terminal branches of the facial nerve to the orbicularis oculi muscles is required; this procedure, and repetitive use of botulinum toxin, may lead to permanent paralysis of the affected muscle.

Essential or Senile Tremor

Essential, familial, or senile tremor is an action tremor, usually bilateral, and resembles an exaggeration of the tremor of anxiety. It is usually most manifest when the arms are held extended and the head is erect. Tremor of the voice and facial muscles and head nodding may accompany it, or it may be the only manifestation. Familial tremor tends to appear in young adulthood. The tremor is often ameliorated by alcohol and is occasionally helped by β-blockers or diazepam (Valium).

▼ *JAMES ELDER (Part I)*

Mr. Elder is a 79-year-old retired minister who remains independent in all daily activities. Recently he has become progressively more forgetful, and he is occasionally unable to manage family finances and the complexities of the professional journals to which he subscribes. He has become severely anxious and recurrently agitated because he and his wife have been forced to sell their home and move into a retirement community under meager financial circumstances. You prescribe trifluoperazine 1 mg bid (Stelazine), which improves his anxiety considerably. After the move his wife notes that he is inanimate in facial expression, slow, slightly tremulous while eating, and excessively sleepy and uninterested.

> **BOX 46-8**
> **Parkinsonism and Cerebellar Disease Compared**
>
> Parkinsonism
> *Major features*
> Slowness and poverty of movements
> Cogwheel rigidity
> Postural instability
> Tremor at rest; pill-rolling
>
> *Associated features*
> Low volume voice
> Diminished facial animation
> Festinating gait
>
> Cerebellar Lesions
> *Major features*
> Poorly coordinated movements of normal speed
> Normal (decreased?) tone
> No tremor at repose
>
> *Associated features*
> Terminal, right-angle action tremor
> May have titubation when erect

Antipsychotic Drugs

Dopamine blocking medications, such as the phenothiazines trifluoperazine (Stelazine), fluphenazine (Prolixin), thioridazine (Mellaril), thiothixene (Navane), and chlorpromazine (Thorazine), and the butyrophenone haloperidol (Haldol), are antipsychotic medications with considerable risk of involuntary movement as a side effect. Four different neuroleptic side effects, which are not particularly related to the elderly, may occur as an idiosyncratic reaction shortly after the drug is administered or may have their onset months or even years later:

1. *Acute dystonias,* such as acute torticollis or oculogyric crisis, after administration of phenothiazines,

particularly if given intravenously or intramuscularly. The dyskinesia disappears with time and may respond to the administration of 1 mg of benztropine (Cogentin) or 50 mg of diphenhydramine (Benadryl).

2. *Akathisia,* which is a continual motor restlessness, may begin during the first month of therapy. It usually ceases after drug cessation or with the use of antiparkinsonian anticholinergic medications.

3. *Parkinsonian akinesia and rigidity* (extrapyramidal syndrome, EPS) may begin within the first month of the initiation of these medications. It usually diminishes with reduction of dose or with institution of antiparkinsonian anticholinergics.

4. *Tardive dyskinesia (TD)* is a syndrome of repetitive rhythmic mouth, lip, and tongue movements (sometimes like chewing or smacking of the lips) and is often associated with facial grimacing, head bobbing, tongue thrusting, or twisting movements of the neck and trunk. It is most common in older women who have received prolonged antipsychotic therapy. The diagnosis rests on the recognition of the involuntary movements. Tardive dyskinesia may abate after cessation of the antipsychotic medication and should be considered a long-lasting rather than a necessarily permanent condition, although it does sometimes persist. The risk should be balanced against the need for the medication, especially in women. Drug therapy is not particularly helpful, although there are some reports of benefit from the use of valproate (Depakote) and baclofen (Lioresal).

▼ *JAMES ELDER (Part II)*

You discontinue the trifluoperazine, resulting in improvement in the sleepiness and tremor, but other parkinsonian manifestations continue and no improvement in mentation occurs.

STUDY QUESTIONS

■ *Could the phenothiazine have caused these persistent parkinsonian manifestations, as his wife believes?*

■ *What further medication is reasonable to attempt if the parkinsonian symptoms persist?*

▼ *JAMES ELDER (Part III)*

You examine Mr. Elder 4 weeks after the trifluoperazine has been discontinued. Although he converses sociably, his lack of facial animation is striking and his voice is weak. He walks stiffly, swinging his arms little. Tremor is slight, and he walks with a bent posture. Standing next to him, after warning him and with your hand behind him, you press sharply on his sternum and he staggers backward without being able to correct himself. Formal testing with the Mini–Mental Status results in a score of 21/30, consistent with only mild dementia, but you are impressed by the extremely small size of his handwriting in the voluntary sentence. Diagnosing parkinsonism, you institute amantadine 100 mg bid. He becomes more animated and speedier, but during the third week of therapy he becomes markedly hallucinated, with unpleasant images of animals in his bedroom causing considerable fright. You replace the amantadine with carbidopa-levodopa 25/100 bid and slowly increase it to qid, causing marked reduction of all parkinsonian signs and symptoms but no improvement in memory or clarity of thought. You alter it to 50/200 bid, and the benefits continue.

SUMMARY

Parkinson's disease is an important problem in old age and must be specifically sought when there are suggestive symptoms. There is reasonable consensus about the appropriate approach to medication at this time. There are a number of other causes of parkinsonism, as well as other types of involuntary movement, which all must be considered in the differential diagnosis and for which specific treatment strategies are sometimes useful.

POSTTEST

1. Which one of the following statements is true?
   a. If carbidopa-levodopa (Sinemet) is needed as often as every 2 hours, the dose is too low.
   b. Amantadine (Symmetrel) should be continued when carbidopa-levodopa (Sinemet) is initiated.
   c. Bromocriptine (Parlodel) is indicated when levodopa treatment starts to fail.
   d. The "on-off" phenomenon is treated by avoidance of dopamine therapy.
2. Which one of the following statements is false?
   a. Amantadine (Symmetrel) maximizes available dopamine.
   b. Selegiline (Eldepryl) generally causes significant relief of symptoms.
   c. Cryothalamotomy helps refractory tremor in some Parkinson's patients.
   d. Titubation suggests a cerebellar lesion.

3. Which of the following statements is false?
   a. Cerebellar tremor characteristically involves a right angle, end-action tremor.
   b. Drug therapy for cerebellar tremor is generally successful.
   c. Familial tremor characteristically onsets in young adulthood.
   d. Antipsychotic-induced tardive dyskinesia is more common in women.
4. Match the medication with the syndrome it may help:
   1. Tardive dyskinesia   A. Benztropine (Cogentin)
   2. Oculogyric crisis   B. Clonazepam (Klonopin)
   3. Essential (familial) tremor   C. Alcohol
   4. Blepharospasm   D. Valproate (Depakote)

REFERENCES

1. Parkinson J: *An essay on the shaking palsy,* London, 1817, Sherwood, Neely, & Jones.
2. Calne BB: Treatment of Parkinson's disease, *N Eng J Med* 329:1021-1026, 1993.
3. Parkinson's disease: one illness and many syndromes? [editorial], *Lancet* 339:1263-1264, 1992.
4. Jankovic J, Shoulson I, Weiner WJ: Early stage Parkinson's disease: to treat or not to treat, *Neurology* 44(suppl 1):S4-S7, 1994.
5. Calne BB, Duvoisin RC, Koller WC: Individualizing therapy in patients with disabling Parkinson's disease symptoms, *Neurology* 44(suppl 1):S8-S11, 1994.
6. Tanner CM, Melamed U, Lees AJ: Managing motor fluctuations, dyskinesias, and other adverse effects in Parkinson's disease, *Neurology* 44(suppl 1):S12-S16, 1994.
7. Parkinson's Study Group: Effect of deprenyl on the progression of disability in early Parkinson's disease, *N Engl J Med* 321:1364-1371, 1989.
8. Tetiad JA, Langston JW: The effect of deprenyl (selegiline) on the natural history of Parkinson's disease, *Science* 245:519-528, 1989.
9. Olanow CW et al: The role of surgery in Parkinson's disease, *Neurology* 44(suppl 1):S17-S20, 1994.

PRETEST ANSWERS
1. c
2. d

POSTTEST ANSWERS
1. c
2. b
3. b
4. 1–d
   2–a
   3–c
   4–b

CHAPTER 4 7

Lower Respiratory Infections

ALICE K. POMIDOR

OBJECTIVES

Upon completion of this chapter, the reader will be able to:

1. Diagnose acute bronchitis and prescribe appropriate therapy.

2. Explain how basic mechanisms of disease in chronic obstructive pulmonary disease (COPD) present as clinical symptoms.

3. Implement stepwise escalation of therapy to treat symptoms and prevent disease progression in COPD.

4. Assess individual risk factors for pneumonia.

5. Choose appropriate empirical antibiotic therapy for pneumonia according to risk factor assessment.

6. Screen for tuberculosis correctly using the two-step Mantoux test.

7. Interpret tuberculin skin test results accurately and recommend appropriate treatment.

8. Prescribe effective prophylactic and supportive therapy for influenza.

9. Organize an office-based influenza immunization program.

PRETEST

1. Which one of the following groups of organisms is most likely to be responsible for acute bronchitis?
   a. *Streptococcus pneumoniae, Haemophilus influenzae, Moraxella catarrhalis*
   b. Rhinovirus, parainfluenzae
   c. *Enterococcus, Escherichia coli*
   d. *Staphylococcus aureus, Haemophilus influenzae, Mycoplasma pneumoniae*
2. Signs and symptoms of COPD correlate with which one of the following?
   a. Centrilobular emphysema and ventilation/perfusion mismatch
   b. Chronic bronchitis and airway obstruction
   c. Mucus hypersecretion and hypoxemia
   d. Asthma and elevated right-sided heart pressure
3. Which one of the following is true regarding the initial signs and symptoms of pneumonia in the older person?
   a. The symptoms are usually obvious on examination.
   b. Symptoms should always include shortness of breath.
   c. The only symptoms may be weakness, confusion, or tachypnea.
   d. Symptoms of pneumonia can easily be distinguished from congestive heart failure.

Lower respiratory infections (LRI) in older adults are a significant source of both morbidity and mortality in the United States. Common LRI syndromes include acute bronchitis, chronic obstructive pulmonary disease (COPD) and its acute exacerbations, influenza, pneumonia, and tuberculosis (TB). These syndromes are frequently difficult to distinguish from one another when they develop in frail elders, and they may progress from less serious airway disease to potentially fatal parenchymal involvement before the clinician can identify and treat the original disease. Patients are often believed to have bronchitis or cancer and may die without the primary etiologies of tuberculosis (TB) or bronchopneumonia ever being discovered.

Elderly persons are particularly vulnerable to respiratory diseases. For example, the U.S. TB case rate was 20.6 per 100,000 population in persons aged 65 and older in 1987 but only 4.6 per 100,000 population in young adults.[1] COPD was the fourth leading cause of death in that same year for persons age 65 and older, accounting for 64,477 deaths. Pneumonia and influenza together were the fifth leading cause of death in 1987 for persons age 65 and older, accounting for 60,571 deaths.[2] More so than with many other illnesses, treatment decisions and outcomes depend heavily on epidemiological factors such as age, functional status, and general health.[2a] Physicians need to be comfortable with the detection, management, and control of the spectrum of lower respiratory infections.

> *In persons age 65 and older, COPD is the fourth leading cause of death and pneumonia and influenza together are the fifth leading cause.*

▼ LARRY BURKE (Part I)

Larry Burke is a 66-year-old former smoker who became short of breath while playing golf and had to quit playing after nine holes instead of his usual 18. He has taken theophylline for years for chronic bronchitis, occasionally requiring nebulizer treatments for acute exacerbations. His only other long-term medication is albuterol by metered dose inhaler as needed, which he used last night and this morning. He recently visited his grandchildren, who both had runny noses. Mr. Burke felt well until yesterday morning, when he noticed that his thick morning sputum was yellow instead of the usual white. Today he has a headache and is unusually tired. He coughs intermittently throughout the interview. He denies fever, chills, or chest pain. He quit smoking 2 years ago, although he admits to a 40-year history of smoking during his career as an electrical engineer.

ACUTE BRONCHITIS
Pathogenesis

Acute bronchitis is an inflammation of the tracheobronchial tree typically resulting from viral infection with adenovirus or influenza, although respiratory syncytial virus and parainfluenza are sometimes acquired from exposure to children.[3] Cough is usually present, and mucoid sputum is produced in about half of the cases.[4] In older adults the most common early symptoms are anorexia, malaise, and headache; chest pain and fever can be present in severe infection. Lung findings are often unremarkable but can include rhonchi and wheezing, especially in patients with underlying chronic lung disease.

▼ LARRY BURKE (Part II)

Mr. Burke has normal vital signs, a few scattered rhonchi that clear with cough, and no wheezing on auscultation. He is sent home with the recommendation that he rest, continue to use his inhaler as needed, take guaifenesin every 4 hours, drink plenty of fluids, and call if he has any further difficulty. Two days later his wife calls to report that he seems more short of breath, is producing much more sputum, and now has a temperature of 100° F. On examination Mr. Burke appears mildly ill with a respiratory rate of 20, widely scattered rhonchi that do not clear on cough, and wheezing that does clear after one albuterol nebulizer treatment.

Diagnosis

Secondary bacterial infection is common following influenza and in patients with chronic lung disease or immunocompromising illnesses. Because symptoms of pneumonia and bronchitis are similar, a chest x-ray examination should be performed in patients who appear ill or do not respond to initial treatment. Sputum gram stain is helpful in guiding therapy, but sputum is often unobtainable and may be contaminated by oral colonization in patients with chronic lung disease. The most common causative bacteria are *Haemophilus influenzae* and *Streptococcus pneumoniae;* in patients with COPD *Moraxella catarrhalis* is also frequently found.[4,5]

▼ *LARRY BURKE (Part III)*

Mr. Burke's chest film shows increased lucency and flattening of both hemidiaphragms consistent with COPD, but no acute interstitial disease or infiltrate is found. The white blood cell count (WBC) is normal, although mild lymphocytosis is noted. Sputum is of good quality (greater than 25 WBCs, fewer than 10 epithelial cells per high power field) but is read as "normal oropharyngeal flora." Mr. Burke is sent home and prescribed trimethoprim-sulfamethoxazole twice a day for 14 days, with albuterol inhaler treatments every 4 hours. One week later he is feeling much better but still has a moderately productive cough. The albuterol inhaler treatments are discontinued. On follow-up 2 weeks later, Mr. Burke says he feels his usual self again.

Treatment

Patients should be treated with general supportive therapy, including rest, fluids, antipyretic-analgesic agents, and cough suppressants if appropriate. When possible, antibiotic selection should be guided by results of the sputum Gram stain and culture, but empirical coverage of the most common causative organisms can usually be achieved with amoxicillin, second-generation cephalosporins, erythromycin, tetracyclines, or trimethoprim-sulfamethoxazole.[3] Use of broad-spectrum antibiotics like the newer, more expensive macrolides and quinolones is generally unnecessary unless dictated by local bacterial

resistance patterns or an unusually immunocompromised host. For patients with severe chronic bronchitis, prophylaxis with low-dose tetracycline or trimethoprim-sulfamethoxazole may be prescribed during winter months or when an exacerbation would be life threatening.

> *In acute bronchitis, empirical treatment with simple broad-spectrum antibiotics is usually sufficient.*

Prevention

Use of the influenza and pneumonia vaccines is highly recommended for patients over age 65, especially those with chronic disease. Further details of these vaccines are discussed later in this chapter.

CHRONIC OBSTRUCTIVE PULMONARY DISEASE
Pathogenesis

The term "COPD" generally includes asthma, chronic bronchitis, and emphysema. Normal aging is associated with panlobular emphysema—a decrease in supporting elastic lung structure with resultant loss of alveoli. However, in the absence of lung disease, normal respiratory reserves are more than adequate to cope with these changes. Symptomatic disease results from centrilobular emphysematous damage to alveoli, generally resulting from smoking or occupational exposures that cause asthma and chronic bronchitis. Asthma is bronchial hyperreactivity, accompanied by mucosal edema and increased secretions. The essential characteristics of chronic bronchitis are excessive bronchial mucus production and a chronic cough that persists for at least 2 successive years in the absence of any specific disease. Mucus hypersecretion and inflammation of the bronchial mucosa produce nonuniform airway obstruction. This airway obstruction first leads to hypoxemia and later causes retention of CO_2. Chronic hypoxemia may cause or exacerbate pulmonary hypertension and lead to elevated right-sided heart pressures.[6]

The postbronchodilator forced expiratory volume in 1 second (FEV_1) is the most clinically useful predictor of outcome in chronic bronchitis, and it correlates closely with other indicators of disease severity such as resting heart rate, dyspnea, and hypercapnia. Once mild dyspnea develops (FEV_1 = 1 to 2 liters), most patients progress to severe dyspnea (FEV_1 <1 liter) within 6 to 10 years. For patients reaching the latter stage, the death rate is about 10% per year; most middle-aged adults with severe dyspnea do not survive to become truly old.[7]

> *Severely dyspneic COPD patients have a 10% per year death rate; few survive into truly old age.*

▼ LARRY BURKE (Part IV)

In the following 3 years Mr. Burke has several acute exacerbations of his chronic bronchitis and now has an FEV_1 of 1.6 liters. You had begun giving him ipratropium (Atrovent), three puffs four times a day. He was never successfully weaned from theophylline therapy. Yesterday he became too short of breath to play golf at all, even with use of a cart. Today he denies chest pain or fever but describes an increased cough with greenish sputum production and swelling of both feet. Because of trouble breathing, he had to sit up in a chair part of last night. He has been using his albuterol inhaler every 4 hours for the last 2 days and admits that he has been "sneaking puffs" at least twice a day for almost 2 weeks now. Mrs. Burke says that Mr. Burke is hardly eating and becomes irritable when she reminds him to eat and rest. Mr. Burke is pale, with bluish lips and nail beds. His temperature is 98.9° F, heart rate 118, blood pressure 180/80, and respiratory rate 30. He has 3+ pitting edema of both legs to the midcalf. He has a fourth heart sound on cardiac auscultation and coarse wheezing rhonchi throughout his lung fields, both of which are unusual for him. The rhonchi do not clear with aerosolized albuterol. His chest x-ray film shows hyperlucency, borderline cardiomegaly, flattening of both hemidiaphragms, and blunting of both costophrenic angles, but no identifiable infiltrate. Arterial blood gases show a pH of 7.51, Pco_2 of 48, Po_2 of 52, and oxygen saturation of 84%.

STUDY QUESTION

- *Given these findings, what will your management strategies be?*

Diagnosis

One of the most common complications of an acute exacerbation of chronic bronchitis is dyspnea secondary to congestive heart failure. Although failure of the right side of the heart may be present at baseline because of pulmonary hypertension, heart failure of the left side can also be triggered by the additional hypoxemia of an acute infection.[7] Since rhonchi and adventitious sounds are frequently present with COPD, lung auscultation is typically not diagnostic. A fourth heart sign on cardiac examination and the presence of pedal edema may both be helpful diagnostic signs. Chest x-rays are only minimally useful, since fibrotic changes and high intrathoracic pressures can mask the usual appearance of pulmonary edema. Demonstration of a pleural effusion may aid in diagnosis, however, and the presence of pneumonia

should be excluded. Serial arterial blood gas measurements at this stage of illness can help establish a baseline from which to measure acute decompensation and to consider when home oxygen therapy may be indicated (Box 47-1).

Treatment

Long-term therapy for elderly patients with COPD is directed toward controlling symptoms, maximizing independent self-care, and reducing the frequency of hospitalization. Acute exacerbations often represent opportunities to adjust therapy, so that patients can return to baseline functioning or actually increase physical activity. Anticholinergic drugs, β-adrenergic drugs, bronchodilators, corticosteroids, and oxygen should be progressively employed in a stepwise fashion (Table 47-1).

Typically, management of an acute exacerbation requires several steps: (1) verifying compliance with existing therapy, (2) monitoring the adequacy of existing therapy (e.g., with a theophylline level), (3) escalating existing therapy to maximal dosages, (4) adding new therapeutic agents directed at the presenting symptoms or apparent precipitating event, and (5) changing the mode of delivery of therapy, for example, from oral to intravenous agents. Hospitalization is generally advisable if new oxygen therapy is prescribed or escalation of oxygen supplementation to levels that must be closely monitored is necessary. Questionable compliance, intravenous therapy, and use of nebulizer treatments more often than every 4 hours are indicators of the need for hospitalization.

▼ LARRY BURKE (Part V)

Mr. Burke is started on 2 liters of oxygen by nasal cannula and hospitalized for close observation, diuretic treatment, intravenous corticosteroids, and antibiotic therapy. He improves steadily on intravenous ampicillin-sulbactam. By day 5 he has

---

BOX 47-1
Indications for Home Oxygen Therapy

Resting arterial oxygen tension (Pao_2) 55 mm Hg or less*
Resting arterial oxygen saturation (Sao_2) 88% or less*
Resting Pao_2 56 to 59 mm Hg with evidence of cor pulmonale, polycythemia, congestive heart failure, or sleep and mentation disturbances
Exercise Pao_2 55 mm Hg or less even if resting Pao_2 >55 mm Hg or Sao_2 >89%
Hypoxic organ dysfunction improved by oxygen therapy

*Meets Medicare criteria for reimbursable oxygen supplementation.

Table 47-1   Stepwise Escalation of Maintenance Therapy for Patients with COPD

Medication*	Dosage	Frequency
Ipratropium bromide by metered dose inhaler with spacer	2-6 puffs	4 times per day
β₂ agonists (albuterol, metaproterenol)	2-6 puffs	3-6 times per day
Theophylline, slow-release, titrated to plasma level of patient response, usually 8-20 μg/ml†	100-600 mg	2 times per day
Corticosteroid inhalation (beclomethasone, triamcinolone)	2-4 puffs	4 times a day
Prednisone, acute short-term course	40-80 mg initial dose	Daily for 7 days and taper off over 1-2 weeks
Prednisone, long-term	Lowest possible dose (usually 5-10 mg)	Every other day
Oxygen, continuous by nasal cannula	Lowest liter flow to raise Pao₂ to 60-65 mm Hg or Sao₂ to 90%-94%	
Oxygen, during exercise or sleep	Raise baseline flow by 1 liter per minute	

*First-line medications are listed first.
†May be eliminated based on patient response and relative toxicity.

been weaned to oral furosemide 20 mg daily, prednisone 40 mg per day, amoxicillin–clavulanic acid 500 mg three times a day, and 1.5 liters per minute oxygen by nasal cannula, in addition to his regular medications of theophylline, ipratropium, and albuterol. His resting Po₂ on room air is still only 55 mm Hg with a percent oxygen saturation of 87. He is discharged home with an oxygen concentrator as well as a portable unit, an air compressor for home nebulizer treatments, and visiting nurse and physical therapy referrals. He is scheduled for a follow-up visit in the office in 1 week. Mrs. Burke reports that her husband is much less irritable and has promised to eat properly once he gets home.

Prevention

Smoking cessation is the most important step in minimizing ongoing damage from chronic bronchitis. Proper nutrition, hydration, and exercise also help maximize function for as long as possible. Use of continuous oxygen therapy to prevent further hemodynamic deterioration from hypoxemia improves survival and provides symptomatic relief, particularly in patients with nighttime hypoxemia and cor pulmonale.[5] Prevention of pneumonia may be enhanced through annual influenza vaccination and use of the pneumococcal vaccine.

> *Multiple preventive steps (smoking, nutrition, hydration, exercise, oxygen, immunization) can help maximize function in the patient with COPD.*

PNEUMONIA
Pathogenesis

Despite improvements in diagnosis and treatment, mortality from pneumonia remains exceedingly high in older persons, ranging from 15% to 70%, depending on the etiology and the population at risk.[8-12] The incidence varies by setting, ranging from 25 to 44 cases of pneumonia per 1000 persons per year in the community to 68 to 114 cases per 1000 persons per year in chronic care facilities.[11] Comorbidity is also high; 80% to 90% of elderly pneumonia patients have one or more concomitant illnesses such as diabetes mellitus, cardiovascular disease, COPD, chronic congestive heart failure, or alcoholism.[13] These diseases lower host defense mechanisms by several routes, most notably through impairment of alveolar macrophage activity. Under such circumstances, bacteria may reach the lower bronchial tree by aspiration, inhalation, inoculation, direct spread from contiguous sites, and hematogenous spread.[8,11,12,14] Aspiration is believed to be the most common route of infection in elderly patients. Rather than the massive intake of regurgitated gastrointestinal contents most often noted clinically, the usual mechanism is inapparent introduction of oropharyngeal secretions into the lung while swallowing, lying supine, or sleeping.[14]

Colonization of the oropharynx with potentially pathogenic bacteria such as gram-negative bacilli occurs frequently in older persons. In one study only 8% of a control population of hospital workers were colonized, compared with 19% of persons 65 years or older living independently, 23% of nursing home residents, 42% of chronically hospitalized patients, and 60% of elderly patients in an acute ward of a chronic disease hospital.[15] Risk factors for colonization include chronic illness, inability to walk without assistance, urinary incontinence, and difficulty in performing activities of daily living (ADLs).[8,11,12,14,15] The increased incidence of colonization, combined with the known decline in aging host defenses (cell-mediated immunity, antibody response, cough reflex, and mucociliary clearance),[11,12,14,15] places aged individuals at far greater risk for infection and adverse outcomes.

The organisms that most commonly cause pneumonia vary directly depending on the patient's setting and functional status. In the community, *S. pneumoniae* is still most frequently recovered, probably followed by *H. influenzae*.[8,9,12,16,17] One large prospective study that routinely tested all patients for atypical etiologies found that *Legionella pneumophila* and *Chlamydia pneumoniae* were the third and fourth most common etiologies.[16] These findings contrast with most previous series describing various gram-negative bacilli and *Staphylococcus aureus* as the next most common organisms[8-12]; they remain to be confirmed by other investigators using similar diagnostic methods. *Moraxella catarrhalis* is now also being appreciated as a common pathologic organism, although it has been recovered for years as "normal flora."[17,18]

In hospital-acquired bacterial pneumonia, gram-negative bacilli predominate, particularly *Klebsiella pneumoniae*.[9,11,12,16,17] Other enteric gram-negative bacteria follow, alone or in combination with *H. influenzae*, *S. pneumoniae*, *Staphylococcus aureus*, or anaerobes. Aspiration pneumonia has accounted for 50% of the cases in some series,[11] but the true incidence is unknown. Nursing home-acquired pneumonias have isolates similar to those of hospital-acquired pneumonias and are also associated with a high rate of previous antibiotic use, leading to a high incidence of resistant organisms.[8,9,11,12,14,19]

▼ AGNES SEARS (Part I)

Agnes Sears is a 78-year-old woman living independently at home alone who has been coming to see you for many years. She comes to your office complaining of being too tired to finish her usual daily activities and of a dry cough at night for the past 3 nights. She denies having excessive sputum production, fever, chills, or chest pain but does admit to some chest tightness. Mrs. Sears has a history of hypertension, chronic stable angina, and osteoarthritis. She has never received pneumococcal or influenza vaccinations. Her usual medications include slow-release diltiazem, diclofenac sodium, and hydrochlorothiazide.

▼ RICHARD WILSON (Part I)

Richard Wilson is an 87-year-old man who became your patient when he moved to a nursing home 3 months ago. He is moderately demented, ambulates poorly because of Parkinson's disease, and requires assistance for all ADLs except feeding. He ordinarily is pleasant and recognizes his family. The nurse has called to report that he became quite agitated this morning, is incontinent, refuses to eat, and is yelling at passersby. His chronic diagnoses include benign prostatic hypertrophy, hypertension, constipation, diabetes mellitus (diet-controlled), and congestive heart failure. His long-term medications are carbidopa-levodopa, selegiline, diltiazem, and furosemide. He is too agitated to permit measurement of accurate vital signs, but the nurse notes that he has been less alert for the past 2 days, has been eating poorly, and is breathing more heavily at a rate of 28 to 32.

STUDY QUESTIONS

- *What diagnoses, aside from pneumonia, should be considered here?*

Diagnosis

The presentation of pneumonia in the elderly is frequently nonspecific, without the expected classic findings of productive cough, fever, chills, and pleuritic chest pain found in the rapid-onset lobar pneumonia typical of younger adults.[8,10-12,14] Instead, the elderly patient may report poor appetite and weakness or appear to suffer from exacerbation of an underlying chronic disease. This slower, more insidious onset is frequently seen in older adults and does not necessarily imply an atypical etiology, as such a presentation would in younger adults. In one recent study, acute mental status abnormalities were associated with community-acquired pneumonia in 66% of older adults versus only 30% of younger patients[20]; mortality more than doubled when such mental status changes were present.[21]

Nonspecific presentation and insidious onset, sometimes with delay in the development of radiological signs, characterize pneumonia in the elderly.

▼ AGNES SEARS (Part II)

Mrs. Sears is mildly obese and appears dehydrated, pale, and somewhat short of breath. Her temperature is 99° F, blood pressure 132/76, respiratory rate 28 and shallow at rest, and heart rate 102. Her lungs have fine crackles at both bases and expiratory wheezes throughout, but only rare rhonchi and no egophony or tactile fremitus. She does have dullness to percussion in the right lower lobe. Cardiovascular examination reveals a regular rhythm and a 2/6 systolic ejection murmur. After an albuterol nebulizer treatment only a few scattered wheezes remain, but coarse rhonchi are now present, and the fine crackles persist. She denies having fallen but is unsteady on her feet and has not eaten much for the past few days because she has felt too weak to cook.

▼ RICHARD WILSON (Part II)

Mr. Wilson remains agitated after he arrives at the emergency room and is sedated with 1 mg of haloperidol intramuscularly. Afterward, he remains agitated but sleepy. His temperature is 97.2° F, blood pressure 90/50, and heart rate 112. His respiratory rate is 32 and shallow. His lungs have coarse rhonchi and crackles halfway up on both sides posteriorly as well as at the left axilla, with dullness at the right base. Cardiovascular examination shows an intermittent S_3 gallop, 2/6 systolic murmur, and mild bilateral pitting edema in the lower legs. No chest pain or productive cough is observed or elicited. Abdominal examination findings are benign.

Findings

Physical examination in the older patient with pneumonia usually reveals tachypnea and tachycardia, both the most sensitive and least specific signs of illness. A respiratory rate above 28 is probably the earliest clue.[10-12] A twofold increase was observed in the mortality rate among patients with a severe vital sign abnormality.[21] Fever may be blunted or absent in a significant proportion of patients (20% to 68%), even in the presence of bacteremia.[12,14,21,22] Shallow respiration and crepitations in the lung bases are common findings in normal older adults because of decreased pulmonary compliance.[12] Because of these nonspecific features, pneumonia may be difficult to distinguish from acute bronchitis. Pneumonia should be suspected when the patient appears to have significant dyspnea or functional impairment.

 Tachypnea and tachycardia are generally found in older patients with pneumonia.

▼ AGNES SEARS (Part III)

Initial laboratory data on Mrs. Sears reveal a white blood count of 9700/mm³ with 72% neutrophils and 11% bands. Arterial blood gases on room air include a pH of 7.46, Po_2 of 69 mm Hg, Pco of 45.4 mm Hg, and an O_2 saturation of 92%. Sputum produced after the nebulizer treatment reveals greater than 25 WBCs and fewer than 10 epithelial cells per high power field on Gram stain, with encapsulated gram-positive diplococci. The chest x-ray examination is notable for findings of minor emphysematous changes and an almost com-plete right lower lobe infiltrate. Two blood cultures and a sputum culture are ordered.

▼ RICHARD WILSON (Part III)

Sputum for analysis is ordered on Mr. Wilson but is unobtainable. The WBC count is 3200/mm³ with 60% neutrophils and 25% bands. Arterial blood gases on 4 liters by nasal cannula reveal a pH of 7.32, Po_2 of 55 mm Hg, Pco_2 of 38 mm Hg, and O_2 saturation of 89%. Diffuse interstitial infiltrates are seen throughout on chest x-ray, as well as an obscured left heart border. The BUN is 38, and the creatinine is 1.6. Two blood cultures are ordered. Despite the inability to obtain a sputum specimen, intravenous antibiotics and parenteral fluid support are ordered immediately.

Confirming a diagnosis of pneumonia in older adults usually depends on the chest x-ray, although an infiltrate may be obscured by pulmonary edema or not apparent until 24 to 48 hours after rehydration.[8,11,12,14] A normal or mildly elevated total WBC count accompanied by a left shift in the differential is characteristic but nonspecific, as is arterial hypoxemia.

Arterial blood gases are frequently helpful in assessing the severity of illness. An elevated Pco_2 may indicate that the patient's respiratory effort is fatiguing. An arterial Po_2 that is lower than expected—after allowing for age and comorbid chronic illnesses—may help determine whether the patient can be observed carefully on an ambulatory basis or must be hospitalized. In particular, patients with underlying chronic lung disease or congestive heart failure can decompensate rapidly and may require early admission for close observation, oxygen, and supportive therapies.

 Arterial Po_2 is helpful in determining which patients should be considered for hospitalization with pneumonia.

Analysis of an adequate sputum specimen is essential (fewer than 10 epithelial cells and greater than 25 WBCs per high power field), although success in obtaining a specimen is more often the exception than the rule. For patients who cannot produce an expectorated specimen and who are immunocompromised, not responding to therapy, or relapsing after an initial response, collection of a specimen by transtracheal aspiration or bronchoscopy may be indicated.[11,12,14] Blood cultures have a diagnostic yield of 10% to 20%, depending on the organism.[8,10-12]

Alternative tests can be used to identify suspected non-bacteriological and atypical etiologies. These tests include direct fluorescent antibody stains for *Legionella pneumophila,* the two-step intermediate purified protein derivative (PPD) for *Mycobacterium tuberculosis,* and acute and convalescent serum titer comparisons to look for a fourfold rise in antibodies to *L. pneumophila, Mycoplasma pneumoniae, Chlamydia pneumoniae,* influenza, or other viral agents. Counterimmunoelectrophoresis has been used to detect *Streptococcus pneumoniae* and *Haemophilus influenzae* but is reported to give high false-negative and false-positive rates.[10]

▼ RICHARD WILSON (Part IV)

*Mr. Wilson is started on ceftazidime and tobramycin for their synergistic effect and fluid resuscitation for his septic shock, with simultaneous treatment of his congestive heart failure. His BUN and creatinine are holding at their baseline values. During the first 24 hours his P*o$_2$ *improves to 60 with a saturation of 91%, but Mr. Wilson remains delirious. By the end of the second day therapy is clearly failing. Permission to perform bronchoscopy is obtained, and metronidazole is added to the regimen after the specimen is obtained. Tuberculin skin testing is performed, and specimens are sent for acid-fast bacillus stain and culture. After another 48 hours of therapy, Mr. Wilson has ceased to deteriorate and is becoming more coherent, although he remains incontinent. Blood cultures reveal* Klebsiella pneumoniae, *which is found in addition to* Bacteroides fragilis *and* Pseudomonas aeruginosa *on the bronchoscopy specimen. After an additional 7 days of IV therapy Mr. Wilson is switched to oral ciprofloxacin and metronidazole and discharged to the nursing home, still on oxygen, with orders for gradual rehabilitation. You plan to visit him within a week.*

Treatment

The treatment of bacterial pneumonia is frequently empirical in the initial stages of illness and therefore must be chosen according to the organisms most likely to be present in the community, hospital, or nursing home settings and according to the patient's functional status (Table 47-2).

> *The essential principle of pneumonia management is early, aggressive, empirical treatment, selected on the basis of the most likely organisms for the setting in which the pneumonia developed.*

Healthy ambulatory patients are often successfully treated as outpatients with coverage based on the most common organisms in that population. Hospitalization is necessary when the patient's functional status decompensates or aggressive intravenous or oxygen therapy is indicated. Patients who are already hospitalized at the time of onset of the pneumonia are almost always immunocompromised and require much more aggressive antibiotic treatment because of the severity of the most likely organisms in that setting.

Nursing home patients comprise two distinct groups: those who are reasonably healthy and those who are frail. "Healthy" individuals with less functional impairment and few comorbid illnesses can often be safely treated in the chronic care facility, depending on the availability of adequate nursing observation, physician monitoring, and supportive therapies. Frail, often immunocompromised individuals should be treated similarly to those with hospital-acquired pneumonias and may require hospitalization.[22a] Patients with high-risk etiologies for pneumonia (staphylococci, gram-negative bacilli, aspiration, or postobstruction) have a substantially higher mortality rate than patients with all other etiologies (44.4% versus 13%).[21] One study found that in 92 episodes of lower respiratory tract infection in nursing home residents with a mean age of 86 years, those who died were 14 times more likely to be in the most dependent group rather than the least dependent group.[23] Risk of death was also 2.7 times higher for patients over 90 years of age and 5.8 times higher for those whose body mass index was in the lowest quartile. Mortality was lowest when therapy was initiated with broad-spectrum oral antibiotics (trimethoprim-sulfamethoxazole, cefaclor, ciprofloxacin, amoxicillin-clavulanate). Provided that proper support is available (laboratory studies, oxygen, radiology, blood gases, frequent physician assessment), treating low-risk patients in the nursing home setting is cost effective and may avoid the iatrogenic effects of hospitalization.

> *Low-risk patients in the nursing home can be effectively treated there, provided there is appropriate support.*

Special caution should be exercised when using certain antibiotics. Aminoglycosides are well recognized for their nephrotoxic and ototoxic side effects; they should be used only for their synergistic effects in empirical therapy for life-threatening disease. Erythromycin has multiple drug interactions, such as elevating the serum theophylline level, and significant gastrointestinal intolerance; and substitution with a second-generation macrolide such as clarithromycin or azithromycin may avoid some of these difficulties. Finally, despite the excellent serum levels and broad spectrum of coverage achieved with ciprofloxacin, clinicians must remember that cover-

Table 47-2 Empirical Antibiotic Treatment of Pneumonia

Clinical Features	Most Likely Organisms	Preferred Agents	Dosage	Alternatives*	Dosage	Oral Therapy
Community Setting						
Healthy, ambulatory, nonsmoker	Streptococcus pneumoniae	Penicillin G	400,000 U IV q4h	Erythromycin	500 mg IV q6h	Pen VK 500 mg q6h Erythromycin 500 mg q8h
COPD, alcoholism, smoker, post influenza	Haemophilus influenzae, Moraxella catarrhalis	Cefuroxime	750 mg–1.5 g IV q8h	Ampicillin-sulbactam Ciprofloxacin	1.5 g IV q6h 400 mg IV q12h	Cefuroxime 500 mg q12h Amoxicillin-clavulanate 500 mg q8h Trimethoprim 160 mg/sulfamethoxazole 800 mg q12h
Smoker, ambulatory	Legionella pneumophila	Erythromycin	500 mg IV q6h	Ciprofloxacin Rifampin	400 mg IV q12h 300 mg IV q12h	Azithromycin 500 mg on day 1, then 250 mg qd Clarithromycin 500 mg q12h
Atypical	Chlamydia pneumoniae	Erythromycin	500 mg IV q6h	Doxycycline	100 mg IV q12h	Doxycycline 100 mg q12h Clarithromycin 500 mg q12h
Hospital and Nursing Home Settings						
Good functional status, few underlying diseases	Streptococcus pneumoniae, Haemophilus influenzae	Cefuroxime	750 mg–1.5 g IV q8h	Ampicillin-sulbactam	1.5 g IV q6h	Amoxicillin-clavulanate 500 mg q8h Cefuroxime 500 mg q12h
Immunocompromised, poor functional status, chronic alcoholism, neoplasia	Klebsiella pneumoniae, gram-negative bacilli	Ceftriaxone	1-2 g IV q12h-q24h	Ceftazidime Ciprofloxacin	1-2 g IV q8h 400 mg IV q12h	Not recommended but may attempt Cefixime 400 mg q24h Ciprofloxacin 750 mg q12h
Post influenza, alcoholism, neoplasia	Staphylococcus aureus	Nafcillin	500 mg–1 g IV q4h	Vancomycin Ciprofloxacin Imipenem	0.5-1 g IV q12h 400 mg IV q12h 500 mg IV q6h-q12h	Dicloxacillin 500 mg q6h Ciprofloxacin 750 mg q12h
Swallowing disorder or suspected aspiration related to abnormal mental status	Oral flora, including anaerobes, Pseudomonas aeruginosa	Ceftazidime plus Tobramycin	1-2 g IV q8h 1-1.5 mg/kg IV q8h-q24h, adjusted for renal function	Clindamycin Aztreonam Ciprofloxacin	600 mg IV q8h 1-2 g IV q8h-q12h 400 mg IV q12h	Not recommended but may attempt Metronidazole 500 mg q6h plus Ciprofloxacin 750 mg q12h

*Ofloxacin 400 mg IV or PO can be substituted for ciprofloxacin wherever noted except for coverage of Pseudomonas aeruginosa.

age for *S. pneumoniae* is generally not considered adequate, and the incidence of delirium from this drug is quite high compared with other antibiotics.[17] Guidelines for empirical oral antibiotic therapy of lower respiratory infections can be found in Table 47-2.[22a]

Prevention

Prevention of pneumonia may be achieved in part by vaccination against influenza and pneumococcus. Approximately 80% to 90% of the excess deaths attributed to pneumonia and influenza are among persons over age 65. There is convincing evidence that polyvalent pneumococcal vaccine is effective in preventing invasive pneumococcal infections in immunocompetent older persons.[24] There is equally compelling evidence that influenza vaccine reduces hospitalization rates not only for pneumonia and influenza but also for all acute and chronic respiratory conditions and congestive heart failure.[22] The Immunization Practices Advisory Committee of the Centers for Disease Control and Prevention has concluded that both vaccines are efficacious and should be administered to all persons over age 65.[25] Every patient contact, including routine office care, nursing home monthly visits, and hospital discharges, should be seen as an opportunity for vaccination.[26]

TUBERCULOSIS

▼ *RICHARD WILSON (Part V)*

Mr. Wilson's initial 5 tuberculin unit (TU) injection of PPD has an 8 mm area of induration after 48 hours. He receives his second 5 TU PPD skin test the day before hospital discharge, which is read at the nursing home 48 hours later as 19 mm of induration. His previous two-stage PPD skin test on admission to the nursing home had shown only 2 mm of induration. Discharge chest x-ray shows that the diffuse bilateral infiltrates and pulmonary edema have largely cleared, but a right lower lobe infiltrate is still present. No apical scarring or hilar lymphadenopathy is noted. Acid-fast bacillus (AFB) stains performed on his bronchoscopy specimens are negative, and cultures are still pending.

Pathogenesis

Reactivation accounts for 80% of active cases of TB today.[1] Elderly persons remain the major reservoir for tuberculous disease in the United States, since these individuals were infected 50 to 70 years ago when many people were infected by the time they were 30 years old. These persons survived the initial infection but continue to harbor dormant bacilli. Although 90% to 95% of active tuberculosis among the aged occurs in community dwellers, the annual incidence is higher among nursing home residents (39.2 compared with 21.5 per 100,000). A positive dermal reaction is seen in 30% to 50% of all

residents on admission to the chronic care facility.[27] Nursing home patients face two important risks: (1) persons with dormant disease may undergo recrudescence of the infection and become infectious; and (2) persons who were never infected or who have outlived their bacilli (5% reversion rate per year) may become infected for the first time or develop new primary TB infections. One study found that the prevalence of positive TB tests nearly doubled among initial nonreacters who were tested again 6 months or more after admission to a nursing home.[1]

Diagnosis

The U.S. Public Health Task Force and the American Geriatrics Society recommend two-step skin testing by the Mantoux method for screening.[28,29] For the Mantoux test 0.1 ml of PPD containing 5 TU is administered intradermally with a disposable tuberculin syringe on the volar or dorsal surface of the forearm. The bevel of the needle should face upward, and the injection should produce a pale discrete 6 mm to 10 mm wheal. The test should be read 48 to 72 hours after placement by palpating the margin of induration. Erythema surrounding the induration should not be considered in evaluating test results. If the first Mantoux test is negative, a second test should be performed 1 to 2 weeks later to optimize the "booster effect" seen in older adults. Guidelines for interpreting the skin test are provided in Table 47-3.

Screening for TB should be with the two-step Mantoux method.

Chest x-ray examinations are indicated when (1) the patient has pulmonary symptoms compatible with active TB; (2) the tuberculin skin test is positive; (3) a history of TB exists but documentation of treatment or follow-up is unclear, or (4) extrapulmonary TB is suspected. In elderly patients evidence is mounting that pulmonary TB is not restricted to upper lobe involvement and may involve the middle and lower lobes or pleura.[27] A positive AFB smear or culture remains the standard for definitive diagnosis of TB. Newer serological tests, enzyme-linked immunosorbent assays, and DNA probe techniques are under development.[30]

▼ *RICHARD WILSON (Part VI)*

Mr. Wilson's conversion to a positive skin test since his entry into the nursing home makes it most likely that he has acquired a new primary infection. His chest x-ray is already abnormal because of his acute bacterial pneumonia, so it is not helpful in confirming or excluding the diagnosis. Repeat chest

Table 47-3   Interpretation of Tuberculin Skin Testing and Guidelines for Prophylaxis

Skin Induration (mm)	Age (Years)	Risk Factors	Result	Recommended Treatment
<5	All adults	None	Negative	None
<5	All adults	Immunocompromised	Inconclusive	Retest with anergy battery
5-9	34 or less	None	Negative	None
5-9	35-64	Entering long-term care facility (LTCF)	Negative	None
5-9	65 or older	None, or entering LTCF	Inconclusive	Give second injection of 5 TU PPD 1-2 weeks after first injection to stimulate "booster effect" and read skin test again
5-9	All adults	Known or suspected HIV; close contact of infectious case; chest x-ray positive for previous untreated TB	Positive	Chemoprophylaxis
10-14	35 or older	None	Negative	None
10-14	34 or younger	Foreign-born from country with high TB prevalence; medically underserved low-income population—African-Americans, Native Americans, Hispanics, homeless	Positive	Chemoprophylaxis
10-14	All adults	New converter with increase of 6 mm in past 2 years; IV drug user still HIV-negative; comorbid illnesses: malignancy, chronic renal failure, diabetes mellitus; immunosuppression; body weight approximately 10% less than ideal; secondary illnesses: silicosis, post gastrectomy or jejunoileal bypass	Positive	Chemoprophylaxis
15 or more	34 or younger	None	Positive	Chemoprophylaxis
15 or more	35 or older	None	Positive	None—risk of active disease does not outweigh risk of treatment
15 or more	All adults	New converter if increased 6 mm or more in last 2 years	Positive	Chemoprophylaxis

x-ray will be necessary in 6 to 8 weeks. AFB staining of the bronchoscopic specimen is negative, so Mr. Wilson probably has infection without active disease. Until culture results are available, Mr. Wilson is started on isoniazid for chemoprophylaxis and pyridoxine for prevention of isoniazid-associated neuropathy. Baseline liver function tests are performed. In addition, the medical director of Mr. Wilson's nursing home orders all nonreactors, both patients and staff, to be retested. Isolation is not necessary, since chemotherapy is being promptly initiated and the patient's recent contacts are being evaluated. The medical director notifies the acute care hospital and Mr. Wilson's family, so that they can also be evaluated.

Treatment

Tuberculosis is both treatable and curable when therapy is based on two principles: (1) the treatment regimen must include at least two drugs to which the organism is susceptible, and (2) treatment must continue beyond the time of microbiological eradication and amelioration of symptoms.[27] Active disease develops in 8% of women and 12% of men who are new converters and are left untreated in the nursing home.[1] The early intensive phase of therapy is designed to kill mycobacterial organisms as rapidly as possible in order to minimize infectivity and drug resistance; the continuation phase serves to eliminate any residual mycobacteria.[27] Several treatment regimens are described in Box 47-2. Since most older adults acquired their infection before the advent of modern chemotherapy, primary drug resistance of tubercle bacilli should be infrequent.[1,27] Older adults suspected of harboring drug-resistant TB organisms should be treated in consultation with clinicians experienced in this area.[31]

Patients with active pulmonary tuberculosis should be monitored with monthly sputum examinations until cultures are negative—a process that takes 3 months in over 90% of patients. Evaluation with repeat chest x-ray is also

9-Month Regimens

INH 300 mg plus RIF 600 mg daily for 9 months, *or*

INH 300 mg plus RIF 600 mg daily for 1-2 months
(until smears are negative), followed by INH 900
mg plus RIF 600 mg twice per week for 8 months

6-Month Regimens

INH 300 mg plus RIF 600 mg plus PZA 15-30
mg/kg body weight (to a maximum of 2 g) daily for
2 months, followed by INH 300 mg plus RIF 600
mg daily for 4 months, *or*

INH 300 mg plus RIF 600 mg plus PZA 15-30
mg/kg body weight (to a maximum of 2 g) daily for
2 months, followed by INH 900 mg plus RIF 600
mg twice a week for 4 months

INH, Isoniazid; *RIF,* rifampin; *PZA,* pyrazinamide.
*Pyridoxine (vitamin B$_6$) 50 mg daily should be taken with any of the
above.

recommended after 2 to 3 months of treatment and at completion of the drug program. Older adults face an increased risk of isoniazid-induced hepatitis; because of this, authorities disagree about indications for the use of isoniazid for prophylaxis.[1,27] Conservative monitoring dictates liver function tests at baseline and after 1, 3, and 6 months of treatment. If symptoms of hepatitis occur or the serum glutamic-oxaloacetic transaminase (SGOT) rises to five times above normal, isoniazid therapy should be discontinued. When symptoms resolve and the SGOT returns to normal, rechallenge with isoniazid at a lower dose may be initiated with careful monitoring for liver abnormalities. If symptoms or SGOT elevation recurs, isoniazid therapy must be terminated and an alternative regimen chosen.[27]

Prevention

Recommendations for chemoprophylaxis according to recently published guidelines from the Centers for Disease Control and Prevention (CDC)[32] are also noted on Table 47-3. Recommendations for the surveillance, containment, assessment, and reporting of tuberculous infection in long-term care facilities by the CDC's Advisory Committee for Elimination of Tuberculosis were recently summarized by Yoshikawa.[33] Clinicians working with chronic care facilities should become familiar with these guidelines.

INFLUENZA
Pathogenesis

Influenza virus infection causes three syndromes: an uncomplicated rhinotracheitis, a respiratory viral infection followed by bacterial pneumonia, and viral pneumonia, each of which has an incubation periods of 1 to 2 days. In each syndrome the respiratory tract epithelium is stripped down to the basal layer by day 3 of infection, begins to regenerate by day 5, but does not begin to function defensively again until day 14. The function of phagocytic alveolar macrophages is also severely impaired.[34] During this interval of lost pulmonary defense mechanisms, elderly adults are at particularly high risk for exacerbation of underlying chronic illnesses and life-threatening secondary infections. During influenza epidemics 80% to 90% of the 10,000 to 50,000 excess deaths occur in persons 65 years of age or older, particularly among those with underlying cardiac or pulmonary disease.[35] The attack rate has been as high as 50% in nursing home populations whose immunization rate is below 70%.[36]

Diagnosis

The typical syndrome is acute onset of fever, malaise, headache, and myalgia with respiratory illness occurring during the winter months in older as well as younger adults. Surveillance cultures and antibody titers are performed in public health institutions but are not generally used elsewhere. Older adults may initially demonstrate lower respiratory tract symptoms.[35,36]

Treatment

The goals of treatment are to restrict infection to the upper respiratory tract if possible, shorten the symptomatic period, prevent secondary complications, and provide supportive therapies to optimize survival until host defenses are able to regenerate. Resting, keeping warm, and drinking plenty of fluid help limit the spread of infection. Resting reduces oxygen demand and thus airflow, decreasing the chance of viral spread from the upper to the lower respiratory tract. Keeping warm helps maintain lower respiratory tract epithelium at core body temperature or higher, inhibiting virus replication, which is optimal at 35° C. Increasing hydration promotes mucus secretion, contributing to airway defenses.[34]

Rimantadine and amantadine interfere with viral replication; they are effective prophylactic and therapeutic agents against influenza A but not influenza B. The drugs are 70% to 90% effective when given prophylactically and can shorten the duration of fever and severity of symptoms if treatment is initiated within 48 hours after onset of symptoms. The two agents have important pharmacokinetic differences: 90% of rimantadine is metabolized hepatically before renal excretion, whereas over 90% of amantadine is excreted unchanged by the kidneys.[35] Even at the 100 mg dose of amantadine, adverse reactions occur in up to one third of nursing home patients, including psychosis, ataxia, hallucinations, seizures, congestive heart failure, postural hypotension, and falls. Hopefully, fewer adverse reactions will be associated with rimantadine, but this difference remains to be proven. Generally, restricting the dosage to 100 mg or less per day is advisable for either agent. Treatment of acute disease for 3 to 5 days is recommended.[35,36]

Prevention

Annual vaccination is crucial to the prevention of disease in older adults, yet only 30% to 40% of noninstitutionalized elderly persons receive vaccine yearly.[36] Therefore efforts must be made to increase the rate of immunization in both ambulatory and institutional populations during November, since most community outbreaks follow shortly thereafter and occur for a 6- to 10-week period. When the vaccine is administered during an outbreak, 2 weeks of adjunctive therapy with rimantadine or amantadine provides protection until vaccine-induced antibodies appear. Vaccination rates of 80% or greater among nursing home residents and staff appear to generate sufficient group immunity so that only sporadic cases are likely to occur.[35] Influenza vaccination should be routinely ordered during October and November in chronic care facilities so that the staff has ample time to obtain permission for the vaccination. Randomized, double-blind, crossover studies have demonstrated that side effects are no more frequent among vaccine recipients than among saline placebo recipients.[37] Systemic antibodies prevent lung infection but not upper respiratory infection and contribute to recovery from both upper and lower respiratory tract infections. Local IgA antibody prevents infection of the upper respiratory tract. Systemic cell-mediated immunity has no role in preventing upper or lower tract infection but is essential for recovery from both.[34]

The third edition of the *Guide for Adult Immunization*[35] issued by the American College of Physicians advocates an organized program for office-based immunizations. In practice, the program has achieved immunization rates of 70%. Box 47-3 details the procedures necessary to implement a population target–based approach that is physician specific for monitoring of performance. The key point is that the influenza vaccine should be offered in a positive manner by mail or by telephone call to all eligible persons in addition to those already scheduled for appointments during vaccination months. When tested in over 100 group and solo practices in New York, the highest immunization rates were achieved in practices with active physician support, use of a physician-

BOX 47-3
Office-Based Immunization
Program Procedures

1. Using computerized billing records, generate an alphabetical list of all patients eligible to receive the vaccine by reason of diagnosis or age.
2. Ensure that the primary care physician for these patients reviews the list for accuracy.
3. The total number of patients eligible after review is the target for the practice.
4. Enter the target total on simple posters that can be incrementally filled in as progress is made toward the target.
5. By mail or telephone, invite all eligible patients to receive the vaccine. Use the alphabetical list generated previously. Remind patients that the cost of the vaccine is now covered by Medicare.
6. Display the posters prominently in the office. Each physician should have his or her own poster.
7. Tally the number of vaccinated persons as they receive the vaccine.
8. Monitor performance by plotting weekly cumulative influenza immunization rates for each physician.

specific monitoring system, and involvement of the office staff.[35] Now that influenza vaccination is reimbursed by Medicare, few barriers remain to general use of one of the most effective prophylactic interventions available for older adults.

SUMMARY

Lower respiratory infections are extremely common in elderly patients in all health care settings, and they cause significant mortality and morbidity. Aggressive, early, empirical treatment can be lifesaving in pneumonia. Many pneumonias can be successfully treated in the nursing home setting. TB is increasingly prevalent, especially in the nursing home, and all clinicians should be familiar with the correct screening, diagnostic, and treatment methods. The patient with COPD requires detailed chronic management efforts if long-term morbidity is to be reduced. All health professionals should make a concentrated effort to increase the immunization rates for influenza (and pneumonia).

POSTTEST

1. An 86-year-old woman from a nursing home is seen in the emergency room. She has known congestive heart failure, diabetes mellitus, and dementia. Her vital signs are unstable, and she is lethargic. After obtaining initial diagnostic studies consistent with pneumonia, you would order which one of the following?
   a. Penicillin
   b. Erythromycin and nafcillin
   c. Nothing; wait until cultures are back
   d. Ceftazidime and an aminoglycoside

2. Which one of the following skin test results for tuberculosis is positive?
   a. Age 36, 13 mm induration
   b. Age 27, 7 mm induration but 12 mm erythema
   c. Age 65, 8 mm induration after step one injection of the Mantoux, 16 mm induration after step two
   d. Age 84, 6 mm induration 2 years ago, 11 mm induration now

3. Which one of the following statements is true regarding rimantadine and amantadine?
   a. They are only 50% effective for prophylaxis.
   b. They must be initiated within 48 hours to shorten the acute course of influenza.
   c. They have the same pharmacokinetics.
   d. They have virtually no central nervous system side effects.

REFERENCES

1. Dutt AK, Stead WW: Tuberculosis, *Clin Geriatr Med* 8(4):761-775, 1992.
2. Bentley DW, Mylotte JM: Epidemiology of respiratory infection in the elderly. In Niederman MS, ed: *Respiratory infections in the elderly,* New York, 1991, Raven Press.
2a. Yoshikawa TT: Antimicrobial therapy for the elderly patient, *J Am Geriatr Soc* 38(12):1353-1372, 1990.
3. Stockley RA: Airways infection. In Niederman MS, ed: *Respiratory infections in the elderly,* New York, 1991, Raven Press.
4. Perlman PE, Ginn DR: Respiratory infections in ambulatory adults: choosing the best treatment, *Postgrad Med* 87(1):175-184, 1990.
5. Heath JM: Outpatient management of chronic bronchitis in the elderly, *Am Fam Physician* 48(5):841-848, 1993.
6. Morris JF: Pulmonary diseases. In Cassel CK et al, eds: *Geriatric medicine,* ed 2, New York, 1990, Springer-Verlag.
7. Allen SC: Aging and the respiratory system. In Brocklehurst JC, Tallis RC, Fillit HM, eds: *Textbook of geriatric medicine and gerontology,* ed 4, Edinburgh, 1992, Churchill Livingstone.
8. Esposito AL: Pneumonia in the elderly, *Am Fam Physician* 40(5S):23S-32S, 1989.
9. Garb JL et al: Differences in etiology of pneumonias in nursing home and community patients, *JAMA* 240(20):2169-2172, 1978.
10. Marrie TJ et al: Community-acquired pneumonia requiring hospitalization: is it different in the elderly? *J Am Geriatric Soc* 33(10):671-680, 1985.
11. Niederman MS, Fein AM: Pneumonia in the elderly, *Geriatr Clin North Am* 2(2):241-269, 1986.
12. Verghese A, Berk SL: Bacterial pneumonia in the elderly, *Medicine* 62(5):271-285, 1983.
13. Cunha BA, Gingrich D, Rosenbaum GS: Pneumonia syndromes: a clinical approach in the elderly, *Geriatrics* 45(10):49-52, 55, 1990.
14. Yoshikawa TT, Norman DC: Pneumonia. In *Aging and clinical practice: infectious diseases,* New York, 1987, Igaku-Shoin.
15. Valenti WM, Trudell RG, Bentley DW: Factors predisposing to oropharyngeal colonization with gram-negative bacilli in the aged, *N Engl J Med* 298(20):1108-1111, 1978.
16. Fang GD et al: New and emerging etiologies for community-acquired pneumonia with implications for therapy: a prospective multicenter study of 359 cases, *Medicine* 69(5):307-316, 1990.
17. Marrie TJ: Pneumonia, *Clin Geriatr Med* 8(4):721-734, 1992.
18. Williams EA, Verghese A: Newer or emerging pulmonary pathogens in the elderly. In Niederman MS, ed: *Respiratory infections in the elderly,* New York, 1991, Raven Press.
19. Bartlett JG et al: Bacteriology of hospital-acquired pneumonia, *Arch Intern Med* 146(5):868-871, 1986.
20. Esposito AL: Community-acquired bacteremic pneumococcal pneumonia, *Arch Intern Med* 144(5):945-948, 1984.
21. Fine MJ et al: Prognosis of patients hospitalized with community-acquired pneumonia, *Am J Med* 88(5):5-1N to 5-8N, 1990.
22. Nichol KL et al: The efficacy and cost effectiveness of vaccination against influenza among elderly persons living in the community, *N Eng J Med* 331(12):778-784, 1994.
22a. Yoshikawa TT: Treatment of nursing home–acquired pneumonia, *J Am Geriatr Soc* 39(10):1040-1041, 1991.
23. Mehr DR, Foxman B, Colombo P: Risk factors for mortality from lower respiratory infections in nursing home patients, *J Fam Pract* 34(5):585-591, 1992.
24. Shapiro ED et al: The protective efficacy of polyvalent pneumococcal polysaccharide vaccine, *N Engl J Med* 325(21):1453-1460, 1991.
25. Recommendations of the Immunization Practices Advisory Committee: Prevention and control of influenza. I. Vaccines, *MMWR* 38:297-311, 1989.
26. Fedson DS et al: Hospital-based pneumococcal immunization, *JAMA* 264(9):1117-1122, 1990.
27. Yoshikawa TT: Tuberculosis in aging adults, *J Am Geriatr Soc* 40(2):178-187, 1992.
28. Clinical Practice Committee of the AGS: The American Geriatric Society statement on two-step PPD testing for nursing home patients on admission, *J Am Geriatr Soc* 36(1):77-78, 1988.
29. U.S. Public Health Service: Tuberculosis in adults, *Am Fam Physician* 50(4):811-815, 1994.
30. Barnes PF, Barrows SA: Tuberculosis in the 1990s, *Ann Intern Med* 119(5):400-410, 1993.
31. Iseman MD: Treatment of multidrug-resistant tuberculosis, *N Engl J Med* 329(11):784-791, 1993.
32. The use of preventive therapy for tuberculous infection in the United States: recommendations of the Advisory Committee for Elimination of Tuberculosis, *MMWR* 39(RR-8):9-12, 1990.
33. Yoshikawa TT: Elimination of tuberculosis from the United States, *J Am Geriatr Soc* 39(3):312-314, 1991.

34. Small PA: Influenza: pathogenesis and host defense, *Hosp Pract* 25(11):51-54, 57-62, 1990.
35. ACP Task Force on Adult Immunization and Infectious Diseases Society of America: *Guide for adult immunization,* ed 3, Philadelphia, 1994, American College of Physicians.
36. Cate TR: Influenza in the elderly. In Niederman MS, ed: *Respiratory infections in the elderly,* New York, 1991, Raven Press.
37. Margolis KL, Nichol KL, Poland GA, et al: Frequency of adverse reactions to influenza vaccine in the elderly: a randomized, placebo-control trial, *JAMA* 264(9):1139-1141, 1990.

PRETEST ANSWERS
1. a
2. b
3. c

POSTTEST ANSWERS
1. d
2. c
3. b

CHAPTER 48

Urinary Tract Infections

GARFIELD C. PICKELL

OBJECTIVES

On completion of this chapter, the reader will be able to:

1. Define the factors predisposing the elderly to urinary tract infection (UTI).

2. Describe the treatment options for asymptomatic bacteriuria.

3. Prescribe empirical treatment for uncomplicated UTI.

4. Describe the presentation and evaluation of urosepsis.

5. Prescribe empirical initial treatment of the acutely ill uroseptic patient.

6. Describe the special features of catheter-associated infections and the techniques of aseptic indwelling catheter care.

7. Describe the place of antibacterial suppressive therapy in prevention.

1. UTIs caused by antibiotic-resistant organisms are associated with all of the following except:
   a. Indwelling catheterization
   b. Nursing home–acquired infection
   c. Nephrolithiasis
   d. Community-acquired infection
   e. Antibacterial suppression therapy
2. Which of the following statements regarding asymptomatic bacteriuria are true:
   a. Asymptomatic bacteriuria should always be treated with a broad-spectrum antibiotic.
   b. Treatment should be undertaken in patients with asymptomatic bacteriuria and new systemic symptoms.
   c. Patients with asymptomatic bacteriuria generally have below average renal function for their age.
   d. Sulfonamide, cotrimoxazole, or nitrofurantoin should be used as suppression therapy or for recurrent symptomatic infections.

Bacteriuria and symptomatic UTIs become dramatically more common with advancing age and debility.

Bacteriuria is present in 15% to 20% of elderly community-dwelling women and 5% to 10% of elderly men. This increases to 20% to 25% of both sexes living in nursing homes and 30% to 50% of elderly hospitalized patients.[1] Morbidity and mortality from UTIs increase as well, since urosepsis accounts for up to 56% of sepsis in the elderly, with a mortality rate as high as 25%.[2]

Multiple factors predispose the elderly to UTIs:

- Incomplete bladder emptying from prostatic obstruction, cystocele, neurological degeneration, immobility, and anticholinergic medications
- Urinary incontinence and declining perineal hygiene
- Decline in cell-mediated immunity and humoral antibody response
- Loss of prostatic antibacterial secretions
- Postmenopausal mucosal atrophy and rise in vaginal pH
- Decrease in bladder epithelium mucopolysaccharides, allowing bacterial adherence to epithelial cells
- Increased hospitalizations with exposure to virulent organisms, bladder catheterization, and other urinary tract instrumentation
- Indwelling bladder catheters

A rational approach to UTI in the elderly is based on the progressive complexity categorized in Box 48-1.

▼ WILMA CARTER (Part I)

Ms. Carter is an 81-year-old, generally healthy woman who lives at home with her husband. She remains quite active, undertakes all of her own activities of daily living, and is an enthusiastic gardener. She comes to your office complaining of a 2-day history of urgency incontinence with no other new symptoms. Urinalysis demonstrates 2+ bacteria and 15 to 20 WBCs per high-power field. You begin treatment with norfloxacin 400 mg bid for 10 days. She is instructed in double

---

BOX 48-1
Progressive Complexity of UTIs in the Elderly

Asymptomatic bacteriuria
  Without pyuria
  With pyuria
Uncomplicated infection
  Lower tract
  Upper tract
  Treatment failures and recurrences
Complicated infection
  Structural and functional abnormalities
  Catheter associated
  Urosepsis

---

voiding. Urine culture results return 2 days later showing $>10^5$ colonies of Escherichia coli *per milliliter. Follow-up urine 2 weeks later is clear.*

At an incidental office visit 3 months later, urinalysis demonstrates 3+ bacteria and 3 to 5 WBCs per high-power field. Culture grows $>10^5$ colonies of Acinetobacter spp per milliliter. No further action is taken.

Incidental urinalysis 6 months later is clear of abnormalities. Another incidental urinalysis and culture a year later demonstrate 3+ bacteria, 3 to 5 WBCs per high-power field, and $>10^5$ colonies of E. coli per ml.

She remains well.

STUDY QUESTIONS

- Should this current infection be treated?
- Was pyuria present on either follow-up cultures?

ASYMPTOMATIC BACTERIURIA

The significance of asymptomatic bacteriuria is controversial. It is not associated with the development of renal failure. It is, however, clearly associated with increased mortality. This may be simply a correlation between increasing debility and the probability of acquiring bacteriuria.[3]

Most authorities recommend that asymptomatic bacteriuria not be treated routinely, since the risks and costs appear to outweigh the benefits. Bacteriuria clears spontaneously or is intermittent in many patients. Long-term eradication of bacteria by treatment is usually unsuccessful, and it is universally unsuccessful in the presence of a catheter or chronic prostatic disease. Antimicrobial treatment also provokes the emergence of resistant organisms and puts the patient at risk of adverse drug effects.[4]

Pyuria is indicative of inflammation, usually caused by infection. Patients with obstructive uropathy, renal calculi, neurogenic bladder dysfunctions, indwelling catheters, or bacteriuria with pyuria should probably receive long-term suppression. This will not eradicate the bacteriuria but will decrease the incidence of pyelonephritis and urosepsis.[5] The antibacterial agent chosen should be well absorbed, be inexpensive, not alter intestinal flora significantly, have a low incidence of side effects, have a low incidence of resistant organisms, and be excreted in the urine. The most appropriate agents appear to be trimethoprim-sulfamethoxazole ½ or 1 tablet daily, nitrofurantoin 50 mg daily, norfloxacin 400 mg daily, or mandelamine 100 mg daily. Nitrofurantoin is well absorbed, is excreted in the urinary tract in high concentrations, is inexpensive, and still has a low grade of bacterial resistance after 40 years of use; therefore it is still the first choice of agent for suppression.[6] Acidifying agents such as vitamin C or cranberry juice are of equivocal benefit.

CASE DISCUSSION

Ms. Carter is a fit, active woman in whom treatable conditions should be aggressively addressed. Empirical treatment was appropriate based on microscopy, and follow-up was appropriate. Neither the follow-up nor an incidental urinalysis later showed pyuria. Even though significant numbers of an organism were grown on the incidental test, her bacteriuria was truly asymptomatic; therefore no treatment was indicated.

▼ ETHEL HARDING (Part I)

Mrs. Harding is an 84-year-old patient with advanced dementia of Alzheimer's type. She lives at home with her daughters who care for her. She is now virtually bed bound and barely able to make her needs known. However, she recognizes her daughters, and they have determined to give her as good a life as possible in the home setting for as long as possible. One of her daughters calls your office because Mrs. Harding has vomited twice, which is unusual for her. She seemed perfectly well yesterday and, until this episode, was eating well. She varies a little in how "good" she is from day-to-day, and to-

day is one of her "bad" days, although she is barely more confused than usual.

STUDY QUESTIONS

- *What is the most likely diagnosis?*
- *Is empirical management justified, and what treatment would you choose?*

SYMPTOMATIC URINARY TRACT INFECTION

The presentation of UTI in the elderly is often atypical and nonspecific. There may be no fever, leukocytosis, or symptoms referable to the urinary tract. Early the patient may have constitutional symptoms such as a decrease in level of functioning, lethargy, anorexia, general malaise, or altered mental status. The most prominent symptoms may be gastrointestinal or respiratory. These features often result in a delay in diagnosis, with the development of urosepsis and increased mortality.

Acute onset vomiting in an elderly patient? Consider UTI first (especially if the patient is female).

Symptomatic patients usually have bacteriuria ($>10^5$ colonies per ml) or pyuria (>10 WBCs per high-power field). Urine for culture should be obtained by straight catheterization in elderly women because of the difficulty of obtaining clean-catch specimens, uncontaminated by vaginal or perineal flora.

UNCOMPLICATED INFECTIONS

Treatment should be started empirically, with a broad-spectrum oral antibiotic. Trimethoprim-sulfamethoxazole, norfloxacin, nitrofurantoin, or amoxicillin-clavulanate is a suitable initial choice. However, bacterial resistance to all of the commonly used agents is increasing, and it is now necessary to match specific bacterial sensitivities when cultures are available.[7] Treatment regimens of 1 to 3 days are not satisfactory in the elderly; they should be treated for 10 days.

If the posttreatment urinalysis demonstrates clearing of pyuria, follow-up cultures are unnecessary; they may lead to the futile pursuit of asymptomatic bacteriuria.

Treatment failures and recurring symptomatic infections suggest chronic prostatitis, bladder dysfunction, nephrolithiasis, persistent low-grade pyelonephritis (upper tract infection), or bladder residual. These patients should be evaluated for structural and functional abnormalities. The intravenous pyelogram (IVP) with a voiding cystourethrogram remains the most useful procedure, but in patients with significantly impaired renal function it can be replaced with a radionuclide renal scan and ultrasound. Elderly men should be evaluated for prostatic obstruction and infection. Postvoiding residual is assessed by straight catheterization. Many causes of incomplete bladder emptying and incontinence are readily treatable, preserving the patient from the consequences of recurrent infection, incontinence, and indwelling catheters.

If the workup for complicating factors is negative, most persistent infections will be cleared by a 6-week course of appropriate antimicrobials. Institutionalized patients occasionally require more aggressive treatment with carbenicillin, ceftriaxone, or aminoglycosides because of multiple resistant organisms, including methicillin- and aminoglycoside-resistant *Staphylococcus aureus* (MARSA). This is a problem even if the patient is asymptomatic because of the risk of the infection's spread to other institutionalized patients, the need for its isolation, and the difficulty with its eradication.

Patients with frequent recurrences of UTI may respond to long-term low-dose suppression.

▼ ETHEL HARDING (Part II)

Since it is the first day of a 3-day weekend, it is impractical to obtain a urinalysis. However, you believe that a urinary infection is so likely based on the symptoms that you treat empirically with trimethopim-sulfamathoxazole, which rapidly improves Mrs. Harding's symptoms. She is treated with clear liquids until 12 hours after the last episode of vomiting. Although she had not noticed it previously, her daughter confirms that her urine smelled "dreadful" and was cloudy, rather than dark, before treatment. You press extra fluids to encourage a good urinary flow and insist on completion of a 10-day course of your antibiotic of choice.

CASE DISCUSSION

Vomiting or new-onset nausea is a common presentation for UTI, and empirical treatment can be justified in certain clinical situations. The consequences of potential overtreatment here are not significant enough to outweigh the extreme difficulties that would be caused by urosepsis in this situation.

▼ WILLIAM JONES (Part I)

You are covering the ER at your local county hospital. Mr. Jones was seen in the ER 3 days ago for urinary retention, and an indwelling Foley catheter was placed pending Medicare approval for a transurethral prostatic resection. He is a physically healthy, mildly demented, 80-year-old man who lives with his daughter and son-in-law. He has a history of hypertension but is not taking medication. His family brings him to the ER at 9 AM today, more confused and disoriented than usual and lethargic. Family members indicate that he
becomes somewhat confused and restless at night, and he apparently pulled out his Foley catheter during the night.

Physical examination of Mr. Jones demonstrates a lean but lethargic, elderly man with a dry mouth and decreased skin turgor. He is disoriented to person, place, and time. He is confused. Pulse is 110, respirations 25, temperature 102.5° F, BP 105/70 lying and 80/40 sitting. The chest is clear. The heart is regular with a rapidly collapsing peripheral pulse and peripheral vasodilation. The abdomen is soft, with no tenderness, masses, or organomegaly. He has no costovertebral angle tenderness. Rectal examination demonstrates a large, boggy prostate. The stool is heme negative. Catheterization produces 120 ml of cloudy urine; specific gravity is 1.028, there are >100 RBCs per high-power field and >100 WBCs per high-power field. Gram stain demonstrates many gram-negative rods; specimen is sent for culture.

The chest x-ray is clear. ECG demonstrates sinus tachycardia and is otherwise unremarkable. The WBC count is 9500/mm³ with 64% polys and 20% bands. Hgb is 14 g/dl, blood urea nitrogen is 28, and creatinine level is 2.1. Other laboratory work is unremarkable.

STUDY QUESTIONS

- Is this an emergency?
- What empirical treatment would you prescribe?
- Could this illness have been avoided?

COMPLICATED INFECTIONS

Elderly patients with acute pyelonephritis who appear to be acutely ill or who have structural abnormalities such as stones, urinary retention, or indwelling catheters should be hospitalized and treated aggressively. Debilitated patients are likely to become bacteremic and suffer septic shock, and they are more likely to be infected with resistant organisms. Initial empirical treatment is directed toward the usual enteric bacteria, *Proteus* and *Pseudomonas aeruginosa*. The traditional choice is IV ampicillin and an aminoglycoside. Reasonable choices of single agents that avoid the toxicity of aminoglycosides are amoxicillin-clavulanate, ceftriaxone, ticarcillin-clavulanate, and aztreonam. Ofloxacin is effective in patients who can reliably take oral medications. When cultures and sensitivities are available, the patient can be switched to an appropriate single agent. In 3 to 5 days, when the patient is afebrile and doing well clinically and pyuria is clearing, the switch can be made to a single oral agent, which should then be continued for at least 2 weeks. Follow-up cultures should be done, but only the original infecting organism should be re-treated, since asymptomatic bacteriuria with other organisms develops quickly in many debilitated patients. However, patients with urinary tract structural or functional abnormalities, recurrences, or indwelling catheters should remain indefinitely on suppression. This reduces the probability of recurrent pyelonephritis and urosepsis.[5]

If urosepsis is suspected (presentation can be obscure), the correct management is early, aggressive treatment with empirical broad-spectrum antibiotics, usually in the hospital.

Because of the risk of nephrotoxicity, aminoglycosides should be discontinued as soon as an appropriate single agent can be chosen. In the elderly it is prudent to administer aminoglycosides once a day (e.g., gentamicin 2 to 3 mg/kg q24h) and of course always to monitor renal function.

CATHETER-ASSOCIATED INFECTIONS

The urinary tract is the most common site of in-hospital acquired infection in the elderly, and bladder catheterization is the major route of entry. Bacteriuria occurs at about 10% per day in acutely hospitalized catheterized patients, and it is present in over 90% of such patients at 30 days. All elderly patients should be screened for UTI when their catheters are removed or before discharge from the hospital.[8] Long-term indwelling catheters are associated with multiple organisms and an increased incidence of unusual and resistant organisms.

Indwelling catheters should be used only when absolutely necessary and for as short a time as possible in circumstances such as the following:

- Acutely ill patients requiring intake and output monitoring
- Perioperative care
- Irremediable obstruction and urinary retention
- Intractable urinary incontinence; here catheters should be used only for the short term when needed to facilitate the healing of decubitus ulcers or in terminal patients when the benefits clearly outweigh the costs

Avoid indwelling catheters; they are the most potent source of urosepsis. Intermittent catheterization is much safer.

Bacteriuria is ubiquitous and inevitable in patients with indwelling catheters. It can be managed conservatively in relatively healthy, stable patients. However, symptomatic infection with fever, altered mental status, leukocytosis, or gross pyuria should be treated promptly and aggressively to avoid sepsis. Patients with catheters who have had recurring symptomatic infections or sepsis should receive long-term suppression.

Indwelling catheters should be managed aseptically with a closed-drainage system (Box 48-2). All of the interventions attempted to date, including systemic antimicrobial prophylaxis, antibiotic irrigations, silicone- and iodine-impregnated catheters, bladder irrigation with antiseptics, and daily care of the urethra-bladder junction, have proved ineffective in preventing bacteriuria in long-term catheterization. Aseptic measures are nonetheless important in preventing infection in patients with short-term catheterization and in preventing transmission of infection between patients.

Because bacteriuria is inevitable in patients with long-term indwelling catheters, and because it increases the risk of sepsis, every effort should be made to manage the patient's urinary tract problems by other means.

With optimal medical management the rate of long-term indwelling catheterization in nursing facilities can be as low as 1.5% of patients.[9]

Condom catheters offer little advantage over indwelling catheters and are associated with bacteriuria of the *Proteus* and *Providencia* species.

BOX 48-2
Recommendations for Catheter Care

Catheterize only when absolutely necessary and remove the catheter as soon as possible.

The catheter should be inserted only by adequately trained personnel.

Follow strict aseptic technique with iodine prep. The catheter should be secured to the patient to prevent traction.

Provide twice daily perineal care with an antiseptic.

Use a sterile closed-drainage system. This should never be opened except at the bag drain.

Use irrigation only when infection is already present, and sterile techniques *must be used* whenever the collecting system is opened.

Aspirate urine for culture by needle through the distal catheter, prepped with iodine.

Maintain nonobstructed downhill flow.

Change contaminated systems immediately.

Do not routinely change the catheter. With chronic indwelling catheters, replacement is done only for malfunction or obstruction. Silastic or silicone catheters are used. Separation of catheterized patients, particularly bacteriuric from nonbacteriuric patients, should be practiced.

Modified from Stamm WE: *Ann Intern Med* 82:386-390, 1975.

▼ WILLIAM JONES (Part II)

Mr. Jones is considered uroseptic, with bacteremia provoked by pulling out his Foley catheter in the presence of a UTI. He receives fluid replacement with half-normal saline, and he is started on IV amoxicillin-clavulanate 2 g q6h and given a single dose of gentamicin 2 mg/kg.

The next day Mr. Jones is alert and oriented and responds appropriately to simple questions and instructions. He is clinically improved with a temperature of 99.5° F. He is eating and drinking well. Urine culture grows >10⁵ colonies of Escherichia coli, sensitive to all antibiotics tested. He is continued on IV amoxicillin-clavulanate alone.

Seven days later Mr. Jones is clinically well with normal findings on the complete blood cell count and renal function tests. He undergoes transurethral prostatic resection and is discharged home feeling well. Urinalysis on discharge demonstrates only 15 to 20 RBCs per high-power field.

CASE DISCUSSION

In this case the second ER visit shows an obviously ill man. Lesser symptoms, perhaps without the high fever or orthosta-sis, would nonetheless have justified the same aggressive empirical treatment, since he was in considerable danger.

SUMMARY

UTIs are common in the elderly, increasing in frequency and severity with increasing age and debility. Asymptomatic bacteriuria should generally not be treated except in patients with recurrent symptomatic infections, urosepsis, significant pyuria, or severe debilitation. Infections often manifest themselves subtly with nonspecific systemic signs or symptoms or mental status changes and may progress to urosepsis before being recognized. Symptomatic infections require aggressive antibiotic treatment and evaluation for and correction of structural and functional urinary tract abnormalities. Indwelling urinary catheters are particularly hazardous in the debilitated elderly and should be used judiciously, cared for fastidiously, and monitored closely.

POSTTEST

1. Which of the following is true regarding indwelling catheters?
   a. The catheter should be changed every 2 months.
   b. Routine catheter irrigation is desirable.
   c. Asymptomatic bacteriuria should receive routine suppressive therapy.
   d. The sterile, closed-drainage system should never be opened except at the bag drain.
2. Which of the following is not true regarding urosepsis?
   a. Initial treatment should include one or two broad-spectrum antibiotics.
   b. Complications such as obstruction, calculi, or abscess should be considered in the patient not responding within 72 hours.
   c. A patient can be changed to oral antibiotics when the culture and sensitivity results are available.
   d. Long-term suppression may be indicated for bacteriuria persisting after urosepsis.

3. Which of the following is not associated with increased risk of UTI?
   a. Immobility
   b. Acute hospitalization
   c. Male gender
   d. Incontinence
4. An ideal antibiotic for treating UTI is all of the following except:
   a. Inexpensive
   b. Completely absorbed in the gastrointestinal tract
   c. Metabolized by the liver
   d. Effective against most gram-negative organisms
   e. Associated with a low incidence of resistant organisms
   f. Infrequent and mild in its side effects
   g. Taken once a day

REFERENCES

1. Kaye D: Urinary tract infections in the elderly, *Bull NY Acad Med* 56:209-220, 1980.
2. Kunin CM: The concepts of "significant bacteriuria" and asymptomatic bacteriuria, clinical syndromes and the epidemiology of urinary tract infections. In Kunin DM: *Detection, presentation and management of urinary tract infections*, ed 4, Philadelphia, 1987, Lea & Febiger.
3. Dontas AS et al: Bacteriuria and survival in old age, *N Engl J Med* 304:939-943, 1981.
4. Boscia JA et al: Epidemiology of bacteriuria in an elderly ambulatory population, *Am J Med* 80:208-214, 1986.
5. Fierer J, Ekstrom M: An outbreak of *Providencia stuartii* urinary tract infections: patients with condom catheters are a reservoir of the bacteria, *JAMA* 245:1553-1555, 1981.
6. Parson CL, Schmidt JD: Control of recurrent lower urinary tract

infection in the post menopausal woman, *J Urol* 128:1224-1226, 1982.

7. Nicolle LE et al: Bacteriuria and mortality in an elderly population, *N Engl J Med* 309:1420-1425, 1983.

8. Warren JW: Catheters and catheter care, *Clin Geriatr Med* 2:857-871, 1986.

9. Sant GR: Urinary tract infection in the elderly, *Semin Urol* 5 (2):126-133, 1987.

10. Stamm WE: Guideline for prevention of catheter-associated urinary tract infections, *Ann Intern Med* 82:386-390, 1975.

PRETEST ANSWERS

1. d
2. b

POSTTEST ANSWERS

1. d
2. a
3. c
4. c

CHAPTER 49

The Acute Abdomen

PATRICK P. COLL

OBJECTIVES

On completion of this chapter, the reader will be able to:

1. List the most common causes of acute abdominal disease in an older patient.

2. Appreciate the importance of considering an intraabdominal process in all acutely ill older patients.

3. Know the appropriate use of diagnostic tests and the indications for surgery.

1. Which of the following is the most common cause of acute abdominal disease in patients over 70 years old?
   a. Appendicitis
   b. Acute mesenteric ischemia
   c. Diverticulitis
   d. Cholecystitis
   e. Perforated duodenal ulcer

The acute abdomen in the older patient is a common and life-threatening condition (Box 49-1). It can prove a diagnostic challenge even for the most astute clinician. Its presentation may be atypical as is common for many acute illnesses in older patients. Early and accurate diagnosis helps reduce mortality. The single best way to ensure this is to consider the possibility of an intraabdominal process in all older patients seeking treatment for an acute illness. Older patients tolerate surgery well, and it should not be rushed, postponed, or not considered on the basis of a patient's age.

▼ WILMA WRIGHT (Part I)

You receive a call from the nurse practitioner at a local nursing home who reports that your 78-year-old patient, Mrs. Wright, has been complaining of abdominal pain for 24 hours. She has not eaten all day and recently vomited. She is in the nursing home following a hip fracture a month before. She is usually mentally alert without any evidence of dementia. Before her fracture, her physical function was very good. Up to this particular incident she is reported to have been making excellent progress with her activities of daily living while at the nursing home. Her only significant medical history is diabetes mellitus, for which she has been taking an oral hypoglycemic agent. She is delirious and has cold, clammy extremities. Her temperature is 99.3° F, blood pressure 60/40 mm Hg, and pulse 120 beats per minute. The nurse practitioner's examination of the abdomen is reported as showing diffuse tenderness, most marked in the right upper quadrant, with bowel sounds present. Rectal examination is normal, and the stool is heme negative.

STUDY QUESTIONS

▪ *What are potential causes of this situation?*
▪ *How should you proceed?*

Any acute illness in an older patient may represent an intraabdominal catastrophe. A high index of suspicion is warranted because of the potential for atypical presentation and the serious consequences of any acute abdominal process in an older patient. An accurate history is of paramount importance but may not be forthcoming

---

BOX 49-1
Causes of an Acute Abdomen in an Older Patient

Cholecystitis and cholangitis
Large bowel obstruction (hernia, adhesions, tumor, volvulus)
Small bowel obstruction (hernia, adhesions)
Peptic ulcer disease
Diverticulitis
Appendicitis
Mesenteric ischemia
Ruptured aortic aneurysm
Pneumonia
Myocardial infarction

---

from the patient. Important aspects of the history include duration and location of pain, presence or absence of vomiting, whether the patient is passing flatus, and what abdominal surgery has previously been performed. If the patient is incapable of giving an accurate history, it should be obtained from a family member or other caregiver. Physical signs are conspicuous by their absence in some older patients with acute abdominal disease.[1] Peritonitis is less likely to cause rebound tenderness; evidence of muscle guarding on gentle palpation of the abdominal wall may be the only sign of its presence. Pyrexia and tachycardia are also less likely to be present. Important aspects of the physical examination include careful inspection of the inguinal and femoral areas for the presence of an incarcerated hernia, listening for bowel sounds, and a rectal examination to rule out fecal impaction and gastrointestinal bleeding. Selected clinical tests, directed by the history and physical examination, will assist with diagnosis (Table 49-1).

CASE DISCUSSION

Mrs. Wright is critically ill, and the most likely cause is an acute abdominal process. The differential diagnosis includes acute cholecystitis, a perforated abdominal viscus, appendicitis, and acute mesenteric ischemia. She has cardiovascular shock, which is probably the result of hemorrhage or sepsis. It is important that she be transferred to an acute care hospital

Table 49-1   Tests in the Older Patient with Acute Abdomen

Tests	Signficance
CBC with differential	WBCs may not be elevated with an acute process. A significant left shift is a more consistent finding. Low Hct may accompany a perforated peptic ulcer.
BUN, creatinine	Decrease in BP may lead to renal failure. Dehydration and GI bleed increase BUN.
Electrolytes	Vomiting and diarrhea may cause low K. Low Na accompanies many acute illnesses in the elderly. Low HCO_3 may indicate metabolic acidosis.
Liver function	May be increased with cholelithiasis, hepatitis, and cholangitis.
ECG	Inferior wall MI in particular may present with abdominal pain.
Erect and supine abdominal x-ray	Free air under diaphragm indicates a ruptured viscus. Air fluid levels indicate obstruction. Large amounts of stool suggest impaction.
Arterial blood gases	Hypoxemia may accompany shock and metabolic acidosis may occur with sepsis.
Abdominal ultrasound	Most useful for diagnosis of biliary disease. Useful for finding pancreatic cysts and aortic aneurysms.
CT scan and laparoscopy	Reserved for continuing diagnostic uncertainty.

unless there are specific preexisting instructions not to hospitalize. In the course of the transfer, oxygen is administered by Ventimask and intravenous fluids are started. The lack of a significant fever does not rule out an infective process. Acute myocardial infarction (MI), a ruptured aortic aneurysm, and pneumonia should be considered in the differential diagnosis.[2,3] MI or cerebral thrombosis can sometimes complicate sepsis and shock in an elderly patient.

STUDY QUESTION

- *You attend and manage her care in the emergency room. What investigations should be requested and what management decisions should be made at this stage?*

CHOLECYSTITIS

Cholecystitis is the most common cause of acute abdomen in the older patient, accounting for up to 33% of acute abdominal presentations. The prevalence of gallstones increases with age. Complications from gallstones are more common in older patients, the most common of these being ascending cholangitis, empyema of the gallbladder, perforation of the gallbladder, and pancreatitis. Perforation of the gallbladder occurs in up to 10% of cases of acute cholecystitis. However, many perforations are walled off and few progress to produce peritonitis.[4] Abdominal ultrasonography usually confirms the diagnosis. It has a high sensitivity and specificity for the presence of gallstones in the gallbladder and gallstones in, or dilation of, the biliary tree. Markedly elevated levels of bilirubin are usually indicative of a gallstone in the common duct. High amylase levels usually indicate pancreatitis from obstruction of the pancreatic duct.

The optimal timing for surgery in acute cholecystitis is controversial. Study results indicate that early, as opposed to immediate or late, surgery is the best course to follow.[5] Prolonged hospitalization and immobility before surgery increase the risk of pulmonary embolism, malnutrition, and the development of pressure sores.

> *In the vaguely, nonspecifically, but clearly "ill" older patient, always consider an intraabdominal catastrophe: watch and wait a little but not too long.*

BOWEL OBSTRUCTION

About 25% of acute abdomens in older patients are caused by a bowel obstruction.[6] The common causes are an incarcerated hernia, carcinoma, adhesions, or a volvulus.[7] Fecal impaction may be severe enough in an older patient to result in bowel obstruction: it should always be considered in the differential diagnosis. Management involves making the patient NPO (nothing by mouth) by placing a nasogastric tube and providing intravenous fluids. A surgical intervention may be required.

APPENDICITIS

Appendicitis is common in older patients, accounting for up to 14% of cases of acute abdomen.[6] Older patients have a higher mortality rate from appendicitis than do younger; mortality rates as high as 15% have been reported. This is due to a combination of factors, including late presentation, inaccurate diagnosis, and the high prevalence of perforation at the time of presentation. This propensity to earlier perforation is due to a decreased blood flow to the appendix in the older patient, combined with the narrower lumen and thinner wall. Older patients with appendicitis are less likely to have classic right lower quadrant abdominal pain and are more likely to have diffuse abdominal pain, abdominal guarding, and an abdominal mass. Laparoscopy may aid in the diagnosis, although most cases are confirmed only at laparotomy. Management is removal of the appendix.

PEPTIC ULCER DISEASE

The incidence of gastric and duodenal ulcer disease increases with age. Older patients are more likely to be taking both prescription and over-the-counter antiinflammatory agents, which predispose them to peptic ulcer disease. Smoking and heavy alcohol intake remain major risk factors in older patients. Empirical antiulcer therapy without endoscopy is common in younger patients but is not recommended for older patients because of the greater risk of the presence of a malignant gastric ulcer.

DIVERTICULITIS

The presence of diverticula in the large bowel increases with age and most commonly affects the sigmoid colon. Thirty percent of persons 60 years of age or older in the United States have evidence of diverticulosis. This increase in diverticula is associated with long-term low-fiber diets. Diverticula are uncommon in countries where dietary fiber is high. Diverticulitis, caused by inflammation in one or more diverticula, is thought to occur when there is a small perforation of a diverticulum. The most common presentation is pain in the left lower quadrant, with fever and a tender mass in the same area. All of these findings are more likely to be absent in an older patient. A perforation may lead to generalized peritonitis. The diagnosis is most often made clinically. Initial management in the patient without evidence of peritonitis is to rest the bowel and supply adequate hydration. Antibiotics are given to cover aerobic and anaerobic gram-negative organisms. Surgery is required if there is evidence of an abscess or peritonitis.

MESENTERIC ISCHEMIA

Acute mesenteric ischemia is a disease of old age, with more than two thirds of recognized cases occurring in persons over 70 years. The mortality rate is extremely high, over 80%. The diagnosis is difficult, and this to a large extent is responsible for the high mortality rate. Findings suggestive of the condition are pain that is more severe than would be suspected from the abdominal examination, a history of arteriosclerosis, and postprandial abdominal pain. Other common findings are diarrhea that is usually heme positive and leukocytosis. Management includes active fluid resuscitation and laparotomy, with resection of all ischemic tissue.

> *Suspect mesenteric ischemia or ischemic colitis in the atherosclerotic and the embolically prone elderly patient. These conditions have a high mortality and are difficult to diagnose.*

CASE DISCUSSION

Initial management in the emergency room should continue to address adequate oxygenation and fluid resuscitation of the patient. A surgical consultation should be obtained at this stage.

▼ WILMA WRIGHT (Part II)

Results of laboratory work are as follows:
WBC 22,640/ml; differential: polys 52%, band 24%, lymph 12%, mono 6%; Na 135 mg/dl; K 4.7 mEq/dl; Cl 100 mg/dl; HCO_3 24 mg/dl; BUN 24 mg/dl; creatinine 0.7 mg/dl; bilirubin, total 1.4 mg/dl; bilirubin, direct 0.9 mg/dl; alkaline phosphatase 335 U/L; AST 537 U/L; ALT 453 U/L; LDH 628 U/L; amylase 4,490 U/L; pH 7.349; Po_2 106 mm Hg; Pco_2 48.9 mm Hg.
Her x-ray examination and ECG are normal.

STUDY QUESTIONS

- *What is the management now?*
- *What is the differential diagnosis at this stage?*

The operative risk and mortality must be considered in decisions regarding surgery. The patient's wishes should be considered and advance directives must be honored. If there is a health care proxy or an individual with a durable power of attorney, he or she has an obligation and right to be involved in the decision-making process if the patient is unable to do so. The role of the family (or anyone else who knew the patient well before the patient's being unable to participate in the decision) is to assist, based on their knowledge of what the patient's wishes would have been; their personal opinion is not being sought (many families and physicians make this mistake). If there is any doubt or conflict, treatment must be in the direction of preserving life and function. Patients should not be rushed to surgery unless the condition is immediately life threatening. Cardiovascular status should be stabilized, electrolyte abnormalities corrected, acid-base balance corrected, renal function optimized, and pulmonary function assessed if necessary. This is particularly important for older patients, who are at increased risk of perioperative complications not because of age but because of the higher likelihood of comorbid disease. Other issues in the postoperative period include nutrition, thrombosis prophylaxis, prevention of pressure sores, and rehabilitation and discharge planning. Adequate pain control is important in the immediate postoperative period, since inadequate pain control predisposes to delirium, interfering with rehabilitation. Pain medication on a regular basis rather than as needed (or, if the patient can tolerate it, self-administered analgesic infusion), is preferred for the first few days after surgery.

CASE DISCUSSION

The clinical picture is highly suggestive of obstructive biliary disease. The initial presentation of shock with leukocytosis suggests ascending cholangitis. The very high amylase level indicates acute pancreatitis, most likely caused by a gallstone in the common bile duct.

▼ WILMA WRIGHT (Part III)

You prescribe broad-spectrum antibiotics to cover gram-negative aerobic and anaerobic organisms. Ultrasound of the abdomen is performed and shows an enlarged gallbladder with thickened walls containing many gallstones. The biliary ducts are dilated. A Swan-Ganz catheter is inserted so that fluid resuscitation can be carefully monitored. Mrs. Wright is transferred to the intensive care unit. A cholecystectomy is performed the following day, and she tolerates it well. She is transferred back to the nursing home 1 week after admission.

SUMMARY

Acute abdominal conditions in older age test the clinical skills of all those involved in elderly care. The significance of comorbid illness and of illnesses that complicate the basic process must be appreciated. If there is time (and there usually is), careful preparation for surgery is invaluable. Rigorous postoperative care is also essential. Many other conditions are manifest as abdominal pain, including acute myocardial infarction, pneumonia, and sometimes even more remote processes.

POSTTEST

1. Which of the following statements is true?
   a. Appendicitis is rare in patients over the age of 80 years because most have already had their appendix removed.
   b. Appendicitis in patients over 75 years old rarely produces pain.
   c. A lower right quadrant mass is a more common finding in older patients with appendicitis than in younger patients.
   d. The appendix, when inflamed in older patients, is less likely to perforate because of its thickened wall associated with chronic inflammation.

REFERENCES

1. Telfer S et al: Acute abdominal pain in patients over 50 years of age, *Scand J Gastroenterol* 144:47-50, 1988.
2. Duffy TP: Sounds in the attic, *N Engl J Med* 228:44-47, 1993.
3. Lederle F, Parenti C, Chute E: Ruptured abdominal aneurysm: the internist as diagnostician, *Am J Med* 96:163-167, 1994.
4. Houghton PWJ, Jemkinsom LR, Donaldson LA: Cholecystectomy in the elderly: a prospective study, *Br J Surg* 72:220-222, 1985.
5. Reiss R, Deutsch A, Eliashiv A: Decision-making process in abdominal surgery in the geriatric patient, *World J Surg* 7:522-526, 1983.
6. Reiss R, Deutsch A: Emergency abdominal procedures in patients above 70, *J Gerontol* 40:154-158, 1985.
7. Krauvar D: The geriatric acute abdomen, *Clin Geriatr Med* 9(3):547-557, 1993.

PRETEST ANSWER

1. d

POSTTEST ANSWER

1. c

CHAPTER 50

Polymyalgia Rheumatica

DOUGLAS C. WOOLLEY

OBJECTIVES

Upon completion of this chapter, the reader will be able to:

1. Describe the typical patient with polymyalgia rheumatica (PMR), including age, sex, onset of symptoms, and symptom complexes.

2. Name at least five disorders whose presenting symptoms and signs overlap somewhat with those of PMR, and describe how these might be distinguished from it.

3. Describe the relationship of giant cell arteritis (GCA or temporal arteritis) to PMR, and compare the treatment of the patient with uncomplicated PMR to that of the patient with GCA.

PRETEST

1. All of the following are typical complaints of a patient suffering from PMR except:
   a. Aching and weakness of the muscles of the shoulder and hip girdles
   b. Swollen, tender, stiff wrist joints
   c. Progressive fatigue, malaise, depression, and dependence
   d. Stiffness and soreness, worse in the morning and evening

2. Which one of the following statements is false?
   a. Polymyalgia rheumatica (PMR) is rare before the age of 55.
   b. An erythrocyte sedimentation rate (ESR) over 100 suggests a more active inflammatory disease than PMR.
   c. Temporal artery biopsy is the only tissue biopsy generally useful in PMR management.
   d. More than two thirds of patients with PMR achieve full remission or long symptom-free periods with prednisone.

Although it was first described a hundred years ago, the clinical significance of polymyalgia rheumatica (PMR) has been widely appreciated for only about 40 years. The average age of onset is between 65 and 70; the disease is rare in people under 55. Women are affected twice as often as men, and whites much more often than blacks.[1]

▼ ANNA HEISNER (Part I)

Your patient, Anna Heisner, is a 78-year-old widow who lives in a small house a few doors from her only daughter. She manages her personal care, but because of advanced degenerative arthritis of the low back and knees, she relies on her family for housework and yardwork. She has a history of 2 months of stiffness and pain around her shoulders, low neck, and thighs, which is becoming worse.

STUDY QUESTIONS

- *What is the differential diagnosis?*
- *What specific question should be asked, and what should be sought on examination?*

Faced with presenting symptoms of new or increased pain and stiffness of the shoulders and hips in an older person, since more than half of the aged have documented musculoskeletal disease, it is easy to assume that an existing process has flared up. The primary symptoms of PMR (limb-girdle muscle pain and stiffness) may not be sought. Associated symptoms are often revealed only by specific inquiry: intermittent mild fever, night sweats, modest loss of appetite and weight, fatigue, malaise, and depression. PMR is therefore unrecognized in the majority of its victims.[1]

The symptoms may emerge rapidly, but more typically the presentation is insidious, with gradual progression of proximal muscle pain and stiffness over several weeks.

The course of the disease, if not treated, is chronic and steady over months to years, after which symptoms may remit. However, flare-ups may occur years after the original episode.

The primary symptom of PMR is limb-girdle muscle pain and stiffness; other symptoms are nonspecific, so PMR is often unrecognized.

Early symptoms may be unilateral, but they quickly become symmetrical. Typically, low neck and proximal shoulder muscles are affected before the hip, buttock, and thigh muscles. Patients often restrict activity because of pain and so suffer secondary muscle atrophy, weakness, and growing dependence. They often become depressed.

Examination may confirm weight loss, mild fever, and progressive frailty. Pain may be found on palpation of proximal muscles and of periarticular shoulder, buttocks, hip, and knee tissues, but there may be no evidence of active articular inflammation or new deformities.[2]

The underlying cause of PMR has not been discovered. No infectious agents have been isolated in PMR, and no environmental factors have been convincingly implicated. That PMR is more common in whites suggests possible genetic factors; that it is seen almost exclusively in the elderly suggests mechanisms involving senescence of the immune system.

▼ ANNA HEISNER (Part II)

Ms. Heisner's pain and stiffness ease somewhat during the course of the day but worsen in the thighs and buttocks after prolonged sitting. She has tried ibuprofen, with minimal re-

lief. She is discouraged by her increasing physical limitations. She has lost 10 lb in the past 3 months and experiences frequent night sweats. She does not have headaches, visual or sensory changes, or changes in concentration and memory. She appears pleasant but discouraged. On examination there is evidence of recent weight loss, with new upper arm dependent skin folds. Her vital signs are normal. She requires assistance to mount the step to the examination table. There are no new skin lesions and no pain to palpation over the temples. When asked to move her neck and shoulders through their full range of motion (active ROM testing), she complains of muscle pain, but with strong encouragement she achieves almost complete ROM. Passive ROM testing of the joints (you move the relaxed limb through its range of motion) does not cause pain. Inspection of extremity joints reveals no acute inflammatory changes or new deformities. No new cardiopulmonary or other organ system dysfunction is noted.

STUDY QUESTION

- *What laboratory abnormalities can be anticipated, and will they help the diagnosis?*

Diagnosis of PMR is based on the clinical picture. Laboratory abnormalities are nonspecific but characteristic. An ESR above 40, and often above 100, is typical and may be used to monitor the response to therapy. Normochromic anemia, as seen in other chronic inflammatory diseases, is typical. Nonspecific chronic inflammatory markers, such as increased platelet counts, fibrinogen, and α_2-globulins (acute phase reactants) are common. White blood cell and differential counts are typically normal, as are rheumatological markers such as antinuclear antigen and rheumatoid factor titers. Tests helpful in demonstrating primary muscle inflammation or damage, such as creatine phosphokinase enzyme levels or electromyograms, are normal in PMR.

Pathological investigations in PMR, such as studies of bodily fluids and tissues, are nonspecific; there are a few typical, minor abnormalities.[3] Synovial fluid shows mild nonspecific inflammatory changes. Synovial tissue biopsy shows evidence of nonspecific inflammation with mild lymphocytic infiltrates. Muscle biopsy is generally normal. The exception is biopsy of arterial tissue, particularly the temporal artery, which can be vital in demonstrating the presence of the closely allied and potentially disabling condition of giant cell arteritis (GCA, often called temporal arteritis); this is discussed below.

PMR is diagnosed from the history and physical examination; laboratory studies differentiate some other illnesses.

The diagnosis of PMR is based on recognizing its typical presentation from a careful history and physical; a few laboratory studies differentiate it from a variety of disorders with similar initial symptoms and signs (Table 50-1).

▼ ANNA HEISNER (Part III)

Ms. Heisner's ESR is increased to 85 mm/hr, there is a normochromic, normocytic anemia with hematocrit of 33%, normal white blood cell and differential counts, slight hypoalbuminemia, normal liver and muscle enzymes, and normal renal, metabolic, and urinalysis values. Antinuclear antigen and rheumatoid factor tests are negative. Over the next week she records several oral temperatures elevated to 38° C. Three sets of blood cultures are negative. A purified protein derivative tuberculin (PPD) test is positive (there is known childhood exposure), but chest x-ray examination findings are negative. Cough and sputum production are absent, and sputum samples cannot be obtained.

STUDY QUESTIONS

- *Is the clinical diagnosis established?*
- *What is the initial treatment, and how should the patient be advised?*

The mainstay of therapy for PMR is oral low-dose steroids, starting with 15 to 20 mg of prednisone daily. If the symptoms resolve and the ESR returns to essentially normal within a month, the dose may be tapered slowly. The daily maintenance dose may be as low as 5 mg, but if symptoms or elevated ESR return, higher doses must be given. Prednisone is usually maintained for at least a year and may be needed much longer before being successfully tapered and stopped. More than two thirds of patients achieve full remission or long symptom-free periods without prednisone. However, relapses are common and can be seen as late as 8 years after successful treatment.

Prednisone is usually the mainstay of PMR therapy for at least a year, but watch out for osteoporosis!

Physical therapy, focusing on weak muscles, unsteady gait, and diminished confidence, is important in returning the patient to full functioning.

▼ ANNA HEISNER (Part IV)

The clinical diagnosis of PMR is made. You start 15 mg prednisone daily. A program of home physical therapy is begun

Table 50-1   Differentiating Polymyalgia Rheumatica From Other Conditions

	Pain Pattern	Common Systemic Symptoms	Onset and Course	Anatomy Affected	Laboratory Findings, X-Ray	Age at Onset
PMR	On arising, after prolonged inactivity	Low-grade fevers, fatigue, general malaise, weight loss, depression, headache (TA)	Acute or subacute onset and chronic steady course	Proximal muscles, periarticular tissues of limb girdles	Elevated ESR, normochromic anemia	>55
Osteoarthritis	End of day or after heavy use of joints	Not prominent	Chronic, may emerge after injury	Weight-bearing joints, axial skeleton, distal hand joints; oligoarticular and asymmetrical	Characteristic degenerative changes of joints on x-ray	>40 (unless posttraumatic)
Rheumatoid Arthritis	On arising, after prolonged inactivity	Fever, fatigue, weight loss, malaise, and organ-specific extraarticular symptoms such as shortness of breath	Acute or subacute onset, with chronic and variable course	Wrists, MCP joints, any synovial joints; symmetrical; extraarticular (e.g., heart, lung, eye, integument)	Elevated ESR, +RA, +ANA; normochromic anemia; x-ray: joint changes and deformities; osteoporosis	Childhood to old age
Chronic Infection	Diffuse aching not clearly related to use	Spiking fevers, sweats, chills, malaise, anorexia, nausea, headache, weakness	Acute or subacute with variable course	Nonarticular diffuse aches and stiffness; varies with kind of infection	Elevated ESR, elevated WBC; normochromic anemia; + skin test or serology; + cultures	Childhood to old age
Polymyositis	Muscle pain with use or on palpation	Weakness, malaise, weight loss, occasional fevers	Slowly evolving and chronic steady course	Proximal muscles; abnormal cardiac and lung function	Abnormal muscle biopsy; high muscle enzymes and ESR; abnormal EMG and nerve conduction	All ages
Depression	Highly variable and changeable	Weakness, anxiety, malaise, insomnia, weight and appetite changes	Subacute to slow onset, with variable chronic course	Diffuse aches difficult to characterize; trigger points not prominent	No specific abnormalities	Childhood to old age
Fibromyalgia	On arising and with active use	Insomnia, malaise, weakness, irritable bowel syndrome	Chronic but evanescent	Periarticular muscle insertion sites: "trigger points"	None	Middle age

TA, Temporal arteritis; *ESR,* erythrocyte sedimentation rate; *MCP,* metacarpophalangeal joints; *RA,* rheumatoid factor; *ANA,* antinuclear antigen; *EMG,* electromyography.

to address her mobility and her ability to take care of herself. She is told that she should expect the muscle pain, stiffness, and weakness to improve within the next 2 to 4 weeks. She is cautioned to report worsening symptoms, particularly headaches, visual changes, tenderness around the temples, or renewed fevers. Within 3 weeks she reports significant improvement. Her long-standing knee pain remains, but her shoulders and buttocks are no longer stiff and aching. Her morning mobility has improved. Fevers and night sweats are gone. Three weeks into therapy, the ESR is 60 mm/hr; at 6 weeks, it is 40 and the hematocrit has increased to 37%. You then taper the prednisone to 10 mg a day and a few weeks later to 5 mg, after which the ESR remains low and symptoms are absent. Her respiratory function and a chest x-ray are unchanged. After a full year of therapy, further tapering of the prednisone is attempted. However, the ESR rises and symptoms return, prompting renewal of prednisone at 5 mg a day for another year. Over the next 3 years she experiences more flare-ups and does not have long symptom-free intervals. Although she feels much better than during the pretreatment phase of her disease, she is disappointed that she is still not symptom free for extended periods unless she is on prednisone. Her stamina wanes, and kyphosis from spinal osteoporosis is progressing.

CASE DISCUSSION

This patient demonstrates the characteristically good initial response to prednisone but also the quite frequent reaction of incomplete remission. The long-term use of prednisone is associated with the hazard of osteoporosis and other problems. Considerable clinical skill is required in treatment of PMR. It is best to base decisions about the use of prednisone on the most objective information available: the physical examination and the ESR.

GIANT CELL ARTERITIS

Giant cell arteritis (GCA), a granulomatous inflammation of the aorta, its proximal branches, and the cranial arteries, may be seen at some time in as many as one third of patients with PMR. In addition to characteristic PMR constitutional symptoms, these patients typically have moderate to severe sharp or stabbing headaches, often localized to the temples. Indeed, the condition is often termed temporal arteritis because of the prominence of inflammation of these vessels. Patients with giant cell arteritis often demonstrate more prominent fever spikes and higher ESR than those with uncomplicated PMR. The possible consequences of untreated GCA are considerably more serious than those of uncomplicated PMR and stem from occlusion of the affected arteries by the granulomatous inflammation. Symptoms include headaches and difficulty concentrating resulting from temporal artery involvement, jaw claudication (aching jaw while chewing) because of facial artery involvement, and the most serious complication, possible partial blindness, complete blindness, or double vision resulting from occlusion of ocular arteries.[4]

The arteritis may be widespread. Rarely, it leads to aortic aneurysm and dissection, to coronary artery blockage, or renal and mesenteric artery insufficiency. The diagnosis is established by temporal artery biopsy, in which the characteristic necrotizing granulomatous vasculitis is seen.

> *When giant cell arteritis (GCA) occurs (as it does in one third of PMR patients), prednisone is urgent.*

The serious complications of GCA can be averted if the patient is quickly treated with daily prednisone, ranging in dose from 40 to 60 mg. However, if ischemic complications (such as impaired vision) occur before treatment is begun, they are unlikely to be reversible. Treatment may be required for a year or more before the vasculitis is quiescent. As with PMR, the activity can be followed by monitoring the ESR.

SUMMARY

Polymyalgia rheumatica (PMR) is an increasingly common illness, especially in elderly white women. Early diagnosis is important because of the common complication of temporal arteritis, with the risk of blindness, as well as the other associated giant cell arteritis (GCA) manifestations. PMR is quite frequently a relapsing condition, and patients may well suffer osteoporosis and more from the use of long-term steroids, which are the only currently effective therapy.

POSTTEST

1. Which of the following statements is false?
   a. Blacks are much less often affected by PMR than are whites.
   b. Giant cell arteritis (GCA) is the preferred term for temporal arteritis, since multiple arteries can be involved.
   c. Aortic aneurysm and coronary artery obstruction can occur in GCA.
   d. Impaired vision from temporal arteritis can generally be checked by a prompt increase in the dose of prednisone.

2. Which one of the following statements concerning PMR is true?
   a. Hypochromic, normocytic anemia is common.
   b. Creatine phosphokinase (CPK) is sometimes elevated.
   c. α_2-Globulins are characteristically normal.
   d. Giant cell arteritis (GCA) occurs in up to one third of PMR patients.

REFERENCES

1. Goodwin JS: Progress in gerontology: polymyalgia rheumatica and temporal arteritis, *J Am Geriatr Soc* 40:515-525, 1992.
2. Cohen MD, Ginsburg WW: Polymyalgia rheumatica, *Rheum Dis Clin North Am* 16:325-339, 1990.
3. Healey LA: The spectrum of polymyalgia rheumatica, *Clin Geriatr Med* 4:323-331, 1988.
4. Spiera H: Giant cell arteritis and polymyalgia rheumatica, *Hosp Pract* 25(11):71-88, 1990.
5. Schumacher HR, Klippel JH, Koopman WJ, eds: *Primer on the rheumatic diseases,* ed 10, Atlanta, 1993, Arthritis Foundation.

PRETEST ANSWERS
1. b
2. b

POSTTEST ANSWERS
1. d
2. d

CHAPTER 51

Hypothermia

LEONARD W. MORGAN

OBJECTIVES

On completion of this chapter, the reader will be able to:

1. Define hypothermia and describe its importance in the elderly population.

2. Discuss predisposing factors for developing hypothermia.

3. Describe the signs, symptoms, and stages of hypothermia.

4. Provide treatment appropriate to the level of hypothermia.

5. Describe preventive strategies for hypothermia.

PRETEST

1. All of the following statements about hypothermia are true except:
   a. It occurs in any season.
   b. It can occur at ambient temperatures in the frail elderly.
   c. Secondary hypothermia is more common than primary in the elderly.
   d. Postoperative elderly patients are routinely monitored for hypothermia.

2. Which of the following statements is true regarding hypothermia in the elderly?
   a. Hypothermia evolving over days to weeks is the characteristic presentation in the elderly.
   b. The mortality rate from hypothermia in older persons is decreasing with increasing professional awareness.
   c. Rewarming is the technique that must be initiated first and foremost in all cases.
   d. The threshold temperature for the development of ventricular fibrillation is 30° C (86° F).

Hypothermia is a decrease in the core body temperature below 35° C (95° F) caused by deliberate or accidental conditions. Accidental hypothermia is an underreported and underrecognized cause of death in the elderly. Although severe cases have a high mortality, early recognition and appropriate management give the best prognosis once the condition has developed. A severe cold stressor is not necessary to its development; hypothermia can occur at ambient temperatures in the frail elderly during any season and anywhere.

▼ HILDA BROWN (Part I)

Hilda Brown is a 79-year-old black woman with a 20-year history of diabetes mellitus previously controlled with NPH insulin 35 U in the morning and 15 U in the afternoon. She has been under your care for 10 years. She is found unconscious in her kitchen by her daughter. Her daughter had talked to her earlier today when she complained of nausea, vomiting, and diarrhea. She had given herself her insulin but was unable to take anything except a small glass of juice.

STUDY QUESTIONS

- *What is the differential diagnosis?*
- *If hypothermia is the problem, how would you diagnose it?*

CLASSIFICATION AND PREVALENCE

Hypothermia is classified in three ways: the pathophysiology, the rate of heat loss, and the severity of the body temperature (Box 51-1).

The pathophysiological classification of hypothermia is simply as primary or secondary, based on whether an underlying condition is responsible for its development.[1] In primary hypothermia the patient has normal thermoregulation but is subjected to an overwhelming cold stress. Secondary hypothermia is characterized by abnormal thermoregulation, with the patient subjected to only mild-to-moderate cold stress. Hypothermia in the elderly (especially in the frail and those over 75) is largely of the secondary type.[2] Common causes are endocrine disorders, cerebrovascular disease, neurological problems, Parkinson's disease, and medications.

Hypothermia can also be classified as mild, moderate, or severe based on the core temperature: mild, 32° C (89.6° F) to 35° C (95° F); moderate, 28° (82.4° F) to 32° C (89.6° F); and severe, 28° C (82.4° F) and below.

Hypothermia is also defined, based on rate of heat loss, as acute (1 hour), subacute (several hours), and gradual (days to weeks). Gradual hypothermia is more common in the elderly.

Incidence, prevalence, and mortality figures do not reflect hypothermia's impact as a health care problem because of underrecognition and underreporting.[2,3] During the winter months in Great Britain, studies have shown that as many as 10% of the elderly population had core body temperatures of 35° C (95° F) or less based on urine temperature.[4] In the United States, 7450 deaths from 1976 to 1985 were attributed to cold exposure.[5] More than 50% of these deaths were elderly individuals. There is increasing evidence that the incidence as well as the mortality rate of hypothermia in older persons is growing.

 Hypothermia can occur in an immobilized patient in a hospital bed.

PREDISPOSING FACTORS

External factors influencing the risk of developing hypothermia are the climate and the social circumstances. Internal determinants include the functional level of the thermoregulatory system (Box 51-2).

BOX 51-1
Classification of Hypothermia

Pathophysiology
Primary   *Secondary*

Normal thermoregulation   Abnormal thermoregulation
Overwhelming cold stress   Often mild to moderate cold stress

Severity
Mild   *Moderate*   *Severe*

32°-35° C   28°-32° C   Below 28° C
89.6°-95° F   82.4°-89.6° F   Below 82.4° F

Rate of Heat Loss
Acute   *Subacute*   *Gradual*

Less than 1 hour   Several hours   Days to weeks

Thermoregulatory mechanisms do decline with age.[6] The elderly tend to have a decreased perception of temperature changes and adjust to them less efficiently. Aging is associated with decreases in resting peripheral blood flow, shivering, muscle mass, fat stores, and metabolic rate, all of which contribute to the decline in thermoregulation. Autonomic dysfunction also increases with aging.

Social factors such as poor housing and alcohol abuse also predispose the elderly to hypothermia. Chronic conditions such as diabetes mellitus, dementia, arthritis, cerebrovascular disease, and ischemic heart disease, all of increased incidence with increasing age, contribute to the risk. There is also a special risk for patients during surgery and early in the postoperative period.[7]

ASSESSMENT AND DIAGNOSIS

The symptoms of hypothermia are nonspecific, insidious, and likely to be confused with other conditions or to go unnoticed. As with other illnesses in the elderly, the symptoms are easy to explain away. Conscious elderly patients with hypothermia often lack a sensation of cold, and they may not shiver.[8] With temperatures between 35° C (95° F) and 36.1° C (97° F), most patients have the perception of being cold. Once hypothermia is established, however, the symptoms of being cold may not be recognized. Early *signs* of hypothermia are mental confusion, impaired gait, lethargy, and combativeness.

Suspect hypothermia often; diagnose it with a low-reading thermometer. (Make sure one is available!)

The presentation is unique and depends on both the severity and duration of the hypothermic state and the associated or underlying medical conditions.[4] However, the evolution of clinical signs and symptoms of hypothermia as the core body temperature decreases are somewhat predictable (Fig. 51-1).

▼ HILDA BROWN (Part II)

You evaluate Mrs. Brown in the emergency room: blood pressure, 130/70; pulse, 56; respirations, 10; rectal temperature, 94° F. She is not alert but responds to noxious stimuli with purposeful movements. Her pupils are slightly dilated but react to light. The rest of the HEENT (head, ears, eyes, nose, throat) examination is normal. There are decreased breath sounds and dry rales at the lung bases. Her abdomen is soft but tender in the epigastric area and otherwise unremarkable. On rectal examination there is good sphincter tone and loose stool in the vault, weakly positive for occult blood. The extremities are normal and Babinski's sign is negative. The skin shows some mild patchy ecchymotic areas on her left side from her face to her legs.

STUDY QUESTIONS

- *How would you categorize her hypothermic state?*
- *What is the explanation for these physical findings?*

The physical findings in hypothermia are nonspecific, too. The patient may appear apathetic with slurred speech and a slow gait; shivering may be absent. There may be altered mental status (confusion or even coma), dilated fixed pupils, bradycardia, absent heart sounds, hypotension, and increased muscle tone. The skin may appear cyanotic with generalized edema. Signs of head trauma, insulin injection sites, a smell of acetone or alcohol, and signs of frostbite should be sought.

▼ HILDA BROWN (Part III)

The electrolyte levels are normal, but the blood glucose is 28 g/dl. The arterial blood gases show pH 7.38; P_{O_2} 66; and P_{CO_2} 38. The creatinine phosphokinase and other enzyme levels are essentially within normal limits.

STUDY QUESTION

■ What should your management plan be at this point?

Initial laboratory studies should include a complete blood cell count, platelets, electrolytes, glucose, renal and hepatic function, blood cultures, urinalysis, stool for occult blood, glucose, arterial blood gases, chest x-ray, and electrocardiogram (ECG). In moderate-to-severe hypothermia, muscle enzyme levels will invariably be elevated; the baseline value will be important.

The differential diagnosis in the early stages of hypothermia is extremely broad. The signs, symptoms, and physical findings and laboratory data are nonspecific and may mimic many clinical conditions, which will frequently be concurrent with the hypothermic state. The disaster is to recognize some of the conditions, or one of the conditions contributing to the person's situation, and not to recognize and address the hypothermia. The examining physician must have a high index of suspicion.

The diagnosis is established by determining the core temperature rectally with a low-reading thermometer. This is a specific piece of equipment that should be available in emergency rooms and other situations where patients with this diagnosis are likely to be seen. The ECG can be helpful; the Osborne wave (positive deflection at the junction of the QRS and ST segments) was once thought to be pathognomonic for hypothermia. However, in recent studies it was identified in only one third of hypothermic patients, and it has been seen in other conditions.[9]

▼ HILDA BROWN (Part IV)

You start an IV with D5/normal saline. You follow this with an IV bolus of D5W. The patient is covered with heated sheets and blankets. Within 20 minutes she becomes more alert; she progresses to full alertness over the next 4 hours.

STUDY QUESTION

■ What other methods might be necessary in a more severely hypothermic patient?

▼ JUANITA JONES (Part I)

Juanita Jones is a 72-year-old Hispanic patient of yours, with a long history of diabetes mellitus and congestive heart failure. Recently she has had multiple falls. History, medications review, physical examination, and laboratory data do not identify a specific reason for her falls. She is admitted for acute care following a left intertrochanteric hip fracture. Her orthopedist elects to put her in traction rather than performing a surgical repair. She does relatively well until 3 days after admission to the hospital, when she becomes lethargic. Review of her medications, physical examination, and laboratory results (including blood and urine cultures) is unrevealing. Close review of her vital signs reveals a slow decrease in her temperature over the previous 2 days. A rectal temperature of 94° F (34.4° C) is obtained with a low-reading thermometer; a diagnosis of hypothermia is made.

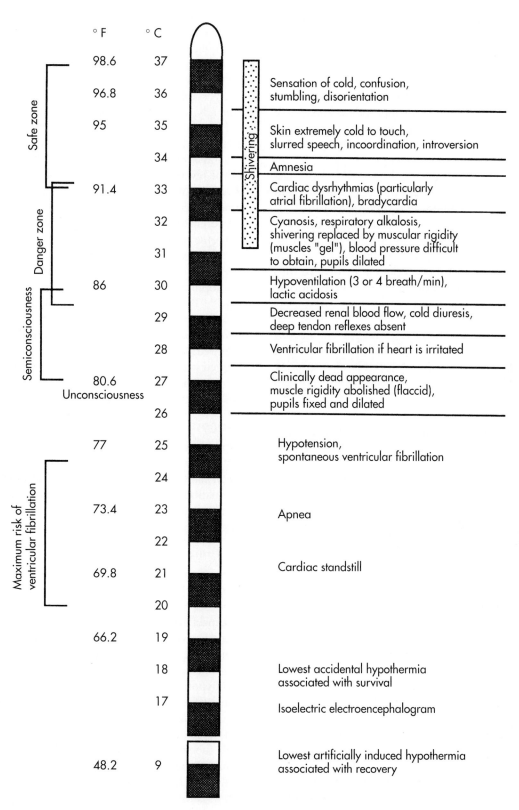

°F   °C

98.6   37   Sensation of cold, confusion,
96.8   36   stumbling, disorientation

95   35   Skin extremely cold to touch,
              slurred speech, incoordination, introversion
        34   Amnesia

91.4   33   Cardiac dysrhythmias (particularly
              atrial fibrillation), bradycardia
        32   Cyanosis, respiratory alkalosis,
              shivering replaced by muscular rigidity
        31   (muscles "gel"), blood pressure difficult
              to obtain, pupils dilated

86   30   Hypoventilation (3 or 4 breath/min),
              lactic acidosis
        29   Decreased renal blood flow, cold diuresis,
              deep tendon reflexes absent
        28   Ventricular fibrillation if heart is irritated

80.6   27   Clinically dead appearance,
              muscle rigidity abolished (flaccid),
        26   pupils fixed and dilated

77   25   Hypotension,
              spontaneous ventricular fibrillation
        24
73.4   23   Apnea
        22
69.8   21   Cardiac standstill
        20
66.2   19
        18   Lowest accidental hypothermia
              associated with survival
        17   Isoelectric electroencephalogram

48.2   9   Lowest artificially induced hypothermia
              associated with recovery

Safe zone
Danger zone
Semiconsciousness
Unconsciousness
Maximum risk of ventricular fibrillation
Shivering

FIG. 51-1   Degrees of hypothermia and associated effects.
(From Matz R: *Hosp Pract* 21:45-64, 1986.)

STUDY QUESTION

■ *What predisposing factors are likely to have been present in this case of postoperative hypothermia?*

MANAGEMENT

Hypothermia is a medical emergency. Successful treatment entails rapid assessment, appropriate supportive therapy, resuscitative measures, and rewarming techniques. Even with appropriate care the mortality rate can be as high as 80%.

The goals of therapy are as follows: (1) restore adequate cardiopulmonary function, fluid, electrolyte, and acid-base balance; (2) minimize additional heat loss; (3) obtain a normal core body temperature within a reasonable time; (4) treat the nonenvironmental precipitating cause(s); and (5) treat coexisting conditions.

The management of hypothermia can be divided into cardiopulmonary resuscitation, supportive care, and rewarming.

Hypothermia is a medical emergency; prevention is the key.

Resuscitation

The level, duration, and comorbidities dictate the intensity of initial treatment.[9] Patients with mild hypothermia and no coexisting condition may not need cardiopulmonary resuscitation; most patients with moderate-to-severe hypothermia do.

The threshold temperature for ventricular fibrillation is 28° C (82.4° F). Patients with moderate-to-severe hypothermia *commonly* have ventricular fibrillation. Resuscitative measures are the same as for cardiac arrest.[4] Patients with a core temperature less than 28° C (82.4° F) who are *not* in ventricular fibrillation are at risk for developing it and must be treated accordingly. Resuscitative measures should continue during rewarming until the patient is in a stable rhythm and until the core temperature rises to 32° C (89.6° F). No patient should be pronounced dead until he or she is adequately rewarmed and resuscitative measures have failed.

Rewarming

Rewarming techniques involve three broad categories: passive external rewarming, active external rewarming, and active core rewarming. Passive external rewarming involves moving the patient to a warm environment (70° F or 21° C) and insulating the patient from additional heat loss. Active external rewarming uses heated materials such as water bottles, water baths, and electric blankets to transfer heat externally to the patient. Active core rewarming uses internal and invasive measures such as gastric or mediastinal irrigation, warmed humidified oxygen,

peritoneal dialysis, or extracorporeal blood rewarming. Rewarming should not be attempted until cardiopulmonary resuscitation measures have been instituted.[4] Rewarming before resuscitative efforts increases metabolic demands at a time when the body is least able to respond.

Patients with mild hypothermia usually have a relatively stable cardiopulmonary status and respond adequately to passive external rewarming.

Patients with moderate hypothermia without cardiac arrest can be treated with a combination of active external and core rewarming techniques.[4] However, active external rewarming must be performed cautiously to prevent afterdrop (reduction of core temperature by cold blood circulating from the periphery) and aftershock (hypotension caused by peripheral vasodilation). The outcome of active external rewarming can be maximized by good oxygenation and fluid and electrolyte support.[10]

Patients with moderate-to-severe hypothermia and cardiopulmonary arrest require active core rewarming.[4,11] External rewarming methods cannot rewarm fast enough to maximize resuscitative efforts. With extracorporeal blood rewarming, cardiac compressions are not required and other resuscitative measures can be performed without interruption, but this procedure requires special skills and facilities, which are not available at many hospitals.

Support

Supportive management includes fluids, electrolytes, and oxygen with cardiac, blood pressure, arterial pH, and rectal temperature monitoring. Rewarming can cause a fluctuation in pH, oxygen tension, and potassium levels, predisposing to cardiac arrhythmias and other life-threatening complications.

Prevention

Prevention is the best approach, but it is difficult to implement. It requires increased awareness of the prevalence of hypothermia and its risk factors. Many health professionals expect hypothermia to have a dramatic presentation related to severe environmental exposure or to alcohol intoxication. Yet it is well established that the elderly are at risk for hypothermia even at ambient temperatures and that hypothermia may develop subtly. An intensive educational effort must extend to all medical personnel managing the elderly and to hospital staff and the public.

The primary care physician should identify patients with subclinical hypothermia (36° C to 35° C) and patients who are at risk, such as those with conditions listed in Box 51-2, and should provide appropriate patient education and anticipatory guidance. Patients at risk are those over 80 and those with multiple medical problems, impaired mental or functional state, poor social support, and the undernourished. The physician should inquire about living conditions, diet, exercise, drugs, alcohol use, and the temperature setting in the patient's home.

Patients at risk for hypothermia should be encouraged to avoid the outdoors during extreme cold. They should be encouraged to wear heavily insulated clothing and a cap or hat if they must go out. They should be instructed on proper diet and the need to maintain the temperature in their homes at 17° C (62.6° F) or above. Support agencies should be recruited to visit isolated elderly during the winter. When such primary prevention fails, prompt recognition and early intervention are literally vital.

All emergency rooms should have a low-reading rectal thermometer, and all patients at risk for hypothermia should be so evaluated. Elderly patients with sepsis and other predisposing illnesses should be monitored for low core body temperatures while in the intensive care unit.

Patients undergoing surgery should be monitored during and after surgery for hypothermia. Strategies to reduce perioperative hypothermia, such as increasing the ambient temperature of the operating room, using preoperative skin-surface warming, covering the patient's head, using warm gowns and drapes, using thermoregulating blankets, warming intravenous fluids and blood, and humidifying and warming ventilatory gases, should be universally implemented.

Finally, more accurate data on the incidence of hypothermia should be obtained and used to develop public policy in this area.

▼ *JUANITA JONES (Part II)*

Mrs. Jones is successfully treated with passive external rewarming. She becomes more alert and is reevaluated for surgical repair of her hip by the orthopedic surgeon, the physical therapist, occupational therapist, and by you, her primary care physician. She undergoes a total hip replacement and has an uncomplicated hospital course. She is discharged to a rehabilitation center for further treatment.

SUMMARY

Hypothermia represents a wide spectrum of illness from quite mild to severe or life threatening. Although the more severe cases have a high mortality, early recognition and prompt treatment are vital. However, preventive approaches must also be implemented. It is important to maintain a high level of clinical suspicion of this problem, which often occurs concurrently in patients who are ill in other ways.

POSTTEST

1. The rewarming method of choice for a patient with severe hypothermia and cardiac arrest is:
   a. External active rewarming
   b. Active core rewarming
   c. Active core rewarming via cardiac bypass
   d. Inhaled heated oxygen
2. The diagnosis of hypothermia is best established by:
   a. The presence of an Osborne wave on ECG
   b. The elevation of pancreatic amylase and muscle enzymes

   c. Ventricular dysrhythmias
   d. A low-reading rectal thermometer
3. Which one of the following statements is false?
   a. Thermoregulatory mechanisms are preserved.
   b. The elderly have a decreased perception of temperature changes.
   c. Aging is associated with a decreased resting peripheral blood flow.
   d. Autonomic nervous system dysfunction increases with age.

REFERENCES

1. Celestino FS: Causes and treatment of hypothermia, *Geriatr Med Today* 9:24-36, 1989.
2. Celestino FS, Van Noord GR, Miraglia CP: Accidental hypothermia in the elderly, *J Fam Pract* 26:259-267, 1988.
3. Moss J: Accidental severe hypothermia, *Surg Gynecol Obstet* 162:501-513, 1986.
4. McAlpine CH, Dall JLC: Outcome after episodes of hypothermia, *Age Ageing* 16:115-118, 1987.
5. Rango N: Exposure-related hypothermia mortality in the United States, 1970-79, *Am J Public Health* 74:1159-1160, 1984.
6. Matz R: Hypothermia: mechanisms and countermeasures, *Hosp Pract* 21:45-64, 1986.
7. Martyn JW: Review article: diagnosing and treating hypothermia, *CMA J* 125:1089-1096, 1981.
8. Sherman FT, Menachem D: Hypothermia detection in emergency departments, *NY State J Med* 374-376, 1982.
9. Fitzgerald FT et al: Accidental hypothermia: a report of 22 cases and review of the literature, *Adv Intern Med* 27:127-150, 1982.
10. Cohen DJ et al: Resuscitation of the hypothermic patient, *Am J Emerg Med* 6:475-478, 1988.
11. Zell SC, Kurtz KJ: Severe exposure hypothermia: a resuscitation protocol, *Ann Emerg Med* 14:339-345, 1985.

PRETEST ANSWERS
1. d
2. a

POSTTEST ANSWERS
1. c
2. d
3. a

Index